HEALTH ISSUES IN THE BLACK COMMUNITY

HEALTH ISSUES IN THE BLACK COMMUNITY

3rd Edition

RONALD L. BRAITHWAITE, SANDRA E. TAYLOR, AND HENRIE M. TREADWELL

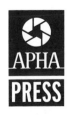

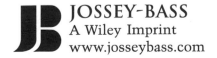

JOSSEY-BASS
A Wiley Imprint
www.josseybass.com

Published by Jossey-Bass
A Wiley Imprint
989 Market Street, San Francisco, CA 94103-1741—www.josseybass.com

Readers should be aware that Internet Web sites offered as citations and/or sources for further information may have changed or disappeared between the time this was written and when it is read.

Limit of Liability/Disclaimer of Warranty: While the publisher and author have used their best efforts in preparing this book, they make no representations or warranties with respect to the accuracy or completeness of the contents of this book and specifically disclaim any implied warranties of merchantability or fitness for a particular purpose. No warranty may be created or extended by sales representatives or written sales materials. The advice and strategies contained herein may not be suitable for your situation. You should consult with a professional where appropriate. Neither the publisher nor author shall be liable for any loss of profit or any other commercial damages, including but not limited to special, incidental, consequential, or other damages.

Jossey-Bass books and products are available through most bookstores. To contact Jossey-Bass directly call our Customer Care Department within the U.S. at 800-956-7739, outside the U.S. at 317-572-3986, or fax 317-572-4002.

Jossey-Bass also publishes its books in a variety of electronic formats. Some content that appears in print may not be available in electronic books.

Library of Congress Cataloging-in-Publication Data

Health issues in the black community/[edited by] Ronald L. Braithwaite, Sandra E. Taylor, and Henrie M. Treadwell.—3rd ed.
    p.; cm.
    Includes bibliographical references and index.
    ISBN 978-0-470-43679-0 (cloth)
      1. African Americans—Health and hygiene. I. Braithwaite, Ronald L., 1945- II. Taylor, Sandra E., 1955- III. Treadwell, Henrie M.
[DNLM: 1. African Americans—United States. 2. Health Status—United States. 3. Health Promotion—United States. 4. Social Problems—United States. WA 300 AA1 H4346 2008]
RA448.5.N4H395 2008
    362.1089'96073--dc22

                                                                                    2009033972

Printed in the United States of America
THIRD EDITION

HC Printing   10 9 8 7 6 5 4 3 2 1

Dedicated to all African Americans awaiting health justice

CONTENTS

PART TWO
SOCIAL, MENTAL, AND ENVIRONMENTAL CHALLENGES

PART THREE
CHRONIC DISEASES

FOREWORD

GEORGES C. BENJAMIN

Achieving and maintaining ideal health is an intricate process. It involves access to and utilization of a range of clinical preventive and health care services, the interaction of one's physical and genetic makeup, our individual behavior, and the social, economic, and physical environment in which we live.

Although access to care, usually in the form of insurance coverage or timely access to health services, plays an important role in achieving health, it is not the primary determinant. In fact, some say it constitutes only 10 percent of the factors that determine our health (Core Functions Project, 1993). Individual behavior plays a much larger role than access and can often explain disease prevalence when people engage in activities that put them at increased risk. Human variation is a powerful modifier of disease prevalence. Mitigating factors can change the course of disease in different individuals and make the link between risk and outcome nonlinear. We have all known people who seem to eat whatever they want without gaining a pound or who smoke but do not get lung cancer. Gene expression likely plays a role, but health is a complex phenomenon often not easily predicted, even in identical twins. Socioeconomic and environmental factors, such as psychological stress, economic distress, toxic environments, and discrimination, which are often disproportionately prevalent in a community, have profound effects on the capacity to achieve health.

Understanding the impact of these factors on inequities in disease prevalence and health outcomes is challenging and has become the focus of an emerging field of research that attempts first to document the presence of health disparities and then to explain the root causes of both poor health and health disparities. One way to approach these causes is to group them into four areas, as suggested above. First, differences in access to preventive, acute, and chronic care, which are driven by insurance status as well as by timely access to providers and other clinical services; second, differences in the quality of care received; third, individual behavioral differences that result in differences in seeking care or in approaches to being healthy; and, finally, differences in social, political, economic, or environmental exposures that result in differences in health status.

Health disparities, particularly those in the black community, have been the focus of analytic work for over one hundred years. W.E.B. Du Bois first reported on them in his 1899 publication, *The Philadelphia Negro: A Social Study*. In his text, Du Bois addressed the need to get to the root causes of these disparities, stating that "we must endeavor to eliminate, so far as possible, the problem elements which make a difference in health among people." To date, our ineffectual efforts to eliminate these disparities have become one of the serious issues of our day and, in the view of many, a national tragedy.

Not only have we failed to eliminate most of these health inequities, but some of them, like the prevalence of HIV and diabetes and the high infant mortality rate in minority communities, have gotten worse. According to the 2000 Census, while the average American could expect to live 77.8 years, the average African American could expect to live only 73.1 years (National Center for Health Statistics, 2007). Eliminating these disparities is a goal we must strive for as a central component of achieving optimal health in our nation.

These are not theoretical concerns. The huge differences in health among various neighborhoods of our nation's capital are prime examples of this phenomenon in action. Why is it that there is a seventeen-year difference in life expectancy for males of different races in communities only twenty-eight miles apart (Murray et al., 2006)? One clue is the fact that the socioeconomic status of these communities mirrors their health status: poor health correlates with high degrees of poverty, inadequate housing, high crime, and poor educational achievement. Clearly the answer is not the unavailability of qualified clinicians, researchers, and medical institutions: the city has three schools of medicine, numerous teaching hospitals, and some of the world's most prominent researchers. Just up the road is the world's top research institute, the National Institutes of Health. The city itself has invested in a large number of health services as well; yet optimal health for all the city's citizens has been elusive. Unfortunately, Washington, D.C., is typical of our national experience.

So how do we change this picture? Certainly we need to ensure universal access to quality, affordable health care for all our citizens as a first step. But to truly be successful we will have to do much more. We need to transform our health system from its current sick-care focus to one that prevents or delays the presence of disease in the first place. We must ensure equal access to high-quality services and ensure the quality and safety of our system for everyone. Such a system must be affordable for both the individual and the nation. We need to make it easy to make healthy choices. Finally, the social determinants that significantly affect our health must be addressed for all.

The United States should work to become a healthier nation than it now is. To do so, we must make eliminating health disparities a priority. Du Bois told us this over one hundred years ago. We should work to achieve health equity, not in another hundred years, but in our lifetime.

REFERENCES

Core Functions Project. (1993). *Health care reform and public health: A paper on population-based core functions.* Washington, DC: Office of Disease Prevention and Health Promotion, U.S. Public Health Service, Department of Health and Human Services.

Murray, C., Kulkarni, S., Michaud, C., Tomijima, N., Bulzacchelli, M., Iandiorio, T., & Ezzati, M. (2006). Eight Americas: Investigating mortality disparities across races, counties, and race-counties in the United States. *Public Library of Science, Medicine, 3*, 1513–1525.

National Center for Health Statistics, Centers for Disease Control and Prevention. (2007, December 28). *National Vital Statistics Reports, 56*(9).

PREFACE

This third edition of *Health Issues in the Black Community* comes eight years following the release of the second edition and, to our chagrin, presents a picture of African American health replete with many of the disparities documented in the first two editions. Following virtually two decades of studies showing stark contrasts between black and white Americans, we are still faced with a situation that portends a lowered health status and overall quality of life for the black community. The third edition not only documents this continuing gap but also calls for all relevant sectors of U.S. society to actively acknowledge the disparities and move toward viable strategies for removing them. The time has come to engage in aggressive steps and to recognize that unless a bold and systematic process is in place to close the unwavering gap, the next edition of *Health Issues* is likely to repeat the litany presented here.

Similar to the first edition of *Health Issues* and its twenty-five chapters, as well as the second edition, containing twenty-six chapters, this edition's twenty-eight chapters provide information on an array of health-related problems affecting the African American population. It presents the impact of existing health conditions on this population and concludes that although some improvements have occurred, they are severely dwarfed by the many adverse conditions that continue to beset the black community.

The purposes of this third edition are the same as those of the previous editions: (1) to provide a forum for debate and discussion on culturally relevant strategies and models for the prevention of disease and the promotion of wellness in black communities; (2) to influence opinion leaders and provide a futuristic perspective on black health issues for students, academicians, public policymakers, and administrators in public health and related disciplines; and (3) to document selected unhealthy conditions and advance viable strategies for ameliorating them. This edition provides a multidisciplinary perspective with an emphasis on a public health approach.

CONTENTS OVERVIEW

This book contains six distinct sections that provide a more comprehensive examination of the topic than previous editions did. Part One, "Health Status Across the Life Span," looks at the population from childhood to old age. The first chapter provides an overview of black health and sets the overall context of the problem. The second chapter gives the historical context and examines racial disparities in health care and their elimination. This section also discusses specific health problems as they relate to the groups affected: African American children, women, men, and the elderly (Chapters Three, Four, Five, and Six, respectively).

Part Two, "Social, Mental, and Environmental Challenges," addresses health-related dynamics in five areas. Chapter Seven examines stigma and mental health. Chapter Eight reviews homicide and violence with a specific focus on black youth. Chapter Nine addresses the supply and demand of organs for transplantation with an emphasis on narrowing the gap between supply and demand. The issue of African Americans and environmental assault is addressed in Chapter Ten, and incarceration and the health of this population is covered in Chapter Eleven.

Part Three, "Chronic Diseases," includes chapters on selected conditions that can have debilitating effects and that are often viewed as critical. Included are hypertension, cancer, diabetes, lupus, and oral health—Chapters Twelve, Thirteen, Fourteen, Fifteen, and Sixteen, respectively.

Part Four, "Lifestyle Behaviors," concentrates on several self-defeating behaviors that adversely affect health status. Chapter Seventeen addresses an ongoing and devastating problem, substance abuse. Chapter Eighteen discusses one of the gravest issues facing the black community, HIV/AIDS, and Chapter Nineteen addresses tobacco use. Chapter Twenty examines alcohol consumption. Nutrition and obesity are discussed in Chapter Twenty-One, and physical activity is the focus of Chapter Twenty-Two.

Part Five, "Alternative Interventions and Human Resources Development," also presents, in part, a new topic for the third edition with the inclusion of chiropractic medicine in Chapter Twenty-Three. Chapter Twenty-Four reflects on the role of black faith communities in health promotion, and Chapter Twenty-Five illuminates the role of community health workers; these two areas were addressed in previous volumes.

The final part of the book (Part Six), "Ethical, Political, and Ecological Issues," reflects on an array of social factors that infringe on health and presents a discussion as to how they can be reversed. They discuss the impact on health of social marketing and the media (Chapter Twenty-Six) and of racism (Chapter Twenty-Seven). Chapter Twenty-Eight describes disparities in health care and suggests how they can be erased.

All chapters are contributions of individual authors and are not intended to constitute a fully integrated work. They are consistent with the editors' intent to provide a reference for the areas addressed. In addition, each chapter presents the views of its particular author(s) and in no way should be construed as representing a consensus of opinion among the contributors or the position of any affiliated organization or agency.

ACKNOWLEDGMENTS

The third edition of *Health Issues in the Black Community* is the result of many dedicated persons' believing in the single mission of uplifting the health status of African Americans. We especially thank our contributing authors, who worked assiduously on the submission and revision of drafts. Recommendations from colleagues facilitated completion of this project and we remain grateful to them as well.

We are particularly indebted to Keisha Harville, who served as coordinating assistant for this effort. The research support of Aba Essuon and Melva Robertson was vital to the completion of this work. Finally, we would like to thank Andy Pasternack and Seth Schwartz from Jossey-Bass and the consummate professionalism of the publisher for all aspects of support.

October 2009, Atlanta, GA
Ronald L. Braithwaite
Sandra E. Taylor
Henrie M. Treadwell

EDITOR BIOGRAPHIES

Ronald L. Braithwaite, PhD, is currently professor in the Community Health and Preventive Medicine Department and professor and director of research in family medicine in the Psychiatry and Family Medicine Department at Morehouse School of Medicine. He received his BA and MS degrees from Southern Illinois University in sociology and rehabilitation counseling and a PhD in educational psychology from Michigan State University. He has done postdoctoral studies at Howard University, Yale University, and the University of Michigan School of Public Health and Institute for Social Research. He has held faculty appointments at Virginia Commonwealth University, Hampton University, Howard University, Rollins School of Public Health of Emory University, and the School of Public Health at the University of Cape Town, South Africa.

His research involves HIV-intervention studies with juveniles and adults in correctional systems, social determinants of health, health disparities, and community capacity building. He also was a senior justice fellow for the Center for the Study of Crime, Culture, and Communities. Dr. Braithwaite currently serves on the National Institute on Drug Abuse—African American Scholars and Research Group. His research also spans the globe to Africa, where he has conducted HIV-prevention projects in Ghana, Kenya, Swaziland, Zimbabwe, Senegal, Gambia, Ethiopia, Malawi, Tanzania, and South Africa.

Sandra E. Taylor, PhD, is a professor and chair in the Department of Sociology and Criminal Justice at Clark Atlanta University. Previously, she headed the W.E.B. DuBois Department of Sociology at Clark Atlanta, where she also served as director of the HIV/AIDS program, a former affiliate site of the Southeastern AIDS Training and Education Center of Emory University's School of Medicine. She has held research appointments with the Nell Hodgson Woodruff School of Nursing and the Rollins School of Public Health of Emory University. Dr. Taylor currently serves as a W.E.B. DuBois Faculty Fellow at Clark Atlanta.

Dr. Taylor has published extensively in the areas of health and illness as well as in aging, race, and gender, including authorship or coauthorship of more than fifty articles and monographs. Among the many journals containing her work are the *Journal of the National Medical Association, Patient Education and Counseling*, the *Journal of Social Behavior and Personality*, the *Journal of Minority Aging*, the *Journal of Social and Behavioral Sciences*, the *Western Journal of Black Studies*, the *Journal of Black Psychology*, and *National Social Science Perspectives*.

She received her PhD in sociology from Washington University and has done postdoctoral studies in social research and HIV/AIDS at the University of Michigan.

She completed her BA in sociology at Norfolk State University and her MA in the same discipline at Atlanta University. She also completed a predoctoral research program in science education at Purdue University.

Henrie M. Treadwell, PhD, is director and senior social scientist for Community Voices, a special policy initiative funded by the W. K. Kellogg Foundation. She is also a full-time research professor in the Department of Community Health and Preventive Medicine at Morehouse School of Medicine. Her work includes the formulation of health and social policy and the oversight of programs designed to address health disparities, the social determinants of health, and reentry into the community by those engaged with the criminal justice system. She is the founder of the Freedom's Voice Symposium and the Soledad O'Brien Freedom's Voice Award, which recognizes mid-career individuals doing significant work to improve global society.

Prior to coming to the National Center for Primary Care, where she is professor in the Department of Community and Preventive Medicine and director, Community Voices: Healthcare for the Underserved and the Men's Health Initiative, Dr. Treadwell served for seventeen years as program director in health at the W. K. Kellogg Foundation, Battle Creek. Her educational background includes a bachelor's degree in biology, University of South Carolina; a master's degree in biology, Boston University; a PhD in biochemistry and molecular biology, Atlanta University; and postdoctoral work, Harvard University School of Public Health. Dr. Treadwell is a member of the editorial board and section editor for the *International Journal of Men's Health and Gender* and is a member of the editorial board of the *American Journal of Men's Health;* she is a past editorial board member of the *American Journal of Public Health.*

AUTHOR BIOGRAPHIES

Jamy D. Ard, MD, is an assistant professor of nutrition sciences and medicine at the University of Alabama at Birmingham. His current research interests include behavioral therapies that are focused on cardiovascular risk reduction with a special interest in the African American population and in developing strategies for behavior modification that are culturally appropriate. Dr. Ard received his BS in biology at Morehouse College and his MD at Duke University Medical Center.

Kimberly Jacob Arriola, PhD, MPH, received her MA and PhD in social psychology from Northeastern University and her MPH in epidemiology from the Rollins School of Public Health at Emory University. With federal funding, she has overseen the development of a culturally sensitive intervention to promote organ and tissue donation among African Americans. Her other primary area of research is improving HIV testing and links to care in correctional settings. She is an associate professor in the Department of Behavioral Sciences and Health Education in the Rollins School of Public Health. She has published both qualitative and quantitative findings from her research.

Mona AuYoung, MPH, MS, ATC, is currently a PhD student in the Department of Health Services at the UCLA School of Public Health. She received her MPH in community health sciences from UCLA, her MS in kinesiology from California State University, Hayward, and her BA in integrative biology from the University of California, Berkeley. Currently, her research focuses on obesity and diabetes prevention, health disparities among ethnic minorities, and public health partnerships with sports philanthropies. She is also a Certified Athletic Trainer who has worked with national, college, and high school sports teams.

Monica L. Baskin, PhD, is an assistant professor in the Department of Health Behavior at the University of Alabama at Birmingham (UAB) School of Public Health (primary appointment) and the Department of Nutrition Sciences in the UAB School of Health Professions (secondary appointment). She is also an associate scientist for the UAB Clinical Nutrition Research Center and the UAB Minority Health and Research Center, a scientist in the UAB Diabetes Research and Training Center, and a member of the UAB Comprehensive Cancer Center. Dr. Baskin received her BA in psychology and sociology from Emory University, and her MS in community counseling and PhD in counseling psychology from Georgia State University. She is a licensed psychologist with extensive training in pediatric psychology. Dr. Baskin's research focuses on behavioral interventions for the prevention and treatment of obesity and cancer, particularly among African Americans. Much of her work links academic partners to community- and faith-based networks.

Rhonda BeLue, PhD, is an assistant professor of health policy and administration and an affiliate of the Center for Family Research in Diverse Contexts and of the Methodology Center at Pennsylvania State University. Dr. BeLue has over ten years of research experience on chronic mental and physical health problems of minority families. Dr. BeLue's research is at the intersection of research and evaluation methodology and community and minority health. She applies systems science and group-based methods to understand the interrelations among community, family, and individual factors in relation to health outcomes in black families. She has served as the principal investigator on a Robert Wood Johnson Foundation–funded project designed to understand the role of health care settings on quality outcomes among minority populations. She is currently funded to conduct research on academic-community partnerships as related to health outcomes in minority communities. Prior to her appointment at Penn State, she was a front line public health worker specializing in community-based participatory research and the evaluation of community-based public health programs.

Jean J. E. Bonhomme, MD, MPH, is medical director of the Alliance Recovery Center, a staff physician at Toxicology Associates of North Georgia, and an assistant professor at Morehouse School of Medicine. He is on the board of directors of the Men's Health Network and is chairman of the Community Health and Men's Promotion Summit. He is cofounder and president of the National Black Men's Health Network (NBMHN), a community-based, nonprofit organization providing preventive health education in minority communities. NBMHN services include education for HIV prevention, antitobacco education for minority youth, veterans' group counseling, nonviolent conflict resolution, minority youth entrepreneurship, prostate-cancer awareness, involved fathers, and substance-abuse awareness among African American youth and adults. He is also on the editorial board of the *Journal of Men's Health and Gender* and the *American Journal of Men's Health.* Dr. Bonhomme is a graduate of the Rollins School of Public Health at Emory University and a graduate of the State University of New York at Stony Brook, School of Medicine. He trained in categorical internal medicine and psychiatry at Emory University Affiliated Hospitals and holds board certification in public health and general preventive medicine as well as certification by the American Society of Addiction Medicine.

L. Ebony Boulware, MD, MPH, is an associate professor with a primary appointment in the Division of General Internal Medicine of the Johns Hopkins School of Medicine and a joint appointment in the Johns Hopkins Bloomberg Department of Epidemiology. She received her MD degree from Duke University and her MPH from the Johns Hopkins Bloomberg School of Public Health. Her current research focuses on identifying patient and physician barriers to the receipt of guideline concordant care for patients with chronic kidney disease and on identifying patient, physician, and population factors affecting kidney transplantation, with special attention to overcoming barriers to organ donation. To carry out her work related to these barriers, she receives funding from the National Institutes of Health and the federal Health Resources and Services Administration.

L. DiAnne Bradford, PhD, is professor of clinical psychiatry and the director of the Minority Mental Health Research Program at Morehouse School of Medicine. Her research experience and publications span psychiatric-drug discovery and development, ethnopsychopharmacology, pharmacogenetics, the etiology of schizophrenia and depression, and African Americans' unique way of reporting symptoms. Dr. Bradford has received numerous research and training grants from the National Institutes of Health. She received her MS and PhD degrees at the Georgia Institute of Technology, postdoctoral fellowships at the Johns Hopkins School of Medicine and the University of Calgary School of Medicine, and her diploma in pharmaceutical medicine from the University of Leiden (the Netherlands).

Gene H. Brody, PhD, is the director of the Center for Family Research at the University of Georgia and a research professor at the Emory University Rollins School of Public Health. Dr. Brody uses longitudinal, epidemiological, and randomized prevention designs to study his primary area of research, the impact of gene X–environment interactions on children's and adolescents' health. His research is currently supported by grants from the National Institute of Child Health and Human Development, the National Institute on Drug Abuse, the National Institute of Alcoholism and Alcohol Abuse, and the National Institute of Mental Health. Dr. Brody received his terminal degree at the University of Arizona.

Robert D. Bullard, PhD, is the Edmund Asa Ware Distinguished Professor of Sociology and founding director of the Environmental Justice Resource Center at Clark Atlanta University. Professor Bullard is the author of fifteen books. His award-winning book, *Dumping in Dixie: Race, Class, and Environmental Quality* (Westview Press, 2000), is a standard text in the field of environmental justice. Some of his related works are *Just Sustainabilities: Development in an Unequal World* (MIT Press, 2003), *Highway Robbery: Transportation Racism and New Routes to Equity* (South End Press, 2004), *The Quest for Environmental Justice: Human Rights and the Politics of Pollution* (Sierra Club Books, 2005), *Growing Smarter: Achieving Livable Communities, Environmental Justice, and Regional Equity* (MIT Press, 2007), and *The Black Metropolis in the Twenty-First Century: Race, Power, and the Politics of Place* (Rowman & Littlefield, 2007). His most recent book is *Race, Place, and Environmental Justice After Hurricane Katrina: Struggles to Reclaim, Rebuild, and Revitalize New Orleans and the Gulf Coast* (Westview Press, 2009). He received his PhD from Iowa State University.

Jeronda T. Burley, MS, MDiv, is currently a doctoral candidate in social work at the Catholic University of America in Washington, D.C. She received her MS from Auburn

University in marriage and family therapy and an MDiv from Howard University in religion. Her research interests are health promotion within faith-based organizations, religion and substance abuse, religion and HIV/AIDS, the black church, and caregiving and religiosity. Mrs. Burley is a research assistant at the Catholic University and an adjunct professor at Prince George's Community College and Bowie State University. She has published articles in social work and public health journals and has presented at numerous local and national conferences.

Kimberly S. Clay, MSW, MPH, PhD, is an assistant professor in the School of Social Work at the University of Georgia. She holds an MSW, MPH, and PhD in health education from the School of Public Health, University of Alabama at Birmingham. Dr. Clay's program of research comprises two complementary lines of work: (1) the assessment of cancer-related quality-of-life and survival disparities among older adults from racially/ethnically diverse populations, and (2) the implementation and evaluation of lifestyle interventions to improve cancer outcomes, survivorship, and symptom control for the aging. She is a former National Cancer Institute Cancer Prevention and Control Research Training Scholar and is currently a fellow with the National Institute of Aging/Hartford Institute of Aging and Social Work. Her research projects include examination of the feasibility and relative clinical effectiveness of a spiritually enhanced exercise program to lessen depression and fatigue in older African American breast-cancer survivors.

Sharon K. Davis, MEd, MPA, PhD, is the founding director of the Social Epidemiology Research Center at Morehouse School of Medicine. Dr. Davis was a senior research scientist at the Harvard School of Public Health and director of its Center for Minority Health Policy Research and Disease Prevention prior to joining Morehouse School of Medicine. She also held a joint academic appointment in the Department of Medicine at Harvard Medical School and was an associate epidemiologist in the Division of Preventive Medicine at the Brigham and Women's Hospital. Dr. Davis received graduate degrees from Northeastern University and from Harvard University Kennedy School of Government. She earned a PhD in health- and social-policy research from Brandeis University and received subsequent postdoctoral training in health-economics and health-services research from the University of California, Berkeley, School of Public Health. She later received additional training in population-based chronic-disease epidemiology at the Center for Research in Disease Prevention at Stanford University School of Medicine. Her research focuses on the influence of biopsychosocial effects on the etiology and amelioration of chronic disease in high-risk sociodemographic groups.

Cristina Drenkard, MD, PhD, is assistant professor of medicine and epidemiology in the Division of Rheumatology at Emory University. She is a rheumatologist with a PhD in clinical epidemiology from Universidad Nacional de Córdoba in Argentina. Dr. Drenkard has extensive experience in the study of clinical outcomes and epidemiology of ethnic minorities with systemic lupus erythematosus (SLE). For nine years, she worked with a large prospective cohort of SLE in Mexico City. Currently, Dr. Drenkard is coprincipal investigator of the Centers for Disease Control and Prevention–funded Georgia Lupus Registry, a population-based registry designed to estimate the incidence and prevalence of lupus and related connective-tissue diseases in Atlanta.

Charmayne Dunlap-Thomas, MS, is a senior program associate in the Division of Rheumatology at Emory University. She has an MS in professional counseling from Georgia State University with years of research experience in the areas of psychology and lupus. She currently assists in the development and implementation of numerous local, national, and international research projects to advance lupus treatment, education, and awareness.

Mesha L. Ellis, PhD, is a research associate at Morehouse School of Medicine. Her research focuses on developmental psychopathology, family functioning, risk behaviors, childhood antisocial-behavior syndromes, and factors affecting utilization of mental health services by underserved youth and families. Specifically, her research examines preventive interventions and the role of temperamental, cognitive, and familial factors in the development and maintenance of childhood antisocial and substance-abusing behavior. Dr. Ellis's research has been published in peer-reviewed journals and books. She recently coedited (along with Joy Asamen and Gordon Berry) *The SAGE Handbook of Child Development, Multiculturalism, and Media.* Currently, Dr. Ellis is an investigator on a supplement to the National Institute on Drug Abuse–funded Morehouse School of Medicine Minority Institutions' Drug Abuse Research Development Program, where she is evaluating intervention engagement among incarcerated youth and adults.

Angelina Esparza, MPH, is the director of the Patient Navigator Program at the American Cancer Society (ACS). Since joining the ACS in 2005, her focus has been on assisting ACS division offices in starting and developing the program. The program has been established in over 130 health care facilities including the National Cancer Institute Comprehensive Cancer Centers, the Commission on Cancer facilities, and public health hospitals. Prior to joining the ACS, Ms. Esparza worked for nine years at the University of Texas M. D. Anderson Cancer Center, Center of Research on Minority Health, in the Department of Health Disparities as the director of community relations and outreach. Ms. Esparza received her BA in psychology/anthropology from the University of Houston, a BS in nursing from the University of Texas–Houston Health Science Center, and an MPH from the University of Massachusetts–Amherst. She has completed much additional training, including holding a prestigious Emerging Leaders in Public Health fellowship at the University of North Carolina Kenan-Flagler Business School and School of Public Health. She has received multiple awards and much recognition for her work in community health as well as her work with underserved populations, including recognition from the mayor of Houston for her contributions to that community.

Aba D. Essuon, MPH, PhD, is a behavioral researcher at the Morehouse School of Medicine. She received a doctorate in chronic and infectious diseases from the University of South Carolina's Arnold School of Public Health in December 2007. Dr. Essuon also holds master's degrees from Emory University's Rollins School of Public Health in behavioral science and from the University of Georgia's Tucker School of Social Work in family-centered practice. She has both qualitative and quantitative HIV/AIDS research experience, which has increased her interest in minority health issues, specifically the disproportionate rates of HIV/AIDS in the African American community. Dr. Essuon has presented HIV/AIDS–related research findings at various national conferences and has given several guest lectures on various HIV/AIDS–related topics at the University of Georgia, the University of South Carolina, and Spelman College.

Caswell A. Evans, DDS, MPH, is the associate dean for prevention and public health sciences at the University of Illinois at Chicago (UIC) College of Dentistry and holds a joint appointment as professor in the UIC School of Public Health. He has been appointed to the Illinois State Board of Health as well as to the Chicago Board of Health. Previously, Dr. Evans served as director of the National Oral Health Initiative, within the office of the U.S. Surgeon General. He was the executive editor and project director for *Oral Health in America: A Report of the Surgeon General*, released in May 2000, and subsequently directed the development of the *National Call to Action to Promote Oral Health*, released in April 2003. Dr. Evans is a past president of the American Public Health Association and the founder of its Faith Community Caucus. He has served on the board of the National Association of County and City Health Officials. He is a diplomate and past president of the American Board of Dental Public Health and a past president of the American Association of Public Health Dentistry. He received his DDS from Columbia University's School of Dental and Oral Surgery in New York City and earned his MPH from the University of Michigan.

Allan J. Formicola, DDS, is former dean of the College of Dental Medicine and currently professor of dentistry at Columbia University. Dr. Formicola's primary research interest is health disparities. Currently, he is the codirector of the Dental Pipeline program (funded by the Robert Wood Johnson Foundation in collaboration with the California Endowment Foundation and the Kellogg Foundation), which has provided funds to almost half of all U.S. dental schools to increase enrollment of underrepresented minority students and to increase service-learning, community-based education in the curriculum. He has recently completed (with Howard Bailit) a major study on the future of dental education for the Josiah Macy Jr. Foundation.

Nicholas Freudenberg, DrPH, is Distinguished Professor of Public Health at Hunter College and the Graduate Center of the City University of New York and is director of the City University of New York's doctoral program in public health. Dr. Freudenberg's research focuses on the social determinants of the health of urban populations. He has worked to develop, implement, and evaluate health programs in schools, communities, churches, and jails and has advocated for municipal policies that promote health. For the past fifteen years, he has implemented and evaluated interventions to reduce drug use, HIV, and recidivism and to improve the health of people leaving New York City jails.

Laura Joslin Frye, MPH, currently works as a management consultant at Public Health Solutions in New York City. Her primary area of interest is working with community-based organizations to measure and then amplify the effects of their programming through monitoring and evaluation and continuous quality improvement. Ms. Frye's interests extend beyond domestic health issues to the international realm. She was a Fulbright scholar to Morocco, where she studied law and women's health, and has worked with Planned Parenthood Association of Thailand. She received her MPH from the Yale School of Public Health in the Department of Social and Behavioral Sciences.

Vanessa Northington Gamble, PhD, MD, is a professor of medical humanities and health policy at George Washington University. Her primary areas of research are the history of U.S. medicine, racial and ethnic disparities in health and health care, cultural competence, and bioethics. Dr. Gamble received her MD and PhD from the University of Pennsylvania.

Gary H. Gibbons, MD, is the endowed director of the Morehouse Cardiovascular Research Institute, a professor of medicine, and chairman of the Department of Physiology at the Morehouse School of Medicine. He also serves as program director of the Center of Clinical Research Excellence and the National Institutes of Health (NIH) T-32 Training Program in Cardiovascular Science. Dr. Gibbons is a board-certified cardiologist with research expertise in molecular vascular biology. He earned his undergraduate degree from Princeton University and graduated magna cum laude from Harvard Medical School. He completed his residency and cardiology fellowship at the Harvard-affiliated Brigham and Women's Hospital in Boston. His research mentors include Victor Dzau, Thomas Smith, A. Clifford Barger, and Eugene Braunwald. Dr. Gibbons has been selected as a Robert Wood Johnson Foundation Minority Faculty Development Awardee, a Pew Foundation Biomedical Scholar, and an Established Investigator of the American Heart Association; he was recently elected a member of the Institute of Medicine of the National Academy of Sciences. Dr. Gibbons directs NIH-funded research in the fields of vascular biology, genomic medicine, and the pathogenesis of vascular diseases and ranks in the top 5 percent of recipients of NIH funding.

Dionne C. Godette, PhD, is assistant professor of health promotion and behavior at the University of Georgia, College of Public Health. She earned her PhD in health behavior and health education from the University of North Carolina at Chapel Hill. Her work seeks to provide a lens for identifying the social determinants of health disparities related to alcohol, tobacco, and other drugs used and experienced by young minorities.

Dr. Godette has published six peer-reviewed articles on these topics and has two articles currently in press. She has also recently coauthored a chapter on network-based approaches for measuring social capital in a book titled *Social Capital and Health* and has another chapter on health disparities in Georgia forthcoming in a book titled *African Americans in Georgia: A Reflection of Politics and Policy in the New South.*

Malika B. Gooden, DC, MPH, a board-certified and licensed chiropractic physician with a focus on integrative medicine, specializes in evaluating and facilitating biomechanical and neurobiological function. She currently collaborates with Chiropractic Physicians of Atlanta Spine Dunwoody in Atlanta. She obtained her DC at Life University, Marietta, Georgia and her MPH in policy and administration from the University of Michigan, and she holds a BS in psychology with a minor in business management. She has been a senior staff specialist with the Ethnic Minority Fellowship Program of the American Nurses Association, a policy intern with the Centers for Disease Control and Prevention (CDC) Liaison Office on Smoking and Health, and a Public Health Fellow in the CDC/Emory University/Morehouse School of Medicine Fellowship Program. Among many achievements, she is a member of the Pi Tau Delta Chiropractic Honor Society and Beta Kappa Chi National Scientific Honor Society.

Ishtar O. Govia, MA, MTS, PhD, is currently carrying out research projects on dyadic and longitudinal modeling of the associations between social relations and health outcomes and on relationships (interpersonal, intragroup, and intergroup) in the contexts of gender, ethnicity, migration, and aging. Dr. Govia holds a BA in liberal studies (St. Thomas University, Florida), an MTS (Harvard Divinity School), and an MA in general psychology (City College of New York). In 2009 she completed her PhD in personality and social-contexts psychology at the University of Michigan, where she studied risk and protective factors in the mental health of black Caribbeans in the United States.

James P. Griffin Jr., PhD, is a faculty member at the Morehouse School of Medicine in the Department of Community Health and Preventive Medicine and in the Department of Pediatrics. He has also served as an adjunct faculty member at Emory University's Rollins School of Public Health. He has been principal investigator for various prevention programs operating in public schools in Atlanta. Dr. Griffin earned his doctorate in psychology with specialized training in behavior modification, school psychology, and community/organizational psychology. He attended West Virginia University in Morgantown (MA) and Howard University in Washington, D.C., and graduated in 1991 from the Department of Psychology at Georgia State University in Atlanta. For the past eighteen years he has focused on the prevention of alcohol, tobacco, and other drug use and on violence prevention.

Anthony Hatch, PhD, is currently an assistant professor of sociology at Georgia State University in Atlanta. His primary areas of research are in critical race theory, medical sociology, and political sociology. His doctoral research investigated the production of racial meanings in biomedical research on metabolic syndrome in the United States. Dr. Hatch was a recipient of an American Sociological Association and National Institute of Mental Health Minority Fellowship between 2004 and 2007. Dr. Hatch earned his PhD in sociology from the University of Maryland at College Park in 2009.

Schnavia Smith Hatcher, MSW, PhD, is an assistant professor in the School of Social Work at the University of Georgia. She received her PhD in social welfare from the University of Kansas, her MSW from the University of Georgia, and her BA in psychology from Spelman College. Most of Dr. Hatcher's research has been concentrated on identifying psychosocial determinants and pathways to the criminal justice system for youth and adults and facilitating the development of proper protocols to respond to health issues within the system; these protocols pertain, for example, to suicide prevention, mental health and substance-abuse treatment, HIV prevention, and continuity of care within the community. Dr. Hatcher also focuses on developing and implementing health-promotion programs for the community in collaboration with faith-based organizations.

Elton D. Holden, DC, a Georgia board-licensed chiropractor, is in private practice at Buckhead Chiropractic Group in Atlanta. He earned his doctorate at Palmer College of Chiropractic West in San Jose, California. Dr. Holden completed a postdoctoral fellowship in San Salvador, El Salvador, where he treated primarily underserved individuals and families. He is committed to applying new scientific information to improve patient care. He is a member of the Gonstead Clinical Studies Society, the Georgia Chiropractic Association, and the International Chiropractic Association.

Kisha Braithwaite Holden, PhD, is associate director for Community Voices: Healthcare for the Underserved and an assistant professor of clinical psychiatry at Morehouse School of Medicine. She earned her doctorate in counseling psychology from Howard University and completed a National Institute of Mental Health–funded postdoctoral research fellowship at Johns Hopkins University in the School of Medicine and School of Public Health. Dr. Holden brings several years of experience as a clinician, evaluator, and researcher conducting community-based studies focused on mental health disparities and depression among African American women. She is committed to promoting the health and well-being of culturally diverse families and the development of strategies for informing mental health policy.

Rhonda Conerly Holliday, PhD, is a developmental psychologist and currently a research assistant professor in the Department of Community Health and Preventive Medicine at the Morehouse School of Medicine. She received her BS degree in psychology from Morris Brown College in Atlanta. She received her master's and doctorate from the University of Alabama at Birmingham and completed postdoctoral training at Emory University's Rollins School of Public Health. Her main research interests are minority health issues and health disparities with a focus on incarcerated populations. In addition to her academic pursuits, Dr. Holliday serves as a volunteer with the American Psychological Association Behavioral and Social Science Volunteer Program, through which she is available to offer technical assistance to community-based HIV/AIDS organizations.

James S. Jackson, PhD, the Daniel Katz Distinguished University Professor of Psychology, is the director and research professor at the Institute for Social Research and a professor in the School of Public Health, University of Michigan. He has conducted research and published in several areas, including international, comparative studies on immigration, race and ethnic relations, physical and mental health, adult development and aging, attitudes and attitude change, and African American politics. He holds BA and MA degrees in psychology and a PhD in social psychology from Wayne State University. He is an elected member of the Institute of Medicine.

Glenn S. Johnson, PhD, is a research associate in the Environmental Justice Resource Center and associate professor in the Department of Sociology and Criminal Justice at Clark Atlanta University. He coordinates several major research activities including work on transportation racism, urban sprawl, smart growth, public involvement, facility siting, toxics, and regional equity. He is the coeditor of *Just Transportation: Dismantling Race and Class Barriers to Mobility* (New Society, 1997), *Sprawl City: Race, Politics, and Planning in Atlanta* (Island Press, 2000), and *Highway Robbery: Transportation Racism & New Routes to Equity* (South End Press, 2004). Dr. Johnson received his BA (1987), MA (1991), and PhD (1996) in sociology from the University of Tennessee at Knoxville.

Camara Phyllis Jones, MD, MPH, PhD, is research director for social determinants of health and equity in the Division of Adult and Community Health, National Center for Chronic Disease Prevention and Health Promotion, Centers for Disease Control and Prevention. Dr. Jones is a family physician and epidemiologist who seeks to broaden the national health debate beyond the provision of health services to encompass attention to the social determinants of health (including poverty) and the social determinants of equity (including racism). Through her research on the impacts of racism on the health and well-being of the nation, she hopes to initiate a national conversation on racism that will eventually lead to a national campaign against racism. Dr. Jones received her BA (molecular biology) from Wellesley College, her MD from the Stanford University School of Medicine, and her MPH and PhD (epidemiology) from the Johns Hopkins School of Hygiene and Public Health. She also completed residency training in general preventive medicine (Johns Hopkins School of Hygiene and Public Health) and in family practice (Residency Program in Social Medicine, Bronx, New York).

Lovell A. Jones, PhD, is presently a professor in the Department of Health Disparities Research as well as the Department of Biochemistry and Molecular Biology at the

University of Texas M. D. Anderson Cancer Center. He has over thirty-five years of experience addressing issues of minority health and the health of the underserved. As a scientist, Dr. Jones has done extensive research into the relationship among hormones, diet, and endocrine-responsive tumors and has presented his work both nationally and internationally. For his work, the National Institutes of Health/National Center on Minority Health and Health Disparities recently awarded him its Director's Award for Excellence in Health Disparities. Dr. Jones is a coauthor of the congressional resolution designating the third full week in April as National Minority Cancer Awareness Week. Dr. Jones's research also involves determining the mechanism by which natural and environmental estrogenic agents may initiate cancers in hormonally responsive tissue. In January 2000, Dr. Jones was named the first director of the congressionally mandated Center for Research on Minority Health.

S. Sam Lim, MD, MPH, is assistant professor of medicine and epidemiology at Emory University and clinical assistant professor of medicine at Morehouse School of Medicine. He went to medical school at the State University of New York in Brooklyn and obtained his MPH in epidemiology from Emory University. He is the chief of rheumatology at Grady Health Systems, where he directs the Grady Lupus Clinic, and he is the principal investigator of the Georgia Lupus Registry, which is funded by the Centers for Disease Control and Prevention. Through these and other avenues, Dr. Lim seeks to improve the treatment and understanding of systemic lupus erythematosus, particularly as it affects black and lower socioeconomic patients.

Shiriki K. Kumanyika, PhD, earned her PhD in Human Nutrition from Cornell University and MPH from the Johns Hopkins School of Hygiene and Public Health. Her research focus is on developing effective approaches to improve population health outcomes related to nutrition and obesity. Dr. Kumanyika is professor of epidemiology (Department of Biostatistics and Epidemiology and Department of Pediatrics [Gastroenterology; Nutrition Section]) and associate dean for health promotion and disease prevention at the University of Pennsylvania School of Medicine. She is founder and chair of the African American Collaborative Obesity Research Network (AACORN), a national organization devoted to improving the quality, quantity, and effective translation of research on weight issues in African American communities. Her publications include the *Handbook of Obesity Prevention* (Springer, 2007), of which she is lead editor.

Jacqueline Martinez, BS, is a senior program director at the New York State Health Foundation. Her primary areas of research are community health workers, social determinants of health, and access to primary care. Ms. Martinez is the former director of the Kellogg Foundation–funded Community Voices initiative and a 1996 National Institutes of Health Fellow. Her works have been published in the *Journal of Health Care for the Poor and Underserved* and the *American Journal of Public Health*. Ms. Martinez received her BS from Cornell University.

Melita Moore, MD, received her BS in 1999 from Hampton University in biology with a minor in Spanish. She received her MD in 2005 from the Ohio State University, College of Medicine and Public Health. Her primary area of research is traumatic brain injury/concussion in athletes. She was also medical director for Active-Release Techniques Corporate Solutions and is a nationally certified massage therapist and full-body-certified active-release-techniques provider. She is a Sports Medicine Fellow with the University of California–Davis Medical Center.

Cassandra Newkirk, MD, MBA, received a BS in black studies from Duke University, her MD from the University of North Carolina at Chapel Hill, and an MBA in health administration from Regis University. She is board certified in psychiatry and neurology and in forensic psychiatry. Her primary area of research is the psychiatric evaluation and treatment of offenders, with a special interest in women who are incarcerated. She has written and lectured on the topic of incarcerated women for the last several years and was a coeditor of *Health Issues of Incarcerated Women*, published in 2006 by Rutgers University Press. Currently she is the vice president for correctional mental health services and chief medical officer for GEO Care, Inc., in Boca Raton, Florida.

Angela M. Odoms-Young, PhD, is an assistant professor in kinesiology and nutrition at the University of Illinois at Chicago. She examined family processes in diverse populations while holding a Family Research Consortium Postdoctoral Fellowship at Pennsylvania State University and the University of Illinois at Champaign-Urbana. She also held a Community Health Scholars Fellowship in community-based participatory research at the University of Michigan School of Public Health. Her research interests include examining social, cultural, and environmental factors that influence weight and weight-related behaviors in African American women and their families; the relationship between diet and religion; and working with lay health advisors in health-promotion efforts. Dr. Odoms-Young earned a BS in foods and nutrition from the University of Illinois at Champaign-Urbana and an MS and a PhD from Cornell University in human nutrition and community nutrition, respectively.

Desirée A. H. Oliver, MPH, PhD, is the project coordinator/research professional at the Center for Family Research at the University of Georgia. Her primary area of research is resilience and protective factors for children's and adolescents' health and behavioral outcomes. Dr. Oliver earned her terminal degree at the University of South Carolina.

Leda M. Perez, PhD, is vice president for Health Initiatives at the Collins Center for Public Policy, where she focuses on policy and practice related to community health, prisoners and prison health, and community health workers. Dr. Perez was director of Community Voices Miami between 1999 and 2008, with funding of $5 million. Her articles have appeared in the *American Journal of Public Health*, the *Journal of Healthcare for the Poor and Underserved*, the *Journal of Correctional Healthcare*, the *American Journal of Health Services*, and the *American Journal of Men's Health and*

Gender. Dr. Perez earned her PhD in interAmerican studies (international studies and development) from the University of Miami.

Rakale Collins Quarells, PhD, is a behavioral scientist and an associate professor of community health and preventive medicine in the Social Epidemiology Research Center at the Morehouse School of Medicine (MSM). She also serves as the track coordinator for the health education and health-promotion track of the master of public health program at MSM. Dr. Quarells joined MSM in July 2000 following the completion of a two-year Postdoctoral Fellowship in Chronic Disease Epidemiology and Prevention at the Stanford Prevention Research Center in the Stanford University School of Medicine. Dr. Quarells received her BS (1991), MS (1993), and PhD (1998) in psychology from Howard University in Washington, D.C.

Megha Ramaswamy, MPH, PhD, holds a PhD in sociology from the Graduate Center, City University of New York. She was an instructor in urban public health at Hunter College, City University of New York. She joined the faculty in preventive medicine and public health at the University of Kansas School of Medicine in July 2009. Her dissertation research was on the relationship among incarceration, gender, and health, in particular the progressive masculinities and social and policy factors that structure health and social risk for young men involved in the criminal justice system.

Ken Resnicow, PhD, is a professor in the Department of Health Behavior and Health Education at the University of Michigan School of Public Health. His research interests include the design and evaluation of health-promotion programs for special populations, particularly cardiovascular and cancer-prevention interventions for African Americans; the relationship between ethnicity and health behaviors; the prevention and treatment of chronic diseases; obesity prevention; substance-use prevention and harm reduction; type 2 diabetes prevention; and comprehensive school health programs. Much of Dr. Resnicow's work is informed by chaos theory and complexity science. Current studies include a National Institutes of Health (NIH)–funded project to test the impact of ethnic and novel motivational tailoring of colorectal-screening materials for African Americans; an NIH-funded project to develop and evaluate two smoking-prevention programs for South African youth; two studies to increase organ-donation rates among African Americans working in Michigan hair salons and churches; a study funded by the Centers for Disease Control and Prevention to improve colorectal-screening rates in members of black churches; and an NIH-funded study to reduce obesity using a technique called Motivational Interviewing in pediatric practices. He has published over 170 peer-reviewed articles and book chapters and has served on numerous advisory panels and review groups.

Joseph Richardson, PhD, is an assistant professor in the Department of African American Studies at the University of Maryland at College Park. He received his doctoral degree in criminology from the Rutgers University School of Criminal Justice.

Dr. Richardson is also a faculty associate for the Maryland Population Research Center, the Consortium for Race, Gender and Ethnicity, and the School of Public Health at the University of Maryland. Dr. Richardson is on the national advisory board for the Juvenile Relational Inquiry Tool, an initiative funded by the federal Office of Juvenile Justice and Delinquency Prevention. He is currently the director of Project CREATE (Cultural Rehabilitative Enrichment Attained Through Education), a health-literacy program for youth offenders detained at the District of Columbia jail, and is funded to conduct research on the health-risk behaviors of those offenders. Dr. Richardson's research interests focus on the social context of youth-offender reentry and the intersection of health-risk behaviors.

Dana H. Z. Robinson, MPH, received her BA in biology and chemistry from Oberlin College and her MPH from the Rollins School of Public Health at Emory University with a concentration in behavioral sciences. After working for four years as a health communication specialist with the Youth Media Campaign, she returned to the Rollins School of Public Health to serve as project director of Project ACTS (About Choices in Transplantation and Sharing), where she educates African Americans about the importance of organ and tissue donation.

Robert G. Robinson, PhD, served as the associate director for health equity at the Office on Smoking and Health, National Center for Chronic Disease Prevention and Health Promotion, Centers for Disease Control and Prevention (CDC) from 1993 to 2006. Dr. Robinson received his BA in 1967, MSW in 1969, MPH in 1977, and PhD in 1983 from the University of California at Berkeley. His primary areas of work are tobacco cessation (which has resulted in the development of Pathways to Freedom, the state-of-the-art material for the African American community), targeted marketing strategies by the tobacco industry, the historical context of tobacco use in the African American community, and the elimination of population disparities (for which he has developed and published a community-focused conceptual model). Prior to joining the CDC in 1993, Dr. Robinson was a researcher with the Fox Chase Cancer Center in Philadelphia. He chaired the nation's first National Black Leadership Initiative chapter, in Philadelphia. In addition, he spearheaded the coalition of multiple community leaders and organizations that defeated the introduction of UPTOWN cigarette, the first tobacco product produced and marketed specifically for the African American community. He was honored with the Robert G. Robinson Nguzo Saba Award in 2005 by the National African American Tobacco Prevention Network.

Sherrill L. Sellers, PhD, is an associate professor in the School of Social Work at the University of Wisconsin–Madison and an associate professor in the Department of Family Studies and Social Work at Miami University (Ohio). She received her PhD from the University of Michigan–Ann Arbor in 2000. Her research focuses on the mental and physical health consequences of social inequalities, with particular interest in race, class, and gender; the intersection of race, genetics, and health; and aging and the life course. She specializes in mixed-model/mixed-method research.

Emilie Phillips Smith, PhD, is a professor of human development and family studies at Pennsylvania State University and director of the Center for Family Research in Diverse Contexts there. She received her PhD in psychology from Michigan State University. She is the coeditor of a book, *Preventing Youth Violence in a Multicultural Society*. Dr. Smith is currently funded to conduct research with community-based after-school programs to foster positive development and prevent problem behavior. She has been involved in local and national initiatives using universal school-based and targeted family intervention and has authored papers on youth and family development and on the roles of identity, race, and ethnicity.

Shedra Amy Snipes, PhD, is currently a National Cancer Institute Career Development Fellow at the University of Texas School of Public Health in Houston. She received her BA in anthropology and human biology from Emory University and her master's and doctoral degrees from the University of Washington in Seattle. Formerly, Dr. Snipes completed extensive training as a W. K. Kellogg Health Scholar in Multidisciplinary Disparities at the University of Texas M. D. Anderson Cancer Research Center within the Department of Health Disparities Research at the Center for Research on Minority Health. Dr. Snipes's overarching interests are biology, culture, folk beliefs, and health-disparities research. In her work thus far, she has amassed data showing numerous occupational-health disparities among Mexican immigrant workers and has also successfully tested the feasibility of collecting longitudinal biospecimens in highly mobile populations. Through grants awarded by the National Science Foundation, as well as the Southwest Agricultural Health and Safety Center of the National Institute of Occupational Safety and Health, Dr. Snipes has collected important information on key factors that are unique to the Mexican farmworker community. Her latest study describes migrant farmworkers in transit from the Texas-Mexico border to find work; it provides useful data on cultural notions associated with pesticide exposure, occupational illness, injury, and health care access among migrant farmworkers.

Gregory Strayhorn, MD, PhD, MPH, is professor of family medicine and former chair of the department at the University of North Carolina School of Medicine. His current scholarly work centers on the management of chronic diseases, with diabetes as a focus. He is currently funded to develop a clinical-data repository for research, chronic-disease management, and quality of care. He is research mentor to the master of science in clinical research fellows and codirector of the family medicine department's research division. Dr. Strayhorn received his MPH, MD, and PhD from the University of North Carolina at Chapel Hill, completed a residency in family medicine, where he served as chief resident during his final year, and was a Robert Wood Johnson Clinical Scholar at the University of North Carolina School of Medicine prior to taking a faculty position there.

Ivory A. Toldson, PhD, is an associate professor of counseling psychology at Howard University, editor-in-chief of the *Journal of Negro Education*, and senior research analyst for the Congressional Black Caucus Foundation. He received a PhD in counseling psychology from Temple University, an MEd in counseling from Pennsylvania State University, and a BS in psychology from Louisiana State University.

Angel O. Torres, MCP, is a geographic-information-system training specialist with the Environmental Justice Resource Center at Clark Atlanta University. He is the coeditor of *Sprawl City: Race, Politics, and Planning in Atlanta* (Island Press, 2000) and *Highway Robbery: Transportation Racism & New Routes to Equity* (South End Press, 2004). Torres received his BS degree (1993) in mathematics from Clark Atlanta University and his MCP degree (1995) from Georgia Institute of Technology, Atlanta.

Adewale Troutman, MPH, MD, earned an MD from the University of Medicine and Dentistry, New Jersey Medical School, an MPH in policy and management from the Mailman School of Public Health at Columbia University, and an MA in black studies from the State University of New York at Albany. He currently serves as an associate professor in the University of Louisville's School of Public Health and Information Sciences and as the director of the Metro Louisville Department of Public Health and Wellness. He is known for his work on creating health equity through social justice and reframing the focus on health inequities to address the social determinants of health. He played a key role in the nationally recognized and award-winning documentary *Unnatural Causes; Is Inequality Making Us Sick?* Dr. Troutman was a coauthor with David Satcher of the landmark article "What If We Were Equal?" in the journal *Health Affairs* (2005). He has significant global health experience and has served as special consultant for the World Health Organization in Japan, Angola, and Uganda. In addition he has worked in Zaire and India under the auspices of the United Methodist Church. Dr. Troutman serves on the board of directors of the National Association of County and City Officials, is a founding member of the Academy for Health Equity, and is a member of the Citizen's Advisory Committee on Healthy People 2020.

Rueben C. Warren, DDS, MPH, DrPH, is the director of the Institute for Faith-Health Leadership and adjunct professor of public health, medicine, and ethics at the Interdenominational Theological Center in Atlanta. He was the director of infrastructure development for the National Center on Minority Health and Health Disparities within the National Institutes of Health in Bethesda, Maryland, from 2005 through 2007. During this appointment he was on leave from the National Center for Environmental Health—Centers for Disease Control and Prevention/Agency for Toxic Substances and Disease Registry in Atlanta, where he served as an associate director with lead-agency responsibility for environmental justice and minority health. From 1988 to 1997, Dr. Warren served as associate director for minority health at the CDC. Most of his published work concerns oral health, public health, environmental health/justice, and most recently spirituality and health.

Melicia C. Whitt-Glover, PhD, is president and CEO of Gramercy Research Group, a private research firm located in Winston-Salem, North Carolina. The mission of Gramercy Research Group is to improve the lives of individuals and communities by addressing health and related issues. Dr. Whitt-Glover received her BA (1993) and MA (1996) in exercise physiology from the University of North Carolina at Chapel Hill, and her PhD in epidemiology (1999) from the University of South Carolina–Columbia. She completed a postdoctoral fellowship at the University of Pennsylvania School of Medicine (2000–2002). Dr. Whitt-Glover's research interests include physical-activity assessment and interventions, cardiovascular disease, obesity, minority health, and community-based participatory research. She is currently serving as co-investigator on several community-based behavior-change interventions focused on increasing physical activity in adults and children.

Donella J. Wilson, PhD, joined the American Cancer Society (ACS) as a scientific program director in January 1993. Before joining the ACS, Dr. Wilson was an associate professor and researcher at Meharry Medical College in Nashville, Tennessee, for eight years. She received her undergraduate degree in biochemistry from Johnston College at Redlands University in California, earned a master's degree in immunogenetics from Texas Southern University, and went on to Purdue University, where she earned another master's and her doctorate in molecular biology. Her postdoctoral studies included work at Washington University in St. Louis and at both Harvard Medical School and MIT/The Whitehead Institute, where she was a Radcliffe College Mary Ingraham Bunting Fellow. In 2003, Dr. Wilson became scientific director of research promotion and communication for the ACS's Research Department. She also works to promote research and increase fund-raising at donor and Relay for Life events, provides scientific consultation and review for research-promotion materials and projects, and manages research-promotion information on the ACS website and other databases. Dr. Wilson has been the recipient of numerous honors and awards for her contributions to biomedical research, and she has served on the Council of the American Society of Cell Biology. She is currently chairperson of their minority affairs committee, successfully submitting a multimillion-dollar grant to NIH on its behalf.

Kamilah M. Woodson, PhD, is an assistant professor and the clinical director at the Howard University School of Education, Department of Human Development and Psycho-educational Studies, in the counseling psychology PhD program. Dr. Woodson works with the DC Baltimore Center for Reducing Health Disparities, with Howard University College of Medicine, and with Howard University Office for Undergraduate Research. She serves on the editorial board of the *Journal of Negro Education* as the book editor, and her research is in the area of health disparities, including factors that affect health-related risk behaviors (HIV/AIDS and substance abuse) among people of color. Dr. Woodson is a graduate of the California School of Professional Psychology, Los Angeles, where she received PhD and MA degrees in clinical psychology; she earned her BA in psychology from the University of Michigan–Ann Arbor.

Antronette K. Yancey, MD, MPH, is currently a professor in the Department of Health Services, UCLA School of Public Health, and is codirector of its Center to Eliminate Health Disparities. Dr. Yancey has authored more than one hundred scientific publications, including briefs, book chapters, health-promotion videos, and, among those, more than seventy peer-reviewed journal articles. She has generated more than $20 million in extramural funds, including four National Institutes of Health independent investigator (R01, R24) grants as principal investigator. She serves on the Institute of Medicine Standing Committee on Childhood Obesity Prevention and Health Literacy Roundtable and on the National Physical Activity Plan steering committee. She chairs the board of directors of the Public Health Institute in Oakland, California. She completed her undergraduate studies in biochemistry and molecular biology at Northwestern University and earned her medical degree at Duke and her MPH at UCLA. Her primary research interests are chronic-disease prevention and adolescent-health promotion.

April M. W. Young, PhD, is vice president for justice initiatives at the Collins Center for Public Policy, an action-oriented think tank based in Florida. She designed the Overtown Men's Health Study, which gathered extensive data on residents of the distressed Miami neighborhood of Overtown. In addition to research on the social determinants of poor men's health, Young works on related issues of juvenile justice, adult incarceration, and community reentry. Young has a PhD in social anthropology from Harvard University and an AB from Princeton University's Woodrow Wilson School of Public and International Affairs.

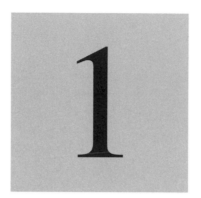

HEALTH STATUS ACROSS THE LIFE SPAN

CHAPTER

AFRICAN AMERICAN HEALTH: AN OVERVIEW

RONALD L. BRAITHWAITE
SANDRA E. TAYLOR
HENRIE M. TREADWELL

In 1980, in response to arguments that the commonly used Gross Domestic Product, a measure of human progress, failed to adequately measure well-being, Mahbub ul Haq, a Pakistani economist, devised the concept for the human development index (Burd-Sharps, Lewis, & Martins, 2008). With the assistance of Nobel laureate Amartya Sen and other economists from Yale University and the London School of Economics, Dr. Haq developed the Human Development Index (HDI). The HDI's success in expanding both the measure and discussion of well-being beyond the confines of income has made it one of the most widely used indices of both global and national well-being. Since its creation in 1990, the HDI has been used by the United Nations Development Program (UNDP) as a means of determining a country's developmental status—developed, developing, or underdeveloped. A country's HDI score and its corresponding developmental status is assessed and reported annually by the UNDP.

The HDI score is computed using variables considered to be standard measures of "human development." The variables are life expectancy at birth, used as an index of population health and longevity; knowledge and education, measured by adult literacy and primary, secondary, and tertiary school enrollment; and standard of living, measured by the Gross National Product per capita at purchasing power parity in U.S. dollars (Burd-Sharps et al., 2008; Sotelo & Gimeno, 2003). The HDI variables are used to generate scale scores between zero and one. The resulting HDI scale score range is divided into three categories—high ($\geq$ 0.80), medium (0.50–0.79), and low ($\leq$ 0.50)—where zero indicates the lowest level of human development and one (1), the highest level of human development (Burd-Sharps et al., 2008). Countries, such as the United States, that have high HDI scores are considered to be developed, and those with medium or low HDI scores are considered to be developing or underdeveloped (third world), respectively.

The HDI is a means by which the United States and other countries assess their global competitiveness, the well-being of their communities, and societal disadvantages (Burd-Sharps et al., 2008). A recent comparison of federal health data from 2005 with those from 2006, using the HDI, revealed a persistently poor international health status for U.S. black males. Despite living in the richest and most medically advanced country in the world, U.S. blacks have a health status comparable to those residing in "medium human development" countries (Gadson, 2006). In 1990, the *New England Journal of Medicine* estimated the life expectancy of U.S. black males to be sixty-five years. In the sixteen years following the 1990 estimate, black male life expectancy rates showed marginal improvement in 2005–6 (68.8 years). In an international life expectancy comparison, the life expectancy at birth for U.S. black males (68.8 years) was less than it was for males in Iran (69.0 years), Colombia (69.3 years), Occupied Palestinian Territories (70.9 years), Ecuador (71.4 years), and Sri Lanka (71.5 years) (see Table 1.1). With a difference of nearly six years from U.S. white males, the life expectancy of U.S. black males is more comparable to the life expectancies of males in Vietnam (68.6 years), El Salvador (67.8 years), and Iraq (67.5 years) than it is to their U.S. white male counterparts (74.6 years) (Gadson, 2006).

In the United States, Northeastern states—such as Connecticut, Massachusetts, New Jersey, Washington, D.C., and Maryland, which have the highest earning potential, education attainment and enrollment, and the second-highest life expectancy of the four U.S. Census regions—have the highest HDI (Burd-Sharps et al., 2008). States such as Mississippi, West Virginia, Louisiana, Arkansas, and Alabama, which are in the Southern region, have the lowest HDI in that the people in this region have, on average, the shortest life expectancy, lower earning potential, and lower levels of educational attainment and enrollment than do Americans in other parts of the country. In general, women have higher educational attainment and a life expectancy five years greater than men; however, the advantages of education and health are overshadowed by women's lower earnings, thus giving men a slightly higher HDI.

Racially and ethnically, Asians outperform all other racial groups in all three human development dimensions. Of all the racial and ethnic groups, Asians have the highest earnings, which are slightly greater than whites, whose HDI ranking too is second to Asians. Asians also rank first and vastly higher than whites in health and educational advantages. Latinos rank third overall. Despite having the lowest educational and income rankings, the overall good health of Latinos gives them an HDI ranking higher than that of blacks. Even though blacks are third in income and education, their poor health status gives them the bottom ranking. The health ranking of blacks has

TABLE 1.1 **Selected Male Life Expectancies at Birth.**

Country	Life Expectancy (yrs)	Country Rank (HDI score)	HDI Category
United States (white)	74.6	12 (0.951)	High
Sri Lanka	71.5	99 (0.743)	Medium
Ecuador	71.4	89 (0.772)	Medium
Malaysia	70.9	63 (0.811)	High
Occupied Palestinian Territories	70.9	106 (0.731)	Medium
Colombia	69.3	75 (0.791)	Medium
Iran	69.0	94 (0.759)	Medium
United States (black)	68.8	12 (0.951)	High
Vietnam	68.6	105 (0.733)	Medium
El Salvador	67.8	103 (0.735)	Medium
Iraq	67.5	N/A	Medium
Nicaragua	67.3	110 (0.710)	Medium

Source: U.S. data from National Center for Health Statistics. (2006). *Health, United States, 2006, with Chartbook on Trends in the Health of Americans.* Hyattsville, MD: Author. International data from United Nations Development Program. (2005). *Human development report 2005: International cooperation at a crossroads—Aid, trade and security in an unequal world.* New York: Hoechstetter Printing; United Nations Development Program. (2007). *Human development report 2007/2008: Fighting climate change—Human solidarity in a divided world.* New York: Palgrave Macmillan.

resulted in life expectancies five years less than those of Native Americans, who have the second-lowest health ranking, and thirteen years less than Asians, who have the highest health ranking.

For the past one hundred years, the U.S. black male has had the shortest life expectancy of any other U.S. racial or ethnic group (Gadson, 2006). Although life expectancy has increased steadily since 1970 for whites and blacks, between 1970 and 2005 the increases in life years have been greater for whites than blacks and for women than men (see Figure 1.1) (U.S. Department of Health and Human Services . . . , 2008).

FIGURE 1.1 *Life Expectancy at Birth, by Race and Sex, 1970–2005.*

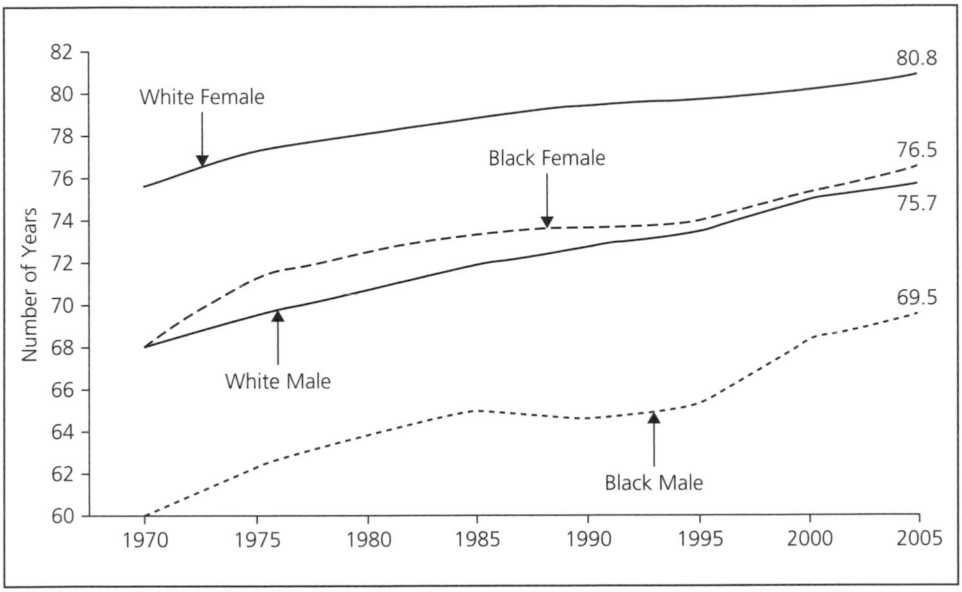

Note: Both racial categories include Hispanics.
Source: Centers for Disease Control and Prevention; National Center for Health Statistics, as referenced in Gadson, 2006.

Between 1970 and 2005 the life expectancy for white females remained the highest in the nation. As reflected in the figure, a white female born in 2005 could expect to live approximately 80.8 years, whereas a black female born in the same year could expect to live an average of only 76.5 years, a difference of 4.3 years. With a difference of 6.2 years, a white male born in 2005 could expect to live 75.7 years, compared to a black male born in the same year with a life expectancy of 69.5 years. In the United States, the black male, from birth to eighty-four years, has the highest mortality rates across all ages and geographic regions, with the greatest racial differences in mortality rates reported for males twenty-five to fifty-four years of age (Gadson, 2006).

In 2005, blacks, with 1,016.5 deaths per 100,000 persons, had a higher overall age-adjusted mortality rate than whites, at 785.3 deaths per 100,000; Native Americans/ Alaska Natives, at 663.4; and Asians/Pacific Islanders, at 440.2 (Kung, Hoyert, Xu, & Murphy, 2008). High rates of U.S. black male mortality are attributed to the racial health disparities that exist for nearly all major chronic diseases. According to the 2000 census, 36.4 million persons, or 12.9 percent of the U.S. population, identified as black or African American (McKinnon, 2001; Centers for Disease Control and Prevention [CDC], 2005). Of those identifying as black or African American, 35.4 million identified as non-Hispanic. This category, non-Hispanic blacks, has a disproportionately greater burden of disease, injury, death, and disability for many health

TABLE 1.2   **Ten Leading Causes of Death (Both Sexes, All Ages).**

Rank	United States	Whites	Blacks
1	Heart disease	Heart disease	Heart disease
2	Cancer	Cancer	Cancer
3	Stroke	Stroke	Stroke
4	Chronic lower respiratory disease	Chronic lower respiratory disease	Diabetes
5	Unintentional accidents	Unintentional accidents	Unintentional accidents
6	Diabetes	Diabetes	Homicide
7	Influenza/Pneumonia	Influenza/Pneumonia	HIV/AIDS
8	Alzheimer's disease	Alzheimer's disease	Respiratory disease (COPD)
9	Kidney diseases	Kidney diseases	Kidney diseases
10	Septicemia	Suicide	Septicemia

Source: CDC. (2005, March). *National Vital Statistics Report*, 53(17); National Center for Health Statistics. (2005, March 7). *National Vital Statistics Reports*.

conditions (CDC, 2005). Although blacks and whites share the top three causes of death and, without regard to ranking, seven of the ten leading causes of death (reflected in Table 1.2), the risk, incidence, morbidity, and mortality rates of disease and injury are often greater for blacks than whites.

HEART DISEASE

Excluding the year 1918, heart-disease–related illnesses have been the leading cause of death in the United States since 1900, killing one American every 34 seconds, or more than twenty-five hundred people daily (American Heart Association, 2005). Heart disease, which is defined as any disorder that prevents the heart from functioning properly, is a general term used to denote various diseases that could affect the heart (U.S. Department of Health and Human Services . . . , 2008). The eight types of heart disease are (1) coronary, a blockage of a coronary artery, which can cause chest pain and heart attack; (2) cardiomyopathy, a disease of the heart muscle, which can cause arrhythmia and/or sudden cardiac death; (3) cardiovascular, any number of specific diseases that affect the heart and/or the blood vessel system leading to and from the heart; (4) ischemic, a disease of the heart characterized by a reduction in blood to organs; (5) congestive heart failure and congestive cardiac failure, diseases resulting from any structural or functional cardiac disorder that impairs the heart's ability to fill with or pump sufficient amounts of blood throughout the body; (6) hypertensive, a disease caused by high blood pressure; (7) inflammatory, a disease involving the inflammation of the heart muscle and/or the surrounding tissue; and (8) valvular, a disease process involving one or more valves of the heart.

With risk factors including obesity, lack of physical activity, smoking, high cholesterol, hypertension, and old age, coronary heart disease is the most common form of heart disease and is the single leading cause of death in America (U.S. Department of Health and Human Services . . . , 2008; American Heart Association, 2005). Heart disease deaths represent nearly 60 percent of the total mortality rate, claiming nearly as many lives annually as the next five leading causes of death combined: cancer, chronic lower respiratory disease, accidents, diabetes mellitus, and influenza and pneumonia. In 2004, coronary heart disease death rates per 100,000 persons were higher for males than females and higher for blacks than whites. Overall, coronary heart disease mortality rates were higher for black males (223.9 per 100,000) than they were for white males (194.2), black women (148.7), or white women (114.7). In 2007, a total of 16 million persons, 8.7 million males and 7.3 million females, were estimated to have a history of heart attack and/or angina pectoris, which are both caused by coronary heart disease. Despite blacks having higher heart disease mortality rates, the prevalence of heart disease and heart-disease–related conditions is higher among whites than blacks. Affecting 12.2 percent of the white population, heart disease in whites is second in prevalence only to Native Americans/Alaska Natives.

CANCER

Cancer is the second leading cause of death in the United States, where black men have the highest cancer death rate per 100,000 persons (see Figure 1.2). The cancer death rates are substantially greater among blacks than whites and among men than women. Cancer incidence among men is highest among blacks (607.3 per 100,000 persons), followed by whites (527.2), Hispanics (415.5), and Asians/Pacific Islanders (325.8). Among the U.S. male population, lung cancer, representing 70.3 percent of all cancer deaths; prostate cancer, representing 25.4 percent; colorectal cancer, 21.6 percent; and liver cancer, 15.1 percent are the top four leading causes of cancer deaths (CDC, 2007). With the exception of Hispanics, lung cancer is the leading cause of cancer death among all male racial groups; however, black males, with a lung cancer death rate of 101.3 per 100,000 persons, are 1.3 times more likely to die from lung cancer than are their white counterparts, with a death rate of 75.2 (see Table 1.3) (Ries et al., 2005). Although prostate cancer is the second leading cause of cancer death for

FIGURE 1.2 *Cancer Death Rates, by Race and Ethnicity, United States, 1998–2002.*

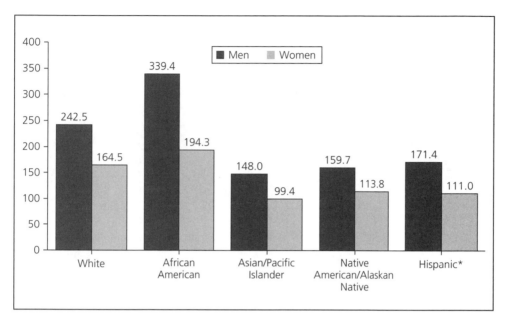

Note: Death rates per 100,000; age-adjusted to the 2000 U.S. standard population.
* Hispanic does not mutually exclude whites, African Americans, Asians/Pacific Islanders, or Native Americans/Alaska Natives.
Source: National Cancer Institute, Division of Cancer Control and Population Sciences. (2005). *Surveillance, Epidemiology, and End Results Program, 1975–2002.*

all U.S. males with the exception of Asians/Pacific Islanders, blacks are disproportionately impacted (CDC, 2007). As shown in Table 1.3, cancer-related mortalities were 1.3 to 2.3 times greater for black males than white males for other cancers, such as of the larynx, stomach, mouth, esophagus, small intestine, and pancreas, and myeloma.

Representing 56.1 percent, the percentage of black male cancer deaths attributed to prostate cancer is 2.4 times that of white males (23.4%), 2.9 times that of Hispanic males (19.3%), and 3.4 times that of Native Americans/Alaska Natives (16.5%). As the third leading cause of cancer death for all male racial groups, colorectal cancer death is 1.4 times greater among black males (9.5 deaths per 100,000) than for white males (6.2) (see Table 1.3) (Ries et al., 2005). Liver cancer, although the second leading cause of cancer death among male Asians/Pacific Islanders, is the fourth leading cause of cancer death among men overall (CDC, 2007). The rate of cancer death among black males (9.5 deaths) is 1.5 times greater than that of white males (6.2).

Overall, within the U.S. female population, white women (405.9 per 100,000 persons) have the highest incidence of cancer, followed by black women (379.7), Hispanic

TABLE 1.3 **Cancer Sites in Which African American Death Rates Exceed White Death Rates for Men, United States, 1998–2002.**

Site	Black Males	White Males	Ratio (Black/White)
All sites	339.4	242.5	1.4
Prostate	68.1	27.7	2.5
Larynx	5.2	2.3	2.3
Stomach	12.8	5.6	2.3
Myeloma	8.8	4.4	2.0
Oral cavity/pharynx	7.1	3.9	1.8
Esophagus	11.2	7.5	1.5
Liver/intrahepatic bile duct	9.5	6.2	1.5
Small intestine	0.7	0.5	1.4
Colon/rectum	34.0	24.3	1.4
Lung/bronchus	101.3	75.2	1.3
Pancreas	15.8	12.0	1.3

Note: Death rates per 100,000; age-adjusted to the 2000 U.S. standard population.
Source: National Cancer Institute, Division of Cancer Control and Population Sciences. (2005).
Surveillance, Epidemiology, and End Results Program, 1975–2002.

women (318.6), Asian/Pacific Islander women (267.4), and Native American/Alaska Native women (242.2) (CDC, 2008a). However, black women presented higher prevalence than white women for colorectal (54.0 vs. 43.3), pancreatic (13.0 vs. 8.9), and stomach (9.0 vs. 4.5) cancers. Breast, lung, and colorectal cancers are the most common cancers among women as well as the leading causes of cancer-related deaths among women. Although breast cancer is the most common form of cancer among women of all races (117.7 per 100,000 persons), it is the second leading cause of cancer deaths for women (24.4 deaths per 100,000). Breast cancer is the first leading cause of death among Hispanic women (15.7) and the second leading cause of death among blacks (32.3), whites (23.8) and Native Americans/Alaska Natives (15.0).

Despite being the second most common cancer among U.S. women (54.2 per 100,000 persons), lung cancer is the leading cause of female cancer deaths (40.9 deaths) (CDC, 2007). Lung cancer is the primary cause of cancer death among white (41.9), black (40.0), Native American/Alaska Native (30.2), and Asian/Pacific Islander women (18.1) and the second leading cause of death for Hispanic women (14.4). Colorectal cancer is the third most prevalent (42.7) as well as the third leading cause of cancer death (15.2 deaths) among U.S. women. Colorectal cancer is the second most common form of cancer among black (50.6), Hispanic (34.2), and Asian/Pacific Islander (32.1) women and the third most common form of cancer among white (41.6) and Native American/Alaska Native (28.7) women.

STROKE

Claiming over 160,000 lives a year, stroke is the third leading cause of death in the United States and the leading cause of serious long-term disability (American Heart Association, 2005). In 2005, strokes accounted for one out of every seventeen deaths. Of the 700,000 annual U.S. strokes, equating to one stroke every 45 seconds, 500,000 are experienced by those who have never had a stroke and 200,000 occur among those with a prior history of stroke. There are three types of stroke—ischemic, hemorrhagic, and transient ischemic attacks—all of which occur more often among people with conditions such as high blood pressure, heart disease, and diabetes. Ischemic stroke, which occurs when oxygenated blood is blocked from the brain, is the most common type of stroke, accounting for 88 percent of all strokes. There are two kinds of hemorrhagic stroke, intracerebral and subarachnoid. Intracerebral hemorrhage, accounting for 9 percent of all strokes, results when blood vessels in the brain leak into the brain, and subarachnoid hemorrhage, accounting for 3 percent of all strokes, results from bleeding under the outer brain membrane. Transient ischemic attack (TIA), sometimes referred to as a mini-stroke, is the mildest of the three types of stroke. The onset of a TIA has the same etiology as any other stroke; however, the effects of a TIA stroke clear within twenty-four hours of the onset.

Although strokes can and do occur at any age, more than three-quarters of all strokes occur in people under the age of sixty-five (American Heart Association, 2005). A person's risk of stroke doubles each decade after age fifty-five. Blacks are twice as likely as whites to experience a stroke. In age-adjusted, first-ever stroke incidence per 100,000 persons, white males had a stroke prevalence of 167, compared to black males, whose prevalence rate was much higher at 323. The age-adjusted prevalence rate for first stroke was again much higher for black women (260) than it was for white women (138). Claiming a life every three minutes, strokes account for more than one out of every fifteen U.S. deaths. In addition to having higher stroke prevalence, blacks are also more likely to die from stroke than are their white counterparts. The higher stroke mortality and morbidity rates experienced by blacks may be directly related to their higher prevalence for stroke-related risk factors, such as hypertension and diabetes.

As of 2004, seventy-three million persons twenty and older were estimated to have high blood pressure in the United States (American Heart Association, 2005). The prevalence of high blood pressure among blacks is among the highest in the world. About 34 percent of the U.S. black population has high blood pressure, which is greater than that of the Hispanic, white, and Native American populations, whose rates are between 24 and 27 percent. High blood pressure rates among blacks have been noted for causing 40 percent of all deaths related to stroke, heart disease, and kidney disease: blacks are 1.8 times more likely than whites to experience fatal strokes, 1.5 times more likely to have fatal heart disease, and 4.2 times more likely to progress to end-stage kidney disease. High blood pressure rates may also be responsible for up to 75 percent of cardiovascular problems in people with diabetes, which is itself a stroke risk factor and the fourth leading cause of death among blacks.

DIABETES

Nationally and among whites, diabetes is the sixth leading cause of death; it is the fourth leading cause of death among blacks (Table 1.2). There are three types of diabetes: type-1, type-2, and gestational diabetes (CDC, 2008b). Type-1 diabetes results when the body's immune system destroys pancreatic beta cells responsible for producing the insulin that regulates blood glucose. Type-1 diabetes usually occurs among children and young adults but can occur at any age. Type-1 accounts for 5–10 percent of all diagnosed diabetes cases among adults. Type-2, also known as adult onset diabetes or non-insulin dependent diabetes mellitus, results when the body gradually loses its ability to meet its demand for insulin. This form of diabetes accounts for 90–95 percent of all diagnosed diabetes cases in adults. Gestational diabetes is a form of glucose intolerance that can be diagnosed during pregnancy. This form of diabetes occurs more often among black, Hispanic, and Native American women. It is also more common among obese women as well as those with a family history of diabetes.

In 2007, the CDC estimated 23.6 million people (7.8% of the U.S. population) to be diabetic, an estimate which includes 17.9 million diagnosed and 5.7 million undiagnosed cases of diabetes (CDC, 2008b). Among those twenty or older, the prevalence of diabetes among blacks was 1.5 times that of whites. Although whites contributed 11.2 million more cases than blacks (14.9 million versus 3.7 million, respectively), the population percentage of blacks aged 20 or older with diabetes was greater than the population percentage of whites in the same age group, 14.7 percent versus 9.8 percent, respectively.

The lifetime risk of developing diabetes for persons born in 2000 was higher for blacks than whites and for women than men (see Figure 1.3). As shown in the figure, the lifetime risk of diabetes for whites was lower than the overall population ("Total") risk, regardless of gender; in contrast, the risk for blacks was higher than the overall population risk for both males and females. The lifetime risk for diabetes among black males exceeded that of white males born in 2000 by more than 10 percent; and the lifetime risk among black women exceeded that of white women by nearly 20 percent.

FIGURE 1.3 *Estimated Lifetime Risk of Developing Diabetes for Individuals Born in the United States in 2000.*

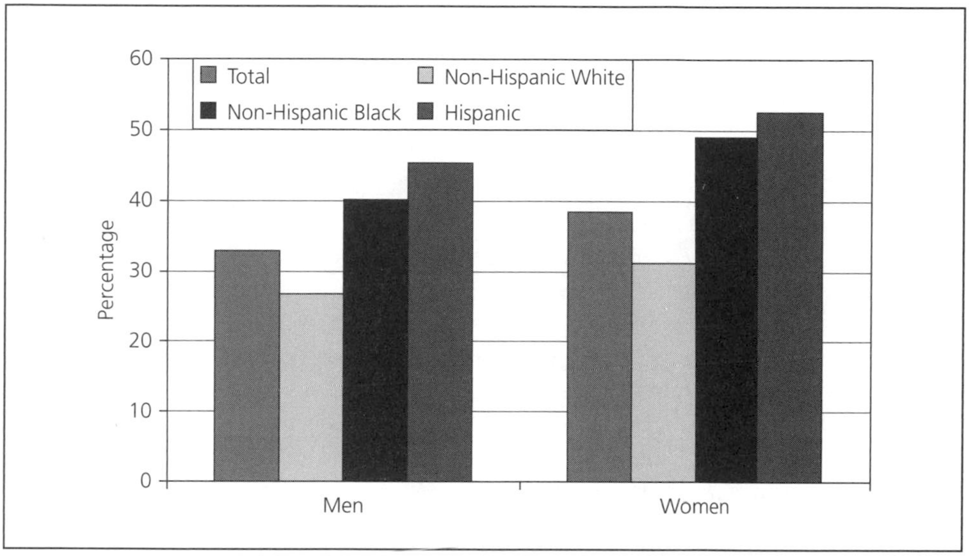

Source: Venkat Narayan, K., Boyle, J., Thompson, T., Sorensen, S., & Williamson, D. (2003). Lifetime risks for diabetes mellitus in the U.S. *JAMA, 290* (2003): 1884–1890.

With the exception of Hispanics, whose risk exceeded blacks' by ≤5 percent, blacks have the highest lifetime diabetes risk.

In addition to being more likely than whites to develop diabetes, blacks are more likely to experience greater diabetes-related disabilities. Diabetes is a leading cause of adult blindness, lower-limb amputation, kidney disease, and nerve damage. Responsible for twelve to twenty-four thousand new blindness cases per year, diabetic retinopathy is the leading cause of new cases of blindness among adults from twenty to seventy-four years (CDC, 2008b). By 2050, it is estimated that diabetic retinopathy will increase from its current prevalence of 5.5 million to between 16 and 18 million (National Center for Chronic Disease Prevention and Health Promotion . . . , 2007). Twenty-three percent of diabetics experience foot problems, including numbness, accounting for more than 60 percent of all nontraumatic lower-limb amputations (CDC, 2008b). Nervous system damage is the major contributing cause of lower-extremity amputation. Approximately 60 to 70 percent of diabetics have mild to severe forms of nervous system damage, which impair such things as sensation in the feet or hands and slow stomach digestion of food. Diabetes is the leading cause of kidney failure, accounting for 44 percent of new cases in 2005 (CDC, 2008b).

Diabetes-related mortality rates are 27 percent greater among blacks than whites (National Center for Chronic Disease Prevention and Health Promotion . . . , 2007).

Two-thirds of those with diabetes die from heart attack or stroke, whereas 65 percent die from cardiovascular disease. Adult diabetics are two to four times more likely than nondiabetic adults to die of heart disease and/or have a stroke. In 2004, heart disease was noted for 68 percent and stroke was noted for 16 percent of diabetes-related deaths among persons sixty-five years or older (CDC, 2008b). Eight percent of diabetics experience congestive heart failure and 9 percent suffer from coronary artery disease.

HOMICIDE

In the United States, homicide is the fifteenth leading cause of death; however, it is among the top five causes of death for ages 1–34 (Kung et al., 2008; Karch, Lubell, Friday, Patel, & Williams, 2008). Homicide is the second leading cause of death for ages 15–24, third for ages 25–34, and fourth for ages 1–14 (Karch et al., 2008). Homicide ranks sixth among the top ten leading causes of death among blacks; for whites, homicide was not among the top ten causes of death. In 2005, blacks accounted for about half of the homicide deaths, and males accounted for 3.5 times more homicide deaths than did females. The trend data reflected in Figure 1.4 depict the population percentage for American males age 14–24, the percentage of male homicide victims by race, and the percentage of male homicide offenders by race from 1976 to 2005.

The graphs in the figure show the 14–24-year-old white male population, as a percentage of total population, to be consistently greater than the black male population within the same age group. Despite having declined from its 1976 high of 8.9 percent of the population to 6.3 percent in 2005, the percentage of white males age 14–24 has always exceeded its black male counterpart, whose percentage has declined from 1976 (1.3%) to 2005 (1.2%). In the twenty-nine years reflected in the figure, both races

FIGURE 1.4 *Young Males as a Percentage of the Population, of Homicide Victims, and of Homicide Offenders, 1976–2005.*

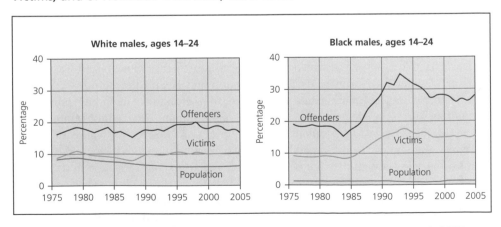

Source: Bureau of Justice Statistics; homicide trends in the United States, by race, July 2007.

experienced population trends as follows: from 1976 to 2005, white males age 14–24 represented population percentages between 6.1 and 8.9 percent. The lowest population percentage for white males (6.1%) began in 1996 and continued through 2001 before increasing to 6.2 percent in 2002, and 6.3 percent in 2005. For black males in the age group, population percentages ranged between 1.1 and 1.4 percent. The lowest population percentage for black males (1.1%) began in 1992 and continued through 2000 before increasing to 1.2 percent in 2001.

Although the white male population was 5.5–6.4 times greater than that of the black male population within the same age group, the percentages of homicide victims and offenders were greater among black males than white males. As shown in Figure 1.5, white males age 14–24 years represented 7.9–10.8 percent of homicide victims and 15.3–20.1 percent of homicide offenders, compared to black males in the same age group, representing 8.2–17.5 percent of homicide victims and 72.3–82.8 percent of homicide offenders. In 2005, blacks age 14–24 years were six times more likely to be the victim of homicide and seven times more likely to have perpetrated a homicide than their white counterparts. Although blacks were less likely than whites to be the victim of sex-related homicides (30.5% black vs. 66.9% white), workplace killings (12.2% black vs. 84.6% white), or homicides by poisoning (16.9% black vs. 80.6% white), they were overrepresented in homicides involving drugs (61.6% black vs. 37.4% white) (U.S. Department of Justice, 2007).

FIGURE 1.5 *Homicide Victimization and Offense, by Race, 1976–2005.*

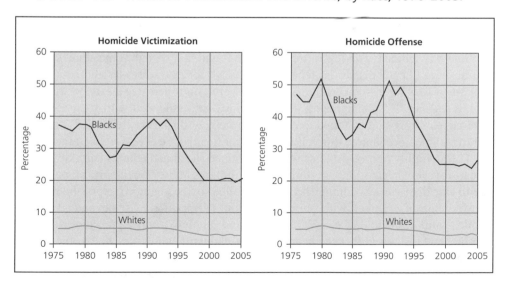

Note: Rates per 100,000 persons.
Source: Bureau of Justice Statistics; homicide trends in the United States, by race, July 2007.

In 2004 black males were more likely than Hispanics or whites to be sentenced for drug-related offenses (23%, 21%, and 15%, respectively) (Sabol, Couture, & Harrison, 2007). By the end of 2005, blacks represented 44.8 percent, Hispanics 20.2 percent, and whites 28.5 percent of the 253,300 state inmates serving time for drug offenses (Sabol & West, 2008). Again, in 2007, blacks had a greater incarceration rate than whites. Black men were incarcerated at a rate of 4,618 per 100,000 compared to white males, with a rate of 773, and black women were incarnated at a rate of 348 compared to white women, at a rate of 95 (Sabol & Couture, 2008). The higher prevalence of incarceration among blacks has contributed to other health disparities, such as HIV/AIDS, which does not rank among the top ten leading causes of death for the nation or among whites but is the seventh leading cause of death for blacks.

CONCLUSION

A review of the nation's top ten leading causes of death revealed periodically higher morbidity and consistently higher mortality rates for blacks. Unlike their white counterparts, blacks were less likely to share in the nation's leading causes of death or to rank those causes in the same order (Table 1.2). When compared to the rankings of the nation's top ten leading causes of death, the rankings for whites deviated from the nation's by one, whereas blacks deviated by four. Three of the leading causes of deaths for blacks—homicide, HIV/AIDS, and respiratory disease (COPD)—did not make the top ten rankings for the nation or for whites. The differences reflected in these rankings may be symptomatic of the health disparities that continue to impact persons of color and those of lower economic status.

After evaluating current peer-reviewed research, the Institute of Medicine found evidence of consistent disparities in health care across a range of illness and health care services among racial and ethnic groups (Smedley, Stith, & Nelson, 2003). The Institute of Medicine's review of the literature found that though some studies argued that observed health disparities tended to diminish for most diseases and even disappear for a few when socioeconomic factors were controlled for, the majority of the studies did not. Despite agreeing that disparities are associated with socioeconomic differences, most studies found that racial and ethnic disparities remained after controlling for socioeconomic differences and other health care access–related factors.

Citing highly rigorous studies which examined racial and ethnic health disparities in cardiovascular care among studies with findings most convincing of persistent health care disparities not diminished by controlled socioeconomic factors, the Institute of Medicine also agrees with popular opinion—disparities exist beyond socioeconomic status (Smedley et al., 2003). Race and ethnicity, rather than disease stage, income, and insurance, dictated heart disease treatment regimens as well as the receipt of appropriate cancer diagnostic tests. With HIV, blacks are less likely than nonminorities, even after controlling for age, gender, education, CD4 cell count, and insurance, to receive antiretroviral therapy, prophylaxis for pneumocystic pneumonia, and protease inhibitors. Racial and ethnic disparities were also observed for a range of other diseases and health service categories, including diabetes care, end-stage renal disease, kidney transplants, pediatric care, maternal and child care, mental health, and many surgical procedures.

The 2007 National Healthcare Disparities Report, which is generated by the Agency for Healthcare Research and Quality on behalf of the U.S. Department of Health and Human Services, noted three major health disparity themes that may help to explain the racial health differences presented in this chapter: (1) overall disparities in heath care quality and access are not declining; (2) despite some progress, many of the larger gaps in quality and access have not been reduced; and (3) being uninsured continues to be a major barrier to disparity reduction (Agency for Healthcare Research and Quality, 2008).

The first conclusion stated in the disparities report was derived from the analysis of sixteen of the forty-two core measures of quality of care, which facilitated cross-racial and -ethnic comparison, where whites were used as the comparison reference group (Agency for Healthcare Research and Quality, 2008). The quality-of-care comparison showed improvements for nearly half of the quality-of-care disparities for Hispanics and a lack of improvement for over 60 percent of quality-of-care disparities among blacks, Asians, and Native Americans/Alaska Natives. The socioeconomic comparison, which focused on the sixteen core measures of quality and six core measures of access supported by reliable estimates of income, found that quality and access to care for the poor had declined by more than 40 percent. As the gap between the "haves" and the "have nots" continues to increase in the United States, the number of persons with limited or no access to quality health care also increases. According to the Gini index, the gap in U.S. incomes increased considerably between 1967 and 2005 (U.S. Census Bureau, 2006).

To date, the Gini index or coefficient is one of the most commonly used measures of income inequality. The Gini coefficient measures income inequality on a scale from zero to one, in which zero represents perfect equality (everyone having the same income) and one (1) represents perfect inequality (one person having all the income). The scale score is then commonly multiplied by 100 to make score interpretation easier (Schiller, 2003). The Gini index is used by the United Nations to rank countries on their income disparities, which range from the lowest level of income disparity, 24.7 in Denmark, to the highest level of disparity, 74.3 in Namibia (United Nations Development Program, 2006). Although most postindustrial nations have a Gini coefficient ranging in the high twenties to the mid thirties, the United States has a Gini rating of 40. From 1967, when the U.S. Census Bureau started measuring the Gini coefficient, to 2005, the Gini coefficient has risen 20 percent for full-time workers and 18 percent for households. Among households, income disparities have risen from 39.7 to 46.9 (U.S. Census Bureau, 2006).

The second conclusion stated in the disparities report is based on the ability to gain access to the health care system and receive care within a timely fashion (Agency for Healthcare Research and Quality, 2008). The conclusion's assessments revealed a 60 percent increase in the core measures used to determine effective access to needed health care for Native Americans/Alaska Natives. For blacks, Asians, Hispanics, and poor populations, there was no improvement in at least half of the core measures used to determine access to needed services. Core measures remained the same or declined 60 percent among blacks and 80 percent among Hispanics. The third conclusion is based on the racially inequitable growth rate of uninsured Americans; being uninsured can lead to a lack of a steady health care provider and delayed care for necessary services. In this assessment both blacks and Hispanics were less likely to have a usual source of care and more likely to delay necessary care than were whites.

Although according to the 2006 U.S. Census data the number of people with health insurance increased from 249.0 million in 2005 to 249.8 million in 2006, there were several decreases in coverage (DeNavas-Walt, Proctor, & Smith, 2007). From 2005 to 2006, the percentage of uninsured people increased from 15.3 percent (44.8 million) to 15.8 percent (47 million), the percentage of those covered by employment-based health insurance decreased from 60.2 to 59.7 percent, and the number of those covered by governmental health programs decreased from 27.3 to 27 percent (DeNavas-Walt et al., 2007). Racially, the percentage of uninsured whites remained constant from 2005 to 2006 at 10.8 percent, whereas the percentage of uninsured blacks increased from 19.0 to 20.5 percent. Economically, the likelihood of having health insurance was directly related to income. Households with annual incomes of less than $25,000 had a health insurance coverage percentage of 75.1, whereas those with annual incomes of $75,000 or more had a coverage percentage of 91.5. Regionally, the uninsured rates are highest in the South (19.0%), followed by the West (17.9%), Northwest (12.3%), and Midwest (11.4%).

In closing, the overall health of black Americans is substantially less than that of white Americans. American blacks have a life expectancy that is unreflective of the developed nation in which they live and more reflective of a developing nation. Their health mortalities and morbidities are also much greater due to continually increasing disparities in poverty, medical coverage, and access to care, which also makes them more susceptible to health conditions (homicide, HIV/AIDS, and respiratory disease) not suffered in the same magnitude by their white counterparts.

REFERENCES

Agency for Healthcare Research and Quality. (2008). *National healthcare disparities report 2007*. U.S. Department of Health and Human Services, AHRQ Pub. No. 08–0041.

American Heart Association. (2005). *Heart disease and stroke statistics—2005 update*. Dallas: American Heart Association.

Burd-Sharps, S., Lewis, K., & Martins, E. (2008). *The measures of America: American human development report 2008–2009*. New York: Columbia University Press.

Centers for Disease Control and Prevention (CDC). (2005). Health disparities experienced by black or African Americans—United States. *MMWR Morbidity Mortality Weekly Report, 54*(1), 1–3.

Centers for Disease Control and Prevention (CDC). (2007). *U.S. Cancer Statistics Working Group. United States cancer statistics: 2004 incidence and mortality*. Atlanta: U.S. Department of Health and Human Services, Centers for Disease Control and Prevention, and National Cancer Institute.

Centers for Disease Control and Prevention (CDC). (2008a). *Statistics about racial or ethnic variations*. Atlanta: Division of Cancer Prevention and Control, National Center for Chronic Disease Prevention and Health Promotion.

Centers for Disease Control and Prevention (CDC). (2008b). *National diabetes fact sheet: General information and national estimates on diabetes in the United States, 2007*. Atlanta: U.S. Department of Health and Human Services, Centers for Disease Control and Prevention.

DeNavas-Walt, C., Proctor, B., & Smith, J. (2007). Income, poverty, and health insurance coverage in the United States: 2006. In *Current population reports* (pp. 60–233). Washington, DC: U.S. Census Bureau, U.S. Government Printing Office.

Gadson, S. (2006). The third world health status of black American males. *Journal of the National Medical Association 98*(4), 488–491.

Karch, D., Lubell, K., Friday, J., Patel, N., & Williams, D. (2008). Surveillance for violent death—National violent death reporting system, 16 states, 2005. *MMWR Surveillance Summary, 2008*, 57 (SS-3), pp. 1–43, 45.

Kung, H., Hoyert, D., Xu, J., & Murphy, B. (2008). Deaths: Final data for 2005. *National Vital Statistics Report 56*(10), 1–121.

McKinnon, J. (2001). *The black population 2000* (Census 2000 brief). Washington, DC: U.S. Department of Commerce, U.S. Census Bureau. Available at http://www.census.gov/prod/2001pubs/c2kbr01-5.pdf

National Center for Chronic Disease Prevention and Health Promotion: NCHS; CDC; ADA; AACE. (2007). *National diabetes fact sheet*. Retrieved January 2009 from http://www.dagc.org/diastatsUS.asp.

Ries, L., Eisner, M., Kosary, C., Hankey, B., Miller, B., Clegg, L., et al. (Eds.). (2005). *SEER cancer statistics review, 1975–2002*. Bethesda, MD: National Cancer Institute. Retrieved January 2009 from http://seer.cancer.gov/csr/1975_2002/ (Based on November 2004 SEER data submission, posted 2005).

Sabol, W., & Couture, H. (2008, June). *Prison inmates at midyear 2007*. Bureau of Justice Statistics Bulletin (NCJ221944). Washington, DC: Bureau of Justice Statistics, U.S. Department of Justice.

Sabol, W., Couture, H., & Harrison, P. (2007, December). *Prisoners in 2006*. Bureau of Justice Statistics Bulletin (NCJ219416). Washington, DC: Office of Justice Programs, U.S. Department of Justice.

Sabol, W., & West, H. (2008, December). *Prison in 2007*. Bureau of Justice Statistics Bulletin (NCJ224280). Washington, DC: Bureau of Justice Statistics, U.S. Department of Justice.

Schiller, B. (2003). *The economy today* (9th ed.). New York: McGraw-Hill.

Smedley, B., Stith, A., & Nelson, A. (Eds.). (2003). *Unequal treatment: Confronting racial and ethnic disparities in healthcare*. Washington, DC: National Academies Press.

Sotelo, M., & Gimeno, L. (2003). What does human development index rating mean in terms of individualism/collectivism? *European Psychologist, 8*(2), 97–100.

United Nations Development Program. (2006). *Human development report 2006: Beyond scarcity: Power, poverty and the global water crisis*. New York: Palgrave Macmillan.

U.S. Census Bureau. (2006). *Historical income tables—Income equality*. Available at http://www.census.gov/hhes/www/income/histinc/p60no231_tablea3.pdf

U.S. Department of Health and Human Services, Health Resources and Services Administration (HRSA), Maternal and Child Health Bureau. (2008). *Women's health USA 2008*. Rockville, MD: U.S. Department of Health and Human Services.

U.S. Department of Justice. (2007). *Homicide trends in the United States*. Washington, DC: Office of Justice Programs, Bureau of Justice Statistics.

CHAPTER

2

"WITHOUT HEALTH AND LONG LIFE ALL ELSE FAILS"

A History of African Americans and the Elimination of Racial Disparities in Health Care

VANESSA NORTHINGTON GAMBLE

ROOTS OF ACTIVITIES TO ELIMINATE DISPARITIES IN HEALTH AND HEALTH CARE

In October 1985, Margaret M. Heckler, secretary of the United States Department of Health and Human Services (DHHS), released the landmark *Report of the Secretary's Task Force on Black and Minority Health* (U.S. Department of Health and Human Services, 1985). The report, also known as the Heckler Report, detailed stark differences between the health status of African Americans, Native Americans, Hispanics, and Asians/Pacific Islanders compared with whites. It concluded that sixty thousand excess deaths occurred each year in minority populations—deaths that probably would not have occurred had the persons been white. The report led DHHS to establish the Office of Minority Health in January 1986 and served as the impetus for the creation of additional offices at the state level. The Heckler Report propelled racial and ethnic health disparities onto the national research and health policy stage. In the years following its release, there has been a dramatic increase in private and public initiatives to eliminate racial and ethnic disparities in health and health care.

Historical analysis makes plain, however, that the roots of these efforts predate the Heckler Report. Beginning at the turn of the twentieth century, African Americans, including physicians, nurses, clubwomen, social scientists, and educators, developed programs and institutions to improve their health status. They frequently argued that these efforts were critical for African Americans' social, political, and economic advancement and indeed for their very survival. As Booker T. Washington, the influential and well-connected principal of Tuskegee Institute, put it, "without health . . . it will be impossible for us to have permanent success in business, in property getting, [and] in acquiring education. . . . Without health and long life all else fails" (Smith, 1995, p. 38). This chapter analyzes twentieth-century efforts initiated by the African American community to improve its health status before the publication of the Heckler Report. Its goals are twofold: (1) to demonstrate the agency of the African American community in the face of a major social problem, and (2) to provide historical context and background to the contemporary campaign to eliminate racial and ethnic disparities in health and health care.

AFRICAN AMERICAN SOCIAL SCIENTISTS AND PHYSICIANS ADDRESS DISPARITIES, 1891–1945

W.E.B. Du Bois: *The Health and Physique of the Negro American* (1906)

The historical record demonstrates that African American scholars and health care professionals frequently combined scholarship with activism to improve the race's health and to contest racist theories about the causes of racial health disparities. In his 1899 monograph, *The Philadelphia Negro*, Dr. W.E.B. Du Bois, the influential sociologist and civil rights activist, urged the following approach to social problems: "We must study, we must investigate, we must attempt to solve" (p. 3). In *The Philadelphia Negro*, the first social study of race in urban America, Du Bois clearly combined passionate advocacy with careful scholarship.

Du Bois examined health briefly in *The Philadelphia Negro* but analyzed it more comprehensively in his 1906 *The Health and Physique of the Negro American*, one of a series of research studies published under the auspices of the historically African American Atlanta University. He used census reports, vital statistics, and insurance company records to document the poor health status of African Americans in comparison to white Americans. A major objective of the monograph was to refute the theories of African American racial inferiority advanced by Frederick L. Hoffman, a statistician at Prudential Life Insurance Company. In his influential 1896 treatise *Race Traits and Tendencies of the American Negro*, Hoffman (1896) argued that the excessive mortality rates in African Americans were caused "not in the conditions of life, but in race traits and tendencies" (p. 95). He viewed immorality, general intemperance, and congenital poverty as race traits. Hoffman (1896) also contended that during slavery, African Americans were healthy and free of disease, but since emancipation, "the colored race is shown to be on the downward grade, tending toward a condition in which matters will be worse than they are now . . . and gradual extinction of the race take [sic] place" (pp. 311–312).

Du Bois agreed that African Americans had higher rates than whites for diseases such as tuberculosis and pneumonia. However, he rejected Hoffman's argument that these disparities reflected racial susceptibilities and contended that they stemmed from social conditions. "The high infant mortality of Philadelphia today," Du Bois (1899) wrote, "is not a Negro affair, but an index of social condition" (p. 89). "With improved sanitary conditions, improved education, and better economic opportunities," he declared, "the mortality of the race may and probably will steadily decrease until it becomes normal" (Du Bois, 1906, p. 90). Previously, in *The Philadelphia Negro*, Du Bois had noted the influence of racial attitudes on the diagnosis of disease. He wrote, "Particularly with regard to consumption [tuberculosis] it must be remembered that Negroes are not the first people who have been claimed as its peculiar victims; the Irish were once thought to be doomed by that disease—but that was when Irishmen were unpopular" (p. 160). Sociologist Tukufu Zuberi (2000) has accurately argued that at the turn of the twentieth century "African American survival depended upon scientific validation of their historical reality and humanity" and that Du Bois's research "provided a fundamental critique to both Social Darwinism and eugenic thought" (p. 85).

The Health and Physique of the Negro American served as the basis for the Eleventh Conference for the Study of Negro Problems. On May 29, 1906, scholars, health professionals, and activists gathered at Atlanta University to review Du Bois's findings. At the end of the meeting they adopted several resolutions. They called for the formation of local health leagues to provide information about preventive medicine and urged existing health organizations to institute programs to address the health care needs of African Americans. Conferees also reaffirmed Du Bois's stance about the primacy of social factors in determining the health status of African Americans. They passed a resolution stating that they "did not find any adequate scientific warrant for the assumption that the Negro race is inferior to other races in physical build or vitality. The present differences in mortality seem to be sufficiently explained by conditions of life" (Du Bois, 1906, p. 110). The conference's final resolution also stressed the connection between research and social reform. It read, "The Conference above all reiterates its well known attitude toward social problems: the way to make conditions better is to study the conditions" (p. 110).

Medicine and Social Activism: The Career of Dr. Virginia Alexander

Throughout her career, Philadelphia physician Virginia Alexander epitomized the conference's final resolution. She researched the links between health and the socioeconomic status of African Americans and crafted a professional life that combined medicine and social activism. Alexander graduated from Woman's Medical College of

Pennsylvania, located in her hometown of Philadelphia, in 1925. After racial discrimination barred her from obtaining an internship in the city, she moved to Kansas City, where she completed an internship at Kansas City Colored Hospital and a year's residency at Wheatley Provident Hospital, another African American hospital. In 1927, after finishing her postgraduate training, Alexander returned to Philadelphia and began a general practice. In 1931, she founded the Aspiranto Health Home, a licensed three-bed maternity hospital. Virginia Alexander viewed her medical practice as inextricably linked to broader social and political concerns (Gamble, 1998).

In the summer of 1935 Alexander led a research investigation of the social, economic, and health problems of North Philadelphia. The study grew out of a 1935 meeting of the Institute of Race Relations, a seminar organized by the Friends Committee on Race Relations to develop scientific strategies to combat discrimination. Alexander, herself a Quaker, was an active member of the race relations committee, and she frequently used her religious connections to lobby white audiences to tackle racial inequities in health care. Alexander's four-part final report, "The Social, Economic, and Health Problems of North Philadelphia Negroes and Their Relation to a Proposed Interracial Public Health Demonstration Center," written in conjunction with Dr. George E. Simpson, clearly reflected the influence of her close friend W.E.B. Du Bois. The first part provided an overview of the health, economic, and social status of African American North Philadelphians. The second part described the results of a survey of the status of five hundred African American families in the area. The third section presented the results of a study of the professional experiences of thirty-nine African American physicians. The last section consisted of an analysis of the policies of local hospitals toward African American patients and physicians. Although Simpson, a white sociology professor at Temple University, collaborated on this study, he contended that his contribution was minimal (George E. Simpson, telephone conversation, March 19, 1998) and that Alexander had conducted the bulk of the research and written the final report.

The report painted a bleak picture of the health of African American Philadelphians. For example, in 1926, African American infants died almost twice as often as white infants, and in 1927, African American Philadelphians died from pneumonia at about four times the rate of white Philadelphians (Alexander & Simpson, 1935). Alexander attributed these sobering statistics primarily to social and political factors such as inadequate housing, education, and unemployment. She found that of the five hundred African American families surveyed, 47 percent had an unemployed head of household and 41 percent of the families were on relief (Alexander & Simpson, 1935). Alexander also pointed to racial discrimination as a contributing factor. Her report documented that many of the city's hospitals maintained separate wards and clinics for African American patients or denied them admission and access to their own physicians. The study also described some of the racism that African American patients faced as they sought treatment. One woman recounted her fears about entering one of the city's hospitals: "I was told to go to Hahnemann for an operation, but I was afraid to go because they always tell you that you need an operation when you don't, and then you can't have any more babies" (Alexander & Simpson, 1935, p. 61). The existence of discrimination in hospitals in Philadelphia had been a major impetus in Alexander's decision to establish her small hospital.

The report recommended the creation of an interracial public health center in North Philadelphia. Alexander saw the center as the beginning of a public health movement for the city's African American population. The center would provide medical care and health education, would offer training for African American physicians and nurses, would serve as a model for the integration of medical facilities, and would promote interracial understanding. Alexander did not view the poor health status of African Americans as a problem that should be addressed by African Americans alone. She strongly believed that any successful campaign to improve the health and health care of African Americans required cooperation between African American and white health professionals. As was true with many of the health activities initiated by African Americans, funds to support these programs were extremely limited. Alexander submitted a proposal to fund the public health center to the Milbank Memorial Fund. The foundation, for unknown reasons, rejected it.

In concert with the recommendations of the Eleventh Conference for the Study of Negro Problems, Alexander used her research findings to inform social activism. Her report revealed that of the fifty African American doctors in North Philadelphia, only five, including herself, had hospital privileges outside of the city's two African American hospitals, and thus few had facilities in which to hospitalize their patients. Alexander called for the admission of African American physicians, interns, and nurses to the staffs of the three municipal hospitals because African American Philadelphians paid taxes to maintain them. Between 1937 and 1940, the municipally operated Philadelphia General Hospital named three African American physicians to its staff. Alexander's research findings had convinced the Friends Committee on Race Relations to take an active role in the successful campaign to push for these appointments (Alexander & Simpson, 1935; McBride, 1989). As her career progressed, Virginia Alexander became increasingly interested in public health. In 1936, at the age of thirty-seven, she left private practice to study public health at Yale—the first African American person to do so.

Tuberculosis: Racial Disparities in the Early Twentieth Century

In her study, Alexander reported that in 1927 the African American tuberculosis death rate in North Philadelphia was six times that of whites. Indeed, in *The Health and Physique of the Negro American*, Du Bois (1906) had warned, "the greatest enemy of the African American race is consumption [tuberculosis]" (p. 73). African Americans recognized the danger posed by the disease and mounted a robust response to fight it. For example, conferees at the Eleventh Conference for the Study of Negro Problems called for an "especial effort . . . to stamp out consumption" and called for "a concerted action to this end" (Du Bois, 1906, p. 110). An analysis of articles written by African American physicians about tuberculosis between 1900 and 1940 provides a lens through which to understand how the African American medical profession conceptualized not only the factors underlying the tuberculosis rates in African Americans but the causes of racial health disparities in general and the actions necessary to decrease them.

African American physicians repudiated theories that attributed tuberculosis's heavy toll on African Americans to biology or racial inferiority, such as those expressed by Dr. J. Madison Taylor, a white physician on the faculty of Temple University Medical School. Taylor (1915) contended that African Americans and whites were totally unlike in racial characteristics and that African Americans were susceptible to tuberculosis because they were structurally maladapted to live in Northern cities. Washington physician Edward Mayfield Boyle (1912) vehemently criticized Taylor's stance because it incorporated beliefs about the inherent inferiority of African Americans into medical discourse. He also pointed out that while suicide and polio affected whites more than African Americans, the medical profession did not consider these higher rates as signs of white inferiority. African American physicians refused to accept pessimistic theories that African Americans were inherently diseased and thus doomed. Dr. John P. Turner, secretary of the Philadelphia Academy of Medicine, an African American medical society, wrote, "The Academy is making [the Negro] realize. . . . that consumption is to a large extent, especially in his case, a result of poor housing facilities and poor economic conditions. We feel that to give the Negro a new vision, a new hope, is to aid him to reduce his mortality through the consciousness that he must not have consumption just because he is a Negro" (Minton, 1924, p. 13). Turner contended that African American physicians had a responsibility to provide African Americans with a more optimistic view of their lives and to demonstrate that tuberculosis could be prevented.

African American physicians believed that the disparities in tuberculosis rates reflected socioeconomic inequalities not physiological inferiority. In a 1905 speech before the American Anti-Tuberculosis League, Dr. John E. Hunter (1905) of the National Association of Colored Physicians and Surgeons stressed the connection between income and health. He argued that African Americans who had been able to move from tenements "by reason of industry, education, and morality have lived above the environments that are conducive to tubercular tendencies, have a very low death rate from tuberculosis" (p. 251). Seeking to investigate the links between tuberculosis and race, Philadelphia physician Charles A. Lewis conducted a public health survey of an African American neighborhood in South Philadelphia between 1911 and 1912. He concluded that the high tuberculosis rates in African Americans stemmed from "the deplorable conditions under which Negroes were forced to live because of an economic setup that failed to net them a living wage, which in turn fostered improper nourishment" (McBride, 1981, p. 84).

African American physicians also pointed to racism as a factor in the high tuberculosis rates. Dr. Edward Mayfield Boyle strongly repudiated the views of the Chicago physician H. J. Achard (1912), who believed that the healthy and idyllic conditions in which African Americans had lived under slavery had made them resistant to tuberculosis. However, echoing the views of Frederick L. Hoffman, Achard argued that they were now susceptible to the disease because freedom had led them to lives that included "dirt, irregular living, alternating between stuffing and starving, excesses of various kinds, often indulgence in alcohol, crowded, unventilated quarters and insufficient clothing" (p. 225). Boyle (1912) retorted, "Those who once exercised the right of tutelage over 'body and soul' have. . . . become, in a large measure, the freedmen's oppressors. Whereas during slavery Negroes were engaged . . . [and] counted efficient as workmen, as freedmen they are vigorously opposed in many a line of industry and labor" (p. 347).

African American Physicians Battle Health Disparities, 1900–1940

Between 1900 and 1940, African American physicians proposed several strategies to decrease tuberculosis and other diseases in African American communities. They pushed for the enforcement of sanitation laws to clean up the tenement housing in which many urban African Americans lived and for environmental reforms to improve the sanitation of African American districts. They called for programs to teach personal hygiene, especially to poor African Americans and to recent migrants from the South. At the time, racial discrimination severely restricted access of African American health care professionals and African American patients to medical facilities.

The physicians also called for more training and clinical opportunities for African American health professionals and increased admission of African American patients to hospitals and sanatoria. At the end of the nineteenth century, the African American community had started its own hospitals to address the needs of African American health care professionals and patients. In 1891, Provident Hospital and Nurse Training School, the nation's first African American–controlled hospital, opened in Chicago. Its founder, the prominent Chicago surgeon Daniel Hale Williams (1900), called on the African American community to establish additional hospitals. He urged, "Let us no longer sit idly and inanely deploring existing conditions. Let us not waste time trying to effect changes or modifications in the institutions unfriendly to us, but rather let us seek to promote the doctrine of helping and stimulating our race" (p. 4). By 1919, at least 119 African American hospitals had opened (Work, 1918–1919).

Although African American physicians during the first half of the twentieth century recognized the adverse effects of a segregated medical care system, most did not call for its dismantlement as a solution to the health problems of African Americans. They advocated for programs and facilities that would work within the context of a segregated society, because they believed that integration was not immediately forthcoming and that the health and professional needs of African Americans demanded immediate solutions. Such views were not universal. At a 1938 conference on national health care, Harlem physician Louis T. Wright, board chair of the National Association for the Advancement of Colored People (NAACP), argued, "the health of the American Negro is not a separate racial problem . . . but . . . an American problem that should be adequately and equitably handled by the identical agencies . . . as the health of the remainder of the population" (Interdepartmental Committee . . . , 1938, p. 87). However, the color line in medicine remained in place until the gains made by the post–World War II civil rights movement.

AFRICAN AMERICAN SELF-HELP ACTIVITIES, 1913–1948

From National Negro Health Week to the National Negro Health Movement

At the turn of the twentieth century, the African American community also established self-help activities to address its poor health status. The largest and most significant was National Negro Health Week. The origins of the movement can be traced to 1913, when the National Organization Society of Virginia, under the leadership of Robert Russa Moton, established a health week to call attention to the high morbidity and mortality rates of the state's African American citizens and to develop programs to attack them. The society, an organization dedicated to improving the status of African American Virginians, had become interested in health issues because it believed that the poor health status of African Americans was a "source of economic loss to the race and a hazard to the general welfare of the state" (R. R. Moton, personal communication, c. 1940). The goal of the health week was to teach African Americans about the principles of public health and hygiene in order to help them become stronger and more economically productive citizens. Its activities, conducted with the support of local health departments, included lectures in churches and schools and the formation of brigades to clean neighborhoods.

The Virginia program attracted the attention of Booker T. Washington, who, in addition to his responsibilities at Tuskegee Institute, headed the National Negro Business League. Washington had becoming increasingly interested in public health, influenced in part by the research and activities of Monroe N. Work, a sociologist who directed the institute's Department of Records and Research. Work's affiliation with a 1905 health campaign conducted in Savannah, Georgia, by an African American men's Sunday club had convinced him that "the gospel of health could be carried directly to the colored people and that they were ready to hear and to put into practice what was told them" (Brown, 1937, p. 554). At the annual Tuskegee Negro Conference in 1914, Work, who had assisted W.E.B. Du Bois with the research for *The Health and Physique of the Negro American*, presented some staggering, yet optimistic, statistics about the poor health of African Americans in the South and its economic costs. He estimated that approximately 225,000 African Americans died in the South annually and that 450,000 were seriously ill. Work's data also showed that the annual economic loss to the South from sickness and death among African Americans was over $300,000,000. Work estimated that 45 percent of all the deaths were preventable (Work, 1916).

Work's presentation prompted Washington into action. He called for a national "Health Improvement Week" to be held April 11–17, 1915, because he viewed good health as a critical element of racial advancement. Washington firmly believed that African Americans could be mobilized to "be taught what to do to aid in improving their health conditions" (Brown, 1937, p. 554). In contrast to the fatalistic views of Hoffman, he contended that the morbidity and mortality rates of African Americans could be reduced. Washington sought, and received, cooperation from a broad range of African American community organizations, including those representing the clergy, fraternal organizations, medicine, nursing, and clubwomen. He also urged white support, and a number of health departments around the country endorsed the endeavor.

Booker T. Washington is often portrayed as an unwavering adherent of an accommodationist philosophy that emphasized self-help, racial solidarity, and economic development as more productive strategies for African American advancement than politics, agitation, and the demand for immediate integration. However, such a view obscures the complexity of Washington's ideology. For example, during a 1915 address in Baltimore launching Maryland's health week activities, he criticized segregation and stressed its detrimental impact on African American health: "Wherever the Negro is segregated," he argued, "it means that he will have . . . poor sewerage, poor sanitary conditions generally, and this reflects itself in many ways in the life of my race to the disadvantage of the white race" (Brown, 1937, p. 554).

The first health week proved successful: sixteen states held activities (Smith, 1995). Unfortunately, Washington died shortly after its start. His successor at Tuskegee, Robert Moton, broadened the scope of the health movement by establishing a formal organizational structure to set policies and design activities and by strengthening connections to national organizations, particularly those concerned with health and social welfare, including African American associations such as the National Medical Association, the National Association of Colored Graduate Nurses, and the National Association for Teachers in Colored Schools as well as white associations such as the American Red Cross, the National Tuberculosis Association, and the American Social Hygiene Association. Beginning in 1921, members of the National Negro Health Week Committee met at Tuskegee to develop practical guidance for local health week committees and to outline strategies to cultivate community support for a national African American health movement. The committee decided to honor the memory of Booker T. Washington by annually holding National Negro Health Week around his birthday, April 5.

The committee wrote an annual health week bulletin to guide the effort at the community level and to announce the year's theme. For example, the theme for 1928 was "Concentrated Attack on the Negro Health Hazards in Every Community," and for the following year it was "A Complete Health Examination for Everybody" (Brown, 1937, p. 557). The bulletin also offered suggestions for organizing the health week activities. Monday, for example, was "Home Health Day," and the day's activities focused on improving personal and social hygiene. Friday was designated "School Health Day," at which time children were to be examined and immunized. The bulletin also included recommendations for the effective organization of local health committees. Suggested health week activities included lectures, films, newspaper articles, health clinics, vaccinations, insect and rodent extermination, and street cleaning. The African American community enthusiastically embraced health week. Monroe Work estimated that by 1930 at least 2,500 communities in thirty-two states held health week activities (Smith, 1995).

The National Negro Health Week Committee recognized the limitations of an annual one-week event and wanted to expand it to a year-round activity. However, Tuskegee Institute lacked the funds and personnel to support and coordinate an expansion. Committee members brought the problem of African American health care to the attention of officials from the United States Public Health Service (USPHS) and began to lobby them to assume responsibility for health week in order to give it financial stability, additional resources, and the imprimatur of the federal government. In 1921, Moton persuaded Surgeon General Hugh S. Cummings to endorse health week and to agree to publish the health week bulletin under the auspices of the Public Health Service (Brown, 1937). In 1932, the Public Health Service made an even larger commitment. It established the Office of Negro Health Work, under the direction of Dr. Roscoe C. Brown, an African American dentist. The office served as the center of the federal government's African American health efforts and as the headquarters for National Negro Health Week, which became a year-round activity called the National Negro Health Movement. Its activities included coordinating health week, developing educational materials, and publishing *National Negro Health News*, a quarterly journal on African American health issues. Under Brown's direction, health week activities expanded. In 1948, 12,000 communities participated. Organizers conducted 3,000 clinics, gave 12,000 health lectures, and cleaned up 200,000 homes and lots (Brown, 1949). The creation of the office was a significant accomplishment. It marked the first time since the demise of the medical department of the Freedmen's Bureau that the federal government indicated that it had a responsibility to improve the health of its African American citizens. Historian Susan L. Smith (1995) has concluded, "African American health activists turned National Negro Health Week into a vehicle for social welfare organizing and political activity in a period when the vast majority of African Americans were without formal political and economic power" (p. 34).

African American Women's Health Activism, 1908–1942

African American women played critical roles in efforts to improve the health of the African American community. African American nurses provided health education, promoted health week activities, and facilitated collaborations between women's organizations. The efforts of African American women's organizations in Chicago contributed to the success of the city's 1929 Negro Health Week activities. The women gave health talks, coordinated meetings, recruited volunteers, and served on one of the twelve planning committees. One member of the planning committee, Chicago physician Mary Fitzbutler Waring, served as head of the Department of Health and Hygiene of the National Association of Colored Women's Clubs and fervently urged African American clubwomen to organize health week activities in their communities (Smith, 1995). In Atlanta, the Neighborhood Union, a settlement house established by African American women in 1908, emerged as the focal point for several health efforts, including National Negro Health Week. Under the shrewd and forceful leadership of Lugenia Burns Hope, the wife of the president of Morehouse College, the Neighborhood Union operated a health center; offered classes in nursing, hygiene, and prenatal care; provided health education; sponsored cleanup campaigns; supported local antituberculosis efforts; and investigated local health conditions. It also developed an intricate organizational structure to facilitate community input into its health activities (Rouse, 1989).

African American women associated with the Alpha Kappa Alpha (AKA) sorority conducted what Surgeon General Thomas Parran described as "one of the best jobs of volunteer public health work he [had] ever seen" (Ratcliff, 1940, p. 466). For seven summers, from 1935 to 1942, members of the sorority conducted and financed the Mississippi Health Project to bring much-needed health care to poor African American communities in the state. AKA president Ida L. Jackson, a school teacher from Oakland, California, initiated the project. She had originally planned an educational program in Holmes County, Mississippi, but decided that the population's poor health would impede the success of any education initiatives. In December 1934, Jackson appointed Washington physician Dorothy Boulding Ferebee chairperson of the sorority's health committee and medical director of the Mississippi Health Project.

By spring 1935, AKA members had donated $2,500 for the project, and Ferebee had successfully recruited twelve volunteers from around the nation, including physicians, public health workers, and clerical assistants and had secured the support of the local health officer. However, as the project's July start date approached, a major problem emerged. The women had planned on traveling to Mississippi by train, but a railroad agent, whom Ferebee characterized as "red-necked, caustic, and racially insulting," refused to sell them tickets because he needed them for the "nay-grus" who regularly rode his train (Ferebee, n.d., p. 2). Ferebee decided that they would drive. Such a plan was not without its own difficulties, because, as she later recalled, it involved transporting volunteers and supplies "on a 2,000 mile run over unknown roads, many without restroom facilities or over night [sic] accommodations, or even gas stations willing to serve African American travelers" (Ferebee, n.d., p. 3). It was also dangerous. If they had an accident, they might be denied care because of hospital segregation and the paucity of hospitals for African American patients in the South.

The volunteers found additional challenges when they arrived in Mississippi. Employers refused to allow their African American employees to attend a clinic run by "outside agitators." The plantation owners relented only after Ferebee agreed to conduct the clinics on the plantations under the watchful eyes of the foremen, armed with guns and whipping prods (Ratcliff, 1940). Ferebee creatively used the automobiles as a mobile health clinic. Every morning for six weeks the volunteers set out, and they often covered a hundred miles a day over dirt roads under the hot Mississippi sun as they traveled from plantation to plantation to conduct their "cotton field clinic" in makeshift facilities. In six weeks, Ferebee and her associates had inoculated over 2,600 children and had performed over 200 physical examinations—and put over 5,300 miles on the cars in their medical caravan (Ratcliff, 1940).

For seven summers, Ferebee led a group of AKA volunteers to Holmes and Bolivar counties. After the success of the first clinic, the sorority added additional services, including nutrition and hygiene lectures, syphilis screening, and dental care. By 1940, they had immunized about 14,500 children against diphtheria and smallpox, had treated thousands of adults, had provided venereal disease screening, and had given nutrition and education classes (Ratcliff, 1940). The sorority unsuccessfully lobbied state and federal public health officials to take over the project, which ended in 1942 because of the gas rationing brought on by World War II. Ferebee contended that the Mississippi Health Project had demonstrated that any efforts to improve the health of African American people had to address broader social and economic factors. In 1940, she became president of AKA; during her presidency she increased the organization's lobbying efforts for progressive legislation in the areas of health, child welfare, racial discrimination, and economic security (Smith, 1995).

CONCLUSION: FROM THE MEDICAL CIVIL RIGHTS MOVEMENT TO THE HECKLER REPORT

After World War II, a vigorous medical civil rights movement emerged in the African American community that sought to desegregate medical facilities and associations. Medical civil rights activists accurately charged that a segregated health care system had led to inferior medical care for African Americans and that it could never adequately meet the health and professional needs of African Americans. A casualty of the growing medical civil rights movement, and with it the rejection of separate programs and facilities for African Americans, was the Office of Negro Health Work. Physician-activist W. Montague Cobb (1950) criticized "the idea of a special 'Negro Health Week'" as "outmoded" because it smacked of segregationism (p. 8). In 1950, the Public Health Service closed the office because it was moving toward integration in all its programs. Roscoe C. Brown (1950) declared the National Negro Health Movement so successful that "there is not the same urgency to emphasize separate needs. Rather the trend now is for all groups to work together for mutual welfare" (p. 2). He noted, for example, that the African American infant mortality rate had declined from 180 per 1,000 live births in 1915, to 48 in 1947. Yet, he cautioned that this rate was 60 percent higher than the rate for whites. Brown urged local communities to continue to work to improve the health of African Americans.

Grassroots activism, judicial decisions, and laws such as the 1964 Civil Rights Act and the 1965 Medicare and Medicaid legislation led to the desegregation of American medicine. Yet, during the 1970s and 1980s it became increasingly clear that despite the significant impact of the medical civil rights movement in securing access of African Americans to the nation's medical institutions, disparities continued to persist between the health of white and minority Americans. In January 1984, DHHS secretary Margaret M. Heckler sent *Health, United States, 1983* to the U.S. Congress. This annual report card on the health status of Americans documented significant gains. But Heckler pointed out that it also "signaled a sad and significant fact; *there was a continuing disparity in the burden of death and illness experienced by African Americans and other minority Americans as compared with our nation's population as a whole*" (Heckler's emphasis) (U.S. Department of Health and Human Services, 1985, p. ix). She noted that although there had been steady gains in the health status of minority Americans, "the stubborn disparity remained an affront both to our ideals and to the ongoing genius of American medicine" (p. ix). In response, Heckler established the previously mentioned Secretary's Task Force on Black and Minority Health. To be sure, the task force's final report placed the issue of racial and ethnic disparities in health and health care on a broader national platform and heralded the advent of recent initiatives to address disparities. However, it should not be forgotten that these contemporary activities are built upon a foundation first constructed by African Americans at the turn of the twentieth century, when they not only recognized the poor health status of their community but took the lead in developing programs and activities to improve health and save lives.

ACKNOWLEDGMENT

I wish to thank Paul R. Goldstein for his assistance in the preparation of this chapter. This work was supported in part by a Robert Wood Johnson Foundation Investigator Award in Health Policy. The views expressed imply no endorsement by the Robert Wood Johnson Foundation.

REFERENCES

Achard, H. J. (1912). Tuberculization of the Negro. *Journal of the National Medical Association, 4*, 224–226.

Alexander, V. M., & Simpson, G. E. (1935, October). *The social, economic, and health problems of North Philadelphia Negroes and their relation to a proposed interracial public health demonstration center* (Unpublished manuscript). Virginia M. Alexander Papers, Box 2, Folder 24, University of Pennsylvania, University Archives and Record Center, Philadelphia, PA.

Boyle, E. M. (1912). The Negro and tuberculosis. *Journal of the National Medical Association, 4*, 344–348.

Brown, R. C. (1937). The National Negro Health Week movement. *Journal of Negro Education, 6*, 553–564.

Brown, R. C. (1949). The health status and health education of Negroes in the United States. *Journal of Negro Education, 18*, 377–387.

Brown, R. C. (1950, April–June). The National Negro Health Week movement. *National Negro Health News, 18*, 1 2.

Cobb, W. M. (1950, April 22). 50 years of progress in health. *Pittsburgh Courier*, p. 8.

Du Bois, W. E. B. (1899, reprint 1967). *The Philadelphia Negro: A social study*. New York: Schocken.

Du Bois, W. E. B. (1906). *The health and physique of the Negro American*. Atlanta: Atlanta University Press.

Ferebee, D. B. (n.d.). *The Alpha Kappa Alpha Mississippi Health Project* (Unpublished manuscript). Dorothy Ferebee Papers, Box 183–14, Folder 11, p. 1. Moorland Spingarn Research Center, Howard University Library, Washington, DC.

Gamble, V. N. (1998, May 8). *Taking a history: The life of Dr. Virginia Alexander.* Paper presented at the Fielding H. Garrison Lecture, American Association for the History of Medicine, Toronto, Canada.

Hoffman, F. L. (1896). *Race traits and tendencies of the American Negro*. New York: American Economic Association.

Hunter, J. E. (1905). Tuberculosis in the Negro: Causes and treatment. *Colorado Medical Journal, 7*, 250–257.

Interdepartmental Committee to Coordinate Health and Welfare Activities. (1938). *Proceedings of the National Health Conference, 18, 19, 20*.

McBride, D. (1981). The Henry Phipps Institute, 1903–1937: Pioneering tuberculosis work with an urban minority. *Bulletin of the History of Medicine, 6*, 78–97.

McBride, D. (1989). *Integrating the City of Medicine: Blacks in Philadelphia health care, 1910–1965*. Philadelphia: Temple University Press.

Minton, H. M. (1924). The part the Negro is playing in the reduction of mortality. *Hospital Social Service, 10*, 10–16.

Ratcliff, J. D. (1940, September). Cotton Field Clinic. *Survey Graphic, 29*, 464–467.

Rouse, J. A. (1989). *Lugenia Burns Hope: Black Southern reformer*. Athens: University of Georgia Press.

Smith, S. L. (1995). *Sick and tired of being sick and tired: Black women's health activism, 1890–1950.* Philadelphia: University of Pennsylvania Press.

Taylor, J. M. (1915). Remarks on the health of colored people. *Journal of the National Medical Association, 7,* 160–163.

U.S. Department of Health and Human Services. (1985). *Report of the secretary's Task Force on Black & Minority Health, Vol. I: Executive Summary.* Washington, DC: Author.

Williams, D. H. (1900). The need of hospitals and training schools for the colored people of the south. *National Hospital and Sanitarium Record, 3,* 3–7.

Work, M. N. (1916). *The Negro year book, 1916–1917: An encyclopedia of the Negro* (pp. 341–352). Tuskegee, AL: Tuskegee Institute, Negro Year Book Publishing Company.

Work, M. N. (1918–1919). *The Negro year book, 1918–1919: An encyclopedia of the Negro* (pp. 424–426). Tuskegee, AL: Tuskegee Institute, Negro Year Book Publishing Company.

Zuberi, T. (2000). *Thicker than blood: How racial statistics lie.* Minneapolis: University of Minnesota Press.

CHAPTER

3

THE HEALTH STATUS OF CHILDREN AND ADOLESCENTS

DESIRÉE A. H. OLIVER
GENE H. BRODY

The children are our future. That is a phrase that has been used time and again. If the future does lie in the hands of our children, then it is important to continually assess our ability to keep them healthy and safe from harm. We must recognize the dangers and determine ways to avoid them. The African American community is riddled with health disparities compared to the population as a whole. It is impossible to ignore the term *disproportionate* as it relates to race and ethnic background when describing multiple risk factors and their negative health outcomes. This of course includes the health outcomes of African American children and adolescents. In many areas, the disparities are still quite evident, while in others the gaps have narrowed. This chapter will provide epidemiological statistics specific to the child and adolescent population, and it will detail some of the more common contributing factors and the methods by which some of the negative outcomes can be surmounted. Knowing the problems is only half of the battle. By making a commitment to instill change, we can change the future of the African American community rather than staying the course.

INFANT MORTALITY

Working chronologically through the life of a child, the first obstacle one faces is surviving birth and infancy. Even in the dawn of the twenty-first century, nations measure the health of their people by the mortality rates of their infants. The United States currently ranks twenty-ninth lowest in the world in infant mortality rates. This ranking is due largely to disparities among racial and ethnic groups, particularly African Americans (Martin et al., 2007). Since the year 2000, infant mortality among African Americans has occurred at nearly twice the rate of the national average (Miniño, Arias, Kochanek, Murphy, & Smith, 2002). In 2005 there were 633,134 births to African Americans; 13.6 percent classified as low birthweight. Low birthweight babies are often born premature (before 37 weeks) and generally weigh less than 5.5 lbs. (Martin et al., 2007).

"The question is not whether we can afford to invest in every child; it is whether we can afford not to."
—Marian Wright Edelman

Infant mortality and low birthweight can be attributed to certain lifestyles, behaviors, and conditions that have an effect on birth outcome. Those include smoking, substance use, poor nutrition, lack of prenatal care, medical problems or infections (like STIs), and chronic illnesses such as diabetes and high blood pressure (Office of Minority Health & Health Disparities [OMHD], 2007). While these factors are not solely related to the black or African American race, there are racial disparities among these behaviors and conditions. In order to eliminate disparities in infant mortality, a network between health care experts and minority communities must be formed to encourage healthy behaviors by pregnant women and by parents of infants. Also, more research must be conducted on effective strategies to identify at-risk infants and effective interventions for high-risk infants (OMHD, 2007).

CHILD IMMUNIZATIONS

During infancy and early childhood, immunizations are necessary to prevent illness or early death. The National Immunization Survey demonstrates that vaccination of U.S. preschoolers in 2001 remained near the all-time highs achieved in 2000. However, the results do not imply that coverage is uniformly high in all areas (Rosenthal et al., 2004). In 2000, children living below the poverty level had a lower immunization coverage rate than those not living in poverty (OMHD, 2007). Traditionally, poor immunization coverage among children in low-income families has affected many racial, ethnic, and underserved child populations (OMHD, 2007). However, by the 2007 National Immunization Survey there were no significant differences between ethnic/ racial groups when controlled for income level (Centers for Disease Control and Prevention [CDC], 2008c). Although incidence of vaccine-preventable disease is low, identifying any areas with low childhood-vaccination coverage remains important. This is particularly true in urban areas, because such areas have the highest risk of transmission if disease is introduced (Rosenthal et al., 2004).

UNINTENTIONAL INJURIES

Injury and violence are serious threats to the health and well-being of children and adolescents in the United States. Children and adolescents are among the highest at risk for many injuries that can lead to death or disability (CDC, 2008b). Young African Americans have statistically equal risks for some types of injuries compared to other races, but elevated risks for other types of unintentional injuries.

Vehicular Accidents

As of 2007, the playing field became equal among racial/ethnic groups regarding vehicular accidents and injuries, although this was not always the case. During the year 2005 in the United States, 4,544 teens ages 16–19 died of injuries caused by motor vehicle crashes. In the same year, nearly 400,000 motor vehicle occupants in this age group sustained nonfatal injuries that required treatment in an emergency department (CDC, 2008d). In 2005, teenagers accounted for 10 percent of the U.S. population and 12 percent of motor vehicle crash deaths (Finkelstein, Corso, Miller, & Associates, 2006). In the same year, African American (13.4%) and Hispanic students (10.6%) were more likely than white students (9.4%) to rarely or never wear seat belts, which placed them at an increased risk of sustaining injury or death during a vehicular accident (CDC, 2006a). However, according to the 2007 Youth Risk Behavior Survey (YRBS), the disparity in this risk factor has narrowed; the number of African Americans, whites, and Hispanics that rarely or never wear seatbelts is now statistically equal (12.4%, 10.1%, and 12.9%, respectively) (CDC, 2008a).

Fire- and Water-Related Deaths

Some groups are at an increased risk of fire-related injuries and deaths. These include children age 4 and under (CDC, 1998), African Americans, Native Americans (CDC, 1998), and low-income Americans (Istre, McCoy, Osborn, Barnard, & Bolton, 2001). Along with death by fire, the rates of fatal drowning are notably higher among certain racial and ethnic minority populations in certain age groups (CDC, 2008d). Factors such as physical environment (such as access to swimming pools) and a combination of social and cultural issues (like valuing swimming skills and choosing water-related recreation) may contribute to the racial differences in drowning rates. If minorities participate less in water-related activities than whites, their drowning rates (per exposure) may be higher than currently reported (Branche, Dellinger, Sleet, Gilchrist, & Olson, 2004). Between 2000 and 2005, the fatal unintentional drowning rate for African Americans across all ages was 1.3 times that of whites, and the fatal drowning rate of African American children ages 5–14 was 3.2 times that of whites in the same age range (CDC, 2008d).

Lead Poisoning

Even today, lead exposure continues to affect young children in the United States. Disparities in risk exposure by income and race are well documented and continue to persist (CDC, 2004). A national survey found that children at highest risk for having an elevated blood lead level are those living in metropolitan areas in housing built before 1946, and who are in low-income families of African American and Hispanic origin (CDC, 2004). Because lead exposure disproportionately affects children in low-income families living in older housing, it represents a significant, preventable contributor to social disparities in health, educational achievement, and overall quality of life. Treatment after exposure to lead poisoning is limited. This has caused the Centers for Disease Control and Prevention (CDC) to focus on programs for primary prevention to eliminate sources of lead in children's environments (CDC, 2004).

Unintentional Poisoning

While environmental poisioning affects African Americans more than other populations, unintentional poisioning does not. The CDC reports that among those who died from unintentional poisoning in 2005, whites and African Americans had comparable rates. In fact, even among those who committed suicide by poisoning in 2005, African Americans were 3.6 times less likely than whites to have died by poisioning (CDC, 2008d).

Suicide and Homicide

African Americans have lower risks of suicide. The 2007 YRBS found that while having a slightly higher rate than that of whites, African Americans were not as likely to have attempted suicide as Hispanics (7.7% African American, 10.2% Hispanic, and 5.6% white). They were the least likely to have "made a plan about how to attempt suicide" (9.5% African American, 12.8% Hispanic, 10.8% white), though African Americans were statistically equal in their likelihood to have "seriously considered a suicide attempt" (13.2% African American, 15.9% Hispanic, 14.0% white) (CDC, 2008a). Undoubtedly, among ten-to-twenty-four-year-olds, homicide is the leading cause of death for African Americans (CDC, 2006a).

OVERWEIGHT AND OBESITY

Pediatric overweight and obesity is a major health concern for African American children and adolescents. It is well known that obese children are more likely to become obese adults, and some of the health consequences associated with pediatric overweight and obesity, such as early development of coronary heart disease, high blood cholesterol levels, high blood pressure, gallbladder disease, and type-2 diabetes, are well documented (Urrutia-Rojas & Menchaca, 2006). With the television and fast-food culture that children are part of, it comes as no surprise that the prevalence of overweight and obesity in children and adolescents is higher than it was twenty years ago in all racial and ethnic groups. The rate of childhood overweight and obesity is increasing on a yearly basis, particularly among low-income and minority children

(Urrutia-Rojas & Menchaca, 2006). Of the African American teens surveyed in the 2007 YRBS, 18.3 percent were obese (CDC, 2008a).

African American teens have more risk factors for overweight and obesity than other racial groups (CDC, 2008a). Similar to adults, children's inactivity increases their chances of becoming overweight or obese. A sedentary practice such as watching television or sitting in front of a computer screen for more than two hours a day is associated with being overweight. Each hourly increment of television viewing has been shown to be associated with a 1–2 percent increase in the prevalence of obesity (Urrutia-Rojas & Menchaca, 2006). African American adolescents were more likely than white or Hispanic teens to have used computers or to have watched television three or more hours per day. While all races were equal in their likelihood to not attend physical education classes daily, 68.9 percent of African Americans did not meet recommended levels of physical activity (CDC, 2008a). But inactivity is not the only elevated risk factor. Poor nutrition is also a concern. African American teens are more likely to have drunk fewer than three glasses of milk per day and to have eaten fruits and vegetables fewer than the recommended five times per day (CDC, 2008a).

CHRONIC DISEASES

Diabetes

Parallel to the surge of overweight and obesity in the past ten to fifteen years is the increase in the onset of type-2 diabetes mellitus (T2DM), often referred to as adult-onset diabetes, occurring among children and adolescents (Urrutia-Rojas & Menchaca, 2006). According to the Centers for Disease Control and Prevention, one in three children born in 2000 in the United States will become diabetic (Urrutia-Rojas & Menchaca, 2006). In children, being overweight is the risk factor most strongly associated with the disease. Approximately 85 percent of children diagnosed with diabetes are either overweight or obese at the time of diagnosis. Along with being overweight there are several other factors related to the onset of T2DM in children, including female gender, puberty status, and minority race (Urrutia-Rojas & Menchaca, 2006). While females are nearly twice as likely to develop T2DM than boys, overall T2DM disproportionately affects African American, Native American, and Hispanic children. Alarmingly, it is predicted that nearly half of all African American and Hispanic children will develop diabetes (Urrutia-Rojas & Menchaca, 2006).

Pediatric Hypertension

With the prevalence of childhood overweight over the past two decades, anecdotal evidence suggests that pediatric hypertension may also have become more prevalent than previously reported (Sorof, Lai, Turner, Poffenbarger, & Portman, 2004). The association between being overweight and hypertension in children has been reported in a variety of ethnic and racial groups, with virtually all studies finding higher blood pressure and/or higher prevalence of hypertension in overweight versus lean children

(Sorof et al., 2004). Given the rate of overweight occurring among African American children and adolescents, pediatric hypertension may soon join the list of diseases disproportionately afflicting this population.

Asthma

According to the 2007 Youth Risk Behavioral Survey, African American teens were more likely than their white and Hispanic counterparts to have had asthma in their lifetime (24.0% African American, 18.5% Hispanic, and 19.6% white). African Americans were also more likely to have had asthma at the time of the survey (14.7% African-American, 9.5% Hispanic, and 10.5% white) (CDC, 2008a).

UNINTENDED PREGNANCY, STIs, AND HIV/AIDS

Unintended pregnancy, sexually transmitted infections (STIs), and HIV/AIDS are disproportionately high among youth of color, especially African American and Hispanic youth (Augustine, Alford, & Deas, 2004). The birth rate among fifteen-to-nineteen-year-olds has steadily declined since 1991. And while the rate among African American teens has had the sharpest decline, 37 percent, the rates of pregnancies among African American and Hispanic teens still remain the highest in comparison to all other ethnic and racial minorities (Augustine et al., 2004). Along with pregnancies, sexually transmitted infections also afflict minorities at disproportionate rates. In 2001, chlamydia rates among females ages 15–19 years were seven times higher in African Americans (8,483 per 100,000) than in whites, and in males the rate was twelve times higher in African Americans (1,500 per 100,000) than in whites. Also, 75 percent of all gonorrhea cases occur among African Americans (Augustine et al., 2004). The disparities with African American teens are far more damaging than just an increased number of curable infections. HIV/AIDS is growing at a disproportional rate among African American adolescents (Glenn & Wilson, 2008). Among pediatric AIDS cases, African American and Hispanic children made up more than 80 percent of all cases reported in 2000 (National Center for Health Statistics, 2002). Furthermore, females again are most at risk. In 2001, African Americans and Hispanics made up 84 percent of all AIDS cases among females ages 13–19 years and 62 percent of all male AIDS cases within the same age group (Augustine et al., 2004).

These trends are clearly a reflection of more risky behaviors among this population combined with sexual networks consisting of high prevalence rates. The 2007 YRBS found that African American teens were more likely than Hispanics and whites to have ever had sex, to be currently sexually active, to have had their first sexual encounter before age 13, and to have had four or more sexual partners (see Table 3.1) (CDC, 2008a). These behaviors persist, even though the risk of contracting HIV/AIDS is a cause of concern for African American teens. The risk is not invisible to this population. Urban adolescent minorities, for example, worry about HIV but have equal or greater concerns about money, health, school, pregnancy, and getting into a fight (Augustine et al., 2004). While African American teens are more likely than whites or

TABLE 3.1   **Black Students Were More Likely to Have . . .**

	Black (%)	Hispanic (%)	White (%)
Ever had sex	66.5	52.0	43.7
First sex before age 13	16.3	8.2	4.4
Four or more partners	27.6	17.3	11.5
Sex in last 3 months	46.0	37.4	32.9

Source: CDC, 2008a.

Hispanics to have been tested for HIV (CDC, 2008a), their efforts to protect themselves are lower. Discussing sexual risks with a partner appears to occur only rarely; 66 percent of African American females felt their partners would feel hurt or be suspicious of them if they asked about HIV risk factors (Augustine et al., 2004). Unplanned sex acts without prior discussion and negotiation lead to infrequent condom use and risk for HIV/AIDS. Of African American females ages 13–19, 26 percent felt they had little control over condom usage, and 75 percent said their partner would not use a condom if he knew she took oral contraceptives (Augustine et al., 2004).

This uprising trend in HIV infection among young African Americans continues despite the fact that 89 percent of schools have educational programs on HIV/AIDS (Glenn & Wilson, 2008). These programs may be put in schools to appease governmentally enforced educational standards; however, it appears that social, economic, and cultural barriers limit the ability of many youth of color to receive accurate and adequate information on preventing unintended pregnancy, STIs, and HIV/AIDS (Augustine et al., 2004). African American youth were more likely than Hispanics and whites to have never been taught in school about AIDS or HIV (CDC, 2008a). Furthermore, the programs that exist do not appear to be efficacious. There is a distinct need for comprehensive and accurate information and for culturally competent, confidential, and affordable services (Augustine et al., 2004). Programs have failed to develop a curriculum based on the cultural competencies of vulnerable populations such as adolescents at risk for HIV (Glenn & Wilson, 2008). Curriculums for youth of color should be based on longitudinal epidemiological research with African American youth that identifies processes which protect youth from engaging in risky behaviors. This is the approach prescribed by the Institute of Medicine (1994).

SUBSTANCE USE

Substance use increases rapidly during early adolescence, and rates of conduct problems such as delinquent and disruptive behavior almost double between ages 9 and 15.

Onset of these behaviors in early adolescence can be significant predictors of school failure, criminal justice system involvement, and drug abuse (Brody, Kogan, Chen, & McBride Murry, 2008). In addition, intoxication can increase the likelihood of teen pregnancy and the contraction of HIV or STIs, among other risks (CDC, 2006b). African American adolescents are less likely to use alcohol, tobacco, and marijuana than are white or Hispanic adolescents. There are few efficacious prevention programs designed to deter substance use for African American youth. One notable exception is the Strong African American Families program, which has been shown to enhance a protective factor that deters both substance use and conduct problems (Brody et al., 2008).

DELINQUENCY AND CRIMINALITY

The same disproportionate representation of racial and ethnic minorities found in U.S. prisons is also apparent in all stages of the juvenile justice system (National Council on Crime and Delinquency [NCCD], 2007). While the last ten years showed a decline in the custody rates for youth in the United States (Davis, Tsukida, Marchionna, & Krisberg, 2008) and among custody populations of most racial and ethnic groups, the biggest decline occurred among whites (18%), with African Americans and Hispanics experiencing smaller declines (11% and 2%, respectively). Consequently, these declines did not affect the overall disproportion among youth of color in custody (Sickmund, Sladky, & Kang, 2008). Despite being less than 15 percent of the total youth population, African Americans represented 58 percent of youth admitted to state adult prison (NCCD, 2007), account for almost 40 percent of the placement population, and have consistently had the highest rates of placement of all groups (see Figure 3.1) (U.S. Census Bureau, 2006). Nationwide, in every offense category, including person, property, drug, and public order, African American youth were disproportionately detained; and in comparison to white youth, African American youth were

FIGURE 3.1 *Black Youth as Proportion of Total Youth . . .*

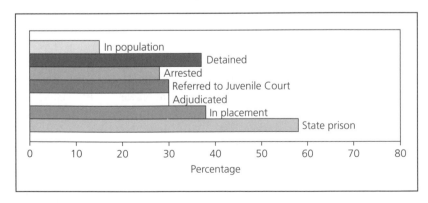

Source: NCCD, 2007.

overrepresented in the detained population in forty-five states (NCCD, 2007). It is not clear whether this overrepresentation is the result of differential police policies and practices (targeting patrols in certain low-income neighborhoods, policies requiring immediate release to biological parents, and group arrest procedures); location of offenses (African American youth use or sell drugs on street corners, while white youth use or sell drugs in homes); different behavior by youth of color (whether they commit more crimes than white youth); different reactions of victims to offenses committed by white youth versus youth of color (whether white victims of crimes disproportionately perceive the offenders to be youth of color); or racial bias within the justice system (NCCD, 2007).

While public attention has tended to focus on the disproportionate number of youth of color in confinement, this overrepresentation is often a product of actions that occur at earlier points in the juvenile justice system, such as the decision to make the initial arrest, the decision to hold a youth in detention pending investigation, the decision to refer a case to juvenile court, the decision to waive a case to adult court, the prosecutor's decision to petition a case, and the judicial decision and subsequent sanction (NCCD, 2007). In 2003, although white youth made up 67 percent of the juvenile court referral population, they made up 60 percent of the detained population. In contrast, African American youth made up 30 percent of the referral population and 37 percent of the detained population (Figure 3.1) (NCCD, 2007). Furthermore, in 2004, the majority of juvenile arrests were white youth; however, African American youth were disproportionately arrested in twenty-six of twenty-nine offense categories documented by the FBI (NCCD, 2007).

EDUCATIONAL DEFICIT AND TRUANCY

There is a well-documented achievement gap in educational performance between African Americans and whites that affects every economic level. Not enough African Americans at any socioeconomic level are faring as well in school as they should (Swain, 2006). Despite more than thirty years of attention and debate on the topic, evidence suggests that disproportionate representation of minorities in special education remains as well (Skiba, Knesting, & Bush, 2002). The debate about minority disproportionality in special education is often framed in terms of test bias. Critics question whether aptitude and achievement tests are constructed in such a way as to be inherently biased against certain groups, yielding inaccurate scores or inaccurate predictions. The administration and interpretation of tests without bias is also of concern (Skiba et al., 2002). But this is far from just a special education issue. Even in top school districts, African American students lag behind. By senior year, the average African American high school student functions at a skill level four years behind the skill levels of white and Asian students (Swain, 2006).

One contributing factor is the social environment in schools. The nature of the schools in which minority students find themselves has a greater influence on sustaining or dissuading students' commitment to education than do their cultural backgrounds

(Mateu-Gelabert & Lune, 2007). Schools can often feel unsafe in minority neighborhoods. Minority students were more likely than white students to have been threatened or injured with a weapon on school property or to have not gone to school because they felt unsafe at school or on the way to and from school (CDC, 2008a). In order to succeed, these students have to develop strategies to remain committed to education while surviving day to day in an unsafe, academically limited school environment characterized by ineffective control and nonengaging classes (Mateu-Gelabert & Lune, 2007). For decades, society has signaled to African Americans that it is okay for them to be less competitive than other groups. These cultural norms and lowered expectations are partially responsible for the fact that African Americans lag behind other racial and ethnic groups in academic achievement (Swain, 2006).

This trend continues even in college. It has been found that African American students exhibit considerably lower performance in college than white students (Swain, 2006). There are a number of possible factors that contribute to this disparity. One study showed that African American students who took the SAT had not followed the same academic track as white students, taking fewer literature and honors writing courses. The white test-takers were far more likely to have completed courses in geometry and higher-level mathematics such as trigonometry and calculus. Racism and the difficulty of adjusting to the social environment are common explanations for the discrepancy among college students. Misinformation about affirmative action can lead some to genuinely believe that traditionally white professional schools are obligated to take them, regardless of their less-than-stellar performance. This perception affects how hard students train. Some have internalized white racist notions of African American inferiority, but something other than white racism and subpar schools must be contributing to African American underachievement (Swain, 2006).

Not all smart students are college bound. When the children of more-affluent African Americans fail to reach their potential, it may be for reasons that cannot be easily dismissed as racism. A part of the problem must lie in parental expectations and societal messages that reinforce the negative stereotypes that African Americans are less capable and less likely to benefit from the application of higher standards imposed by teachers and institutions (Swain, 2006). Teachers, guidance counselors, and concerned adults need to encourage students to stay in school, work hard, and avail themselves of resources to improve their life chances. Having just one adult in the life of a child who genuinely cares can make a dramatic difference in the student's likelihood of success. Words of encouragement, when offered sincerely, are priceless. Teachers and counselors often unintentionally reinforce African American students' affirmations that they are not able to make it academically, and when difficulties do arise, parents are quick to blame teachers and the educational system rather than properly attributing lapses to what is not being said and done at home. Middle-class parents can hire private tutors; they can restrict the amount of time their children watch television and play sports; they can monitor peer-group associations; and they can make sure that their offspring take full advantage of enrichment opportunities offered by schools and other institutions (Swain, 2006).

Parental support and the home environment have just as much influence as the school environment. One study of 374 African American students attending a rural public school addressed future education orientation. Gender and current level of achievement distinguished adolescents with differing levels of future education orientation, but the study found the strongest predictors of future education orientation to be self-efficacy, ethnic identity, and maternal support (Kerpelman, Eryigit, & Stephens, 2008). Longitudinal studies and research that integrates quantitative and qualitative methods are needed to further clarify the nature and importance of future education orientation for African American youth (Kerpelman et al., 2008).

FOSTER CARE

The foster care and juvenile justice systems are populated largely by the same types of children, with minorities, especially African Americans, and low-income youth represented disproportionately to the general population (see Figure 3.2) (Goldstrom, Jaiquan, Henderson, & Male, 2000). The admission of these children into care often comes about because of a breakdown in parenting or because of neglect, abuse, and family discord (Rutter, 2000), or because of poverty-stricken or otherwise unsuitable home environments. While children of all races and ethnicities have been equally likely to be abused or neglected since the early 1980s, African American children, and to some extent other minority children, have been significantly more likely to be represented in foster care (Government Accountability Office [GAO)], 2007). Nationally, African American children made up less than 15 percent of the overall child population in the 2000 U.S. Census, but they represented 27 percent of the children who entered foster care during fiscal year 2004, and they represented 34 percent of the children remaining in foster care at the end of that year (GAO, 2007). The growing number of African American children in foster care may be a reflection of the simultaneous

FIGURE 3.2 *Percentage of Children in Foster Care.*

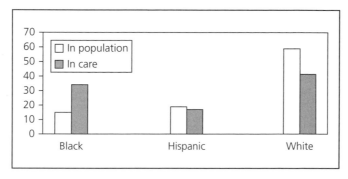

Source: GAO, 2007.

impact of parental substance use, poverty and homelessness, family violence, and AIDS on at-risk families (Leslie et al., 2000).

Foster care and juvenile justice youth often have histories of prenatal exposure to drugs and alcohol (Hartney, Wordes, & Krisberg, 2002). Studies of children exposed to cocaine during pregnancy indicate certain behavioral and developmental differences during early infancy and childhood. These differences can evolve into parenting challenges which increase the risk of maltreatment (Bartholet, 1999). Therefore, it is no surprise that parental drug abuse and alcohol addiction have especially triggered an explosion in child abuse and neglect. Children whose parents abuse drugs and alcohol are almost three times more likely to be abused and more than four times more likely to be neglected than children of parents who do not abuse alcohol and other drugs (Children's Defense Fund, 2005). Many alcoholics and addicts neglect their children because they can think of only one goal, getting their next high. It is common for children to end up "parenting" their own parents, taking care of them and running the household (Bartholet, 1999).

By the very nature of their involvement with CPS (Child Protective Services), these youth are at an increased risk for many negative health outcomes and behaviors. The children of drug-abusing parents are at greater risk than their peers for engaging in alcohol and drug use, delinquency, and having poor school performance, as well as depression and other psychiatric disorders (Bartholet, 1999). Having a history of maltreatment was found to be a precursor to excessive drinking, drug use, and a wide range of problems and disorders in adolescence and adulthood (Bensley, Van Eenwyk, & Simmons, 2000; Bissada & Briere, 2002). Youths who have been abused or neglected and in out-of-home care are among those at highest risk for not only HIV but STDs and pregnancy as well (Auslander, Slonim-Nevo, Elze, & Sherraden, 1998; Becker & Barth, 2000). Youth in foster care and the juvenile justice system are already likely to be suffering from inadequate health care (GAINS Center, 1999), significantly more medical problems (Goldstrom et al., 2000), and high prevalence of co-occurrence of two or more mental health problems, often including substance abuse (Hartney et al., 2002), compared to demographically similar youth outside of the systems.

Poverty can also play a role, considering that children who live in families with annual incomes less than $15,000 are twenty-two times more likely to be abused or neglected than children living in families earning $30,000 or more (Children's Defense Fund, 2005). A higher rate of poverty, challenges in accessing support services, and racial bias were identified as factors contributing to the higher proportion of African American children entering foster care. Thirty-three states surveyed cited high rates of poverty among African Americans as a factor influencing children's entry into foster care (GAO, 2007). Studies have shown that families living in poverty have difficulty accessing needed services that can help support families and keep children who may be vulnerable to abuse and neglect safely at home. However, research suggests that poverty does not fully account for differing rates of entry into foster care. Bias or cultural misunderstanding, and distrust between child welfare decision makers and the families they serve, also contribute to the removal of children from their homes (GAO, 2007).

Another dilemma is that once African American children are removed from their homes, they tend to stay in foster care longer. Their lengths of stay in foster care average nine months longer than those of white children; this may be due to the challenges in accessing services such as substance abuse treatment and subsidized housing (GAO, 2007). Other contributing factors include difficulties finding appropriate permanent homes, in part because of the challenges in recruiting adoptive parents, especially for youth who are older or have special needs, and because African Americans are more likely to rely on relatives to provide foster care. Although this type of foster care placement, known as kinship care, can be less traumatic for children and reduce the number of placements and chance of their reentry into foster care, it is also associated with longer lengths of stay. These relatives may be less willing to terminate the parental rights of the child's parents, or to proceed with adoption, or they may need the financial subsidy they receive while the child is in foster care (GAO, 2007).

Researchers and officials stress that there is no single strategy to fully address the issue but that strategies to increase access to support services, reduce bias, and increase the availability of permanent homes all hold some promise for reducing disproportionality (GAO, 2007). Reportedly, federal policies that provide for family support services and promote adoption were generally considered helpful in reducing the proportion of African Americans in foster care. These policies, such as the requirement to recruit minority adoptive parents and providing subsidies to families adopting children that states have identified as having special needs, affect a state's ability to find permanent homes for children. Policies that limit the use of foster care funding for family support services and legal guardianship were reported to have a negative effect (GAO, 2007).

POVERTY AND ACCESS TO CARE

One of the most important factors that contribute to the health status of African American children and adolescents is low income. Nationally, African Americans are nearly four times more likely than others to live in poverty (GAO, 2007). As alluded to in the previous sections, poverty can affect the health and well-being of African Americans in multiple ways. Income level has been associated with infant mortality. The rate of sudden infant death syndrome (SIDS) may be higher among those at poverty level; and income may contribute to preterm and low birthweight (OMHD, 2007). Mothers lacking much-needed prenatal care can also contribute to infant mortality. Continuing medical care and necessary vaccinations for growing children require some form of health insurance to be affordable. Healthier, more nutritious food choices come with a steep price tag. Poverty status can affect the performance of students from poor families; few will have parents able and willing to work in the schools and participate in parent-teacher conferences; and what most people take for granted is often not available to the poor, such as having proper clothes for the weather, hygiene products, or alternative forms of transportation to school (Swain, 2006). Families living in poverty have greater difficulty accessing housing, mental health, and other services needed to keep families stable and children safely at home (GAO, 2007).

The inflated costs of health care have made nongroup coverage unaffordable for most low-income families, leaving more than nine million children uninsured in the United States (National Conference of State Legislatures [NCSL], 2008). This is of particular importance to the African American community since the U.S. surgeon general reports that low-income people of color have more illness and less access to adequate health care than the rest of the U.S. population (U.S. Department of Health and Human Services [DHHS], 2001). Youth of color as well as young people in foster care and the juvenile justice system especially have higher rates of medical indigence and confront even more financial, cultural, and institutional barriers to obtaining healt care (Hartney et al., 2002). Need-based health care programs, such as Medicaid and the State Children's Health Insurance Program (SCHIP), help to provide coverage for millions, especially children. SCHIP, a state-federal partnership, was created to bridge the safety-net gap for low-income children who do not qualify for Medicaid but remain in families that cannot afford insurance. Enrollment in these programs provides simple preventative care such as immunizations and regular check-ups to ensure proper growth and development (NCSL, 2008). These services are centered on a child's health care needs; however, they also provide limited access to comprehensive and adolescent-appropriate health services. Adolescence is a particularly difficult developmental stage, which requires special emphasis on health care provision and intervention (Hartney et al., 2002). Research shows that early intervention makes a measurable improvement in the future health of these children (NCSL, 2008). Furthermore, the lack of adequate early intervention contributes to longer stays in foster care and deeper involvement in the juvenile justice system (Hartney et al., 2002).

Despite the availability of such programs, six and a half million children living in families with household incomes below 200 percent of the federal poverty level, which makes them eligible for Medicaid or SCHIP, are not enrolled. As of 2008, declining state budgets and a lack of federal action to reauthorize SCHIP have diminished the capacity for states to pass large health reform and to offer coverage to additional children. In addition, a directive issued by the Centers for Medicare and Medicaid Services (CMS) on August 17, 2007, made it more challenging for states to raise the eligibility levels of their programs (to include families with incomes above 250% of the federal poverty guidelines) without meeting several additional criteria (NCSL, 2008).

When additional health care services are needed, use of public emergency medical services (EMS) is a way to obtain guaranteed medical services with little or no money. The available literature suggests that children account for approximately 4–10 percent of all EMS use, relying on EMS as a mode of transport to emergency departments 5–7 percent of the time (Shah et al., 2008). Furthermore, study results show that demographic characteristics associated with EMS use include African American race and urban residence (Shah et al., 2008). Despite previous studies indicating higher EMS use rates by African Americans under the age of twenty-four years, no similar studies have been performed for the pediatric populations (Shah et al., 2008). Future study is required to examine the demographic, socioeconomic, and health care factors behind the increased EMS utilization rate observed among the African American pediatric population (Shah et al., 2008).

PROTECTIVE FACTORS

The needs and concerns of minority children often seem insurmountable. Environmental conditions, such as living in noisy, high crime areas in overcrowded homes with depressed parents can affect a child's ability to function and even the decision of whether to stay in school. There is often a need for children to escape these bad home situations. They may seek work outside the home as soon as they reach a certain age, or they may turn to teenage marriage, childbirth, and eventually the responsibilities of being a single parent (Swain, 2006). Researchers continue to identify ways to minimize or counteract the negative effects of adverse experiences that may manifest as health and behavioral problems (Masten & Reed, 2002; Scales & Leffert, 1999). Exposure to protective factors can decrease the odds of participating in risky behaviors; lessen the chances of experiencing negative outcomes from participation in risky behaviors; or buffer against being exposed to risk factors or exhibiting risky behaviors (Jessor, Turbin, & Costa, 1998). Protective factors have not been studied as extensively or rigorously as risk factors; however, identifying and understanding protective factors are equally as important as researching risk factors (DHHS, 2001; Resnick, Ireland, & Borowsky, 2004).

It is important to recognize that protective factors can stem from multiple levels of influence (Mancini & Huebner, 2004). The Search Institute has worked to define protective factors from multiple sources, including relationships, opportunities, skills, and other strengths that can promote young people's healthy development (Benson, Roehlkepartain, & Sesma, 2004). Some protective factors that have been especially effective for African American youth to possess include having hope for the future, high self-esteem, parental relationships, and adult mentors. During adolescence, individuals make their first choices in pursuit of a purpose. Having a sense of purpose is related to being future oriented or having hope for the future, and in turn, hope for the future has been associated with improved parent-child relationships; increased self-esteem; decreased emotional or behavioral problems, such as depression and sexual risk taking; and reduced violence (Scales & Leffert, 1999). Higher self-esteem in early adolescence was found to decrease the likelihood of pregnancy among African American and Hispanic teen females (Berry, Shillington, Peaks, & Hohman, 2000) and was positively related to safe sex attitudes among incarcerated youth, along with greater hopefulness (Chang, Bendel, Koopman, McGarvey, & Canterbury, 2003).

The support of family and adult mentors are other protective factors for African American youth. Having a natural mentor has been associated with lower levels of problem behaviors (Zimmerman, Bingenheimer, & Notaro, 2002) and is a predictor of having fewer sexual partners among African American males in particular (Reininger et al., 2005). In addition to having positive role models, the family environment can also promote successful child outcomes through closeness, communication, and the ability to adapt to change (Johnson-Garner & Meyers, 2003; Werner, 1995). Every child needs love, affirmation, and acceptance. Provision of these needs is what is meant by the term "support" (Scales & Leffert, 1999). Being supported addresses the need for young people to experience care and love from their families, neighbors, and many others (Search Institute, 1997). Researchers have consistently found that an individual's feelings of being supported, connected, and cared about by someone in his or her life are strongly related to a variety of positive outcomes: lower substance use; higher self-esteem, self-concept, and perceived competence; less anxiety and depression; less delinquency and school misconduct; less casual, unprotected sexual intercourse; and higher school engagement, academic achievement, and aspirations (Scales & Leffert, 1999; St. Lawrence, Brasfield, Jefferson, Alleyne, & Shirley, 1994; Willis, Resko, Ainette, & Mendoza, 2004).

The adolescent's perception of the parent as the provider of support, in particular, facilitates the adolescent's ability to grow into a healthy, independent adult (Parker & Benson, 2004). Most parents are able to provide some type of protection to offset the biological, behavioral, and environmental risks that their children face. However, some parents are unable to give their children the opportunities or settings needed for successful development (Jenson & Fraser, 2006). If they are not receiving the proper support and reinforcements during development, they may be more susceptible to engaging in risky health behaviors that can have life-altering consequences. Research has concentrated heavily on the family environment as the primary influence on the health and well-being of children, along with other environments such as peer influences and school context (Earls & Carlson, 2001). Studies suggest that the family, and more specifically the parent, plays an important role in helping adolescents avoid many risk behaviors (Cohen, Richardson, & LaBree, 1994; Dishon, Reid, & Patterson, 1988; Jaccard & Dittus, 1991; Metzler, Noell, Biglan, Ary, & Smolkowski, 1994; Miller, Levin, Whitaker, & Xiaohe, 1998; Patterson, DeBaryshe, & Ramsey, 1989).

Given the home environments of many African American youth, a major step toward bettering the health status of these children and adolescents is to strengthen the African American family. The historical African tradition of the village raising a child has all but vanished. African American children are often being raised by a matriarchal head of household, who is often a grandmother instead of the biological mother, with no male role model in the home. The problem is cyclical in nature. The plight of the single African American mother, the incarceration rates of the African American male, the epidemic of substance abuse, poor education, low income, and many other conditions create cycles that are hard to disrupt. The cycle must be broken through a combination of behavioral, environmental, and political interventions. By saving the parents and supporting the African American family, we can protect our African American children.

REFERENCES

Augustine, J., Alford, S., & Deas, N. (2004). *Youth of color: At disproportionate risk of negative sexual health outcomes.* Washington, DC: Advocates for Youth.

Auslander, W. F., Slonim-Nevo, V., Elze, D., & Sherraden, M. (1998). HIV prevention for youths in independent living programs: Expanding life options. *Child Welfare, 77*(2), 208–221.

Bartholet, E. (1999). *Nobody's children: Abuse and neglect, foster drift, and the adoption alternative.* Boston: Beacon Press Books.

Becker, M. G., & Barth, R. P. (2000). Power through choices: The development of a sexuality education curriculum for youths in out-of-home care. *Child Welfare, 79*(3), 269–282.

Bensley, L. S., Van Eenwyk, J., & Simmons, K. W. (2000). Self-reported childhood sexual and physical abuse and adult HIV-risk behaviors and heavy drinking. *American Journal of Preventive Medicine, 18*(2), 151–158.

Benson, P. L., Roehlkepartain, E. C., & Sesma, A., Jr. (2004). Tapping the power of community: The potential of asset building to strengthen substance abuse prevention efforts. *Search Institute Insights & Evidence, 2*(1), 1–14.

Berry, E. H., Shillington, A. M., Peaks, T., & Hohman, M. M. (2000). Multi-ethnic comparison of risk and protective factors for adolescent pregnancy. *Child and Adolescent Social Work Journal, 17*(2), 79–96.

Bissada, A., & Briere, J. (2002). Child abuse: Physical and sexual. In J. Worell (Ed.), *Encyclopedia of women and gender*. San Diego: Academic Press.

Branche, C. M., Dellinger, A. M., Sleet, D. A., Gilchrist, J., & Olson, S. J. (2004). Unintentional injuries: The burden, risks, and preventive strategies to address diversity. In I. L. Livingston (Ed.), *Policies and issues behind disparities in health* (2nd ed., pp. 317–327). Westport, CT: Praeger.

Brody, G. H., Kogan, S. M., Chen, Y.-F., & McBride Murry, V. (2008). Long-term effects of the Strong African American Families Program on youths' conduct problems. *Journal of Adolescent Health, 43*(5), 474–481.

Centers for Disease Control and Prevention (CDC). (1998). Deaths resulting from residential fires and the prevalence of smoke alarms—United States 1991–1995. *Morbidity/Mortality Weekly Report, 47*(38), 803–806.

Centers for Disease Control and Prevention (CDC). (2004). *Preventing lead exposure in young children: A housing-based approach to primary prevention of lead poisoning*. Atlanta: Author.

Centers for Disease Control and Prevention (CDC). (2006a). Web-based injury statistics query and reporting system (WISQARS). Retrieved February 2006 from http://www.cdc.gov/injury/wisqars/index.html

Centers for Disease Control and Prevention (CDC). (2006b). Youth risk behavior surveillance—United States, 2005. *Morbidity/Mortality Weekly Report, 55*, 1–112.

Centers for Disease Control and Prevention (CDC). (2008a). *Health risk behaviors by race/ethnicity—National YRBS: 2007* (Fact sheet). Atlanta: Author.

Centers for Disease Control and Prevention (CDC). (2008b). Injuries among children and adolescents. Retrieved November 18, 2008, from http://www.cdc.gov/ncipc/factsheets/children.htm

Centers for Disease Control and Prevention (CDC). (2008c). National, state, and local area vaccination coverage among children aged 19–35 months—U.S., 2007. *Morbidity/Mortality Weekly Report, 57*(35), 961–966.

Centers for Disease Control and Prevention (CDC). (2008d). Web-based injury statistics query and reporting system (WISQARS). Retrieved March 14, 2008, from http://www.cdc.gov/injury/wisqars/index.html

Chang, V. Y., Bendel, T. L., Koopman, C., McGarvey, E. L., & Canterbury, R. J. (2003). Delinquents' safe sex attitudes: Relationships with demographics, resilience factors, and substance use. *Criminal Justice and Behavior, 30*(2), 210–229.

Children's Defense Fund. (2005). Child abuse and neglect fact sheet. Retrieved October 8, 2005, from http://www.childrensdefense.org/child-research-data-publications/data/child-abuse-and-neglect-fact-sheet-pdf.pdf

Cohen, D., Richardson, J., & LaBree, L. (1994). Parenting behaviors and the onset of smoking and alcohol use: A longitudinal study. *Pediatrics, 93*, 368–375.

Davis, A., Tsukida, C., Marchionna, S., & Krisberg, B. (2008). *The declining number of youth in custody in the juvenile justice system*. Woodland Hills, CA: National Council on Crime and Delinquency.

Dishon, T., Reid, J., & Patterson, G. (1988). Empirical guidelines for a family intervention for adolescent drug use. *Journal of Chemical Dependency Treatment, 2*, 181–216.

Earls, F., & Carlson, M. (2001). The social ecology of child health and well-being. *Annual Review of Public Health, 22*(1), 143–167.

Finkelstein, E. A., Corso, P. S., Miller, T. R., & Associates. (2006). *Incidence and economic burden of injuries in the United States*. New York: Oxford University Press.

GAINS Center. (1999). *The courage to change: A guide for communities to create integrated services for people with co-occurring disorders in the justice system*. Rockville, MD: Substance Abuse and Mental Health Services Administration.

Glenn, B. L., & Wilson, K. P. (2008). African American adolescent perceptions of vulnerability and resilience to HIV. *Journal of Transcultural Nursing, 19*(3), 259–265.

Goldstrom, I., Jaiquan, F., Henderson, M., & Male, A. (2000). *The availability of mental health services to young people in juvenile justice facilities: A national survey*. Rockville, MD: U.S. Department of Health and Human Services.

Government Accountability Office (GAO). (2007). *African American children in foster care: Additional HHS assistance needed to help states reduce the proportion in care* (No. GAO-07-816). Washington, DC: United States Government Accountability Office.

Hartney, C., Wordes, M., & Krisberg, B. (2002). *Health care for our troubled youth: Provision of services in the foster care and juvenile justice systems of California*. Woodland Hills, CA: National Council on Crime and Delinquency.

Institute of Medicine. (1994). *Reducing risks for mental disorders: Frontiers for preventive intervention research*. Washington, DC: National Academies Press.

Istre, G. R., McCoy, M. A., Osborn, L., Barnard, J. J., & Bolton, A. (2001). Deaths and injuries from house fires. *New England Journal of Medicine, 344*, 1911–1916.

Jaccard, J., & Dittus, P. (1991). *Parent-teen communications: Toward the prevention of unintended pregnancies*. New York: Springer Verlag.

Jenson, J. M., & Fraser, M. W. (Eds.). (2006). *Social policy for children and families: A risk and resilience perspective*. Thousand Oaks, CA: Sage.

Jessor, R., Turbin, M., & Costa, F. (1998). Protective factors in adolescent health. *Journal of Personality and Social Psychology, 75*, 788–800.

Johnson-Garner, M. Y., & Meyers, S. A. (2003). What factors contribute to the resilience of African-American children within kinship care? *Child & Youth Care Forum, 32*(5), 255–269.

Kerpelman, J. L., Eryigit, S., & Stephens, C. J. (2008). African American adolescents' future education orientation: Associations with self-efficacy, ethnic identity, and perceived parental support. *Journal of Youth and Adolescence, 37*(8), 997–1008.

Leslie, L. K., Landsverk, J., Ezzet-Lofstrom, R., Tschann, J. M., Slymen, D. J., & Garland, A. F. (2000). Children in foster care: Factors influencing outpatient mental health service use. *Child Abuse & Neglect, 24*(4), 465–476.

Mancini, J. A., & Huebner, A. J. (2004). Adolescent risk behavior patterns: Effects of structured time-use, interpersonal connections, self-system characteristics, and socio-demographic influences. *Child and Adolescent Social Work Journal, 21*(6), 647–668.

Martin, J. A., Hamilton, B. E., Sutton, P. D., Ventura, S., Menacker, F., Kirmeyer, S., et al. (2007). Births: Final data for 2005. *National Vital Statistics Reports, 56*(6), 1–104.

Masten, A. S., & Reed, M. G. (2002). Resilience in development. In C. R. Snyder & S. J. Lopez (Eds.), *The handbook of positive psychology*. New York: Oxford University Press.

Mateu-Gelabert, P., & Lune, H. (2007). Street codes in high school: School as an educational deterrent. *City & Community, 6*(3), 173–191.

Metzler, C., Noell, J., Biglan, A., Ary, D., & Smolkowski, K. (1994). The social context for risky sexual behavior among adolescents. *Journal of Behavioral Medicine, 17*, 419–438.

Miller, K., Levin, M., Whitaker, D., & Xiaohe, X. (1998). Patterns of condom use among adolescents: The impact of mother-adolescent communication. *American Journal of Public Health, 88*, 1542–1544.

Miniño, A. M., Arias, E., Kochanek, K. D., Murphy, S. L., & Smith, B. L. (2002). Infant, neonatal, and postneonatal mortality rates by race and sex: United States, 1940, 1950, 1960, 1970, and 1980–2000 (Table). In Deaths: Final Data for 2000. *National Vital Statistics Reports, 50*(15), 1–120; table p. 17.

National Center for Health Statistics. (2002). *Health, United States, 2002, with chart book on trends in the health of Americans*. P. N. Pastor, D. M. Makuc, C. Reuben, & H. Xia (Eds.). Hyattsville, MD: Author.

National Conference of State Legislatures (NCSL). (2008, October). Children's health reform. Retrieved November 2008 from http://www.ncsl.org/default.aspx?tabid=14477

National Council on Crime and Delinquency (NCCD). (2007). *And justice for some: Differential treatment of youth of color in the justice system*. Oakland, CA: Author.

Office of Minority Health & Health Disparities (OMHD). (2007). Eliminate disparities in infant mortality. Retrieved November 2008 from http://www.cdc.gov/omhd/amh/factsheets/infant.htm

Parker, J. S., & Benson, M. J. (2004). Parent-adolescent relations and adolescent functioning: Self-esteem, substance abuse, and delinquency. *Adolescence, 39*(155), 519–530.

Patterson, G., DeBaryshe, D., & Ramsey, E. (1989). A developmental perspective on antisocial behavior. *American Psychology, 44*, 329–335.

Reininger, B. M., Evans, A. E., Griffin, S. F., Sanderson, M., Vincent, M. L., Valois, R. F., et al. (2005). Predicting adolescent risk behaviors based on an ecological framework and assets. *American Journal of Health Behavior, 29*(2), 150–161.

Resnick, M., Ireland, M., & Borowsky, I. (2004). Youth violence perpetration: What protects? What predicts? Findings from the National Longitudinal Study of Adolescent Health. *Journal of Adolescent Health, 35*, 424.e1–424.e10.

Rosenthal, J., Rodewald, L., McCauley, M., Berman, S., Irigoyen, M., Sawyer, M., et al. (2004). Immunization coverage levels among 19- to 35-month-old children in 4 diverse, medically underserved areas of the United States. *Pediatrics, 113*(4), e296–e302.

Rutter, M. (2000). Children in substitute care: Some conceptual considerations and research implications. *Children and Youth Services Review, 22*(9/10), 685–703.

Scales, P. C., & Leffert, N. (1999). *Developmental assets: A synthesis of the scientific research on adolescent development.* Minneapolis: Search Institute.

Search Institute. (1997). 40 developmental assets (Table). Minneapolis: Author.

Shah, M. N., Cushman, J. T., Davis, C. O., Bazarian, J. J., Auinger, P., & Friedman, B. (2008). The epidemiology of emergency medical services use by children: An analysis of the National Hospital Ambulatory Medical Care Survey. *Prehospital Emergency Care, 12*(3), 269–376.

Sickmund, M., Sladky, T. J., & Kang, W. (2008). Census of juveniles in residential placement databook. Retrieved June 25, 2008, from http://www.ojjdp.ncjrs.gov/ojstatbb/cjrp/

Skiba, R. J., Knesting, K., & Bush, L. (2002). Culturally competent assessment: More than nonbiased tests. *Journal of Child and Family Studies, 11*(1), 61–78.

Sorof, J. M., Lai, D., Turner, J., Poffenbarger, T., & Portman, R. J. (2004). Overweight, ethnicity, and the prevalence of hypertension in school-aged children. *Pediatrics, 113*(3), 475–482.

St. Lawrence, J., Brasfield, T., Jefferson, K., Alleyne, E., & Shirley, A. (1994). Social support as a factor in African-American adolescents' sexual risk behavior. *Journal of Adolescent Research, 9*, 292–310.

Swain, C. M. (2006). An inside look at education and poverty. *Academic Questions, 19*(2), 47–53.

Urrutia-Rojas, X., & Menchaca, J. (2006). Prevalence of risk for type 2 diabetes in school children. *Journal of School Health, 76*(5), 189–194.

U.S. Census Bureau. (2006). *American Community Survey, 2006.* Washington, DC: U.S. Department of Commerce, Economics and Statistics Administration.

U.S. Department of Health and Human Services (DHHS). (2001). Youth violence: A report of the Surgeon General. Retrieved June 25, 2008 from http://www.surgeongeneral.gov/library/youthviolence/toc.html

Werner, E. E. (1995). Resilience in development. *Current Directions in Psychological Science, 4*(3), 81–85.

Willis, T. A., Resko, J. A., Ainette, M. G., & Mendoza, D. (2004). Role of parent support and peer support in adolescent substance use: A test of mediated effects. *Psychology of Addictive Behaviors, 18*(2), 122–134.

Zimmerman, M. A., Bingenheimer, J. B., & Notaro, P. C. (2002). Natural mentors and adolescent resiliency: A study with urban youth. *American Journal of Community Psychology, 30*(2), 221–243.

CHAPTER

4

THE HEALTH STATUS OF BLACK WOMEN

SANDRA E. TAYLOR
KISHA BRAITHWAITE HOLDEN

A synthesis of selected publications on the health of black women demonstrates the lack of positive change for this group over the past decade. While the status of black women's health has been examined through a host of conditions and recommendations for reversing trends, there has been virtually no significant improvement in key indicators for this vulnerable group. Additionally, critical health issues continue to affect black women at a magnitude that renders this group at crisis levels compared to other racial/gender categories. Alongside this is the plethora of chronic as well as acute illnesses affecting black women disproportionately. The various health conditions discussed in the chapter on black women in this book's second edition (Taylor, 2001) still remain and in some instances have worsened. The gender gap is especially apparent when considering specific health outcomes. The health of black women has been found to be poorer than that of white women as well as white and black men for certain health measures after controlling for socioeconomic and background factors (Read & Gorman, 2006).

Black women's health lags behind that of white women despite some narrowing of this gap over the years. Still, the overall gap is approximately five years between these two groups, and the mortality rate of white women continues to surpass that of black women. For example, life expectancy in 2001 was 79.9 years for white women and 74.7 years for black women (CDC, 2007b).

Correlates of the health status of black women, specifically socioeconomic status, including income and occupation, help place this group's status in context. The fact that a disproportionate number of black women, compared to white women, have lower income and education levels presents a barrier to health. Black women's health has been discussed in various contexts but often within that of self-empowerment. Studies show that vulnerable populations can benefit from measures that promote health improvement from within, thereby emphasizing the role of individual behaviors. Other contexts important to the health of black women include the cultural environment and psychosocial factors. The sparseness of empirical literature directly related to black women's health (despite repeated recommendations for such by researchers and practitioners alike) prohibits a fuller understanding of ways to improve health outcomes for this group that encompass the myriad of factors affecting health. Consequently, disparities are not diminished, and the desired progress has been elusive.

While this chapter discusses some of the health disparities that most prominently affect black women, it only begins to sketch the many conditions faced by this population. And though the chapter briefly reviews data on the causes of death for black women, it does so only for the four leading causes: heart disease, cancer, stroke, and diabetes. The data in Table 4.1 show ranked causes of death for the year 2004.

DISEASE, HYPERTENSION, AND STROKE

Heart disease (or cardiovascular disease) claims more American lives than any other disease. Heart disease mortality differs substantially among women of different racial and ethnic groups, and studies show that black women bear a particular burden in dealing with cardiovascular disease.

Research consistently shows that black women are less likely than other groups of women or men to be referred for diagnostic procedures or to have access to lifesaving therapies for heart attack. Of the four race/gender groups, black women are least likely to receive reperfusion or therapy to restore blood flow to the artery (either thrombolytic drugs or primary angioplasty), followed by black men. White men are most likely to be recipients of this lifesaving therapy, just ahead of white women (Canto et al., 2000).

Because heart disease poses a particular risk to black women, several national organizations have taken the lead in improving health outcomes related to cardiovascular diseases. As would be expected, the American Heart Association and the National Heart, Lung, and Blood Institute have launched specifically tailored initiatives to address women and heart disease. Other organizations are banding together in a coalition to promote the passage of a bill to improve the prevention, diagnosis, and treatment of heart disease, stroke, and other cardiovascular diseases through education for women and their health care providers.

Hypertension (or high blood pressure) is a grave risk factor for heart disease and stroke. Black women have higher rates of hypertension, tend to develop it at an earlier age, and are less likely than either white women or males to receive treatment to control it. Research shows that management of chest pain in patients with hypertension

TABLE 4.1 Ranked Cause of Death for U.S. Black and White Females, All Ages, 2004.

Rank	Cause of Death (All Females, All Ages)	Percentage	Cause of Death (White Females, All Ages)	Percentage	Cause of Death (Black Females, All Ages)	Percentage
1	Heart disease	27.2	Heart disease	27.3	Heart disease	26.9
2	Cancer	22.0	Cancer	22.0	Cancer	21.3
3	Stroke	7.5	Stroke	7.5	Stroke	7.4
4	Chronic lower respiratory diseases	5.2	Chronic lower respiratory diseases	5.7	Diabetes	5.1
5	Alzheimer's disease	3.9	Alzheimer's disease	4.1	Kidney disease	3.0
6	Unintentional injuries	3.3	Unintentional injuries	3.3	Unintentional injuries	2.9
7	Diabetes	3.1	Diabetes	2.8	Chronic lower respiratory diseases	2.4
8	Influenza and pneumonia	2.7	Influenza and pneumonia	2.8	Septicemia	2.3
9	Kidney disease	1.8	Kidney disease	1.7	Alzheimer's disease	2.2
10	Septicemia	1.5	Septicemia	1.4	Influenza and pneumonia	2.1

Source: CDC, 2007b.

varies by gender, race, and ethnicity. As with heart disease, women and blacks have been found to receive fewer medications to treat hypertension than their counterparts. Additionally, it has been found that men's diagnoses of cardiovascular conditions are more definitively categorized (such as "angina"), while women receive a vaguer diagnosis (such as "chest pain") (Hendrix, Mayhan, Lackland, & Egan, 2005).

While some studies have concluded that there *may* be an increase in hypertension among black women which is associated with experiences of racism in certain subgroups, others point to more definitive evidence of this relationship. Cozier and others (2007) sought to assess whether racism is associated with hypertension through an analysis of data from the Black Women's Health Study. An analysis of personally mediated racism and institutionalized racism resulted in 2,316 incident cases of hypertension reported during 104,574 person-years of observation from 1997 to 2001, with a majority of the women reporting experiences of racism.

Also using data from the Black Women's Health Study, Cozier and others (2007) found a significant inverse association between median housing values and hypertension. This finding is not surprising given that a lowered socioeconomic status can be a stressor. This study corroborates the expectation and shows that the reported association was evident even at higher individual levels of income and education.

The inverse relationship that would be expected between measures of socioeconomic status and prevalence of health problems is clearly evidenced in a condition highly related to heart disease and hypertension: stroke. As the third leading cause of death for all women as well as the third leading cause for black women, stroke tends to be more severe in black women than for white women. This is partially explained by black women's overrepresentation in lower socioeconomic categories. Hence, interventions that target the behaviors and overall cultural context of low-income women separate from those of higher-income categories are increasingly viewed as critical in improving health outcomes related to stroke.

A recent cross-sectional study analyzing data from the Behavioral Risk Factor Surveillance Survey (BRFSS) found that knowledge of heart attack and stroke symptoms varies significantly among black women, depending on socioeconomic variables (Lutfiyya, Cumba, McCullough, Barlow, & Lipsky, 2008). These investigators showed that, consistent with previous literature, black women scoring low on questions about heart attack and stroke knowledge were more likely to be uninsured and to be in lower-income categories. By increasing knowledge about these conditions through tailoring interventions that meet black women where they are, one might expect to see enhanced outcomes for this group. Some studies show limited success with community and business venues in increasing knowledge about stroke warning signs, risk factors, and related health; for example, with an intervention done in a beauty salon (Kleindorfer et al., 2008). This stroke education project was designed to introduce an innovative intervention to black women by working through parlors; the intervention improved the women's knowledge on certain variables (including stroke warning) but not on others (such as risk factors).

CANCER

Cancer is the second leading cause of death among black women and is the most commonly diagnosed. Although more white women than black are diagnosed with breast cancer, black women are more likely to die from the disease. Cervical cancer, however, occurs most often among women of color, and these women continue to die at rates higher than whites. Black women are more likely to die from all cancers as a factor of late diagnosis, often given that the disease has done irreparable damage at the time of detection. In other cases, delays in follow-up tests and incomplete follow-up accounted for the disparity. More than one-fourth of black women who have abnormal results from mammography or clinical breast exams have not resolved the diagnosis with follow-up six months later, and black women with prior breast abnormalities were about half as likely to follow up on the abnormal results within the recommended time (three to six months).

Breast Cancer

Breast cancer is the second leading cause of cancer death among black women. Breast cancer survival rates continue to be lower for black women than for white women despite efforts to close this gap. A recent study using data from the National Cancer Institute (NCI) Surveillance, Epidemiology, and End Results (SEER) program for 1995–2004 (Baquet, Mishra, Commiskey, Ellison, & DeShields, 2008) found that the invasive breast cancer age-adjusted incidence for black women was significantly higher than for whites and that the age-adjusted mortality rate for black women was twice that of white women. Moreover, the study found that black women were more likely to be diagnosed with regional or distant disease, have a lower relative five-year survival rate, and have a higher likelihood of being diagnosed with tumors carrying a poorer prognosis. Studies also show that black women are also more likely than white women to receive mastectomy versus breast-conserving surgery and radiation (Mandelblatt et al., 2002).

Cancer screening is important for early detection, and mammography is credited for saving lives, albeit fewer black women have benefited. Early detection programs are particularly important, and those that attempt to reach underserved and low-income women are crucial in closing the black-white gap. The creation of the Centers for Disease Control and Prevention's National Breast and Cervical Cancer Early Detection Program, started in 1990, substantially increased the percentage of women in low-income households who reported having had a recent mammogram (Centers for Disease Control and Prevention [CDC], 2005).

High-fat and high-caloric diets and a sedentary lifestyle increase risk for breast cancer recurrence, comorbid conditions, and premature death. Studies show that as much as 82 percent of black women are overweight, making them more vulnerable than their white counterparts, particularly relative to survival (from National Health and Nutrition Examination Survey [NHANES]). And when black women do survive, their quality of life tends to be less robust than that of white women. Some studies have suggested that black women gain more weight than white women after a breast cancer diagnosis. Health promotion initiatives (especially weight loss programs) for women with breast cancer have been around for years; however, few are targeted expressly to black women. One intervention designed to promote the health of black breast cancer survivors targets weight loss as critically important in combating recurrence and proposes a culturally tailored weight loss program to address needs. The study describing the program's overall purpose and design points to the importance of lifestyle interventions and concludes, through feasibility and impact data, that the positive results of the tested weight loss intervention may well be viable for black women (Stolley, Sharp, Oh, & Schiffer, 2009).

Psychosocial factors also play a role in the incidence and prevalence of breast cancer. For example, racism, whether perceived or real, has been shown to adversely affect cancer survivors. Using data from the Black Women's Health Study, one study found that perceived experiences of racism are associated with increased incidence of breast cancer among black women and that the association is more substantial among younger women (Taylor et al., 2007). These investigators examined a total of 593 incident cases of breast cancer and found positive relationships (albeit weak) between "everyday discrimination" (operationalized in terms of how one is treated or regarded) and "major discrimination" (a more institutionalized or structural construct). The higher risk for younger women could well be a factor of greater consciousness of insidious racism on the part of this group (Taylor et al., 2007; Williams, 2002).

Although breast cancer survivors of diverse racial and ethnic groups tend to have similar general stories of survivorship, their specific experiences can be delineated. Some investigators posit that the "illness experience" may be different in light of unintentional racism encountered in treatment, care, support, or the work environment. Coggin and Shaw-Perry (2006) suggest that socioeconomic status does not protect black women from the burden of racial inequity, thereby presenting an additional stressor as this group of women navigates the lack of parity relative to affordable housing, educational and income opportunities, quality medical care, and adequate health insurance.

High levels of stress from perceived or actual racism, as well as stress from any event, are related to an overall diminished health status. In evaluating the associations among health status, well-being, and perceived stress in a sample of urban black women, Young and others (2004) showed that the perceived-stress scores of the women negatively correlated with health status dimensions and well-being. This finding, consistent with the literature on the impact of stress on well-being, points to the far-reaching potential of health promotion strategies that emphasize stress reduction. Because cultural beliefs and attitudes including spirituality and religiosity affect health outcomes generally and those of cancer survivors in particular, interventions targeting faith become especially important toward meeting the needs of black cancer survivors.

MATERNAL AND REPRODUCTIVE HEALTH

Women of color face several maternal and reproductive health issues; some of the more common and selected concerns are cervical cancer and uterine fibroids. Understanding maternal and reproductive issues among black women is particularly significant since black infants born in America are twice as likely as white infants to die before they reach their first birthday (Children's Defense Fund, 2004); it is of paramount importance that research and clinical work be conducted if we are to deter the host of issues that contribute to infant mortality. In 2004, the lowest infant mortality rate observed in the United States was among Asians and Pacific Islanders, who had a rate of 4.67 per 1,000 live births, which pales in comparison to the infant mortality rate of 13.60 per 1,000 live births for blacks (Matthews & MacDorman, 2007).

Just as breast cancer affects black and other ethnic women disproportionately, so too does cervical cancer. There is higher incidence, higher mortality, and poorer survival rates compared to whites. Disparities related to cervical cancer are evident by the following examples highlighted by the Centers for Disease Control and Prevention (CDC, 2005):

- In 2001, black women had the highest age-adjusted mortality rate from cervical cancer (4.8 per 100,000), followed by Hispanic women (3.4 per 100,000).

- From 1992 to 2000, black women were less likely to survive cervical cancer five years after diagnosis compared with white women (blacks 62.6%; whites 73.3%).

- In 2001, cervical cancer incidence was highest among black women (11.9 per 100,000) and Hispanic women (11.8 per 100,000).

Uterine fibroids are the most common pelvic tumor in women and are approximately three times more common in black women than white women. Research on fibroid tumors (or uterine leiomyoma) has not provided consistent explanations as to why the black-white disparity is so large. Risk factors include African ancestry, family history, obesity, and hypertension, among others. The incidence of uterine fibroid tumors increases as women age and may occur in more than 30 percent of women ages 40–60 (Evans & Brunsell, 2007). Symptoms of fibroids include heavy bleeding or painful periods; bleeding between periods; feeling of fullness in the pelvic area (lower abdomen); urinating often; pain during sexual intercourse; lower back pain; and reproductive problems such as infertility, having more than one miscarriage, or having early onset of labor during pregnancy. There are several pharmacological and surgery options available for the treatment of fibroids.

OBESITY AND DIABETES

Black women compose the highest risk category in the United States for being overweight or obese. Obesity is a risk factor for a number of diseases, including the top critical health conditions affecting this population. It has risen to epidemic proportions in this country and is strongly associated with diabetes in black women. The relationship between overall obesity and a host of health conditions is consistently documented by empirical studies. Research on specific types of obesity (such as abdominal obesity or areas of fat distribution) corroborates the strong association between obesity, regardless of type, and health threats. Krishnan, Rosenberg, Kjousse, Cupples, and Palmer (2007) examined the association of body mass index (BMI), abdominal obesity, and weight gain with the risk of type-2 diabetes, observing at every level of BMI an increased risk relative to higher waist-to-hip ratios. Central obesity, like overall obesity, is thus a strong risk factor and should be recognized as such. Data from NHANES show that approximately 82 percent of black women are overweight or obese compared with 58 percent of white women.

Countless weight loss programs have been developed in response to the high rates of overweight and obese black women. In comparison to white women, black women are less likely to participate in weight loss programs, are more likely to drop out after participation in a structured program, and lose less weight than white women. The literature discusses biological, environmental, and cultural factors in its discussion of these occurrences. Kumanyika and others (2007) appropriately argue the importance of creative interventions on overweight or obesity that directly consider the specific needs and perspectives of black women. Espousing a paradigm that reaches beyond the general population, they demonstrate the impracticability of designing interventions that are incongruent with these specific needs. Instead, interventions addressing alternative ways to meet needs and expanded perspectives on food and its symbolism, on activity, and on weight issues are suggested.

Black women are disproportionately affected by diabetes (both type-1 and type-2, the most common type), and the prevalence of this disease continues to be high. It is the fourth leading cause of death among this group and tends to be at least twice as high among black and other ethnic women than white women (CDC, 2007a). According to recent data, of the sixteen million Americans with diabetes, more than half are women. Data from 1980 to 2006 show that age-adjusted prevalence of diagnosed diabetes increased among all racial/gender groups examined, and that prevalence of diagnosed diabetes was highest among black females (Agency for Healthcare Research and Quality [AHRQ], 2008).

Efforts to promote enhanced care for black women with diabetes, including improvements to insulin and glucose therapies and improvements in glycemic control, have been intensified toward reducing some of the complications accompanying the disease (AHRQ, 2008). It has long been recognized that black women with diabetes could benefit from self-management of the disease that takes into account their multifaceted existence. Studies point to the importance of interventions that recognize the influences of spirituality, general life stress, multi-caregiving responsibilities, and the psychological impact of diabetes in providing a heightened quality of life for this group (Samuel-Hodge et al., 2000).

LUPUS

Lupus is an autoimmune disease that can affect various parts of the body, including the skin, joints, heart, lungs, blood, kidneys, and brain. Normally the body's immune system makes proteins, called antibodies, to protect the body against viruses, bacteria, and other foreign materials (called antigens). In an autoimmune disorder like lupus, the immune system cannot tell the difference between foreign substances and the person's own cells and tissues. The immune system then makes antibodies directed against cells and tissues, which cause inflammation, pain, and damage in various parts of the body. Approximately 1.5–2 million Americans have a form of lupus, but the actual number may be higher. More than 90 percent of people with lupus are women. Symptoms and diagnosis occur most often when women are in their child-bearing years, between the ages of fifteen and forty-five years (Lupus Foundation of America, 2009).

Lupus is three times more common in black women than in white women. Compared to white women, it is also more common in women of Hispanic, Asian, and Native American descent. For reasons that are not fully understood, black and Hispanic women tend to develop symptoms at an earlier age than other groups. Data show that death rates are more than five times higher for women than for men and more than three times higher for blacks than for whites.

There are four types of lupus: discoid, systemic, drug-induced, and neonatal lupus. Discoid (cutaneous) lupus is always limited to the skin. It is identified by a rash that may appear on the face, neck, and scalp. Discoid lupus is diagnosed by examining a biopsy of the rash. In discoid lupus the biopsy will show abnormalities that are not found in skin without the rash. Discoid lupus does not generally involve the body's internal organs. Systemic lupus is usually more severe than discoid lupus and can affect almost any organ or organ system of the body. For some people, only the skin and joints will be involved; in others, the joints, lungs, kidneys, blood, or other organs or tissues may be affected. Drug-induced lupus occurs after the use of certain prescribed drugs. The symptoms of drug-induced lupus are similar to those of systemic lupus. The drugs most commonly connected with drug-induced lupus are hydralazine (used to treat high blood pressure, or hypertension) and procainamide (used to treat irregular heart rhythms). Drug-induced lupus is more common in men, who are given these drugs more often. However, not everyone who takes these drugs will develop drug-induced lupus; only about 4 percent of the people who take these drugs will develop the antibodies suggestive of lupus. Of those 4 percent, only an extremely small number will develop overt drug-induced lupus. The symptoms usually fade when the medications are discontinued. Neonatal lupus is a rare condition acquired from the passage of maternal autoantibodies, specifically anti-Ro/SSA or anti-La/SSB, which can affect the skin, heart, and blood of the fetus and newborn. It is associated with a rash that appears within the first several weeks of life and may persist for about six months before disappearing.

Physicians use a variety of medicines to treat their patients who have lupus, which can be complicated due to the complex nature of the disease. Some of the medications reduce inflammation, which causes pain, fever, and swelling, while others suppress the overactive immune system. They range in strength from mild to extremely potent, and often several of these medicines are used in combination to control the disease. Utilizing a holistic approach that includes physical, spiritual, and emotional components may be a viable adjunct to traditional pharmacological methodologies.

HIV/AIDS

Black women bear an alarmingly disproportionate burden of HIV/AIDS. It is the sixth leading cause of death among American women ages 25–34 but the leading cause of death for black women in this same age group. In 2004, HIV/AIDS was the third leading cause of death for black women ages 35–44; for women ages 45–54, it was the fourth. (CDC, 2006). For women of all races and ethnicities, the largest number of HIV/AIDS diagnoses was for women ages 15–39. The rate of AIDS diagnosis for black women in 2005 was approximately twenty-three times the rate for white women and four times the rate for Hispanic women (CDC, 2007a). CDC data further show that a direct relationship exists between poverty and HIV/AIDS, and that black women are disproportionately represented among categories of absolute poverty. The socioeconomic problems associated with poverty exacerbate the condition of black women living with HIV/AIDS. These problems, including limited or no access to quality health care, a heightened level of substance abuse, and the exchange of sex for drugs and other needs, create situations leading to additional health conditions, many of which are related to mental functioning. As such, black women often reach out to religion or other faith-based mechanisms for solace. The role of spirituality in coping with HIV/AIDS has been explored through an array of methods and findings and tends to point to faith as a buffer in dealing with the virus (Braxton, Lang, Sales, Wingood, & DiClemente, 2007).

DOMESTIC AND INTIMATE PARTNER VIOLENCE

Women who are victims of intimate partner violence have been found to exhibit higher levels of anxiety and depression than women not suffering from abuse (Ramos, Carlson, & McNutt, 2004). In a study of black and white women in a primary health care setting, these investigators found that both groups of women showed more similarities than differences in the associations between most abuse experiences, but black women reported more excessive jealousy by partners. Jealousy in relationships has been linked to power and manipulation, and the perpetuation of violence toward a partner has been discussed in relation to deriving a sense of personal control. Based on a national sample including black and white women, a related study shows that having a violent partner undermines personal control for women but not for men (Umberson, Anderson, Glick, & Shapiro, 1998). The authors found that men scored higher on personal control scores than women, and that blacks scored lower than whites. Hence, black women are found to be more vulnerable, with abuse adversely impacting them more.

Further, the role of perceived racism has been linked to intimate partner violence. Some evidence has been established to demonstrate a relationship between perceived racial discrimination and intimate partner violence and how these exposures interact to affect the mental and physical health of black women. Waltermaurer, Watson, and McNutt (2006) found these exposures to be strongly related to women who both reported and showed higher prevalences of anxiety and nonspecific health symptoms compared with women who reported either or neither exposure.

MENTAL HEALTH

Black women are not frequently confronted with isolated stressors but with a constellation of issues that can engender anxiety, such as balancing work and home life demands, healing from adverse life events, managing personal relationships, nurturing identity development, and creating a purpose in life that motivates them toward positive goals and an orientation for achievement and success. Consequently, it is crucial to heighten the awareness of prevalence and predictors of mental health and substance abuse disorders among black women—and the myriad of social determinants that relate to black women's access to and utilization of behavioral health services. Additionally, it is essential that culturally relevant strategies and models for the prevention of mental illnesses and for the promotion of overall wellness among black women from diverse sectors of the community—including underserved, underrepresented, and uninsured populations—receive adequate consideration on a national level.

Stress, an experience resulting from a process or transaction between person and environment in which the stimulus (event or condition) demands adjustment and may cause physical, mental, or emotional strain, contributes to one's mental health and general health. Stress can be viewed as a stimulus, a response, or an interaction of the two, and as a combination of psychological, physiological, and social components. For women in general, and black women in particular, stress can have a deleterious effect on health. Stress may be associated with the following issues:

- Health concerns and chronic diseases

- Individual or personal concerns (such as negative cognitions, identity, self-perception, body image)

- Interpersonal and intimate relationships (issues of commitment, intimacy, trust, communication, fidelity)

- Family relationships and daily demands

- Unresolved pain and trauma (such as sexual, emotional, and physical abuse)

- Negative life events (such as the death of a loved one or being the victim of crime)

- Confronting historical negative stereotypes and media images about black women

- Sociopolitical stressors, including racism and sexism

- Economic and financial concerns

- Community concerns (such as poor environmental conditions)

- Handling multiple expectations of others

Chronic stress can contribute to depression, one of the most prevalent mental health problems in the United States, and is associated with considerable impairment in functioning. Depression among black women is underrecognized and undertreated (Levin, 2008). Furthermore, although blacks are less likely than whites to have a major depressive disorder, when they do, it tends to be more chronic and severe, and they are much less likely to undergo treatment (Williams et al., 2007). This may be due to stigma and less trust within the medical community, poor or no insurance coverage for mental health services, problems accessing culturally responsive mental health professionals, and overreliance on family, friends, or religious communities for support. Nevertheless, there is a dearth of research concerning depression among diverse black women. Women are twice as likely as men to suffer from depression; one of four women is likely to suffer from a serious depressive episode at some time in her life (Peden et al., 2000). According to the U.S. Department of Health and Human Services, Office on Women's Health (2007), black women tend to have lower rates of major depression than white women, and higher rates of phobias. Research and clinical programs have not consistently nor systematically examined the epidemiology of depression in a comprehensive context that evaluates the interaction that may exist between psychological, interpersonal, and sociocultural variables specific to the experiences of diverse (low-, middle-, and upper-income) black women—variables that can influence their mental health, emotional conditions, and overall well-being.

The reported incidence of mental illnesses among black women is unclear. This may be due to a variety of reasons, including controversy regarding misdiagnosis; the lack of clinical research within this population; limited knowledge of the epidemiology of mental illnesses relative to black women; published statistics that combine the incidence of depression for both sexes within the black population; and the general underrepresentation of reporting mental illnesses due to the low number of blacks who seek formal treatment for mental health problems. Depression often coexists with eating disorders (Bulk, 2005), anxiety disorders (Devanem, Chiao, Franklin, & Kruep, 2005), and substance abuse or dependency (Kessler et al., 2003). Depression also often coexists with other serious medical illnesses, such as heart disease, stroke, cancer, HIV/AIDS, diabetes, Parkinson's disease, thyroid problems, and multiple sclerosis, and may even make symptoms of the illness worse (Cassano & Fava, 2002). Research has shown that treating depression along with the coexisting illness helps to ease both conditions (Katon & Ciechanowski, 2002).

VULNERABLE POPULATIONS

Older Women

Triple jeopardy has been used to describe low-income black women at retirement age. These women are especially vulnerable to a larger set of health disparities. Apart from the fact that advanced age carries a unique set of health challenges for all racial/gender groups, black women continue to be most vulnerable. For example, older black women (ages 65 and older) have been found to underestimate their risk of getting breast cancer and tend to be the least likely to have had a recent mammogram or breast exam in comparison to their younger counterparts (Jones et al., 2003). Moreover, older black women tend not to receive preferred breast cancer treatment (Mandelblatt et al., 2002).

A recent investigation using data from the Health and Retirement Study underscores the role of gender relative to the dispensation of retirement. Hogan and Perrucci

(2007) show that both black and white women, in comparison to their male counterparts, are less likely to retire (after controlling for employment, age, insurance, assets, and spousal employment or retirement status). They further show that after controlling for gender differences in employment earnings and in retirement decisions, white women actually receive more total income (including Social Security, pension, and asset) than white men. While black men showed no significant net effect compared to white men, black women were found to receive the least, a finding consistent with how they have fared on other measures. While persons generally tend to covet the retirement years and look forward to a period of rest beyond protracted work in relative financial security, black women continue to struggle with burdens that block their chances of attaining a heightened quality of life, even during their "golden years."

Included among the major factors leading to more deleterious health outcomes for older black women is the experience of widowhood. In an investigation of mental and physical health decline among older adults, Kelley-Moore and Ferraro (2005) discuss various domains of health over time and their multidimensional and complex relationships; they conclude that widowhood accelerates health decline for older black adults but not for whites. Given that more women are widowed than men, black women are once again disadvantaged with respect to health outcomes. Research pointing to the disproportion in the number of other conditions affecting older women also includes a condition that has not been given adequate attention: chronic pain.

While chronic pain does not single out any one group, it does disproportionately affect older adults and places a particular burden on persons who do not have resources to alleviate the condition. The socioeconomic status of older black women can position this group as especially vulnerable. Baker, Buchanan, and Corson (2008) discuss the importance of understanding disease processes as well as physical and mental health outcomes of older black women who experience chronic pain; they underscore the value of research that focuses on within-group factors impacting a single population. Just as a complex set of factors has been shown to account for many of the health conditions facing black women, chronic pain should be conceptualized along these lines. Chronic pain can lead to or worsen depression, another condition that plagues this group. The research of Black, White, and Hannum (2007) aptly captures depression in a group of older black women as a cultural phenomenon within a framework of meaning constructed by black women from cultural systems rooted in North American society and black tradition. In this context, and consistent with a cross-section of the more generalizable literature, depression was found to be linked with diminishment of personal strength, related to sadness and suffering, and was believed to be preventable or resolvable through personal responsibility.

Homeless Women

A growing number of black women contribute to the population of Americans who lack living quarters. These women often have children, which places them at an even greater need. Shelters and other resources serving this population have not been able to keep pace with the need. While the data on homelessness for black women are unclear, it would appear that structural circumstances, including an inadequate public welfare system, are related more to homelessness in this group than in other groups.

Imprisoned Women

The multiple health issues of incarcerated women, including addictive behaviors and sexual and reproductive health as well as serious and chronic mental and physical conditions, cannot be omitted from any discussion of prison life. For black women, who constitute a disproportionate number of women behind bars, this situation is exacerbated by perceptions of unequal treatment by prison staff. In light of the dramatic rate of increase of women inmates over the past decade compared to men, and in view of the special needs of women (such as reproductive health), there is a dire need for the health care system to assess current policy in rendering services.

The disproportion of incarcerated black women is reflected in statistics that show black women to be seven times more likely to be incarcerated in their lifetime than white women and two times more likely than Hispanic women (Braithwaite, Arriola, & Newkirk, 2006). The health of this population differs significantly from women in the general population and is a price paid not only by the inmates themselves but also by the inmates' children, who are often left with a plethora of complexities with which to deal.

SUMMARY

While the overall health of Americans is improving and life expectancy is increasing, blacks face significant health challenges and disparities relative to other ethnic groups; limited access to health care places an immense burden on the social and economic realities that are central to existence and the ability to thrive. The overwhelming incidence among blacks of preventable chronic diseases, such as diabetes, stroke, heart disease, and cancer, not only contributes to high morbidity and mortality rates but also threatens the health and survival of families. In nearly all measures and indicators of health, blacks lag behind their white counterparts.

Women of color, and black women in particular, are faced with many challenges throughout their lives—during adolescence, adulthood, and senior years. Individual, familial, and community responsibilities and other stressors heighten this population's risk and vulnerability for health problems. Physiological, psychological, sociocultural, interpersonal, and spiritual discord also contribute to black women's challenges. There is a need to carefully scrutinize health issues from a holistic and contextual perspective; the goal should be to significantly improve awareness and understanding of the complexities behind optimal health for black women and building stronger and healthier black families.

A number of promising strategies have been launched throughout the literature on enhancing outcomes for black women's health. Needed, however, are approaches that systematically and methodically detail paths to enhanced health. If we assume that such approaches promote an increased understanding of disparities between black and white women, then perhaps we will be on the right path to actually closing the gap. This is appropriately argued by Hogue (2002) in a call for the ultimate elimination of black women's health disparities. The Centers for Disease Control and Prevention's Healthy People 2010 initiative is designed to achieve two overarching goals: (1) increase quality and years of healthy life, and (2) eliminate health disparities. In order to achieve these targets, addressing the multifaceted issues that relate to black women's health from research, clinical, programmatic, and policy perspectives must be prioritized, and intensified, on national and international levels.

REFERENCES

Agency for Healthcare Research and Quality (AHRQ). (2008, November). *Women with diabetes: Quality of health care, 2004–2005* (AHRQ Publication No. 08–0099). Rockville, MD: Author.

Baker, T., Buchanan, N., & Corson, N. (2008, June). Factors influencing chronic pain intensity in older black women: Examining depression, locus of control, and physical health. *Journal of Women's Health, 17*(5), 869–878.

Baquet, C., Mishra, S., Commiskey, P., Ellison, G., & DeShields, M. (2008, September). Breast cancer epidemiology in blacks and whites: Disparities in incidence, mortality, survival rates and histology. *Journal of the National Medical Association, 100*(5), 480–488.

Black, H., White, T., & Hannum, S. (2007). The lived experience of depression in elderly African American women. *Journals of Gerontology Series B: Psychological Sciences and Social Sciences, 62*, S392–S398.

Braithwaite, R., Arriola, K., & Newkirk, C. (2006). Health issues among incarcerated women. New Brunswick, NJ: Rutgers University Press.

Braxton, N. D., Lang, D. L., Sales, M. J., Wingood, G. M., & DiClemente, R. J. (2007). The role of spirituality in sustaining the psychological well-being of HIV-positive black women. *Women and Health, 46*(2–3), 113–129.

Bulk, C. (2005). Anxiety, depression, and eating disorders. In C. Fairburn and K. Brownell (Eds.), *Eating disorders and obesity* (pp. 193–198). New York: Guilford Press.

Canto, J. G., Allison, J. J., Kiefe, C. I., Fincher, C., Farmer, R., Sekar, P., et al. (2000). Relation of race and sex to the use of reperfusion therapy in medicare beneficiaries with acute myocardial infarction. *New England Journal of Medicine, 342*(15), 1094–1100.

Cassano, P., & Fava, M. (2002). Depression and public health, an overview. *Journal of Psychosomatic Research, 53*(4), 849–857.

Centers for Disease Control and Prevention (CDC). (2005). Cancer awareness: Promising intervention strategies. Retrieved February 2009 from http://www.cdc.gov/omhd/highlights/2005/HJan05.htm

Centers for Disease Control and Prevention (CDC). (2006). Cases of HIV infection and AIDS in the U.S. by race/ethnicity, 2000–2004. *HIV/AIDS Surveillance Supplemental Report, 12*(1), 1–36.

Centers for Disease Control and Prevention (CDC). (2007a). *HIV/AIDS Surveillance Report, 2005, 17*(1), 1–46.

Centers for Disease Control and Prevention (CDC). (2007b). *Leading causes of death in females—United States, 2004.* Retrieved February 2009 from http://www.cdc.gov/women/lcod.htm

Children's Defense Fund. (2004). Black child health fact sheet. Retrieved February 2009 from http://cdf.convio.net/site/PageServer?pagename=policy_ch_blackfactsheet

Coggin, C., & Shaw-Perry, M. (2006, December). Breast cancer survivorship: Expressed needs of black women. *Journal of Psychosocial Oncology, 24*(4), 107–122.

Cozier, Y., Palmer, J., Wise, L., Rosenberg, L., Horton, N., & Fredman, L. (2007, April). Relation between neighborhood median housing value and hypertension risk among black women in the United States. *American Journal of Public Health, 97*(4), 718–724.

Devanem, C. L., Chiao, E., Franklin, M., & Kruep, E. J. (2005, October). Anxiety disorders in the 21st century: Status, challenges, opportunities, and comorbidity with depression. *American Journal of Managed Care, 11*(Suppl. 12), S344–S353.

Evans, P., & Brunsell, S. (2007, May). Uterine fibroid tumors: Diagnosis and treatment. *American Family Physician, 75*(10), 1503–1508.

Hendrix, K. H., Mayhan, S., Lackland, D. T., & Egan, B. M. (2005). Prevalence, treatment, and control of chest pain syndromes and associated risk factors in hypertensive patients. *American Journal of Hypertension, 18*(8), 1026–1032.

Hogan, R., & Perrucci, C. (2007, September). Black women: Truly disadvantaged in the transition from employment to retirement income. *Social Science Research, 36*(3), 1184–1199.

Hogue, C. J. (2002). Toward a systematic approach to understanding and ultimately eliminating African American women's health disparities. *Women's Health Issues, 12*(5), 222–237.

Jones, A. R., Thompson, C. J., Oster, R. A., Samadi, A., Davis, M. K., Mayberry, R. M., et al. (2003). Breast cancer knowledge, beliefs, and screening behaviors among low-income, elderly black women. *Journal of the National Medical Association, 95*(9), 791–805.

Katon, W., & Ciechanowski, P. (2002). Impact of major depression on chronic medical illness. *Journal of Psychosomatic Research, 53*(4), 859–863.

Kelley-Moore, J., & Ferraro, K. (2005, December). A 3-D model of health decline: Disease, disability, and depression among black and white older adults. *Journal of Health and Social Behavior, 46*(4), 376–391.

Kessler, R. C., Barker, P. R., Colpe, L. J., Epstein, J. F., Gfroerer, J. C., Hiripi, E., et al. (2003, February). Screening for serious mental illness in the general population. *Archives of General Psychiatry, 60*(2), 184–189.

Kleindorfer, D., Miller, R., Sailor-Smith, S., Moomaw, C. J., Houry, J., & Frankel, M. (2008). The challenges of community-based research: The beauty shop stroke education project. *Stroke: A Journal of Cerebral Circulation, 39*(8), 2331–2335.

Krishnan, S., Rosenberg, L., Kjousse, L., Cupples, L. A., & Palmer, J. R. (2007). Overall and central obesity and risk of type 2 diabetes in U.S. black women. *Obesity, 15*(7), 1860–1866.

Kumanyika, S. K., Whitt-Glover, M. C., Gary, T. L., Prewitt, T. E., Odoms-Young, A. M., Banks-Wallace, et al. (2007, October). Expanding the obesity research paradigm to reach African American communities. *Preventing Chronic Disease, 4*(4), A112.

Levin, A. (2008). Depression care for black women may hinge upon cultural factors. *Psychiatry News, 43*(15), 11.

Lupus Foundation of America. (2009). *Fact sheet.* Retrieved February from 2009 http://www.lupus.org/newsite/index.html

Lutfiyya, M. N., Cumba, M. T., McCullough, J. E., Barlow, E. L., & Lipsky, M. S. (2008). Disparities in adult African American women's knowledge of heart attack and stroke symptomatology: An analysis of 2003–2005 Behavioral Risk Factor Surveillance Survey data. *Journal of Women's Health, 17*(5), 805–813.

Mandelblatt, J. S., Kerner, J. F., Hadley, J., Hwang, Y. T., Eggert, L., Johnson, L. E., et al. (2002). *Cancer, 95,* 1401–1414.

Matthews, T. J., & MacDorman, M. F. (2007). Infant mortality statistics from the 2004 Period Linked Birth/Infant Death data set. *National Vital Statistics Reports, 55*(14), 1–32.

Peden, A. R., Hall, L. A., Rayens, M. K., & Bebee, L. A. (2000). Negative thinking mediates the effect of self-esteem on depressive symptoms in college women. *Nursing Research, 49,* 201–207.

Ramos, B. M., Carlson, B. E., & McNutt, L. (2004). Lifetime abuse, mental health, and African American women. *Journal of Family Violence, 19*(3), 153–164.

Read, J., & Gorman, B. (2006, March). Gender inequalities in U.S. adult health: The interplay of race and ethnicity. *Social Science & Medicine, 62*(5), 1045–1065.

Samuel-Hodge, C., Headen, S., Skelly, A., Ingram, T., Keyserling, E., Jackson, E. J., et al. (2000). Influences on day-to-day self-management of type 2 diabetes among African-American women: Spirituality, the multi-caregiver role, and other social context factors. *Diabetes Care, 23*(7), 928–933.

Stolley, M. R., Sharp, O. K., Oh, A., & Schiffer, L. (2009). A weight loss intervention for African American breast cancer survivors, 2006. *Preventing Chronic Disease, 6*(1), 8–26.

Taylor, S. E. (2001). The health status of black women. In Ronald L. Braithwaite & Sandra E. Taylor (Eds.), *Health Issues in the Black Community* (2nd ed.) (pp. 44–61). San Francisco: Jossey-Bass.

Taylor, T. R., Williams, C. D., Makambi, K. H., Mouton, C., Harrell, J. P., Cozier, Y., et al. (2007). Racial discrimination and breast cancer incidence in U.S. black women: The black women's health study. *American Journal of Epidemiology, 166*(1), 46–54.

Umberson, D., Anderson, K., Glick, J., & Shapiro, A. (1998). Domestic violence, personal control, and gender. *Journal of Marriage and the Family, 60*(2), 442–452.

U.S. Department of Health and Human Services, Office on Women's Health. (2007). *Minority women's mental health fact sheet.* Retrieved February 2009 from http://www.womenshealth.gov/minority/africanamerican/mh.cfm

Waltermaurer, E., Watson, C., & McNutt, L. (2006, December). Black women's health: The effect of perceived racism and intimate partner violence. *Violence Against Women, 12*(12), 1214–1222.

Williams, D. R. (2002). Racial/ethnic variations in women's health: The social embeddedness of health. *American Journal of Public Health, 92*(4), 588–597.

Williams, D. R., Gonzalez, H. M., Neighbors, H., Nesse, R., Abelson, J. M., Sweetman, J., & Jackson, J. S. (2007). Prevalence and distribution of major depressive disorder in African Americans, Caribbean Blacks, and non-Hispanic whites. *Archives of General Psychiatry, 64*(3), 305–315.

Young, D. R., He, X., Genkinger, J., Sapun, M., Mabry, I., & Megan, J. (2004). Health status among urban African American women: Associations among well-being, perceived stress, and demographic factors. *Journal of Behavioral Medicine, 27*(1), 63–76.

CHAPTER

5

THE HEALTH STATUS OF BLACK MEN

JEAN J. E. BONHOMME
APRIL M. W. YOUNG

In the United States, African American men are clearly in the midst of a health crisis. The health status of African American men is compromised by broad social policy phenomena such as exceptional rates of incarceration, lack of access to primary and preventive health care, adverse neighborhood conditions, unfavorable socioeconomic experiences, and maladaptive behavioral and attitudinal factors. In addition, multiple studies have established that the experience of race has very real and measurable health implications that doubtlessly contribute to elevated morbidity and mortality among black men.

AFRICAN AMERICAN MEN'S HEALTH STATUS

In the 1980s, the average life expectancy for African American males was under sixty-five years, too low to collect Social Security or Medicare. While overall mortality and morbidity rates have since improved in the United States, black men are still more likely to die of common diseases such as cardiovascular disease, diabetes, and major cancers than their white counterparts. In 2004, life expectancy for African American men was 69.5 years, substantially lower than the 75.7-year life span a white man in the United States can anticipate (National Center for Health Statistics, 2009). In particular geographic regions, African American men's lives remain significantly shorter than the national average. For instance, the Fulton County Department of Health and Wellness stated that in 2007 the average life expectancy of an African American male in Fulton County (which comprises most of the city of Atlanta, Georgia) remained only about sixty-four years.

Why Men's Health Matters

The health status of African American males has received surprisingly little attention given that in many respects it is the poorest of any large population group in the United States. African American men's health status is often dismissed inappropriately as irrelevant to the well-being of other demographic groups in America. Many people seem concerned that addressing the health of men might take away from efforts to address the health challenges facing women and children. Seeing the health of the genders like opposite ends of a seesaw, they appear to believe that for one to rise, the other must fall. However, the genders are so highly interrelated and interact on so many levels that the overall health of any community or ethnic group depends upon a positive balance between the genders. The health challenges of African American men affect African American women in so many ways that achieving optimal overall health in African American communities is not a matter of either one gender or the other; it is both or neither. Overall, the complex nature of the African American men's health crisis calls for a multi-dimensional approach in which broadened, inclusive notions of health are embraced by health practitioners, policy analysts, community redevelopment advocates, neighborhood-based service providers, and men themselves.

Gender Disparities in Morbidity and Mortality

Men's health and longevity outcomes are noticeably poorer than women's. According to the Centers for Disease Control and Prevention (CDC), the all-causes male-to-female mortality ratio is 1.6 to 1 (Bonhomme, 2007). All ten leading causes of death, as defined by the CDC, affect men more than women. Death rates are conspicuously higher in men for heart disease (1.8 to 1), accidents and adverse events (2.4 to 1), and chronic liver disease and cirrhosis (2.3 to 1). The single greatest ratio disparity is suicide (4.3 to 1). The all-causes mortality ratio for African Americans to whites is 1.5 to 1. Furthermore, eight of the ten leading causes of death afflict African Americans more than whites. Notable racial disparities include heart disease (1.5 to 1), stroke (1.8 to 1), diabetes (2.4 to 1), and kidney disease (2.5 to 1). Two major causes of death that affect African Americans less than whites are chronic obstructive pulmonary disease (0.8 to 1) and suicide (0.5 to 1). Though suicide is less common overall among blacks, the rate among African American males is much more polarized toward youth than it is for other demographic groups. Overall, homicide ranks thirteenth among causes of death in the United States. Yet, for African American males, homicide ranks fifth and is the second leading cause of death between the ages of fifteen and twenty-four years.

In 1920 there was only one year's difference between the genders in average life expectancy in the United States (Bonhomme, 2007). Today, the average difference overall is between five and six years, and about seven or eight years for African Americans. This raises the question of whether we are viewing inherent life expectancy differences between the races and genders or instead different rates of increase in life expectancy over the course of the twentieth century. This in turn raises another question: how did the interventions that led to the overall increase in population life expectancy differ between the genders?

Effects of Poor Health Among Males on Their Community

The impaired health status of African American men has demonstrable negative effects on the health of African American women and children. Following widowhood, a woman typically suffers considerable bereavement, often involving the loss of a long-term companion. The surviving spouse faces an increased risk of dying over the months that follow, and older women typically face limited prospects for remarriage. In the event of preventable disability or chronic illness, a considerable burden of care usually falls to the woman. In disability or chronic illness limiting the ability to work, a family may face increased health care expenses in the face of diminished earnings.

There are demonstrable economic effects on the African American community and the whole of society owing to preventable illness and death among African American men. These include lost time from work, reduced work productivity, and disability. Men who were formerly actively providing for their families may become financially dependent on them instead. Men who were formerly taxpayers may be reduced to financial dependency on other taxpayers. Chronic illnesses short of outright disability may interfere with the ability to maintain gainful employment; for example, excessive absence or lateness due to episodic pain. Poverty is strongly associated with widowhood, and the financial repercussions of unnecessary and preventable morbidity and mortality among African American males are faced by children as well. Just as one cannot effectively weed half a garden, if we fail to contend with the health challenges facing both genders, we cannot do a thorough job of addressing the health needs of either gender. Though it is frequently overlooked, African American men's health must be considered a vital aspect of the health of the African American community as a whole.

Financial hardship among women resulting from widowhood may exceed that caused by divorce. Termination of marriage is correlated with higher poverty rates as shown by both cross-sectional and longitudinal data (Morgan, 1989). Forty percent of widows, as opposed to just over 25 percent of divorced women, fall into poverty for at least some time during the first five years after the end of marriage (Morgan, 1989). Over half of the elderly widows currently living in poverty were not poor before the deaths of their husbands (U.S. Administration on Aging, 2001). Fiscal implications for society include health care and other social programs, such as housing assistance (U.S. Administration on Aging, 2001). Women's all-causes death rates increase in widowhood. A twofold increase in mortality has been observed in the first month after widowhood (Jones, 1987).

Healthy Fatherhood and the Health of Children

The health status of fathers has long been dismissed as irrelevant to the well-being of children. Maternal and child health is the accepted catchphrase, as opposed to the more inclusive concept *parental* and child health. However, paternal health likely impacts the type and frequency of birth defects in offspring. Advanced paternal age has been associated statistically with greater rates of preauricular cyst, nasal aplasia, cleft palate, hydrocephalus, pulmonic stenosis, urethral stenosis, and hemangioma among offspring (Savitz, Schwingl, & Keels, 1991). Smoking among fathers is similarly associated with cleft lip (with or without cleft palate), hydrocephalus, ventricular septal defect, and urethral stenosis among offspring (Savitz et al., 1991). Paternal alcohol use is associated with increased risk of ventricular septal defect among offspring (Savitz et al., 1991). Women have usually been well informed that advanced age is associated with specific risks of health problems among their offspring. However, more recent research has demonstrated a statistically significant monotonic association between advancing paternal age and risk of adult schizophrenia and schizophrenia spectrum disorders among offspring. This analysis controlled for maternal age and other potential confounders (Brown et al., 2002). Paternal exposures clearly may impact the health of children adversely. Offspring of military fathers who served in Vietnam and Cambodia were found to be at increased risk of childhood leukemia (Wen et al., 2000). Data from three case-control studies conducted by the Children's Cancer Group were analyzed. Cases of acute myelogenous leukemia (AML) and acute lymphocytic leukemia (ALL) were compared with 1:1 matched controls. Statistically significant associations with AML were demonstrated, which were especially strong among children under two years of age (Wen et al., 2000).

Sexually Transmitted Infections and HIV

Direct implications of men's health problems are clearly evident in areas of reproductive and sexual health. A significant proportion of human immunodeficiency virus (HIV) cases among African American women is linked to heterosexual transmission. The CDC estimates that 1 in 50 African American men in the United States is HIV-positive, placing African American women at considerable risk. As a result, 1 out of 160 African American women is believed to be HIV-positive. Other sexually transmitted infections may lead to serious obstetrical and gynecological complications for women. Human papilloma virus (HPV) infection is the principal cause of cervical cancer. Herpes simplex virus (HSV) infection may lead to major obstetrical hazards. *Chlamydia* may cause pelvic inflammatory disease and possible infertility among women. These and other sexually transmitted infections cannot be prevented from adversely affecting women and children if they are not controlled effectively among men.

Depression and Men's Mental Health

Twice as many women as men in the United States are diagnosed with major depression, but the suicide rate among men is four times greater than for women (Kilmartin, 2005). Among African Americans, suicide appears to be less frequent overall but with a major caveat. In most demographic groups, the typical suicide victim is a middle-aged or elderly male. Among African Americans, however, suicide is centered among youth. It is likely that depression in men is greatly underrecognized (Kilmartin, 2005). Substance abuse is a well-known association of mood disorders, and men are believed to abuse alcohol and drugs at least twice as often as women. Depression in male subjects may be missed because interviewers are not attuned to male-specific styles of expression. Typical male socialization stresses avoidance of introspection and denial of awareness of helpless feelings. For this reason, many men may not recognize that they may have a mental health problem requiring intervention. A man reporting difficulty concentrating, diminished motivation, distractibility, and sleep disturbance might not even be subjectively aware of underlying feelings of sadness. Culturally, socialization in men demands banning thoughts about emotional problems from consciousness and expects stoicism and dissociation from emotions. A phenomenon known as the "male emotional funnel" may convert many men's vulnerable feelings (such as fear and powerlessness) into anger, and men may act out in response to these feelings. This acting out may take the form of chronic anger, self-destructive behavior, alcohol and drug use, gambling, womanizing, and overworking, all of which may actually be behavioral expressions of underlying depression (Kilmartin, 2005) .

Disparities in Health Care Access

Men participate in preventive health care notably less often than women. Even excluding pregnancy-related visits, the rate of doctor visits for such reasons as annual examinations and preventive services was twice as high for women than for men (Brett & Burt, 2001). Thirty-three percent of men (compared with only 19 percent of women) do not have a regular physician (Sandman, Simantov, & An, 2000). Twenty-four percent of men (compared with only 8 percent of women) have not seen a physician in the past year (Sandman et al., 2000). These gender disparities become increasingly pronounced as age groups become progressively younger (Sandman et al., 2000). African-American and Latino men in the United States, in all income brackets (poor, near-poor, middle, and high income), are only half as likely to have had physician contacts in the past year (U.S. Department of Health and Human Services, 1998) and are appreciably less likely to carry health insurance compared with their respective African American female and Latina counterparts (Kass, Weinick, & Monheit, 1999).

IMPACT OF SOCIAL POLICIES ON BLACK MEN'S HEALTH

The Increasing Significance of Incarceration

U.S. Department of Justice figures for 2006 indicate that one in nine African American men is incarcerated. African American men are jailed at a rate that far exceeds their representation in the population (Justice Policy Institute, 2007). A study of men in one distressed urban neighborhood found that a vast majority of adult men—two in three—reported having been incarcerated (Young, 2006). With figures as startling as these, it is important to consider the impact of imprisonment on the health and well-being of African American men. In correctional settings, men's well-being is jeopardized by exposure to a range of physiological and psychological risks that increase the likelihood of poor health outcomes. Those detained in correctional facilities are frequently subject to communicable infections, injury by violence, sexual trauma, and to under-regulated clinical trials (Young, Meryn, & Treadwell, 2008). Facilities' adherence to correctional health care standards is a matter of ongoing uncertainty and controversy (Gallagher & Dobrin, 2007). Additionally, psychological torment is a pervasive health risk inmates face. They may be subjected to extreme custodial interventions such as "close management" (solitary confinement); injurious chemical, electrical, and manual control techniques; strip searches and invasive body cavity searches; and documented physical torture in some instances. The capacity and opportunity for ex-offenders to address the health implications of prison are hindered by marginal access to primary care and counseling. Chronic conditions that develop while incarcerated, disabilities due to injury sustained in detention, substance dependency, and the psychological effects of confinement pose ongoing health challenges for many men following release. At the same time, their ability to work is severely limited in many states (Collins Center for Public Policy, 2006; New York City Bar . . . , 2008), separating them from the resources they need to improve or manage their health conditions (Western, 2002; Pettit & Western, 2004). Evidence supports that the jeopardy resulting from the experience of incarceration is indeed lasting, extending well beyond the period of confinement. Regarding the immediate postrelease term, a Washington State study found that newly released prisoners were 12.7 times more likely to die in the two weeks following release compared to other state residents in the same demographic groups (Binswanger et al., 2007). Other findings confirm contentions that incarceration has an independent negative effect on health status (Massoglia, 2005; Freudenberg, Moseley, Labriola, Daniels, & Murrill, 2007).

Lack of a National Provision for Access to Health Care for Men

As others have discussed compellingly in this volume, access to health care or the lack thereof figures prominently in the health profiles of demographic groups in the United States. However, that African American men fall into a category of persons—men—for whom there is no national program providing access to primary and preventive health care (Treadwell & Ro, 2003) warrants mention as a factor in the health crisis among African American men. The extent to which lack of access to health care compromises the well-being of African American men is difficult to quantify precisely. Somewhat paradoxically, the lack of access to health care can lead to reduced surveillance capability resulting in a disturbing underdiagnosis of chronic and dangerous conditions. The dearth of data means there are gaps in the health profile for African American men, precluding a full and accurate description of their predicament. For instance, among men in a poor Miami, Florida, neighborhood living largely without routine health care, reported rates of several disorders were significantly lower than national rates for African Americans (Young, 2006). It is reasonable to assume that the sample population, composed 95 percent of African American men, is in no better health than blacks generally in the United States. Given characteristics such as low income, low educational attainment, and low rates of employment—all risk factors for poor health—it is likely that the men from the distressed neighborhood suffer undetected conditions (Young et al., 2007).

War Exposures and the Relevance of Veteran Status

The toll taken by war on African American men's health is an oft-neglected issue. African American males have been overrepresented relative to their numbers in the population in several recent wars. Veterans must first be identified within patient populations in order to receive appropriate assistance (Bonhomme, 2006); however, men who are of age to have been involved in specific wars are rarely asked by medical practitioners if they served in the military or were involved in combat. Outside veterans' health care systems, medical histories usually do not include questions regarding military service or combat experience, although these factors may impact physical and psychological health significantly. For this reason, the medical and psychological issues facing veterans may go completely unrecognized and untreated. Veterans may appear hard to reach, as many perceive themselves as having been let down by government programs supposedly instituted to help them. In dealing with combat veterans, trust can be a major issue. Often, war veterans have lost close friends suddenly and traumatically, and they may fear that in getting close to people again they risk further pain and loss. Some African American veterans have had experiences of discrimination based not only on race but also on their status as veterans; so, not being open about their military history may have worked to their advantage. War veterans often need to discuss their experiences openly in order to overcome psychological trauma, but such experiences may be extremely painful to think about, let alone discuss (Bonhomme, 2006).

NEIGHBORHOOD CONDITIONS AND HEALTH

Exposures in Resource-Strained Settings

Frequently, the communities in which African American men reside are characterized by limited civic, economic, and social resources (Menchik, 1993). Though the majority of African American men live in major metropolitan areas, the districts of the cities in which they are concentrated are more likely to be resource-poor (U.S. Census Bureau; http://www.census.gov/apsd/www/statbrief/sb95_5.pdf). Many indicators can qualify an urban setting as blighted or distressed: the income level of its residents, the condition of its housing stock, the types of available services and businesses, crime rates, and the state of its civic infrastructure. Recognizing that urban distress not only describes a condition of place but also names an experience in which residents abide day to day (Young, 2006), its health implications beg attention. Also, given the known obstacles to accessing health care among low-income groups and among men, we can expect that in distressed urban settings men will face particular jeopardy due to unmet health needs. Common features of poor urban settings are likely to register particularly strongly on African American men's mental health. Income shortfalls and unreliable employment along with tenuous lodging terms or substandard housing conditions can make utter financial ruin and homelessness imminent and constant threats in the lives of men and their families. Proximity to illicit activity—whether one is a participant or bystander—can mean heightened risk of violence and exposure to the criminal justice apparatus (U.S. Department of Housing and Urban Development, 2001).

While social networks in distressed settings are often of necessity strong and extensive, the nature of contemporary urban life, especially where poverty is present, can fracture central household structures, isolating men from their primary family units for long periods. In addition to facing their own difficulties, men may routinely witness the subjection and hopelessness of others around them. The results can be psychological and physiological stress; physical injury; self-medication with tobacco, alcohol, or illegal drugs; sexual risk taking; and various forms of abusive or self-endangering acting out. It is important that health practitioners and others in positions to be of assistance to African American men are aware of economic and social data on the areas in which their patients or clients live.

Life Expectancy and Lowered Expectations

African American men's lower life expectancy may have a sinister effect on the general consciousness and expectations in communities. The relative rarity of the elderly African American man as a presence in the social environment may lead people (including African American men themselves) to expect these men to live shorter lives than other demographic groups. In settings in which early death is common due to violence or illness, a sense of the imminence of demise may be magnified and quite explicit. In such contexts, one would anticipate that self-caretaking behaviors would be compromised. Indeed, risky behaviors and clearly self-destructive activity may occur more frequently. Much of the analysis of this issue is based on powerful anecdotal accounts from urban core neighborhoods (Stewart, Schreck, & Simmons, 2006).

The literature on civilian lives and consciousness in theaters of war is probably relevant to invoke as well (Krippner & McIntyre, 2003). The answer to this complex predicament is multilayered. Reducing racial health disparities and disproportionate mortality among African American men; raising the visibility of mature, healthy African American men; addressing violent, crime-ridden communities; and cultivating a deeper love of self are steps to establishing longevity as both a value and a virtue that African American men can see as realistically within their reach.

THE REALITY OF RACE: STRESS AND HEALTH

Evidence

Since 2000, findings from more than one hundred studies documenting the damaging effects of racism on the body have supported recasting racism as a public health problem (Drexler, 2007). Most of the studies regard racism as a stressor whose impact is chronic and pervasive, elevating blood pressure (Brondolo et al., 2008), heart rate, and cortisol levels; suppressing immune system response; and inspiring health-averse behaviors like overeating and smoking. Though the studies center explicitly on physiological phenomena, mental health is critical to the discussion of racism's consequences. Psychological mechanisms and processes line the pathways by which experiences of discrimination inscribe their deleterious effects on the body. The stress, fear, depression, rage, and frustration that are the response to racism all have psychological dimensions that we understand to then manifest physiologically as the fight-or-flight hormonal cascade and elevated cardiovascular values. These data suggest the need to further examine responses to racial discrimination. Developing positive mental health strategies to cope with or counter the psychological and physiological assault of racism is crucial to addressing the health crisis among African American men.

Commonalities Across Social Class

The most affluent African Americans in the United States are sicker than the poorest whites (Drexler, 2007). This enduring fact was evidence for researchers in the period approaching the new millennium that racism had discrete influence on health outcomes, even across socioeconomic class lines. The work of social psychologist Claude Steele on the phenomenon he has named "stereotype threat" (Steele, 1999) has shown that social class does not insulate privileged African Americans from the physiological response to experiences of race. African American college students taking a challenging exam who believed their performance might comment negatively on their capabilities, thereby possibly confirming stereotypes of lesser competence, experienced elevated blood pressure and heart rate. When their race was not made salient, they not only scored better on the exam but also did not have the physiological anxiety response. Given the well-developed body of evidence confirming racism's ill effects on health, the contribution of discrimination to the African American men's health crisis should be a matter of priority in policy reform efforts and health advocacy.

DEFINING BARRIERS TO MEN'S PARTICIPATION IN HEALTH CARE

As we describe the various indicators that make up the dimensions of the health crisis among African American men, it is important to also consider men's consciousness and their capacity to exercise agency in matters of health. Obstacles men face to accessing needed care are not only structural. Behaviors and attitudes about health, health care institutions, and beliefs about the nature of masculinity can create barriers that contribute to poor health outcomes. Addressing these behavioral and attitudinal barriers will be key to improving the health and well-being of African American men.

Behavioral Barriers

African American men are less likely than white men, white women, or African American women to make use of health services. The reasons, like many behavioral dynamics, are complex and challenging to tease apart. For example, many men in the Overtown neighborhood of Miami, Florida, tend to use hospital emergency rooms for health concerns that likely would be more appropriately addressed in a primary care setting. Nearly two in three reported the emergency room as their sole health care facility (Young et al., 2007). Inadequate access to care is certainly a causal factor, though lack of familiarity with more appropriate alternatives, a preference for the treatment interventions likely to be pursued in an emergency setting, and habit also contribute to Overtown men's reliance on the emergency room. Findings that men tend not to seek medical care in response to pain or feeling ill are especially striking. Only 18 percent of males stated that they would seek help promptly if they were in pain or feeling ill. Surprisingly, 24 percent stated that they would delay seeking health care as long as possible, with 17 percent stating that they would wait for a week or more (Sandman et al., 2000). Men's demonstrably low rate of involvement in preventive health care is likely related to traditional male gender role socialization. Characteristics inherent in traditional male socialization which appear to be related to lower rates of utilization of therapeutic counseling services include achievement orientation, restricted emotional expression, instrumental nature, self-reliance, and poorer tolerance for same-sex affection (Campbell, 1996). Gender role training encourages males to develop stoic attitudes toward pain and fear. Attitudes and behaviors such as not running from danger, not resting when fatigued, and not "giving in" to pain are often culturally prized among males. As a result, many boys have been habituated from childhood to disregard and minimize the signals of their own bodies, including those signals that result from illness.

When a boy skins his knee at age 8, he typically gets told, "brave boys don't cry." If he gets hurt playing high school football, he may be told to "take one for the team." By the time he is fifty and having chest pain, he may say, "it's just indigestion." Many males have been socialized during childhood to expect that if pain is ignored, it will simply go away with time, a view that is often confirmed by the rapid resolution of childhood's minor ailments and injuries. However, in middle age, the rules of the game change, with mild symptoms possibly indicating early progressive disease that may quickly go from manageable to incurable. Many men believe that "a man takes care of his own problems," and through maladaptive self-reliance they may fail to seek outside help even when a problem is recognized. This excessive, pathological, unhealthy stoicism may well affect African American men out of proportion to the general male population owing to their tragic history of deep involvement in painful, arduous types of heavy labor. Male socialization may reduce adaptive responses to pain, injury, and fear, including seeking health care when ill, in turn leading to poorer health outcomes. Many men reported that they would not respond to pain by seeking health care (Sandman et al., 2000). Men's general inattention to their own pain and illness understandably perplexes women, but in some respects it is a logical extension of men's cultural gender role expectations. Fatalistic attitudes are yet another attitudinal barrier, as many African American men believe that "when it's your time to go, it's your time to go." Many individuals who have had unfavorable life experiences, such as persons of low socioeconomic status, tend to feel that nothing they can do will make any difference in their fate. A study found that subjects who considered heart disease, arthritis, or difficulty sleeping to be a normal part of aging ("fatalistic") were found in multivariate analyses to be less likely to have received preventive medical services in the previous year. Those who felt nothing could be done to improve those conditions ("nihilistic") were less likely to have a regular physician (Goodwin, Black, & Satish, 1999). Albert Bandura (1977) introduced the concept of self-efficacy, defining the barrier posed by individuals not believing that they can actually perform a health-promoting behavior such as diet change, smoking cessation, abstinence from drugs or alcohol, and so on.

Health Care System Structural Barriers

Barriers to men's participation in health care are interwoven in the structure of the health care system itself. For instance, work hours for men often eclipse the hours when health care is available, leading to scheduling conflicts in pursuing health care. Men are less likely than women to carry health insurance and are often less eligible for social programs that subsidize health care, creating substantial economic barriers. In contrast to the health care structure for women, there are no targeted health specialties for men comparable to obstetrics and gynecology and women's health. When a girl reaches the threshold of womanhood, the pediatrician typically hands off her care to the obstetrician-gynecologist, maintaining a beneficial continuity of care. Gender-targeted medical specialties may help habituate women into regular physician contact early in life. By contrast, the pediatrician has no corresponding specialist for males to hand the young male off to, and his contact with the health care system is often lost. The comparative lack of male-targeted specialties and health care programs may hamper men's ability to identify as participants in health care, seeing nothing in the health care system with a male face on it. Men's health problems are often fragmented across different specialties, rendering cohesive interventions unnecessarily difficult. When a man recognizes a problem, he may be confused as to where to take it.

SOCIOECONOMIC EXPERIENCES: EMPLOYMENT

Men's relationships to employment and the conditions under which they often must labor can play an important role in their health and psychological well-being (Doyal, 2001). Lack of job security, low wages, and dangerous working conditions often characterize the employment to which many African American men have access. Men are disproportionately represented in manual labor jobs, in which workplace conditions by their very nature may reinforce men's stoic acculturation. Lifting heavy loads or working in the burning heat or the freezing cold necessitates high tolerance for discomfort, forcing men to detach from their feelings just to get through the workday. In turn, these men may ignore pain and discomfort caused by illness as well. Over 90 percent of workplace fatalities occur among men, and African American men are disproportionately represented in manual labor jobs that are physically painful and hazardous. Traditionally, some dirty, dangerous jobs were actually referred to as "negro work" (Braithwaite, 2001).

Work undoubtedly has a great influence on mental health and a man's sense of well-being. Unfortunately, the influence can be negative quite frequently. A lack of esteem, authority, or control on the job can lead to anxiety or depression. Humiliating circumstances at work or demeaning hierarchies can erode a man's sense of self-worth, diminish his social esteem as a breadwinner and provider, and thwart his ambitions for himself and his family. Employment is also a critical determinant of health care access for men, more so perhaps than for other groups. Because there is no national provision for primary and preventive health care for men in the United States, one of the only sources of health coverage for men is employer-based private insurance plans. A small proportion of the jobs available to entry-level and lower-wage earners offer affordable health insurance plans to employees (Maxwell & Paringer, 2004). African American men tend to be concentrated at the lower end of the labor market spectrum, so their access to employer-provided health plans is more constrained.

DISCRIMINATION IN HEALTH PRACTICES

African American males frequently express considerable distrust of the health care system. Such distrust has been engendered and exacerbated by misguided medical experimentation and substandard treatment by the health care system. Many scholars trace current-day misgivings about medicine among African Americans to the infamous Tuskegee Syphilis Trials. (See, for instance, information in the U.S. National Archives and at http://www.archives.gov/southeast/exhibit/6.php.) However, contemporary examples suggest that it is unnecessary to go so far back in the history of medicine for instances of discriminatory practices. U.S. researchers found that Hispanic men were less likely to receive colorectal cancer screening, cardiovascular risk-factor screening, and vaccinations. African American men consistently received worse care for end-stage renal disease (Felix-Aaron et al., 2005). Examining a number of studies and findings, a researcher has recently concluded that controlling for prognostic factors, there are no racial differences in treatment response to traditional lung cancer chemotherapy, radiation therapy, and surgery. However, compared to whites, a remarkable proportion of African Americans with lung cancer do not receive potential curative treatments and optimal therapies (Brawley, 2006). Evidence of medical discrimination based on race and socioeconomic status has emerged in other nations as well. Swedish researchers found that socioeconomic disadvantage and the perception of discrimination relate independently to the likelihood of refraining from seeking medical services (Wamala, Merlo, Bostrom, & Hogstedt, 2007).

Regardless of its origin, distrust of the health care system often becomes a self-fulfilling prophecy by promoting delay in seeking health care. As a result, the individual becomes more likely to present in an advanced state of disease, with a higher likelihood of an unfavorable outcome. African American men can and should be enlisted in projects to make medical institutions and health practitioners more responsive to their needs. By participating in movements to develop cultural competence among health providers, making use of community-based health facilities for a range of community activities, and getting involved in health-related outreach efforts, African American men can help to break down barriers between themselves and medical institutions.

KNOWLEDGE AND AWARENESS OF HEALTH CHALLENGES

Informational barriers have been a substantial impediment to better health outcomes for African American men. There is a pervasive lack of awareness concerning men's health challenges. For instance, many people say *"prostrate"* cancer, even though prostate cancer is the most diagnosed cancer among African American men and men's second leading cancer killer. In a convenience street sampling, about 50 percent of men could not say what the prostate gland does or where it is located. Considerable public ignorance on the health challenges facing African American men exists, and this lack of awareness crosses the gender divide. Interestingly, we have encountered women who actually come to prostate cancer screenings asking for prostate exams.

EDUCATIONAL ATTAINMENT

Much evidence substantiates that health outcomes tend to improve as education levels rise in populations. Among African American men, educational attainment lags behind that of many other demographic groups (educational attainment available at http://www.census.gov/prod/2003pubs/c2kbr-24.pdf). The gap likely accounts in part for the health disparities that disfavor African American males. Educational settings, as well as the home, are locations in which we form central notions of health and amass much of the baseline health information that will guide conscious decisions about our health. The fact that African American males separate sooner from educational institutions than other groups (Sum, Khatiwada, McLaughlin, & Tobar, 2007) argues for enhancing the health components of school curricula in the earlier grade levels to reach boys. It also makes the case for designing creative outreach programs that can deliver critical health information about men's health in a variety of settings in communities.

INCOME

Like education, income is positively correlated with better health outcomes (College Board, 2005; Menchik, 1993). The fact that African American men abide at the lower end of the income continuum in the United States may also account in part for their poorer health relative to other demographic groups. Lack of financial resources has pervasive and ominous practical effects in men's lives. Economic want can preclude access to health care specifically, and can also hinder health-promoting behaviors on a daily basis. With limited resources, the capacity to make beneficial food choices, to maintain a safe and secure living environment, and to undertake restorative leisure activities is diminished. The impact of such day-to-day constraints may compromise well-being and contribute significantly to poor health outcomes among African American men.

RECOMMENDATIONS AND POTENTIAL SOLUTIONS

It is important to cultivate prevention and health-promoting behaviors among African American men. Approaches to community planning and redevelopment that encourage active living and that make available fresh, nutritious food are critical to improving African American men's health. Recreational opportunities should be available across the life span from youth through the senior years. Organized occasions for men to socialize safely and soberly, particularly in the senior years, can reduce isolation and diminish detrimental, health-compromising behaviors like drinking and smoking.

In addition, African American men should be encouraged to make use of primary care where possible. Regular thorough physical examinations, age-appropriate screenings, and diligent monitoring of health indicators are critical. Men should also pay close attention to oral health (Meurman, Sanz, & Janket, 2004). They should be familiar with mental health services and should confidently avail themselves of them when necessary. Where primary care, dental services, and mental health support are not currently accessible to African American men, vigorous advocacy is warranted to achieve availability. To accomplish these ideals is a complicated undertaking requiring comprehensive planning and programming, and innovative collaborative efforts across a range of organizations. Given the magnitude of the challenge, the African American men's health crisis calls for ambitious and visionary approaches.

HEALTH AS A CIVIL RIGHTS ISSUE

To speak of health as a civil right is transformative. In the contemporary U.S. context in which health is arguably a commodity, access to which is determined by socioeconomic standing and purchasing power, the notion of reimagining and re-presenting health as an entitlement to which all Americans should be able to lay equal claim is eminently political. The re-presentation of health as a civil right has been a compelling development in health advocacy and policy reform efforts.

The same approach may hold great promise as a grassroots strategy to involve African American men in seeking better health outcomes for themselves. Routine physical examinations, age-appropriate yet uncomfortable screenings, and health-promoting behavior modification may be a "tough sell" to African American men who live pressured lives and manage many competing priorities. However, if African American men are able to envision themselves as engaged in a struggle of broader relevance with wider implications—a struggle for the right to live longer and live healthier—health may then assume the position of a moral imperative in their lives. An understanding of how their health prospects are determined in large measure by their racial group affiliation can make poor health outcomes a black man's issue, so to speak. Representing health as a civil rights issue has resonance with powerful social movements of the 1960s and taps a collective memory of the mythic leaders with whom many African American men readily identify.

Using the approach at a grassroots level, health policy advocates organized men in the distressed neighborhood of Overtown in Miami, Florida. The men responded well to a quote by sixteenth U.S. Surgeon General David Satcher: "Health is a civil rights issue. We need a movement if we are to eliminate disparities." The men incorporated these words into their mission, accompanied by a photograph of Dr. Satcher, a distinguished fellow African American with whom they identified. They formed the Overtown Grassroots Men's Health Team to advocate for access to health care for poor and working poor men.

Approaching health as a civil right has not been systematically tested as a strategy to enlist African American men in the project to achieve better health outcomes for themselves. However, because of its promise, it warrants consideration by those in positions to influence thinking by and about African American men concerning their health and well-being.

THE GLOBAL CAUSE

To advance men's health as a global priority entails proliferation of male-focused approaches in clinical care, expansion of research on men's health and well-being, and development of a consciously international discourse within the field of men's health. An influential men's health movement with worldwide relevance will be made up of strong, successful local efforts to improve awareness, advocacy, and outcomes. These efforts must be clearly recognizable as consistent with global men's health priorities and must be deliberately drawn into a global discussion.

Garnering political will within nation-states to provide access to care for poor men in particular is a daunting undertaking. However, a globally collaborative approach to policy reform may hold promise. For instance, working with other national, regional, and international organizations, Community Voices: Healthcare for the Underserved has argued for recognition of underserved men throughout the world as an important untapped "resource." With appropriate support, many socially marginalized men can realize their potential as valuable members of their communities. Providing systematic access to primary and preventive health care, mental and oral health services, and where appropriate, drug therapies, will enable employment, support of families, and relief of the burden on states of male morbidity and early mortality.

Similarities in the predicament across contexts should encourage global collaboration and the wide dissemination of lessons from efforts to cultivate better health outcomes among men in localities around the world. Inadequate health-seeking behaviors are typical of men in general worldwide, and correlate with poorer health outcomes. For instance, Aboriginal and Torres Strait Islander men in Australia have a lower average life expectancy than Australian men overall—fifty-nine years compared to seventy-six years (Australian Government, Department of Health and Ageing, 2008). Predictably, men in Australia underutilize health services (Australian Indigenous HealthInfoNet, 2009). The *Vienna Declaration on the Health of Men and Boys in Europe* (available at http://www.emhf.org/resource_images/viennapush.pdf), a document ratified in 2005 that states the principles and conditions necessary to improve male health outcomes, has been introduced to men in distressed urban neighborhoods in the United States. It has functioned as a tool to organize local men's advocacy for access to health care and male-appropriate approaches to outreach and provision. The *Vienna Declaration* insists upon men's health as a priority but at the same time situates it within the context of family and community well-being.

RACISM: SOCIAL REALITY AS HEALTH RISK

Health advocates, researchers, and practitioners working with or treating African American men should be aware of the health risks that racism poses. The evidence is clear and compelling that dangerous cardiovascular dynamics result from experiences of racism. Elevated heart rate, cortisol levels, and blood pressure occur when African Americans are exposed to explicitly racist events, and cardiovascular stress has been observed in some situations in which race is more subtly salient. Given the reality of racism in African American men's lives, health practitioners should be extra vigilant for the indicators of cardiovascular health, monitoring them with increased frequency. Health practitioners working with African American men may also make their patients aware of findings about the health implications of racism, encouraging the men to be especially mindful of their own apparent stress responses. It is important that stress management be a cornerstone of each black man's health maintenance plan, which he develops with his health provider. This calls on providers to acknowledge racism as a health risk and to perhaps include behavioral guidance—such as encouraging restorative leisure activity, positive social networks, or mental health intervention if necessary—in their consultations with their African American male patients.

More work is required to develop, test, and disseminate specific strategies for individuals coping with racism. It would appear from the evidence of racism's health implications that improving health outcomes among African American men depends in part upon men's capacity to recognize—and find ways to effectively counteract—the adverse effects of discrimination at the personal level. Individually oriented self-help discourses; movements that galvanize group identity and promote positive personal consciousness about race and masculinity; and other approaches should be tested systematically and rigorously to determine whether they can enhance African American men's psychological and physiological resistance to racism.

RELEVANCE OF SOCIAL HISTORIES AND SOCIAL CONTEXT

Health practitioners and others in positions to be of assistance to men must be aware of economic and social data on the areas where their patients or clients live. Beyond health history and strictly defined physiological risk factors, social background and context can yield information critical to a man's health management plan. For instance, knowing that 47.6 percent of men in central Harlem smoke offers insight into a man's asthma risk beyond what his own personal health history might suggest. Likewise, the fact that a study in which two-thirds of adult men in Overtown (Miami) reported having been incarcerated (Young et al., 2007) would suggest to a health practitioner—particularly a mental health provider—that a man from this neighborhood is likely to have psychological issues associated with extended confinement and the traumatic experiences typical in detention facilities.

CHARACTERISTICS OF SUCCESSFUL OUTREACH TO AFRICAN AMERICAN MALES

Increasing men's participation in preventive health care is possible. In Atlanta, Georgia, eight public health screenings held between 1999 and 2008 evinced extensive participation of African American men. These include Men's Health Day (in 1999), the Health Initiative for Men (HIM) (in 2002), and the Community Health and Men's Promotion Summit (CHAMPS) (annually from 2003 to 2008). Screenings included prostate and colorectal cancer, blood pressure, diabetes, dental health, cholesterol, HIV/AIDS and STDs, body mass index (BMI) readings, disease counseling, health exhibits, seminars, and instruction on healthy lifestyles. Factors contributing to the substantial turnouts of men at these screenings included engaging entire families to bring men in and help them understand health regimens (such as taking medications properly); taking time to explain and promote understanding of disease processes and management; the use of multiple media formats to publicize the event (television, radio, newspapers, posters, and so on); and treating the male individual as a whole person, "not just a prostate."

The Washington, D.C.–based Men's Health Network has pioneered the innovative approach of bringing health screenings to the workplace as a solution to the conflict between work hours and the times that health care is usually offered. Many employers have actually embraced these efforts, perceiving current and future financial benefits from decreases in absenteeism and employee turnover as well as from increases in work productivity.

It is important to recognize that men's inattention to health matters in no way reflects a lack of intelligence. Health care providers and health educators must be careful not to belittle men in attempting to get them to be more active in health care. Men often take meticulous care of their cars (Schardt, 1995). If an engine makes odd noises or burns oil, men are usually right on it. Even well-educated and accomplished men may work long hours, fail to rest, and eat junk food while on the road as part of their drive for achievement, while neglecting their health and ignoring signs of illness. The real issue is cultural role expectations. What have men been taught to consider more important, their work performance or the maintenance of their bodies?

IDENTIFYING AND COMBATING "JOHN HENRYISM"

Health practitioners should be vigilant for signs of high-stress coping among African American men at all socioeconomic levels. "John Henryism," as epidemiologist Sherman James dubbed the phenomenon in the early 1990s, fuels performance under extraordinary conditions. Recognizing analogous circumstances for African American men in the current day, James entered a strong caution in identifying John Henryism

(James, 1994). However, just as the legendary railroad worker fell dead after his successful race against the steam engine, abiding pressures on contemporary black men can be extreme and clearly pose very real threats to physical health.

HOLISTIC NOTIONS OF HEALTH

Arguably, men in general have perceptions of health that are largely condition-oriented and driven by ideas about distinct systems within the body. Instead of holistic and integrated notions of what constitutes health, men may focus on the specific health concerns for which they are typically screened or the conditions publicized in commercial advertising media. A man may generalize the condition of the prostate, blood pressure, or sexual functioning, for instance, to his overall health standing. Because notions of health play a critical role in shaping health-related behaviors, African American men should develop an integrated sensibility about health. This involves understanding the interrelationships among oral health, the wide-ranging aspects of physical, sexual, and reproductive health, mental health, and the various activities, attitudes, and choices that produce or compromise well-being. Accomplishing such an essential shift in thinking requires that practitioners, health policy advocates, coaches, teachers, and others promote well-rounded and holistic ideas about manhood itself and what defines a healthy man.

ENLISTING FAMILY AND COMMUNITY

Women often serve as the "health police" in the family (Feeny, 2002). Having a motivated partner may be central in increasing a man's participation in preventive health care, as women are usually more experienced and knowledgeable in health matters. The best approaches to motivating a man are tactful, nonblaming, and tailored to his individual personality. For example, if he is vain, commenting on his "spare tire" may motivate him to diet, but if he is depressed, any criticism may discourage him and he might start eating more. Appeals to responsibility may be valuable, such as, "It is very important to me that you exercise, eat right, and take care of this health problem. Please make an appointment so I don't have to worry." If he is afraid of receiving bad news if he goes to the doctor, aim to shift his fear from going to not going—speak about how early diagnosis and treatment is the best and only way to avoid a bad outcome. If he likes to be in charge, challenge him to take control; for example, "Your blood pressure was high. What are you going to do about it?"

REDEFINING HEALTH AS A MASCULINE IDEAL

Typically, a great deal of emphasis is placed on male achievement and productivity. For this reason, men's interest in health matters may be stimulated by speaking to their desire for better performance. Consider also the success of Viagra and Propecia, as well as steroid use to build muscle and enhance performance among professional athletes. Most men want to be "better men," and the health care system can use the aspiration for optimal performance to build a bridge to men currently not being served. Fortunately, the relatively new erectile dysfunction drugs have brought to the doctor men who would not otherwise have gone. However, the need for these drugs usually arises late in life, when lifestyle factors like smoking, diet, and exercise are already established. For this reason, sports medicine is being considered as a way to establish a connection between the health care system and younger males as well.

At present, many men see being sick or going to the doctor somehow as a shameful personal failure or a sign of weakness. This paradigm can be reversed by portraying health care as a staunch ally of masculinity while instead portraying illness and infirmity as the true enemy of manliness. Appeals to men to "take charge" of their health as a means to attain, maintain, or regain their maximum productivity, vitality, strength, speed, endurance, virility, stamina, concentration, attractiveness, and all the things that make men "feel like men" are likely to enhance male participation in preventive health care.

As a culture, we need to stop shaming boys and men into the belief that feeling pain or fear is always weak or cowardly if we are to prevent attitudinal barriers to participation in health care among males. These feelings are healthy tools of survival. Nature put pain in place to warn that something is wrong that requires attention. Fear alerts us that something is dangerous and is better avoided. A far better approach to children of both sexes would be to teach that there are times when pain may be safely ignored (such as monitored athletic competition) and specific times when pain urgently needs to be addressed.

ADDRESSING DISTRUST OF THE HEALTH CARE SYSTEM

The health care provider can play an important role in facilitating African American men's success in health matters. Distrust of the health care system can be reduced by the peer-to-peer approach, using male African American health care providers to deliver treatment and African American male public figures to do public service announcements and other forms of outreach. Health care providers must be careful to listen when a man expresses concern or pain, or the man may learn that it doesn't help to seek aid. In many respects, provider deafness promotes patient muteness. Providers must strive to recognize the unique cultural hurdles African American men must overcome in the act of seeking health care. Caregivers should be receptive and nonjudgmental toward a patient's attempts to communicate, even if they are clumsy and inexperienced at first.

THE COST-EFFECTIVENESS BENEFIT TO SOCIETY

The benefits of improving African American men's health to communities and the nation are manifold. Rising health care costs can be reduced or controlled through preventing costly, advanced disease. Economic costs of preventable male illness, including lost time from work, disability, and diminished income, can be reduced, while work productivity can be increased. African American longevity figures and health care outcomes compared with other ethnicities may be improved.

Increased attention to African American men's health ultimately holds the potential to bolster and uplift the health status of the African American community as a whole. A tetrad approach is essential to achieve optimal community health, including children's health, women's health, men's health, and minority health as coequal partners. While African American men's health currently receives the least attention of any other major population group, failure to address the health needs of any of these groups impairs the ability to fully address the needs of the others. Increased attention to African American men's health is in no way antagonistic to meeting the health needs of other groups. Addressing the compelling, unmet health needs of African American men should be welcomed as a logical complement to African American women's and children's health, a vital step towards building a complete and inclusive health care system, and an essential means of achieving optimal overall health in African American communities.

REFERENCES

Australian Government, Department of Health and Ageing. (2008). *Developing a men's health policy for Australia: Setting the scene.* Retrieved March 2009 from http://www.health.gov.au/menshealthpolicy

Australian Indigenous HealthInfoNet. (2009). *What are male health issues?* Available at http://archive .healthinfonet.ecu.edu.au/html/html_population/mens_health/reviews/mens_health_what.htm#what

Bandura, A. (1977). Self-efficacy: Towards a unifying theory of behavioral change. *Psychological Review, 84*(2), 191–215.

Binswanger, I., Stern, M. F., Deyo, R. A., Heagerty, P. J., Cheadle, A., Elmore, J. G., & Koepsell, T. D. (2007, January 11). Release from prison—A high risk of death for former inmates. *New England Journal of Medicine, 356*(2), 157–165. (Erratum in *356*(5), 536).

Bonhomme, J. J. (2006, June 23). Address to the Massachusetts Medical Society. Winter St., Waltham, MA.

Bonhomme, J. J. (2007). Men's health: Impact on women, children and society. *Journal of Men's Health & Gender, 4*(2), 124–130.

Braithwaite, R. (2001).The health status of black men. In R. Braithwaite & S. Taylor (Eds.), *Health issues in the black community,* 2nd ed. (p. 70). San Francisco: Jossey-Bass.

Brawley, O. W. (2006). Lung cancer and race: Equal treatment yields equal outcome among equal patients, but there is no equal treatment. *Journal of Clinical Oncology, 24*(3), 332–333.

Brett, K. M., & Burt, C. W. (2001). Utilization of ambulatory medical care by women: United States, 1997–98. *Vital and Health Statistics, 13*(149), 1–46.

Brondolo, E., Libby, D. J., Denton, E., Thompson, S., Beatty, D. L., Schwartz, J., et al. (2008). Racism and ambulatory blood pressure in a community sample. *Psychosomatic Medicine, 70,* 49–56.

Brown, A. S., Schaefer, C. A., Wyatt, R. J., Begg, M. D., Goetz, R., Bresnahan, M. A., et al. (2002). Paternal age and risk of schizophrenia in adult offspring. *American Journal of Psychiatry, 159*(9), 1528–1533.

Campbell, J. L. (1996). Traditional men in therapy: Obstacles and recommendations. *Journal of Psychological Practice, 2*(3), 40–45.

College Board. (2005). *Education pays: Update: The benefits of higher education for individuals and society.* Retrieved March 2009 from http://www.collegeboard.com/prod_downloads/press/cost05/education_pays_05pdf

Collins Center for Public Policy. (2006). Florida's restrictions on employment opportunities for people with criminal records. Miami, FL: Author.

Doyal, L. (2001). Sex, gender, and health: The need for a new approach. *British Medical Journal, 323,* 1061–1063.

Drexler, M. (2007, July 15). How racism hurts—Literally. *Boston Globe.* Retrieved March 2009 from www.boston .com/news/globe/ideas/articles/2007/07/15/how_racism_hurts____literally/

Felix-Aaron, K., Moy, E., Kang, M., Patel, M., Chesley, F. D., & Clancy, C. (2005). Variation in quality of men's health care by race/ethnicity and social class. *Medical Care, 43*(3 Suppl.), 172–181.

Freudenberg, N., Moseley, J., Labriola, M., Daniels, J., & Murrill, C. (2007). Comparison of health and social characteristics of people leaving New York City jails by age, gender, and race/ethnicity: Implications for public health interventions. *Public Health Reports, 122,* 733–743.

Gallagher, C. A., & Dobrin, A. (2007). Can juvenile justice detention facilities meet the call of the American Academy of Pediatrics and National Commission on Correctional Health Care?: A national analysis of current practices. *Pediatrics, 119*(4), e991–e1001.

Goodwin, J., Black, S. A., & Satish, S. (1999). Aging versus disease: The opinions of older black, Hispanic, and non-Hispanic white Americans about the causes and treatment of common medical conditions. *Journal of the American Geriatric Society, 47*(8), 973–979.

James, S. A. (1994). John Henryism and the health of African Americans. *Culture, Medicine and Psychiatry, 18*(2), 163–182.

Jones, D. R. (1987). Heart disease mortality following widowhood: Some results from the OPCS Longitudinal Study, Office of Population Censuses and Surveys. *Journal of Psychosomatic Research, 31*(3), 325–333.

Justice Policy Institute. (2007). *The vortex: The concentrated racial impact of drug imprisonment and the characteristics of punitive counties.* Washington, DC: Author.

Kass, B. L., Weinick, R. M., & Monheit, A. C. (1999, February). *Chartbook #2: Racial and ethnic differences in health 1996* (p. 9). Rockville, MD: Agency for Healthcare Research and Quality. Retrieved March 2009 from http://www.meps.ahrq.gov/data_files/publications/cb2/cb2.shtml.

Kilmartin, C. (2005). Depression in men: Communication, diagnosis and therapy. *Journal of Men's Health & Gender, 2*(1), 95–99.

Krippner, S., & McIntyre, T. M. (2003). *The psychological impact of war trauma on civilians.* New York: Praeger.

Massoglia, M. (2005, August 12). *Health consequences of incarceration.* Paper presented at the annual meeting of the American Sociological Association, Philadelphia. Retrieved October 23, 2008, from http://www.allacademic.com/meta/p31988_index.html

Maxwell, N., & Paringer, L. (2004, July). *Employer-based health insurance and worker skills.* Conference paper presented at ERIU Research Conference, Ann, Arbor, MI. Retrieved March 2009 from http://eriu.sph.umich.edu/pdf/wp34.pdf

Menchik, P. L. (1993). Economic status as a determinant of mortality among African American and White older men: Does poverty kill? *Population Studies, 47,* 427–436.

Meurman, J. H., Sanz, M., & Janket, S.-J. (2004). Oral health, atherosclerosis, and cardiovascular disease. *Critical Reviews in Oral Biology & Medicine, 15*(6), 403–413.

Morgan, L. A. (1989). Economic well-being following marital termination: A comparison of widowed and divorced women. *Journal of Family Issues, 10*(1), 86–101.

National Center for Health Statistics. (2009). *Health, United States, 2008.* Hyattsville, MD: Author.

New York City Bar Association Task Force on Employment Opportunities for the Previously Incarcerated. (2008). *Legal employers taking the lead: Enhancing employment opportunities for the previously incarcerated.* New York: Author.

Pettit, B., & Western, B. (2004). Mass imprisonment and the life course: Race and class inequality in U.S. incarceration. *American Sociological Review, 69,* 151–169.

Sandman, D., Simantov, E., & An, C. (2000). *Out of touch: American men and the health care system. Commonwealth Fund Men's and Women's Health Survey findings.* New York: Commonwealth Fund. Retrieved March 2009 from http://www.cmwf.org/usr_doc/sandman_outoftouch_374.pdf

Savitz, D. A., Schwingl, P. J., & Keels, M. A. (1991). Influence of paternal age, smoking, and alcohol consumption on congenital anomalies. *Teratology, 44*(4), 429–440.

Schardt, D. (1995, June). For men only—Mortality of men. *Nutrition Action Healthletter.* Retrieved March 2009 from http://www.findarticles.com/p/articles/mi_m0813/is_n5_v22/ai_16995315

Steele, C. M. (1999, August). Thin ice: Stereotype threat and Black college students. *Atlantic.* Retrieved March 2009 from http://www.theatlantic.com/doc/199908/student-stereotype

Stewart, E. A., Schreck, C. J., & Simmons, R. L. (2006). I ain't gonna let no one disrespect me: Does the code of the street reduce or increase violent victimization among African American adolescents? *Journal of Research in Crime and Delinquency, 43*(4), 427–458.

Sum, A., Khatiwada, I., McLaughlin, J., & Tobar, P. (2007). *The educational attainment of the nation's young Black men and their recent labor market experiences: What can be done to improve their future labor market and educational prospects?* Northeastern University Center for Labor Market Studies.

Treadwell, H., & Ro, M. (2003). Poverty, race, and the invisible men. *American Journal of Public Health, 93,* 705–707.

U.S. Administration on Aging. (2001). *Meeting the needs of older women: A diverse and growing population.* Washington, DC: Author. Retrieved March 2009 from //www.menshealthnetwork.org/library/AOAolderwomenneeds.pdf (Information available via e-mail at aoainfo@aoa.gov)

U.S. Department of Health and Human Services. (1998). *Health, United States, 1998, with socioeconomic status and health chartbook.* Hyattsville, MD: National Center for Health Statistics (Fig. 43, p. 133). Retrieved March 2009 from http://www.cdc.gov/nchs/data/hus/hus98.pdf

U.S. Department of Housing and Urban Development. (2001). *In the crossfire: The impact of gun violence on public housing communities.* Retrieved March 2009 from http://www.ncjrs.gov/pdffiles1/nij/181158.pdf

Vogin, G. D. (2002). Helping men get healthy. *WebMD Feature Archive.* Retrieved March 2009 from http://women.webmd.com/feature/men-in-your-life

Wamala, S., Merlo, J., Bostrom, G., & Hogstedt, C. (2007). Perceived discrimination, socioeconomic disadvantage and refraining from seeking medical treatment in Sweden. *Journal of Epidemiology and Community Health, 6,* 409–415.

Wen, W. Q., Shu, X. O., Steinbuch, M., Severson, R. K., Reaman, G. H., Buckley, J. D., et al. (2000). Paternal military service and risk for childhood leukemia in offspring. *American Journal of Epidemiology, 151*(3), 231–240.

Western, B. (2002). The impact of incarceration on wage mobility and inequality. *American Sociological Review, 67,* 526–546.

Young, A. M. W. (2006). *Overtown Men's Health Study report.* Miami, FL: Collins Center for Public Policy, 2006.

Young, A. M. W., Meryn, S., & Treadwell, H. (2008). Poverty and men's health. *Journal of Men's Health, 5*(3), 18–48.

Young, A. M. W., Perez, L. M., Northridge, M. E., Vaughn, R. L., Braithwaite, K., & Treadwell, H. M. (2007). Bringing to light the health needs of African American men: The *Overtown Men's Health Study. Journal of Men's Health & Gender, 4*(2), 140–148.

CHAPTER

6

HEALTH AND BLACK OLDER ADULTS

Insights from a Life-Course Perspective

SHERRILL L. SELLERS
ISHTAR O. GOVIA
JAMES S. JACKSON

For the most part, black people living in the United States have been portrayed in the scientific literature in a simplistic and undifferentiated manner. An underlying assumption of prior research has been that there is extensive homogeneity in values, motives, social and psychological statuses, and behaviors among black persons living in the United States (Jackson, 1991). Though categorical treatment based on race may produce some group uniformity in attitudes and behaviors, a rich heterogeneity exists among blacks in these same status, attitudinal, and behavioral dimensions, as well as in their national and ethnic groups of origin (Jackson, 2000; Jackson et al., 2004). Recent studies show that older black Americans are a diverse and heterogeneous population possessing a wide array of group and personal resources (Chatters, Taylor, Bullard, & Jackson, 2008; Chatters, Taylor, Jackson, & Lincoln, 2008; Farley, 2000; Jackson, Forsythe-Brown, & Govia, 2007).

Older black Americans are one of the fastest growing segments of the population and, along with elders of other ethnic minority populations, in three decades will constitute a fifth of the over-65-year-old group (Siegel, 1999). Projections indicate that the number of black persons aged 65 and older in the United States will increase from 8 to 14 percent by the year 2050 (Angel & Hogan, 2004; Federal Interagency Forum on Aging-Related Statistics [FIFARS] 2008). A large proportion of the future older black Americans of the twenty-first century have already been born. The tail of the baby boom cohort will reach age 65 in fewer than twenty years; a child born in 1998 will reach 65 in 2063.

Human development, aging, and the life course are the central concerns in an approach to understanding ostensible health–race effects. Ethnic and racial groups have divergent life experiences in part because of differences in sociostructural, socio-economic, and cultural conditions (Dressler & Bindon, 2000; Jackson & Antonucci, 2005). These different experiences have significant influences, both positive and negative, on individual, family, and group well-being and health at all stages of the life course, ultimately influencing the adjustment to major life transitions (such as loss of spouse, retirement, and disability) in older ages.

A life-course framework is needed to explore how social, historical, and cultural context influences and interacts with individual and group resources to both impede and facilitate the quality of life and health of successive cohorts of black Americans over the group life course, and in the nature of their individual human development and aging experiences (Baltes, 1987; Burton, Dilworth-Anderson, & Bengtson, 1991; Smith & Kington, 1997a).

HEALTH STATUS OF BLACK OLDER ADULTS[1]

By the year 2050 an unprecedented proportion of the total U.S. population will be over the age of 65 (FIFARS, 2008; United Nations, 2007). The 2006 estimate of persons 65 and older was 12 percent, but by the year 2020, it is expected to increase to over 16 percent, and to experience a further 4 percent increase by the year 2050. This increase is largely due to a decline in mortality rates among large birth cohorts born immediately after World War II, and declines in fertility rates among the general American population.

Although non-Hispanic whites 65 and over are expected to remain the largest group of elderly by the year 2050, their proportion within the total U.S. aged population is anticipated to decrease from almost 81 percent today to 61 percent, whereas all other ethnic groups are anticipated to demonstrate large increases in their numbers of adults 65 and older. Specifically, the proportion of black elderly is expected to increase from 8 percent to 12 percent (FIFARS, 2008). Though some of this increase can be

---

[1] This chapter focuses on physical health. See Mills and Edwards (2002) for a review of research on mental health and older black Americans. Other important studies in this area include, but are not limited to, Brown, Milburn, & Gary, 1992; Cook, Black, Rabins, & German, 2000; and Turnbull & Mui, 1995.

attributed to changes in general population fertility, the increases for black elderly are also thought to be rooted in their relatively better material and social advantages in comparison to past birth cohorts.

Nonetheless, comparative mortality statistics suggest that blacks encounter disadvantages over the life course. The infant mortality rate for blacks is 13.6 deaths per 1,000 live births, the highest of any census-defined race/ethnic group (National Center for Health Statistics [NCHS] 2007). Although the average life expectancy at birth increased more for blacks than whites in the United States between 1990 and 2004, national data from 2005 indicate that the average life expectancy for blacks is still significantly lower than for whites—approximately 78.3 years for whites, compared to 73.2 years for blacks, with an almost five-year difference between white men (75.7) and black men (69.5), and a four-year difference between white women (80.8) and black women (76.5) (NCHS, 2007).

Across the life span, blacks in the United States face numerous health disadvantages. For example, hypertension disproportionately affects them. According to 2001–2004 age-adjusted estimates of the population of persons 20 years and over, 41.5 percent of the black male population suffered from hypertension, compared to 29.3 percent of the white male population. Similarly, 44.3 percent of the black female population suffered from hypertension, compared to 29 percent of the white female population (NCHS, 2007, Table 70). These health outcome differentials that disadvantage blacks throughout their lives are also seen in cancer rates. Age-adjusted estimates from 2004 highlight that, among men, blacks have 71.4 more deaths per 100,000 than whites; among women, blacks have 24.4 more deaths per 100,000 (NCHS, 2007, Table 38). Perhaps most alarming is the disproportionate risk that blacks in the United States have for HIV when compared with whites. In 2005, the age-adjusted death rate per 100,000 from HIV was 2.2 for whites, while it was 19.4 for blacks (NCHS, 2007, Table 29).

Investigations of causes of death among older blacks in the United States highlight great within-group heterogeneity. As indicated in Table 6.1, heart disease, cancer, and cerebrovascular disease are the top three causes of death among blacks, regardless of age or gender. These findings are similar to those for other racial/ethnic groups in the United States. However, the impact of Alzheimer's disease, diabetes mellitus, and chronic lower respiratory disease as main causes of death is highly associated with age and gender among older blacks.

For Alzheimer's disease, although women and men are at equal risk for developing the disease, female tendencies to have greater longevity than men result in a higher prevalence of the disease among aging women (Alzheimer's Association, 2008). Furthermore, women bear a double burden with Alzheimer's because they are more likely to provide informal caregiving for partners, aging parents, and relatives afflicted with the disease (Alzheimer's Association, 2008). These roles are often associated with role strain and stress (Cannuscio et al., 2002; Cannuscio et al., 2004). Further, recent research highlights the links between depression over the life course and various stages of Alzheimer's disease, suggesting possible differences between women and

TABLE 6.1 **Top 10 Leading Causes of Death Among Blacks in the United States Ages 65 and Older and 85 and Older, by Sex.**

	Ages 65 and older		Ages 85 and older	
	Men	Women	Men	Women
1.	Diseases of heart	Diseases of heart	Diseases of heart	Diseases of heart
2.	Malignant neoplasms	Malignant neoplasms	Malignant neoplasms	Malignant neoplasms
3.	Cerebrovascular diseases	Cerebrovascular diseases	Cerebrovascular diseases	Cerebrovascular diseases
4.	Diabetes mellitus	Diabetes mellitus	Influenza and pneumonia	Alzheimer's disease
5.	Chronic lower respiratory disease	Nephritis	Chronic lower respiratory disease	Diabetes mellitus
6.	Nephritis	Alzheimer's disease	Nephritis	Influenza and pneumonia
7.	Influenza and pneumonia	Chronic lower respiratory disease	Diabetes mellitus	Nephritis
8.	Septicemia	Influenza and pneumonia	Alzheimer's disease	Hypertension
9.	Unintentional injuries	Septicemia	Septicemia	Septicemia
10.	Hypertension	Hypertension	Hypertension	Chronic lower respiratory disease

Source: Federal Interagency Forum on Aging-Related Statistics. (2008). *Older Americans 2008: Key indicators of well-being*. Washington, DC: Government Printing Office. Derived from data presented in Tables 15b and 15c.

men in mechanisms involved in the disease (Geerling, den Heijer, Koudstaal, Hofman, & Breteler, 2008; Wilson, Arnold, Beck, Bienias, & Bennett, 2008).

Chronic respiratory disease is higher on the list of leading causes of death for men than for women, both in the 65-and-older age group and in the 85-and-older age group.

Smoking, a major risk factor in chronic respiratory disease, is more prevalent among men than among women. In addition, more men than women tend to work in occupational contexts in which fuel and other toxic substances are present. These factors likely place black men at greater risks for these diseases when compared to black women.

Table 6.2 draws attention to within-group heterogeneity in the prevalence of chronic health conditions. As would be expected, the prevalence for many chronic health conditions increases with age, such that the prevalence for many diseases is lower in the 65–74 age group and higher in the 85-and-older age group. What is perhaps most striking about the data, however, is the extent to which the prevalence of these diseases is dissimilar within age group by gender. Black men and women clearly demonstrate significant differences in the diseases with which they are afflicted and the increasing or decreasing prevalence of these diseases as they age.

Across the age groups, the prevalence of arthritis and diabetes is higher for women than for men, between 20 to 30 percent higher in the case of arthritis. There have been speculations that the higher prevalence rates of arthritis in women might be due to processes related to levels of estrogen as well as to environmental conditions (Theis, Helmick, & Hootman, 2007). The disadvantage that women face in the prevalence rates of diabetes has been linked to their higher prevalence of obesity, among other factors (Williams, 2002).

Yet, older black men also demonstrate health disadvantages when compared to older black women. Specifically, the prevalence of cancer as a chronic health condition for men far outweighs the prevalence for women within each of the age groups (65 to 74, 75 to 84, and 85 and over), by anywhere between 3 and 24 percent.

The story of sex and age differences in chronic disease among aging blacks is not clear-cut, however. The data in Table 6.2 highlight the complexity of the age–sex interaction among blacks in the United States. For example, both heart disease and coronary heart disease are more prevalent in men ages 65 to 74 and 85 and over, but greater in women ages 75 to 84. A similar pattern is seen in the prevalence of heart attacks, which are more prevalent for men ages 65 to 74 but greater in women ages 75 to 84.

Overall, data suggest that blacks in the United States, especially older blacks, are at disproportionate risk for negative health outcomes when compared to whites (Adelman, 2008; NCHS, 2007; Office of Minority Health and Health Disparities [OMHHD] 2008). A number of factors may contribute to this disparity. A great deal of recent research suggests that discrimination, cultural barriers, and inadequate access to health care are some of the principal factors contributing to ethnic health disparities (Adelman, 2008; OMHHD, 2008). Additional perspectives highlight the role of biological dispositions (Baquet & Ringen, 1987), health behaviors such as dietary habits (Winkleby & Cubbin, 2004), and a failure to receive adequate health care (Williams & Rucker, 2000). The specific mechanisms that produce these distinct outcomes are less clear (Adler & Rehkopf, 2008; LaVeist, 2000; Williams, 1999). Given the complex sociohistorical context of blacks in the United States, and the increasing focus on differential exposure to chronic stress as a key mechanism via which these disparities manifest (Adler & Rehkopf, 2008), it may be less useful in

TABLE 6.2 Prevalence of Chronic Conditions for the Years 2004–2006 Among Black Adults Aged 65 and Older, by Age and Sex.

	Ages 65+ (age adjusted)			Ages 65–74			Ages 75–84			Ages 85 and over		
	All	Men	Women	All	Men	Women	All	Men	Women	All	Men	Women
Heart Disease	25.5	25.5	25.5	23.3	25.1	21.9	27.4	22.9	30.1	29.5	34.6	27.7
Coronary Heart Disease	18.1	17.8	18.4	16.1	16.6	15.7	19.8	16.4	21.9	21.5	26.6	19.6
Heart Attack	9.5	10.7	8.7	8.8	11.3	6.9	9.7	8.0	10.7	11.9	–	–
Stroke	12.6	13.5	12.1	11.1	12.6	10.0	13.9	13.2	14.3	15.6	–	14.7
Cancer, All	12.5	17.6	12.8	10.8	12.9	9.3	12.0	17.3	8.8	20.9	38.4	14.6
Arthritis	52.9	40.2	60.6	47.7	36.7	55.7	59.3	48.0	66.2	56.6	32.2	65.5
Diabetes	27.3	23.5	29.7	29.1	25.8	31.6	28.1	24.0	30.6	17.1	–	18.9

Source: Centers for Disease Control and Prevention, National Center for Health Statistics, National Vital Statistics System

Note: All percents adjusted for income, location, and urbanicity.

determining exact mechanisms to compare between racial and ethnic group outcomes than within groups. For example, black–white comparisons may be less illuminating than the examination of various intra group social and cultural factors as possible sources of risk and resilience for black men, women, and children (Dressler & Bindon, 2000; Jackson & Antonucci, 2005; Jackson & Sellers, 1996; McEwen & Seeman, 1999).

LIFE-COURSE CONSIDERATIONS

Significant improvements in the life situations of blacks (Farley, 1987, 2000), particularly health, have occurred over the last forty years (Jackson, 1981, 1993, 2000). However, recent literature (see, for example, Farley, 2000) documents the negative life events and structural barriers, particularly for poor blacks, that still exist. These problems include the difficulties of single-parent households, high infant morbidity and mortality, childhood diseases, poor nutrition, lack of preventive health care, deteriorating neighborhoods, poverty, adolescent violence, un- and underemployment, teen pregnancy, and drug and alcohol abuse. Though the exact causal relationships are not known (Williams, 1990, 1999; Williams & Collins, 1995), it is clear that these are predisposing factors for high morbidity and mortality across the entire life span (for example, Berkman & Mullen, 1997; Dressler, 1991).

It is important to develop a life-course framework within which the nature of the economic, social, and health status of black Americans can be explained and understood (Jackson, 1991; Jackson, Antonucci, & Gibson, 1990a, 1990b). A life-course perspective illuminates how current and aging cohorts of blacks have been exposed to conditions that will influence profoundly their social, psychological, and health statuses as they reach older ages in the years and decades to come (Baltes, 1987; Barresi, 1987; Jackson & Sellers, 1996). Three themes within a life-course framework are especially relevant for understanding the health and well-being of aging blacks in the United States—period and cohort, socioeconomic status, and race-relevant risk and coping mechanisms (Berkman & Mullen, 1997; LaVeist, 2000; Miles, 1999; Tucker, 2000).

Period and Cohort Influences on the Health of Aging Blacks

A main theoretical focus of a life-course perspective is to explore the intersection of age, period, and cohort-related phenomena as they influence the black American family and individual experience. These studies address how the age cohort into which blacks are born, the social, political, and economic events that occur to blacks born together, and the individual aging process at different points in a person's life course, influence the adaptation and quality of life of individuals, families, and larger groups of black Americans. For example, blacks born before the 1940s faced very different environmental constraints and have experienced a very different set of life tasks, events, opportunities, and disappointments than those born in the 1970s (Smith & Kington, 1997a). Those born in the twenty-first century will experience a new set of challenges and opportunities.

In addition to significant changes in the legal structure, health care advances and delivery, family changes, urban migration, and macroeconomic influences all differed dramatically across birth cohorts, as they will for future cohorts of blacks (Richardson, 1996). For example, blacks born since the struggles of the Civil Rights Movement (CRM) have a very different set of expectations of what life should offer than those who came of age before this point. Although there is overlap across the generations within families, and across birth cohorts, the fact is that the CRM and its corollary events changed irrevocably the level of aspirations and expectations of African Americans, especially those who came of age during and following this period (Jackson & Sellers, 1996). After the CRM, a substantial number of blacks were able to improve their social status through occupational achievement, educational advancement, and home ownership in better neighborhoods. In the past thirty years, relative to whites, blacks have experienced substantial occupational upward mobility (Levy, 1998).

The United States recently witnessed another historic shift, with the election of the nation's first black president. Perhaps the most visible reflection of the changing nature of blacks in the United States is the presidency of Barack Obama, a son of an African father and white mother who identifies with African-American culture but also views himself as a "mutt." The Obama presidency suggests that, as a matter of politics and public policy at least, race is not nearly the defining issue it was a generation ago. It is not clear how these events will impact the health and well-being of blacks in the United States. Early data suggest a renewed sense of pride and optimism. It is quite possible that President Obama's election will have paradoxical consequences similar to the CRM.

The CRM was conducive to upward mobility but constrained by persistent racial prejudices. Thus, the group that came of age after the CRM has been caught in a historical bind. On one hand, the expectation was for continued upward social mobility; on the other, it became clear that the full promise of the CRM was not to be realized. Further, a changing economy not only dampened prospects for upward mobility but also threatened past gains (Hochschild, 1995; Massey, 2007). In parallel, the current economic recession has been especially difficult for black Americans (Austin, 2008b; Rivera, Cotto-Escalera, Desai, Huezo, & Muhammed, 2008). Already-tenuous middle-class status has been strained nearly to the breaking point because of the disproportionate number of blacks who have been adversely affected by the mortgage crisis and other financial catastrophes (Austin, 2008a; Rivera et al., 2008).

In essence, the post-CRM birth cohorts constitute a "disappointment" generation (Jackson, 1993). Not only have their legitimate aspirations not been fulfilled, but the nature of racial oppression has changed dramatically from the pre-CRM period. The struggle for equal opportunity is a very different and more difficult one than the struggle for equal rights under the law (Jackson, 2000). How this may affect the "disappointment" generation as they age is unknown. It may be that the adaptive mechanisms of system-blame, or religious orientations, may not be as effective for a more cynical, though no less disadvantaged, group of blacks in the United States as they grow older. On the other hand, somewhat greater access to health care (through

Medicare, Medicaid, and so on) may eventually offset some of the negative consequences of continued structural barriers to individual and group mobility and achievement.

In a more pessimistic vein, it may be that blacks in the United States who were middle-aged at the time of the CRM have benefited the most from what now appears to be the "radical" changes that occurred during the mid-1960s and 1970s. New cohorts of middle-aged and elderly blacks may exist in an environment of fewer tangible goods and services as well as a more pessimistic and worsening social and psychological atmosphere.

Though several authors have indicated the necessity of considering history and cohort and period effects in the nature of black status (see, for example, Barresi, 1987; Manton & Soldo, 1985), few have actually collected the type of data or conducted the analyses that would shed any light on these processes. For example, in reviewing the material on health, mortality, morbidity, and risk factors, it appears that the examination of black health status has been conducted in a relative vacuum. This has been as much the fault of a lack of good conceptual models of black health status as it has been the lack of quality trend data on sizable numbers of representative samples of black Americans. Nevertheless, models of age-period-cohort effects have recently been developed and applied to aging groups in general (see, for example, Yang, 2007; Yang, Schulhofer-Wohl, Fu, & Land, 2008). One promising direction for future research on the heterogeneity of aging blacks in the United States is to apply these models to blacks, particularly because cohort effects for blacks native to the United States would probably differ from cohort effects of blacks who immigrated to the United States.

Older blacks often arrive in adulthood and older ages with extensive histories of disease, ill health, and varied individual adaptive reactions to their poor health (Smith & Kington, 1997b). The available cohort data for cause-specific mortality and morbidity across the life course over the last few decades indicate that there are accumulated deficits that perhaps place black middle-aged and older people at greater risk than whites of comparable ages (Jackson, 1991). Similarly, the fact that blacks actually outlive their white counterparts in the very older ages suggests possible selection factors at work that may result in hardier older blacks (Gibson & Jackson, 1987, 1992; Manton & Stallard, 1997). These selection factors may act on successive cohorts of blacks in a "sandwich-like" manner, leaving alternate cohorts of middle-aged and older blacks of relative wellness and good functional ability. The cohort experiences of blacks undoubtedly play a major role in the nature of their health experiences over the life course in terms of the quality of health care from birth, exposure to risk factors, and the presence of exogenous environmental factors. Another contributing factor is the stressor role of prejudice and discrimination across the life course, even though it may differ in form and intensity as a function of birth cohort, period, and age (Bulatao & Anderson, 2004, especially Chapter 7; Cooper, Steinhauer, Miller, David, & Schatzkin, 1981; Dressler, 1991; Williams & Williams-Morris, 2000). Further study of age-period-cohort effects is needed. Particularly in light of the increasing differences within aging blacks in the United States, future research needs to disentangle, with the help of longitudinal data, the contributions of each of these components to health outcomes.

Socioeconomic Status and the Health of Blacks over the Life Course

Studies indicate that blacks in the United States are most likely to spend the majority of their childhoods in low-income, single female–headed households (Tucker & Mitchell-Kernan, 1995; Johnson & Staples, 2005). Poverty in turn places black Americans at risk for inadequate diets, fewer educational opportunities, greater exposure to crime, and limited opportunities for occupational advancement (Smith, 2004; Massey, 2007; Thorpe et al., 2008; Wight et al., 2008). Job prospects will be poor in young adulthood and a large proportion of blacks will die or suffer chronic disease prior to reaching middle adulthood. Only a comparative few will have the advantage of intergenerational economic transfers from parental sources (Darity, Dietrich, & Guilkey, 2001). Even for those born into contemporary middle-class homes (an often fragile situation for most blacks), providing a tangible legacy for children, even college funding, is problematic (Darity et al., 2001). Dental visits, preventive health maintenance, well-baby checks, hearing and vision screenings, and the like will go undone. Other "luxuries" of life are difficult to afford (Jackson, 1993), which may translate into adverse health trajectories.

Blacks at every family income level have lower wealth than comparable whites (Darity et al., 2001; Darity, 2005). At the lowest income quintile, whites have ten thousand dollars in wealth whereas comparable black families have one dollar. In every new generation of blacks in the United States, wealth is thus re-created and consumed. This results in structural disadvantage that increases risk for poor health over the life course (Shuey & Willson, 2008).

Data on the statuses of middle-aged and younger minority groups, especially blacks, relative to whites, in housing, income, occupation, health, and education suggest that only small gains can be expected as new cohorts enter older ages (Anderson, Bulatao, & Cohen, 2004; Muhammad, Muhammad, Davis, Lui, & Leondar-Wright, 2004). Further, recent data indicates that the disadvantage of elderly minorities in America, relative to whites, increases when assets and wealth resources are examined. Specifically, this research demonstrated that blacks were about six times more likely than whites to be poor (Butrica, 2008). Racial differences in social and economic status create disparities that affect the health and well-being of aging populations in the United States.

The role of socioeconomic status (SES) has been touted as a major risk factor and implicated in the effects of other risk factors in mortality and morbidity (Williams, 1999; Smith & Kington, 1997a, 1997b). Impressive evidence exists that SES plays a major role in a wide variety of diseases such that increasing SES is associated with better health and lowered morbidity, and vice versa (Adler & Rehkopf, 2008). This effect has been shown at both the individual and ecological levels on blood pressure, general mortality, cancer, coronary heart diseases, cerebrovascular disease, diabetes, obesity, quality of life, and general self-reported health (Hayward, Crimmins, Miles, & Yang, 2000; Huguet, Kaplan, & Feeny, 2008; Shuey & Willson, 2008). What has been examined to a lesser extent is how SES status from conception, birth, or early in the life course affects these health outcomes in adulthood and older ages (Kahn & Fazio, 2005). Perhaps, over the full life course, advantaged blacks would be considerably more similar to their white counterparts than less advantaged blacks to theirs (Jackson, 1993); but current middle-to-high SES blacks would be at an intermediate position, and the full life-course disadvantaged blacks would continue to show worse health status conditions than their comparable low-SES white counterparts (Crimmins, Hayward, & Seeman, 2004).

Research (Skarupski et al., 2005; Williams & Collins, 1995) suggests that this complex effect of SES on health, in which its effects on health disparities cannot be confined to examinations of income and education alone, is one that must be attended to in studies of aging ethnic minorities in the United States. Thus, an emerging theme in some of the empirical literature is that similarity in income and education may serve to equate upper-income race groups, but may have fewer effects on certain health outcomes among lower-income groups (see, for example, Kessler & Neighbors, 1986). Income and other socioeconomic control variables may serve to underequate different race groups at lower income levels and overequate at upper income levels. The causes of these observed effects are not known and may be due to several factors (Williams, 1999). In a racially divided society in which blacks have had to struggle to be successful, perhaps harder than whites in comparable income (or education and occupation) positions, blacks at these upper levels may in fact have more of the underlying factors that are correlated with education, income, or occupation levels than do comparable whites, thus countering the effects of discrimination. Thus, blacks at these upper socioeconomic positions may show equal or superior health outcomes to whites at comparable levels.

Lower socioeconomic status blacks, however, are not as well off as comparable low-income whites, perhaps due to discrimination and lack of resources (Williams & Rucker, 2000; Williams & Williams-Morris, 2000). It is probable that whites at these levels would still maintain an advantage over blacks, with blacks showing decidedly poorer health outcomes. It may also be true that different health outcomes may show differential effects of the interaction between race and SES. On one hand, it may be that SES is less effective in reducing health outcome differentials between blacks and whites in which stress plays a major etiological role (McEwen & Seeman, 1999). On the other hand, health outcomes in which social and economic resources may play a major role (like infectious diseases, HIV/AIDS) may show marked differences between blacks and whites (LaVeist, 2000).

We suggest that controls for socioeconomic status should be progressively more effective in younger age cohorts. Current older blacks, of both upper and lower socioeconomic status, have had longer to suffer the difficulties associated with racial group membership. The older blacks from upper socioeconomic status groups will show continued health deficits and older blacks in lower socioeconomic positions will show continued poorer health outcomes. These differences should be much less prominent in younger age groups which thus may show no appreciable differences when socioeconomic controls are applied at either upper or lower status levels. Geronimus (1991) has proposed a related notion (weathering theory) to account for why younger teen mothers among African Americans may have better birthing and post-partum health experiences than relatively older teen mothers. In addition, the weathering perspective may explain the differences in findings (Williams, 1999) in studies on socioeconomic status and health (Kaplan, 1999). The use of younger age cohorts may have been more likely to show a clear effect of socioeconomic status to eliminate health status differentials; while for the reasons outlined above, the use of older age groups may have been much less effective. The impact of aging and socioeconomic status on the health of black Americans raises a number of intriguing questions and requires additional research (Adler & Ostrove, 1999).

Race-Relevant Risks and Coping Mechanisms and the Health of Aging Blacks

A growing number of researchers have explored the nature of the reactions of blacks to their unequal status in the United States (Brown, Sellers, & Gomez, 2002; Neighbors, Njai, & Jackson, 2007; Sellers & Neighbors, 2008). Specifically, this research has addressed the question of how structural disadvantages are translated at different points in the individual and group life courses into physical and mental health outcomes. This work has focused on such things as self-esteem, personal efficacy, close personal and social relationships, neighborhood, church and family integration, political participation, group solidarity, and physical and mental health (Gibson & Jackson 1992; Neighbors et al., 2007).

A unifying theme in this research is that contemporary cohorts of blacks being born today are at considerable risk. There are economic, political, social, and psychological costs of life among blacks in the United States—lack of perceived control, discouragement, and discrimination that sap energy and thwart aspirations and expectations of a successful life (Sellers & Neighbors, 2008; Williams & Williams-Morris, 2000). When the barriers to educational and occupational mobility and the high probability of exposure to environmental risk factors are considered (Berkman & Mullen, 1997), the early health morbidity, disability, and excess mortality of older black Americans become understandable (LaVeist, 2000; Miles, 1999; Williams & Rucker, 2000).

Yet, older age among blacks does not have to be a time of inevitable poor health (Jackson, 1993; Manton & Stallard, 1997; Rowe, 1985; Smith & Kington, 1997b). Changes in lifestyle, environmental risk reduction, and medical interventions can have positive influences on the quantity and quality of life among middle-aged and older black adults (Williams & Rucker, 2000). Health care has improved significantly for middle-aged and older black adults and consecutive cohorts are better educated and better able to take advantage of available opportunities. Yet, without extensive environmental intervention, it is highly likely that a significant proportion of older black adults of the mid-twenty-first century, born in the mid- to late twentieth century, are at severe risk for impoverished conditions, and poor social, physical, and psychological health in older age. This poor prognosis is predicated less on biological dimensions of racial differences (Neel, 1997) than on the physical, social, psychological, and environmental risk factors correlated with racial and ethnic group membership in the United States (Berkman & Mullen, 1997; Dressler & Bindon, 2000).

One wonders how, in the face of severe structural, social, and psychological constraints, older black Americans do as well as they do. Survey data (for example, Gibson & Jackson, 1987, 1992; Manton & Stallard, 1997) show that many older blacks are free from functional disability and limitations of activity due to chronic illness and disease. Studies that address the coping skills, capacity, and adaptability of blacks in the United States at different points in the life course are particularly important (Jackson, 1991). Over the individual life course blacks may utilize different mechanisms from whites to maintain levels of productivity, physical and mental health, and effective functioning (Williams & Williams-Morris, 2000).

One race-relevant adaptive mechanism may be the use of a system-blame psychological orientation. In the face of significant and severe structural barriers, a cognitive orientation to life that stresses the existence of systematic, systemic blockages to upward mobility may be very important among blacks in understanding why hard work and prodigious individual efforts do not lead to positive outcomes (Sellers & Neighbors, 2008). This perspective, sometimes labeled a fatalistic view, may be even more important at the upper end of the individual life course as both blacks and whites have to come to grips with the failures and missed opportunities of their lives. A coping orientation that employs reasonably accurate assessments of environmental constraints can lead to external attributions of failure and can protect blacks from some of the life disappointments (Neighbors et al., 2007; Williams & Williams-Morris, 2000). This coping strategy may be particularly effective for understanding failure due to racism and discrimination.

Another possible protective mechanism may be the sense of collectivity or group identity and consciousness that places the good of the group on an equal or greater priority status than the good of the self. Thus, even though individual mobility and achievement may not be great, concerns about the group may serve as an important filter for interpreting one's own contributions.

Religious orientation and spirituality seems to serve a similar role for blacks. Recent research suggests that African Americans and black Caribbeans, more than non-Hispanic whites, report higher levels of spirituality (Taylor, Chatters, & Jackson, 2009). Additional studies highlight that organizational, nonorganizational and subjective religious participation are all very high within the black community in the United States, although the levels of such participation differ across gender, marital status, income level, region of residence, and nativity (Taylor, Chatters, & Jackson, 2007a, 2007b). Religion and spirituality might operate as part of a group "world view" that provides a guiding set of values for life and a key coping strategy to deal with the many stresses involved in day-to-day living (Chatters, Taylor, Bullard et al., 2008; Chatters, Taylor, Jackson, et al., 2008). Future research on aging blacks would do well to investigate race-specific coping mechanisms as strategies for maintaining health and well-being.

EMERGING ISSUES IN THE HEALTH OF AGING BLACKS

Four areas are of emerging importance in the study of health among aging blacks in the United States: diversity, the changing context of health care, changes in family structure, and the increasing role of genetics. We believe that one of the key areas deserving increased research and intervention focus in the coming years is the diversity within the population of aging blacks in the United States (Jackson & Antonucci,

2005; Jackson et al., 2007). The increasing diversity along lines of nativity, immigrant ancestry, sex, and age suggests that more nuanced investigation is needed to provide appropriate and meaningful health research and service to the aging. This heterogeneity is intertwined with categorical group membership and experience of racial discrimination. Blacks in the United States vary widely in the nature of their cultural beliefs and health and family practices. However, we believe that there are common themes (Jackson, 2000). These themes include widespread community respect for elders, cultural concerns about family versus institutional sources of care, and an over riding set of expectations regarding the need for respectful delivery of health care to elders.

Related to the burgeoning significance of diversity in research on the health of older blacks, the shifting role of the concept of racial categorization in studying health disparities and inequalities needs more attention. There is a significant body of literature on the use of race and ethnicity as variables in health research (see, for example, Dressler, Oths, & Gravlee, 2005; LaVeist, 2002; Lillie-Blanton & Hudman, 2001). There is also increasing research suggesting the complex ways in which ethnic minority status and health disparities are associated in general, and specifically in the health of aging persons (see, for example, Anderson et al., 2004; Thomas, 2002). Though some genetic and biological factors may vary with the categorization of peoples of African descent (for example, sickle cell anemia, hypertension, lupus), conditions that are largely associated with, though not restricted to, being black in the United States (residential segregation, concentrated poverty, racial discrimination, a lack of access to proper health care) are intricately tied to health disparities that disadvantage blacks. The conditions under which race, ethnicity, and socioeconomic factors may serve as important risk factors and resources in the coping processes and adaptation of blacks in the United States to their environmentally disadvantaged circumstances therefore need to be integrated into models of health and aging (Dressler, 1985, 1991; Wilkinson & King, 1987). Yet, it is also important to examine the contributory role of sociocultural factors to health behaviors within racial and ethnic groups. It is possible that the most important race effects, if they do occur, are probably in the form of interactions with other ethnic, structural, or cultural factors (for example, religion, socioeconomic status, and world views) (Jackson & Antonucci, 2005; Jackson, 2000; Markides, Liang, & Jackson, 1990). Thus, we believe that the development of more encompassing models of aging-related processes is best accomplished by understanding the ways in which ethnicity, culture, and race may contribute to the aging process and service delivery (e.g., Jackson et al., 2007).

Another emerging issue is the changing health care context. It appears that the retirement process may be different for blacks than for whites (Brown, Jackson, & Faison, 2006; Jackson & Sellers, 1996). In contrast to inadequate jobs in the regular labor market, retirement for older blacks may provide a small but secure government income, leading to increased material, psychological, and social well-being (Brown et al., 2006; Chadiha, Brown, & Aranda, 2006). Older black adults are more dependent than whites on government-provided health care resources because their lower earnings and job instability have made many ineligible for private pension plans, made it nearly impossible for them to accumulate personal savings, and made them eligible only for reduced levels of government support. New cohorts of black older adults may find it increasingly difficult to meet rising health care costs due to greater restrictions on public programs and the increased privatization of health care delivery systems.

Changing roles within families is a concern that will impact aging among blacks in the United States in the coming decades. An increasing proportion of grandparents are providing care for grandchildren (Fields, 2003; Harris & Skyles, 2008; Minkler & Fuller-Thomson, 2001). These responsibilities impact the physical and mental health of the caregivers (Hayslip, Shore, Henderson, & Lambert, 1998; Kelch-Oliver, 2008; Leder, Grinstead, & Torres, 2007), often because of the stress involved in child care a second time around (Blustein, Chan, & Guanais, 2004). Recent research suggests that this phenomenon is disproportionately present in the black community in the United States, with the responsibility often falling on the shoulders of aging black women to provide custodial or informal care for grandchildren (Minkler & Fuller-Thomson, 2005). The potential reasons for these arrangements are numerous, ranging from the inability of the parents to secure adequate child care from other avenues, to the high levels of the incarceration of black men. Whatever the reason, the health of aging blacks, especially aging black women, is often compromised (Blustein et al., 2004). Although there are also potential positive health effects of these added responsibilities, often the detrimental effects surpass any benefits for the caretakers. Future research needs to examine the antecedents of this phenomenon and strategies that may buffer the negative health outcomes associated with these scenarios.

Black families, like many other ethnic groups, are becoming increasingly diverse. These changing family structures will undoubtedly impact the understanding of aging with of blacks in the United States. For example, gay and lesbian aging persons are a burgeoning area of study. There has been very limited focus on non-heterosexual aging persons within the black community (Black, Gates, Sanders, & Taylor, 2000; Smith & Gates, 2001; Allen, 2005). Because of the historical stigma attached to these identity statuses within the black community, more attention will need to be paid to these populations and to how discrimination from those both outside and within the ethnic community is associated with health outcomes.

Finally, there is emerging social and scientific research related to assessing the complex relationships between race, ancestral origin, and the genetic components of diseases. Though the application of genomic information to address common diseases is still in its infancy, the use of race as a surrogate marker for describing human genetic variation and to conduct gene expression analysis is becoming common (Bamshad 2005; Carey et al., 2006; Reiner et al., 2005). This reemergence of race in the biological conceptualization of health has been subject to considerable debate (Krieger, 2005). The dangers of conflating race and genetic differences have concerned sociologists, clinicians, and the lay public (Bonham et al., 2009; Frank, 2007). We believe that though some genetic and biological factors may vary with the categorization of peoples of African descent, the more fundamental nature of being black in the United States derives from both self- and other-definitions and continuing discrimination and maltreatment (Cooper, 1984; Dressler & Bindon, 2000; Neel, 1997). Thus, although the genomic era may be a time of great promise for developing new diagnostics tools and drug therapies, the challenge will be to ensure that these advances will be used to improve the health and well-being of all people, regardless of their racial identity.

SUMMARY AND CONCLUSION

The life course of blacks in the United States, perhaps more so than in the majority population, highlights the continuities and discontinuities of a life-span perspective on health. From birth to death, blacks are at greater risk for debilitating social, psychological, and physical conditions that negatively influence the quality of individual and family life and, in many instances, result in "premature" death—greater fetal death rates, greater homicide statistics in adolescence and midlife, and greater risk of death from chronic health conditions early in old age (Miles, 1999; Smith & Kington, 1997b). However, all blacks are not born into such circumstances. Though people argue over its relative proportions, a black middle class exists and some blacks in the United States can look forward to relatively comfortable styles of living over their life courses (Farley, 2000). It is likely that a growing, but still small, group of older blacks will have adequate pensions and financial resources in older age; it is just that this proportion, though larger than in prior years and cohorts, still will be relatively small in comparison to the proportion of older whites in the United States who enjoy these statuses (Friedland & Summer, 2005).

Even with economic and social resources, the pernicious nature of racial discrimination and other structural barriers can negatively influence the aspirations and expectations of youth and young adults—aspirations and expectations that the majority assume as a given right of citizenship (Jackson, 2000). The often-portrayed success stories of black Americans in sports, the arts, and entertainment are exceptions to the working-class, near poverty, and poverty existence of a large proportion of blacks (Jackson, 2000), especially older blacks (Siegel, 1999). Numerous writers have theorized about how responding to the stress of blocked opportunities can affect the well-being of blacks in the United States and a few studies have found associations between aspirations, achievements, and health (Guyll, Matthews, & Bromberger, 2001; Harrell, Hall, & Taliaferro, 2003; Sellers & Neighbors, 2008). These studies hint at potential cohort differences that have yet to be explored.

A life-course perspective suggests the need to consider human development, historical context, and structural position as factors that influence the health of present and future cohorts of aging blacks. Different birth cohorts, historical and current environmental events, and individual differences in developmental and aging processes interact with one another to affect physical and mental health. One of the ways in which this intersectionality is most manifest in the health of aging blacks is in the differences that men and women experience in health outcomes and in the pathways to these outcomes. Racial group membership plays an important part in the health of these elders; cultural resources provide important coping and adaptive mechanisms in alleviating the distinct socioeconomic and psychological disadvantages of categorical racial membership (Jackson, 1993; Williams & Williams-Morris, 2000). The unique social history and the nature of their group and individual developmental experiences all serve to place new elderly cohorts of black Americans from birth to death at disproportionate risk for poor physical and mental health (LaVeist, 2000). Yet, older age among both the general population and that of blacks in the United States is not a time of inevitable and irreversible decline. Removal of known environmental risk factors, and social and medical interventions, can improve the quality of life in the latter stages of the life course (Riley & Riley, 1994; Rowe & Kahn, 1987).

The development of better national health policies—policies that are responsive to life-course considerations and realities of family life in the United States—is essential if we are to improve the health of black American populations, especially older black adults. Individual efforts are not enough to improve the health of aging blacks. Unfortunately, we can predict what the most likely life experiences will be for a sizeable proportion of coming elderly blacks in the United States (Jackson, 2000). Without significant intervention, the health future of older black Americans is clear and it is dismal (Richardson, 1996). Thankfully, there currently exist several interventions, such as the U.S. government's Healthy People 2010 program, to increase quality and years of life and eliminate health disparities, and the Racial and Ethnic Approaches to Community Health program (REACH 2010), which focuses on community-based coalitions to develop strategies that eliminate or reduce health disparities. As programs such as Healthy People 2010 and REACH 2010 suggest, the urgent need to change factors related to the health of future cohorts of black middle-aged and elderly persons can be addressed when research and interventions move in tandem.

REFERENCES

Adelman, L. (Creator and Executive Producer) (2008). Unnatural causes: Is inequality making us sick? In L. Adelman, L. M. Smith, & C. Herbes-Sommers (Producer). USA: California Newsreel.

Adler, N. E., & Ostrove, J. M. (1999). Socioeconomic status and health: What we know and what we don't. *Annals of the New York Academy of Sciences, 896* (December), 3–15.

Adler, N. E., & Rehkopf, D. H. (2008). U.S. disparities in health: Descriptions, causes, and mechanisms. *Annual Review of Public Health, 29*(1), 235–252.

Allen, K. R. (2005). Gay and lesbian elders. In M. L. Johnson, V. L. Bengtson, P. G. Coleman, & T. B. L. Kirkwood (Eds.), *The Cambridge handbook of age and ageing* (pp. 482–493). New York: Cambridge University Press.

Alzheimer's Association. (2008). *Alzheimer's disease: Facts and figures.* Chicago: Alzheimer's Association National Office.

Anderson, N. B., Bulatao, R. A., & Cohen, B. (Eds.). (2004). *Critical perspectives on racial and ethnic differences in health in late life.* Washington, DC: The National Academies Press.

Angel, J. L., & Hogan, D. P. (2004). Population aging and diversity in a new era. In K. E. Whitfield (Ed.), *Closing the gap: Improving the health of minority elders in the new millennium* (pp. 1–12). Washington, DC: The Gerontological Society of America.

Austin, A. (2008b). Subprime mortgages are nearly double for Hispanics and African Americans. *Economic Policy Institute Snapshot for June 11, 2008.* Retrieved February 2, 2009, from http://www.epi.org/economic_snapshots/entry/webfeatures_snapshots_20080611/

Austin, A. (2008a). What a recession means for black America. *Economic Policy Institute Issue Brief, #241* (January 18).

Baltes, P. B. (1987). Theoretical propositions of life-span developmental psychology: On the dynamics between growth and decline. *Developmental Psychology, 23*(5), 611–626.

Bamshad, M. (2005). Genetic influences on health: Does race matter? *The Journal of the American Medical Association, 294*(8), 937–946.

Baquet, C., & Ringen, K. (1987). Health policy: Gaps in access, delivery, and utilization of the pap smear in the United States. *The Milbank Quarterly, 65,* 322–347.

Barresi, C. M. (1987). Ethnic aging and the life course. In D. E. Gelfand & C. M. Barresi (Eds.), *Ethnic dimensions of aging* (pp. 18–34). New York: Springer.

Berkman, L. F., & Mullen, J. M. (1997). How health behaviors and the social environment contribute to health differences between black and white older Americans. In L. G. Martin & B. J. Soldo (Eds.), *Racial and ethnic differences in the health of older Americans* (pp. 163–182). Washington, DC: The National Academies Press.

Black, D., Gates, G., Sanders, S., & Taylor, L. (2000). Demographics of the gay and lesbian population in the United States: Evidence from available systematic data sources. *Demography, 37*(2), 139–154.

Blustein, J., Chan, S., & Guanais, F. C. (2004). Elevated depressive symptoms among caregiving grandparents. *Health Services Research, 39*(6), 1671–1689.

Bonham, V., Sellers, S. L., Cooper, L., Odunlami, A., Frank, D., Gallagher, T., et al. 2009. Physicians' attitudes toward race, genetics and clinical medicine. *Genetics in Medicine, 11*(4), 1–8.

Bowles, J., & Kington, R. S. (1998). The impact of family function on health of African American elderly. *Journal of Comparative Family Studies, 29*(2), 337–347.

Brogden, M., & Nijhar, P. (2000). *Crime, abuse and the elderly.* Portland, OR: Willan Publishing.

Brown, D. R., Milburn, N. G., & Gary, L. E. (1992). Symptoms of depression among older African-Americans: An analysis of gender differences. *The Gerontologist, 32*(6), 789–795.

Brown, E., Jackson, J. S., & Faison, N. A. (2006). The work and retirement experiences of aging black Americans. *Annual Review of Gerontology and Geriatrics: The crown of life: Dynamics of the early postretirement period, 26,* 39–60.

Brown, T. N., Sellers, S. L., & Gomez, J. P. (2002). The relationship between internalization and self-esteem among black adults. *Sociological Focus, 35*(1), 55–71.

Bulatao, R. A., & Anderson, N. B. (2004). *Understanding racial and ethnic differences in health in late life: A research agenda.* Washington, DC: The National Academies Press.

Burton, L. M., Dilworth-Anderson, P., & Bengtson, V. L. (1991). Creating culturally relevant ways of thinking about diversity: Theoretical challenges for the twenty-first century. *Generations: Journal of the American Society on Aging, 15,* 67–71.

Butrica, B. A. (2008). Do assets change the racial profile of poverty among older adults? *The Urban Institute Opportunity and Ownership Facts Newsletter, 8,* 1.

Cannuscio, C. C., Colditz, G. A., Rimm, E. B., Berkman, L. F., Jones, C. P., & Kawachi, I. (2004). Employment status, social ties, and caregivers' mental health. *Social Science & Medicine, 58*(7), 1247–1256.

Cannuscio, C. C., Jones, C. P., Kawachi, I., Colditz, G. A., Berkman, L. F., & Rimm, E. B. (2002). Reverberations of family illness: A longitudinal assessment of informal caregiving and mental health status in the Nurses' Health Study. *American Journal of Public Health, 92*(8), 1305–1311.

Carey, L. A., Perou, C. M., Livasy, C. A., Dressler, L. G., Cowan, D., Conway, K., et al. (2006). Race, breast cancer subtypes, and survival in the Carolina Breast Cancer Study. *The Journal of the American Medical Association, 295*(21), 2492–2502.

Chadiha, L. A., Brown, E., & Aranda, M. P. (2006). Older African Americans and other black populations. In B. Berkman & S. Ambruoso (Eds.), *Handbook of social work in health and aging* (pp. 247–256). New York: Oxford University Press.

Chatters, L. M., Taylor, R. J., Bullard, K. M., & Jackson, J. S. (2008). Spirituality and subjective religiosity among African Americans, Caribbean Blacks, and non-Hispanic Whites. *Journal for the Scientific Study of Religion, 47*(4), 725–737.

Chatters, L. M., Taylor, R. J., Jackson, J. S., & Lincoln, K. D. (2008). Religious coping among African Americans, Caribbean Blacks and non-Hispanic Whites. *Journal of Community Psychology, 36*(3), 371–386.

Cook, J. M., Black, B. S., Rabins, P. V., & German, P. (2000). Life satisfaction and symptoms of mental disorder among older African American public housing residents. *Journal of Clinical Geropsychology, 6*(1), 1–14.

Cooper, R. (1984). A note on the biologic concept of race and its application in epidemiologic research. *American Heart Journal, 108*(3, Part 2), 715–723.

Cooper, R. S., Steinhauer, M., Miller, W., David, R., & Schatzkin, A. (1981). Racism, society and disease: An exploration of the social and biological mechanisms of differential mortality. *International Journal of Health Services, 11*(3), 389–414.

Crimmins, E. M., Hayward, M. D., & Seeman, T. (2004). Race/ethnicity, socioeconomic status and health. In N. B. Anderson, R. A. Bulatao, & B. Cohen (Eds.), *Critical perspectives on racial and ethnic differences in health in later life* (pp. 310–352). Washington, DC: The National Academies Press.

Darity, W., Jr. (2005). Stratification economics: The role of intergroup inequality. *Journal of Economics and Finance, 29*(2), 144–153.

Darity, W., Jr., Dietrich, J., & Guilkey, D. K. (2001). Persistent advantage or disadvantage?: Evidence in support of the intergenerational drag hypothesis. *American Journal of Economics and Sociology, 60*(2), 435–470.

Dressler, W. W. (1985). Extended family relationships, social support, and mental health in a southern black community. *Journal of Health and Social Behavior, 26*(1), 39–48.

Dressler, W. W. (1991). Social class, skin color, and arterial blood pressure in two societies. *Ethnicity & Disease, 1*(1), 60–77.

Dressler, W. W., & Bindon, J. R. (2000). The health consequences of cultural consonance: Cultural dimensions of lifestyle, social support, and arterial blood pressure in an African American community. *American Anthropologist, 102*(2), 244–260.

Dressler, W. W., Oths, K. S., & Gravlee, C. C. (2005). Race and ethnicity in public health research: Models to explain health disparities. *Annual Review of Anthropology, 34*(1), 231–252.

Farley, R. (1987). The quality of life for Black Americans twenty years after the Civil Rights Revolution. *The Milbank Quarterly, 65*, 9–34.

Farley, R. (2000). Demographic, economic, and social trends in a multicultural America. In J. S. Jackson (Ed.), *New directions: African Americans in a diversifying nation* (pp. 11–44). Washington, DC: National Policy Association.

Federal Interagency Forum on Aging-Related Statistics. (2008). *Older Americans 2008: Key indicators of well-being*. Washington, DC: Government Printing Office.

Fields, J. (2003). Children's living arrangements and characteristics: March 2002. In *Current Population Reports, P20–547*. Washington, DC: U.S. Census Bureau.

Frank, R. (2007). What to make of it? The (re)emergence of a biological conceptualization of race in health disparities research. *Social Science & Medicine, 64*(10), 1977–1983.

Friedland, R. B., & Summer, L. (2005). *Demography is not destiny, revisited*. Washington, DC: Center on an Aging Society, Georgetown University.

Geerling, M. I., den Heijer, T., Koudstaal, P. J., Hofman, A., & Breteler, M. M. B. (2008). History of depression, depressive symptoms, and medial temporal lobe atrophy and the risk of Alzheimer disease. *Neurology, 70*(April), 1250–1264.

Geronimus, A. T. (1991). Teenage childbearing and social and reproductive disadvantage: The evolution of complex questions and the demise of simple answers. *Family Relations, 40*(4), 463–471.

Gibson, R. C., & Jackson, J. S. (1987). The health, physical functioning, and informal supports of the black elderly. *The Milbank Quarterly, 65*, 421–454.

Gibson, R. C., & Jackson, J. S. (1992). The black oldest old: Health, functioning, and informal support. In R. M. Suzman, D. P. Willis, & K. G. Manton (Eds.), *The oldest old* (pp. 321–340). New York: Oxford University Press.

Guyll, M., Matthews, K. A., & Bromberger, J. T. (2001). Discrimination and unfair treatment: Relationship to cardiovascular reactivity among African American and European American women. *Health Psychology, 20*(5), 315–325.

Harrell, J. P., Hall, S., & Taliaferro, J. (2003). Physiological responses to racism and discrimination: An assessment of the evidence. *American Journal of Public Health, 93*(2), 243–248.

Harris, M. S., & Skyles, A. (2008). Kinship care for African American children: Disproportionate and disadvantageous. *Journal of Family Issues, 29*(8), 1013–1030.

Hayslip, B., Jr., Shore, R. J., Henderson, C. E., & Lambert, P. L. (1998). Custodial grandparenting and the impact of grandchildren with problems on role satisfaction and role meaning. *Journals of Gerontology Series B Psychological Sciences and Social Sciences, 53B*(3), S164–173.

Hayward, M. D., Crimmins, E. M., Miles, T. P., & Yang, Y. (2000). The significance of socioeconomic status in explaining the racial gap in chronic health conditions. *American Sociological Review, 65*(6), 910–930.

Hochschild, J. L. (1995). *Facing up to the American dream: Race, class, and the soul of the nation*. Princeton: Princeton University Press.

Huguet, N., Kaplan, M. S., & Feeny, D. (2008). Socioeconomic status and health-related quality of life among elderly people: Results from the Joint Canada/United States Survey of Health. *Social Science & Medicine, 66*(4), 803–810.

Jackson, J. S. (1981). Urban black Americans. In A. Harwood (Ed.), *Ethnicity and medical care* (pp. 37–129). Cambridge, MA: Harvard University Press.

Jackson, J. S. (Ed.). (1991). *Life in black America*. Newbury Park, CA: Sage Publications.

Jackson, J. S. (1993). Racial influences on adult development and aging. In R. Kastenbaum (Ed.), *The encyclopedia of adult development* (pp. 18–26). Phoenix, AZ: Oryx Press.

Jackson, J. S. (Ed.). (2000). *New directions: African Americans in a diversifying nation*. Washington, DC: National Policy Association.

Jackson, J. S., & Antonucci, T. C. (2005). Physical and mental health consequences of aging in place and aging out of place among black Caribbean immigrants. *Research in Human Development, 2*(4), 229–244.

Jackson, J. S., Antonucci, T. C., & Gibson, R. C. (1990a). Cultural, racial, and ethnic minority influences on aging. In J. E. Birren & K. W. Schaie (Eds.), *Handbook of the psychology of aging* (3rd ed., pp. 103–123). San Diego: Academic Press.

Jackson, J. S., Antonucci, T. C., & Gibson, R. C. (1990b). Social relations, productive activities, and coping with stress in late life. In M. A. P. Stephens, J. H. Crowther, S. E. Hobfoll, & D. L. Tennenbaum (Eds.), *Stress and coping in later-life families* (pp. 193–212). Washington, DC: Hemisphere Publishing Corp.

Jackson, J. S., Forsythe-Brown, I., & Govia, I. O. (2007). Age cohort, ancestry, and immigrant generation influences in family relations and psychological well-being among Black Caribbean family members. *Journal of Social Issues, 63*(4), 729–743.

Jackson, J. S., & Sellers, S. L. (1996). African-American health over the life course: A multidimensional framework. In P. M. Kato & T. Mann (Eds.), *Handbook of diversity issues in health psychology* (pp. 301–317). New York, NY: Plenum Press.

Jackson, J. S., Torres, M., Caldwell, C. H., Neighbors, H. W., Nesse, R. M., Taylor, R. J., et al. (2004). The National Survey of American Life: A study of racial, ethnic and cultural influences on mental disorders and mental health. *International Journal of Methods in Psychiatric Research, 13*(4), 196–207.

Johnson, L. B., & Staples, R. (2005). *Black families at the crossroads: Challenges and prospects*. San Francisco: Jossey-Bass.

Kahn, J. R., & Fazio, E. M. (2005). Economic status over the life course and racial disparities in health. *Journal of Gerontology Series B Psychological Sciences and Social Sciences, 60*(Supplement Special Issue 2), S76–84.

Kaplan, G. A. (1999). Part III Summary: What is the role of the social environment in understanding inequalities in health? *Annals of the New York Academy of Sciences, 896* (Socioeconomic status and health in industrial nations: Social, psychological, and biological pathways), pp. 116–119.

Kelch-Oliver, K. (2008). African American grandparent caregivers: Stresses and implications for counselors. *The Family Journal, 16*(1), 43–50.

Kessler, R. C., & Neighbors, H. W. (1986). A new perspective on the relationships among race, social class, and psychological distress. *Journal of Health and Social Behavior, 27*(2), 107–115.

Krieger, N. (2005). Stormy weather: Race, gene expression, and the science of health disparities. *American Journals of Public Health, 95*(12), 2155–2160.

LaVeist, T. A. (2000). African Americans and health policy: Strategies for a multiethnic society. In J. S. Jackson (Ed.), *New directions: African Americans in a diversifying nation* (pp. 144–161). Washington, DC: National Policy Association.

LaVeist, T. A. (2002). *Race, ethnicity, and health: A public health reader*. San Francisco: Jossey-Bass.

Leder, S., Grinstead, L. N., & Torres, E. (2007). Grandparents raising grandchildren: Stressors, social support, and health outcomes. *Journal of Family Nursing, 13*(3), 333–352.

Levy, F. (1998). *The new dollars and dreams: American incomes and economic change*. New York: Russell Sage Foundation.

Lillie-Blanton, M., & Hudman, J. (2001). Untangling the web: Race/ethnicity, immigration, and the nation's health. *American Journal of Public Health, 91*(11), 1736–1738.

Manton, K. G., & Soldo, B. J. (1985). Dynamics of health changes in the oldest old: New perspectives and evidence. *The Milbank Memorial Fund Quarterly. Health and Society, 63*(2), 206–285.

Manton, K. G., & Stallard, E. (1997). Health and disability differences among racial and ethnic groups. In L. G. Martin & B. J. Soldo (Eds.), *Racial and ethnic differences in the health of older Americans* (pp. 43–104). Washington, DC: The National Academies Press.

Markides, K. S., Liang, J., & Jackson, J. S. (1990). Race, ethnicity, and aging: Conceptual and methodological issues. In R. H. Binstock & L. K. George (Eds.), *Handbook of aging and the social sciences* (pp. 112–129). San Diego: Academic Press.

Massey, D. S. (2007). *Categorically unequal: The American stratification system*. New York: Russell Sage Foundation.

McEwen, B. S., & Seeman, T. (1999). Protective and damaging effects of mediators of stress: Elaborating and testing the concepts of allostasis and allostatic load. *Annals of the New York Academy of Sciences, 896* (Socioeconomic status and health in industrial nations: Social, psychological, and biological pathways), pp. 30–47.

Miles, T. P. (Ed.). (1999). *Full-color aging: Facts, goals, and recommendations for America's diverse elders*. Washington, DC: The Gerontological Society of America.

Mills, T. L., & Edwards, C. D. A. (2002). A critical review of research on the mental health status of older African-Americans. *Aging & Society, 22*(3), 273–304.

Minkler, M., & Fuller-Thomson, E. (2001). Physical and mental health status of American grandparents providing extensive child care to their grandchildren. *Journal of the American Medical Women's Association, 56*(Fall), 199–205.

Minkler, M., & Fuller-Thomson, E. (2005). African American grandparents raising grandchildren: A national study using the Census 2000 American Community Survey. *Journals of Gerontology Series B Psychological Sciences and Social Sciences, 60*(2), S82–92.

Muhammad, D., Davis, A., Lui, M., & Leondar-Wright, B. (2004). *State of the dream 2004: Enduring disparities in black and white*. Boston: United for a Fair Economy.

National Center for Health Statistics (NCHS) (2007, November). *Health, United States, 2007*. Hyattsville, MD: Public Health Service.

Neel, J. V. (1997). Are genetic factors involved in racial and ethnic differences in late-life health? In L. G. Martin & B. J. Soldo (Eds.), *Racial and ethnic differences in the health of older Americans* (pp. 210–232). Washington, DC: The National Academies Press.

Neighbors, H. W., Njai, R., & Jackson, J. S. (2007). Race, ethnicity, John Henryism, and depressive symptoms: The national survey of American life adult reinterview. *Research in Human Development, 4*(1), 71–87.

Office of Minority Health and Health Disparities. (2008). Black or African American populations. Retrieved December 4, 2008, from http://www.cdc.gov/omhd/Populations/BAA/BAA.htm

Reiner, A. P., Ziv, E., Lind, D. L., Nievergelt, C. M., Schork, N. J., Cummings, S. R., et al. (2005). Population structure, admixture, and aging-related phenotypes in African American adults: The Cardiovascular Health Study. *The American Journal of Human Genetics, 76*(3), 463–477.

Richardson, J. (1996). *Aging and health: Black American elders (Stanford Geriatric Education Center Working Paper Series, Number 4)* (2 ed.). Stanford, CA: Stanford Geriatric Education Center (SGEC), Division of Family & Community Medicine, Stanford University.

Riley, M. W., & Riley, J. W., Jr. (1994). Age integration and the lives of older people. *Gerontologist, 34*(1), 110–115.

Rivera, A., Cotto-Escalera, B., Desai, A., Huezo, J., & Muhammad, D. (2008). *Foreclosed: State of the dream 2008*. Boston: United for a Fair Economy.

Rowe, J. W. (1985). Health care of the elderly. *New England Journal of Medicine, 312*(13), 827–835.

Rowe, J. W., & Kahn, R. L. (1987). Human aging: Usual and successful. *Science, 237*(4811), 143–149.

Sellers, S. L., & Neighbors, H. W. (2008). Effects of goal-striving stress on the mental health of Black Americans. *Journal of Health and Social Behavior, 49*(1), 92–103.

Shuey, K. M., & Willson, A. E. (2008). Cumulative disadvantage and Black-White disparities in life-course health trajectories. *Research on Aging, 30*(2), 200–225.

Siegel, J. S. (1999). Demographic introduction to racial/Hispanic elderly populations. In T. P. Miles (Ed.), *Full-color aging: Facts, goals, and recommendations for America's diverse elderly* (pp. 1–19). Washington, DC: The Gerontological Society of America.

Skarupski, K. A., Mendes de Leon, C. F., Bienias, J. L., Barnes, L. L., Everson-Rose, S. A., Wilson, R. S., et al. (2005). Black-White differences in depressive symptoms among older adults over time. *Journals of Gerontology Series B Psychological Sciences and Social Sciences, 60*(3), P136–142.

Smith, D. M., & Gates, G. J. (2001). *Gay and lesbian families in the United States: Same-sex unmarried partner households: A Preliminary analysis of the 2000 United States census data*. Washington, DC: Human Rights Campaign Report.

Smith, J. P. (2004). Unraveling the SES-health connection. *Population and Development Review, 30* (Supplement on Aging, Health, and Public Policy), pp. 108–132.

Smith, J. P., & Kington, R. (1997a). Demographic and economic correlates of health in old age. *Demography, 34*(1), 159–170.

Smith, J. P., & Kington, R. (1997b). Race, socioeconomic status, and health in late life. In L. G. Martin & B. J. Soldo (Eds.), *Racial and ethnic differences in the health of older Americans* (pp. 105–162). Washington, DC: The National Academies Press.

Taylor, R. J., Chatters, L. M., & Jackson, J. S. (2007a). Religious and spiritual involvement among older African Americans, Caribbean blacks, and non-Hispanic whites: Findings from the national survey of American life. *Journals of Gerontology Series B Psychological Sciences and Social Sciences, 62*(4), S238–S250.

Taylor, R. J., Chatters, L. M., & Jackson, J. S. (2007b). Religious participation among older black Caribbeans in the United States. *Journals of Gerontology Series B Psychological Sciences and Social Sciences, 62*(4), S251–S256.

Taylor, R. J., Chatters, L. M., & Jackson, J. S. (2009). Correlates of spirituality among African Americans and Caribbean Blacks in the United States: Findings from the National Survey of American Life. *Journal of Black Psychology, 35*(3), 317–342.

Theis, K. A., Helmick, C. G., & Hootman, J. M. (2007). Arthritis burden and impact are greater among U.S. women than men: Intervention opportunities. *Journal of Women's Health, 16*(4), 441–453.

Thomas, N. M. (2002). Revisiting race/ethnicity as a variable in health research. *American Journal of Public Health, 92*(2), 156.

Thorpe, R. J., Jr., Kasper, J. D., Szanton, S. L., Frick, K. D., Fried, L. P., & Simonsick, E. M. (2008). Relationship of race and poverty to lower extremity function and decline: Findings from the Women's Health and Aging Study. *Social Science & Medicine, 66*(4), 811–821.

Tucker, M. B. (2000). Considerations in the development of family policy for African Americans. In J. S. Jackson (Ed.), *New directions: African Americans in a diversifying nation* (pp. 162–206). Washington, DC: National Policy Association.

Tucker, M. B., & Mitchell-Kernan, C. (1995). Trends in African American family formation: A theoretical and statistical overview. In M. B. Tucker & C. Mitchell-Kernan (Eds.), *The decline in marriage among African Americans: Causes, consequences, and policy implications* (pp. 3–26). New York: Russell Sage Foundation.

Turnbull, J. E., & Mui, A. C. (1995). Mental health status and needs of black and white elderly: Differences in depression. In D. K. Padgett (Ed.), *Handbook on ethnicity, aging, and mental health.* (pp. 73–98). Westport, CT: Greenwood Press/Greenwood Publishing Group.

United Nations. (2007). *World population ageing 2007.* New York: United Nations.

Wight, R. G., Cummings, J. R., Miller-Martinez, D., Karlamangla, A. S., Seeman, T. E., & Aneshensel, C. S. (2008). A multilevel analysis of urban neighborhood socioeconomic disadvantage and health in late life. *Social Science & Medicine, 66*(4), 862–872.

Wilkinson, D. Y., & King, G. (1987). Conceptual and methodological issues in the use of race as a variable: Policy implications. *The Milbank Quarterly, 65,* 56–71.

Williams, D. R. (1990). Socioeconomic differentials in health: A review and redirection. *Social Psychology Quarterly, 53*(2), 81–99.

Williams, D. R. (1999). Race, socioeconomic status, and health: The added effects of racism and discrimination. *Annals of the New York Academy of Sciences, 896* (Socioeconomic status and health in industrial nations: Social, psychological, and biological pathways), pp. 173–188.

Williams, D. R. (2002). Racial/ethnic variations in women's health: The social embeddedness of health. *American Journal of Public Health, 92*(4), 588–597.

Williams, D. R., & Collins, C. (1995). US socioeconomic and racial differences in health: Patterns and explanations. *Annual Review of Sociology, 21,* 349–386.

Williams, D. R., & Rucker, T. D. (2000). Understanding and addressing racial disparities in health care. *Health Care Financing Review, 21*(4), 75.

Williams, D. R., & Williams-Morris, R. (2000). Racism and mental health: The African American experience. *Ethnicity & Health, 5*(3), 243–268.

Wilson, R. S., Arnold, S. E., Beck, T. L., Bienias, J. L., & Bennett, D. A. (2008). Change in depressive symptoms during the prodromal phase of Alzheimer disease. *Archives of General Psychiatry, 65*(4), 439–445.

Winkleby, M. A., & Cubbin, C. (2004). Racial/ethnic disparities in health behaviors: A challenge to current assumptions. In N. B. Anderson, R. A. Bulatao, & B. Cohen (Eds.), *Critical perspectives on racial and ethnic differences in health in late life* (pp. 450–491). Washington, DC: The National Academies Press.

Yang, Y. (2007). Is old age depressing? Growth trajectories and cohort variations in late-life depression. *Journal of Health and Social Behavior, 48*(1), 16–32.

Yang, Y., Schulhofer-Wohl, S., Fu, W. J., & Land, K. C. (2008). The intrinsic estimator for age-period-cohort analysis: What it is and how to use it. *American Journal of Sociology, 113*(6), 1697–1736.

PART

2

SOCIAL, MENTAL, AND ENVIRONMENTAL CHALLENGES

CHAPTER

7

STIGMA AND MENTAL HEALTH IN AFRICAN AMERICANS

L. DIANNE BRADFORD
CASSANDRA NEWKIRK
KISHA BRAITHWAITE HOLDEN

Stigma is composed of unconstructive attitudes, beliefs, views, and behaviors that affect the person or society, causing fear, rejection, avoidance, prejudice, and discrimination against individuals with mental disorders. Stigma is evident in language, disregard in interpersonal relationships, and private and social behaviors (Gary, 2005). Stigma is a process that involves negative beliefs (frequently based on erroneous or incomplete knowledge), and underlies prejudice expressed as negative attitudes, which ultimately affects the community through discrimination, poor behavioral outcomes, and diminished human capital (Rüsch et al., 2005). It is informative to use a social cognitive model of stigma, as proposed by Rüsch et al. (2005, Figure 7.1), as well as a compilation of core features of Corrigan, Link, and colleagues (Corrigan et al., 2004; Link et al., 2004). Stigma encompasses both public stigma and self-stigma and, when institutionalized, stigma of mental health systems and providers *per se* (Corrigan, 2003; Corrigan et al., 2004).

Prejudice and stereotypes alone cannot account for stigma; it must be energized by social, economical, and/or political power and policies (Rüsch et al., 2005), denoted

FIGURE 7.1 *Underlying Components of Public and Self-Sigma.*

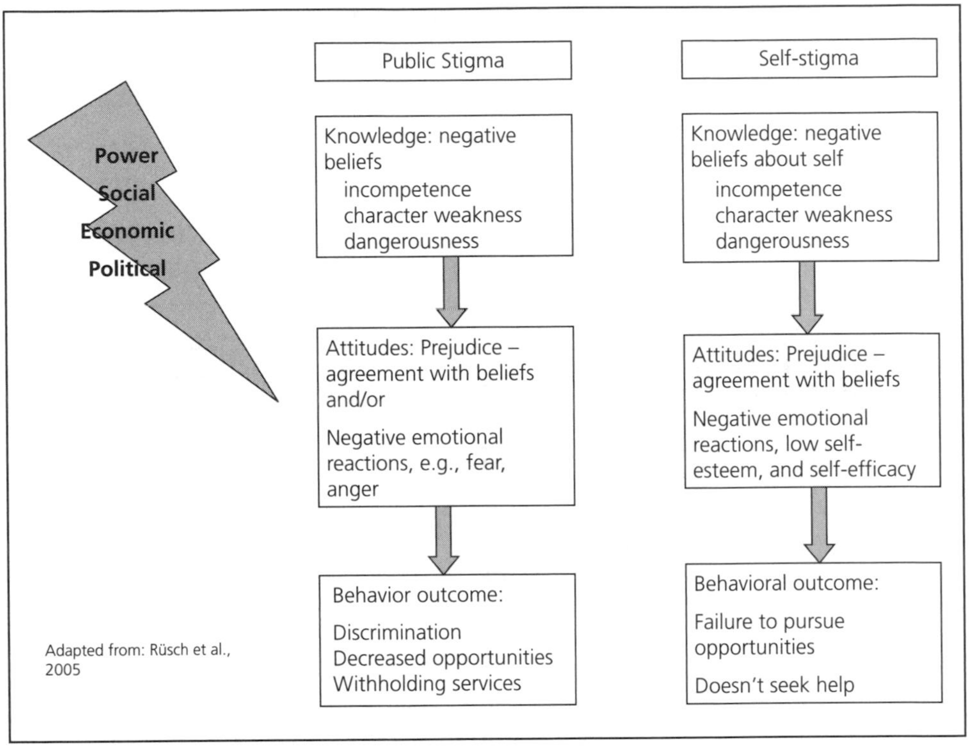

Public Stigma	Self-stigma
Knowledge: negative beliefs incompetence character weakness dangerousness	Knowledge: negative beliefs about self incompetence character weakness dangerousness
Attitudes: Prejudice – agreement with beliefs and/or Negative emotional reactions, e.g., fear, anger	Attitudes: Prejudice – agreement with beliefs Negative emotional reactions, low self-esteem, and self-efficacy
Behavior outcome: Discrimination Decreased opportunities Withholding services	Behavioral outcome: Failure to pursue opportunities Doesn't seek help

Power
Social
Economic
Political

Adapted from: Rüsch et al., 2005

as the lightning bolt in Figure 7.1. Public and self-stigma include *labeling, stereotyping, discrimination, cognitive and actual separation* (e.g., "us" vs "them"), *emotional reactions*, and *loss of status* (Link et al., 2004). Self-stigma can be a restraining influence that obstructs help-seeking behaviors (Corrigan, 2004); promotes avoidance of employment out of fear of failure (Balsa and McGuire, 2003); negatively influence one's confidence and self-esteem (Link et al., 2001; Wahl & Harman, 1989); and prompt withdrawal from interactions with the public for fear of denunciation, potentially heightening social separation, which can impact productivity and quality of life and result in diminished human capital for both consumers and their families (Bolden & Wicks, 2005; Gary, 2005; Rüsch et al., 2005; Wahl, 1999). By defining stigma by its various components—knowledge, beliefs, and attitudes—specific targets for interventions can be identified.

STIGMA AND MENTAL HEALTH

The stigmatization of mental illness is one of the chief reasons people in need of treatment do not readily seek help, or choose to postpone treatment and assistance until an emergency ensues or the disorder grows to be unbearable and incapacitating (US DHHS, 1999). From the model shown in Figure 7.1, it is apparent that the basis of stigma—both public and self—is knowledge. How do we gain knowledge about mental illness? Predominantly through the media, societal myths, and taboos about psychological problems and disorders that cause individuals to be embarrassed about, ashamed of, and uncomfortable with, their mental health status designation or label. Mental health stigma is often nurtured in the media (e.g., in movies and TV programs about killers and violent people with mental illness), sensational media coverage of tragedies perpetrated by people with severe mental illness, causal labels such as "crazy" or "psycho," and jokes about mental illness (Wahl & Harman, 1989). Media analysis of film and print in several countries, including the United States, indicates common misconceptions about the mentally ill (Rüsch et al., 2005), which sadly impacts as early as childhood and adolescence (Adler &Wahl, 1998; Dietrich, Heider, et al., 2006; Wilson et al., 2000).

In surveys and follow-up interviews with members of the families of the mentally ill and with the consumer advocacy group the National Alliance for the Mentally Ill (NAMI), public and self-stigma of mental illness were reported by consumers to damage their self-esteem, contribute to difficulties in making and keeping friends and finding a job, and force them to conceal their mental illness. Encountering public stigma is worrying and discouraging, and provokes anger in the individual consumer. The effects that stigma had on family members included lowered self-esteem and negative impact on family relationships. NAMI members also reported that factual information about the mental illness, including a biological basis for the illness, and involvement with advocacy and family support groups were helpful in dealing with the stigma, and urged public education as a method for reducing stigma (Wahl, 1999; Wahl & Harman, 1989). As a result, NAMI launched its "stigmabusters" program, which is challenging mental health representation in the media and fighting against stigma across the fifty states.

Nevertheless, research on public stigma has shown that

1. schizophrenia (88% of the time) and major depressive disorder (69%) are frequently "labeled" as mental illness;

2. "dangerousness" was frequently attributed to a person with schizophrenia, but less so to a person with depression;

3. dangerousness is directly related to preference for social distance/exclusion;

4. a biological etiology was attributed more frequently to schizophrenia than to depression;

5. a biological etiology was associated with unpredictability and dangerousness and fear, but decreased blame and punishment for an act of violence (Angermeyer & Matschinger, 2003a, 2003b, 2005; Dietrich et al., 2004; Dietrich, Heider, et al., 2006; Dietrich, Matschinger, et al., 2006; Link et al., 1999).

Among some individuals, avoidance of interacting with mental health systems may in part be due to the potential for intensified stereotypes, prejudice, and discrimination

(Lefley, 1989). Stigma among close family members of persons with major depressive disorder, and attribution of the mental illness to cognitive and attitudinal problems—rather than a medical and biological etiology—is directly related to treatment noncompliance in the affected family member (Sher et al., 2005).

The Surgeon General's report on mental illness emphasized stigma as a chief obstacle to consuming and receiving satisfactory mental health services, particularly among racial and ethnic minority populations (USDHHS, 1999; 2001). Racial minority populations, who already face prejudice and discrimination due to their group membership, experience double stigma when confronted with the effects and impact of mental illness (Gary, 2005). The notion of double stigma is conjectured to be an added burden that faces ethnic minority populations in the United States, but may impact disparate cultural groups in particular ways (Gary, 2005). Double stigma among African Americans encompasses lower socioeconomic status, maltreatment, misdiagnosis and distrust of health care systems, with mental health systems and providers characterized by inadequate cultural competence, communication failures, conscious and unconscious stereotyping, and limited access (Gary, 2005). African Americans are reported to experience considerable shame and stigma associated with mental illness, which contributes to greater utilization of primary care, emergency services, and informal resources such as ministers (Snowden, 2001), but there is little empirical evidence to suggest potential interventions to reduce this stigma.

Because stigma is influenced by culture, there is every reason to believe that knowledge, beliefs, and attitudes underlying stigma are likely to be different for whites, African Americans, Asian Americans, and Latinos. Research in depression in African Americans has shown that stigma negatively impacts mental health treatment seeking behavior (Baker and Bell, 1999; Van Hook, 1999) and overall treatment participation and compliance (Bystritsky et al., 2005; Cooper et al., 2003; Gary, 2005). However, there is a paucity of research on identifying key components of stigma regarding depression in African Americans. A nationally representative sample telephone survey (only 81 African Americans, 590 whites) reported racial differences in beliefs regarding perceptions of mentally ill persons (schizophrenia or major depression) as dangerous and violent, as well as the degree to which blame or punishment for inappropriate behavior should be placed on these individuals (Anglin et al., 2006). African Americans were more likely than whites to perceive the person as dangerous, whether the diagnosis was schizophrenia or major depression, but less likely to place blame or think the person should be punished. There is still an enormous gap in knowledge of the characterization of stigma concerning mental illnesses and depression in African Americans.

MENTAL ILLNESS STIGMA IN AFRICAN AMERICANS

The most cohesive body of literature concerning stigma in African Americans (presence/absence rather than characterization) and underlying attitudes and beliefs addresses a single issue: patient attitudes/preferences for conventional depression/anxiety treatment (i.e., psychotropic drug treatment—antidepressants or anxiolytics) versus counseling/psychotherapy, mainly in primary care patients. (Cooper-Patrick et al., 1997) conducted focus groups of African American and white patients with depression, asking probative questions concerning depression treatment relevant to primary care settings. African Americans more frequently commented on spirituality and stigma issues, and were less likely than whites to comment on relationships between physical health and depression or attributes of treatment types. In a subsequent study (Cooper et al., 2000), items identified from these focus groups were given to patients with depression (27 African Americans, 49 whites) to rate their importance. The top thirty items came from the following domains: health care provider's interpersonal skills, primary care provider recognition, treatment effectiveness, treatment problems, patient's understanding of treatment, intrinsic spirituality, and financial access to services. Contrary to the authors' expectations, stigma was not rated as highly as anticipated. However, there were few African Americans in the sample, and the patients had already overcome the barriers of stigma sufficiently to have entered a study on minor depression.

A recent study (Givens et al., 2007) conducted on over 78,000 people (3,596 of whom were African American) with significant levels of depressive symptoms replicated these studies. African Americans (and other minorities) were less likely to believe that medications were effective and that the etiology of depression is biological, or that counseling and prayer are effective treatments. African Americans reported more employment-related stigma associated with depression. Thus, from a variety of studies in primary care patients with either depression or anxiety disorders, it is apparent that African Americans are less likely than whites to find psychotropic medications acceptable, and more likely to prefer counseling (although not more frequently than whites) (Bystritsky et al., 2005; Cooper et al., 2003; Dwight-Johnson et al., 2000; Hazlett-Stevens et al., 2002; Schraufnagel et al., 2006). The unacceptability of psychotropic medication may be based on the erroneous beliefs that antidepressant drugs are addictive (which they are not, and treatment need not be a lifelong commitment), and that antidepressants do not work very well (which they do in the majority of patients, including African Americans) (Brown et al., 1999; Cooper et al., 2003). These reports are in contrast to a Diala et al. (2001) study, which found that African Americans reported more positive attitudes about seeking mental health services than did whites.

But the preponderance of evidence indicates that African Americans find conventional treatments for depression less acceptable than do whites, based partially on erroneous beliefs about antidepressant medications, whereas preferences for alternative and complementary approaches are virtually unexplored. The irony of one of these so-called false beliefs held by African Americans—that antidepressant drugs are not very effective—comes from recent publications on the NIMH-sponsored STAR*D (Sequenced Treatment Alternatives for Depression) study. In fact, the most commonly used second-generation antidepressants, Serotonin-Specific Reuptake Inhibitors (SSRIs), are *not* as effective in African Americans as they are in either whites or Latinos (Lesser et al., 2007). A pharmacogenetic study has shown that an allele associated with good response to the SSRI was seven times more frequent in whites compared with African Americans (McMahon et al., 2006). These findings underscore the fact that drugs, which are discovered and developed in primarily white populations, cannot be assumed to work equally as well in people of Asian and African descent.

Reducing Stigma

Well-controlled research on interventions to reduce stigma toward mental illness in the community is scarce, and has focused on three types of interventions: education (gaining knowledge or dispelling myths); contact (challenging attitudes based on research in decreasing racial prejudice) (Desforges et al., 1991); and protest (suppressing negative attitudes). Both education of and contact with people with a mental illness produced positive changes in attitudes about mental illness, but contact was the more effective intervention (Corrigan, 2002; Corrigan, Green, et al., 2001; Corrigan, River, et al. 2001; Corrigan et al., 2004). In planning research and interventions designed to reduce stigma, it is necessary to differentiate the various components of stigma as well as various mental disorders (Angermeyer & Matschinger, 2003a, 2003b). Although the public may report some perceived differences in attributions between severe mental disorders, e.g., dangerousness in schizophrenia and depression (Angermeyer & Matschinger, 2003a, 2003b, 2005; Dietrich et al., 2004; Dietrich, Matschinger, et al., 2006; Link et al., 1999), they really do not understand the wide ranges of symptoms, prognosis, and characteristics of mental illnesses. Most depression is not severe, seldom associated with violent behavior, and has a good prognosis if adequately treated. The most common depression found in the community is mild to moderate (Bluthenthal et al., 2006), but even moderate depression has a negative impact on functioning (Huang et al., 2006; Kroenke et al., 2001). There is also a need to educate the public

1. in the concept of mental wellness and mental illness as a continuum;

2. the direction and magnitude of mental illness being based on both biological and environmental conditions;

3. a holistic approach to addressing depression and ensuring mental wellness, which embraces spiritual components;

4. the impact of how one feels/thinks on physical symptoms;

5. how environmental issues (stressors of low income and safety issues) can impact depression and vice versa.

Future Targets of Stigma Interventions: Individuals/Patients

Culturally competent educational interventions can reduce the stigma associated with depression. These educational interventions should encompass recognizing the symptoms, the biological etiology, the influence of one's emotions on physical and social well-being, and treatment options. Most primary care practices have health-related continuous videotapes in their waiting rooms. Short videotapes (from 30 seconds to several minutes) of mental health material could be inserted into waiting room video loops, as an effective means of reducing negative attitudes about depression treatment

(Primm et al., 2002). Brochures from groups such as NAMI about depression can be downloaded from the NAMI website, and left in the waiting areas. The primary care center could provide evening programs in which both the consumers and the speakers are African American, or speak directly with the patient about issues directly related to depression in African Americans.

Community

NAMI, at the national level, represents a strong political presence and spearheads national programs to reduce stigma and provide resources, but local NAMI chapters are invaluable in their support of the individual consumers, families, and friends. Local NAMI chapters not only provide social and spiritual support; they also empower members with knowledge. One of the authors (LDB) is an active participant in a local Atlanta NAMI chapter, where she presents the latest information on ethnopsychopharmacolgy and pharmacogenetics, as well as soliciting input on evolving research. Although this is an open meeting, to which any interested party is welcome, this chapter is attended primarily by African Americans and draws attendees far outside the local community. In a recent NIMH-sponsored multicenter study conducted throughout the Southeast (Aliyu et al., 2006), as part of the community outreach, interactions, and collaborations, participants of the study were encouraged to give information about contacting their local community patient advocate groups (e.g., NAMI and Mental Health American of Georgia).

After the Morehouse School of Medicine reported successful interactions with a local chapter, participants and family members attending the meetings, attendees volunteering for the study and agreeing to pilot questionnaires for use in future studies, and centers from other states reported that study participants were reticent about attending meetings that were composed of primarily white attendees. Local chapters of national patient advocacy groups could increase efforts in forming ethnically and culturally compatible groups. Local patient advocacy groups are presently composed of consumers and families of those with severe mental illnesses (e.g., bipolar disorder and schizophrenia), and should consider forming local groups for milder or moderate mental disorders (e.g., depression).

In the African American community, especially in the South, churches hold a central spiritual, social, and political role that is based on the infrastructures and leadership these institutions provided after the emancipation. Religious activity, both personal and public, is associated with better mental and physical health (Ellison, 1995). Churches provide a sense of belonging, social support, and network systems, and are often the first—and last—point of contact for African Americans seeking help for their emotional distress (Neighbors et al., 1998; Snowden, 2001; Cummings et al., 2003). Stronger religiosity reported in African Americans compared with whites underlies the difference in beliefs in the biological basis of depression, and importance of religion in treatment factors (Cooper et al., 2001; Husaini, 1999; Millet et al., 1996).

Pastoral counseling by African American clergy can play an important and solitary role in the treatment of mental health issues in African Americans. In a study of ninety-nine clergy of African American churches in a metropolitan area of a Northeastern state, the clergy spent 14 percent (6.2 hours/week) of their clerical duties involved in counseling; 48.5 percent had training in counseling, mental health, or interpersonal communications and 11 percent had degrees in counseling; 50 percent had participated in counseling-related workshops or seminars within the last two years; and 58 percent reported making referrals (e.g., to physician or medical services, pastoral counseling) (Young et al., 2003). A growing number of African American churches are adding mental health programs to their health ministry, but in order to work effectively, stigma within the church must be addressed. Examples of this within the metro Atlanta area are the joint collaborative efforts of local NAMI chapters, Mental Health America of Georgia, and the Concerned Black Clergy to present consumer-driven mental health programs to clergy, staff, and congregations of local African American churches. It is also important for physicians (psychiatrists, primary care providers) to embrace a culturally competent, holistic approach to treatment of depression, which will include the patient's spiritual beliefs and strengths in making medical decisions and facilitating compliance with treatment (Carter, 2002). Physicians could familiarize themselves with local area churches that offer pastoral counseling for mental health issues, and include those in treatment options.

HEALTH CARE PROFESSIONALS AND STIGMA

The medical profession has played a role in the stigmatization of mental illness. Psychiatry was first recognized as part of the medical profession in the late eighteenth century. The causes of mental illnesses propagated by psychiatrists and non-psychiatrists alike for the next century served to confuse the public about the nature of mental illness. At times, mental illness was thought to be due to unhealthy lifestyles or heredity. The reform movement advocated that persons with mental illness be hospitalized and treated like any other persons with a medical disease (Dain, 1994). Religious groups have attributed mental illness to demonic possession and moral ineptitude, further adding to the etiological controversy.

By the late nineteenth century, American psychiatrists had become pessimistic that psychiatric hospitalization really was of any help to the patients (Dain, 1994). Superintendents, who were mostly psychiatrists, began to see their roles as custodial instead of healing, but did note that the hospital environment provided a place with structure that reduced the violent behavior often displayed by the patients. The hospital as a refuge later lost its luster as funds dissipated with the advent of the Great Depression and World War II, and psychiatric hospitals became places where patients were mechanically restrained as a primary form of treatment. This image further stigmatized people living with mental illnesses in hospitals as being unable to control any of their behaviors without restraints and thus a danger to themselves.

Karl Menninger and other psychoanalysts experienced working with servicemen during World War II and changed their views regarding psychiatric hospitalization. Psychoanalysis had been made popular as an office-based treatment for mental illness in the late nineteenth century by Sigmund Freud. It was Menninger's influence along with others and the presidential commission report on mental illness during the Kennedy administration that led to the deinstitutionalization of persons living with mental illness from public psychiatric hospitals. Services were to be provided in the community for all levels of care, but in most jurisdictions funding has never been adequate to care for those in most need. The perception that people living with mental illness are unable to care for themselves and are violent is perpetrated even more because of inadequate and oftentimes inappropriate care, which can lead to inappropriate behaviors.

There is often open and extreme hostility toward psychiatrists by other physicians (Fink, 1983). If primary care physicians have negative views of the field of psychiatry it is no wonder that their patients do as well. All physicians are exposed to psychiatric training in medical school and during residency training. Family practitioners usually have more exposure during residency training than other primary care specialties (AAFP, 2008), but this does not seem to allay the negative perceptions surrounding psychiatry. One psychiatrist suggests that the negative images of psychiatrists come from the psychiatry teachers, who often reinforce negative stereotypes of psychiatrists such as making jokes about patients (Fink, 1986). The other source of negative stereo-types is non-psychiatry teachers who disparage psychiatry to the students and residents (Fink, 1986). Though Fink's comments were written more than twenty years ago, many primary care physicians continue to be disparaging of psychiatry as a helpful discipline for any except the most severely mentally ill.

There is a culture of medicine that is perpetrated by standardized curriculums which lead to the development of similar sets of beliefs, norms, and values learned in Western medical training (US DHHS, 2001). Therefore, the disparaged ideas surrounding psychiatry become a part of the culture of medicine. Many psychiatrists have often been told that they are not real doctors because they do not touch the patients nor perform procedures as other physicians do. Though training may be similar for many physicians, they all are raised in a family of a particular cultural background and thus bring their own cultural biases into any treatment setting. The professional culture of medicine also influences a sense of emotional distance between clinician and patient.

African Americans and other minorities seek mental health care from primary care providers and other informal sources such as clergy, family, and friends before thinking about seeking help from a mental health professional (US DHHS, 2001). Stigma keeps family, clergy, and friends from recommending that the person acknowledge their problem and seek help. Oftentimes patients do not realize that they are depressed or suffering from any type of mental disorder because their primary complaint is one of physical discomfort such as headache, generalized malaise, difficulty sleeping, and vaguely painful joints and muscles. Culture impacts how patients describe their illness to their physicians (Masand et al., 2005), and in the case of African Americans the notion that they may be suffering from some sort of mental disorder may not have crossed their minds. If so, the stigma of mental illness in the African American community would decrease the likelihood that patients would consider that some or all of their symptoms could be due to a mental disorder.

It is estimated that physicians in primary care settings recognize less than half of patients that exhibit symptoms of depression and anxiety as actually having these disorders (Masand et al., 2005). The culture of the physician matters, as does the culture of medicine, as to how psychiatric symptoms are perceived. Many physicians consider all symptoms as having a physical basis with no consideration given to the possibility of the existence of psychological issues. Others recognize that mental health problems can have a significant impact on physical health (AAFP, 2008).

Primary care physicians and emergency room personnel often make inaccurate diagnoses of depression in African Americans seen and evaluated in these settings (US DHHS, 2001). One can question whether these professionals also have biases and stigma against mental illness or some other variable responsible. It is recognized that patients who present with mental health problems in primary care physicians' offices have subthreshold conditions and thus symptoms that are not quite so obvious (AAFP, 2008), whereas psychiatrists are much more likely to see patients with obvious symptoms. Many patients also downplay emotional issues when talking with their primary care providers because of the stigma surrounding mental disorders, so it is incumbent on the physicians to screen for mental health issues. One study reported that only 20 to 30 percent of patients with emotional problems reported them to their primary care provider (Eisenberg, 1992). Many primary care physicians say they are comfortable treating depression in their patients (Williams et al., 1999) and a large number also prescribe antidepressant medications. The problem with primary care physicians treating depression is the lack of appropriate follow-up in most cases (AAFP, 2008). Recognized best practices for the treatment of depression include psychotherapy and medication and regular follow-up.

One might think that African American physicians would be more sensitive in recognizing signs and symptoms of mental illness in their African American patients because of cultural similarities. Little research has been done in this area but it is noted that physicians trained in the Western medical culture, no matter their culture of origin, will have similar notions regarding mental illness as all physicians practice from the cultural context of their training in medicine. Therefore, African American physicians treating African American patients may do no better than other physicians in making such diagnoses. A study of cardiac patients did not show any difference in the level of care of African Americans utilizing white or African American physicians (Chen et al., 2001).

It is apparent that more research needs to be done to assess the role that stigma plays in the assessment and recognition of mental disorders by primary care physicians, as they play a most important role in assuring that more African Americans receive the treatment now available for mental illness. Stigma must also be addressed directly to the consumer by availability of culturally competent educational programs to primary care patients, churches, and local communities. Because African Americans are more likely to prefer counseling than drug therapy, both public and private insurance policy must provide parity for treatment of both mental and physical health concerns.

ACKNOWLEDGMENTS

Drs. Bradford and Braithwaite received support from the Community Voices Program of the Morehouse School of Medicine (W. K. Kellogg Foundation, PO100563).

REFERENCES

Adler, A. K., & Wahl, O. F. (1998). Children's beliefs about people labeled mentally ill. *American Journal of Orthopsychiatry, 68*, 321–326.

Aliyu, M. H., Calkins, M. E., Swanson, C. L., Jr., Lyons, P. D., Savage, R. M., May, R., Wiener, H., Devlin, B., Nimgaonkar, V. L., Ragland, J. D., Gur, R. E., Gur, R. C., Bradford, L. D., Edwards, N., Kwentus, J., McEvoy, J. P., Santos, A. B., Cleod-Bryant, S., Tennison, C., & Go, R. C. (2006). Project among African-Americans to explore risks for schizophrenia (PAARTNERS): Recruitment and assessment methods. *Schizophrenia Research, 87*, 32–44.

American Academy of Family Physicians. (2008). *Mental health care services by family physicians (position paper)*. Retrieved November 20, 2008, from http://www.aafp.org/online/en/home/policy/policies/m/mentalhealthcareservices.html

Angermeyer, M. C., & Matschinger, H. (2003a). Public beliefs about schizophrenia and depression: Similarities and differences. *Social Psychiatry and Psychiatric Epidemiology 38*, 526–534.

Angermeyer, M. C., & Matschinger, H. (2003b). The stigma of mental illness: Effects of labelling on public attitudes towards people with mental disorder. *Acta Psychiatry Scandanavie 108*, 304–309.

Angermeyer, M. C., & Matschinger, H. (2005). Labeling—stereotype—discrimination: An investigation of the stigma process. *Social Psychiatry and Psychiatric Epidemiology 40*, 391–395.

Anglin, D. M., Link, B. G., & Phelan, J. C. (2006). Racial differences in stigmatizing attitudes toward people with mental illness. *Psychiatric Services, 57*, 857.

Baker, F. M., & Bell, C. C. (1999). Issues in the psychiatric treatment of African Americans. *Psychiatric Services, 50*, 362.

Balsa, A. I., & McGuire, T. G. (2003). Prejudice, clinical uncertainty and stereotyping as sources of health disparities. *Journal of Health Economics 22*(1), 89–116.

Bluthenthal, R. N., Jones, L., Fackler-Lowrie, N., Ellison, M., Booker, T., Jones, F., McDaniel, S., Moini, M., Williams, K. R., Klap, R., Koegel, P., & Wells, K.B. (2006). Witness for wellness: Preliminary findings from a community-academic participatory research mental health initiative. *Ethnic Disparities 16*, S18–S34.

Bolden, L., & Wicks, M. N. (2005). Length of stay, admission types, psychiatric diagnoses, and the implications of stigma in African Americans in the nationwide inpatient sample. *Issues in Mental Health Nursing 26*, 1043.

Brown, C., Schulberg, H. C., Sacco, D., Perel, J. M., & Houck, P. R. (1999). Effectiveness of treatments for major depression in primary medical care practice: A post hoc analysis of outcomes for African American and white patients. *Journal of Affective Disorders 53*, 185.

Bystritsky, A., Wagner, A. W., Russo, J. E., Stein, M. B., Sherbourne, C. D., Craske, M. G., & Roy-Byrne, P. P. (2005). Assessment of beliefs about psychotropic medication and psychotherapy: Development of a measure for patients with anxiety disorders. *General Hospital Psychiatry 27*, 313–318.

Carter, J. H. (2002). Religion/spirituality in African-American culture: An essential aspect of psychiatric care. *Journal of the National Medical Association 94*(5), 371–375.

Chen, J., Rathore, S. S., Radford, M. J., Wang, Y., & Krumholz, H. M. (2001). Racial differences in the use of cardiac catheterization after acute myocardial infarction. *New England Journal of Medicine 344*, 1443–1449.

Cooper, L. A., Brown, C., Vu, H. T., Ford, D. E., & Powe, N. R. (2001). How important is intrinsic spirituality in depression care? A comparison of white and African-American primary care patients. *Journal of General Internal Medicine 16*, 634.

Cooper, L. A., Brown, C., Vu, H. T., Palenchar, D. R., Gonzales, J. J., Ford, D. E., & Powe, N. R. (2000). Primary care patients' opinions regarding the importance of various aspects of care for depression. *General Hospital Psychiatry 22*, 163.

Cooper, L. A., Gonzales, J. J., Gallo, J. J., Rost, K. M., Meredith, L. S., Rubenstein, L. V., Wang, N. Y., & Ford, D. E. (2003). The acceptability of treatment for depression among African-American, Hispanic, and white primary care patients. *Medical Care 41*, 479.

Cooper-Patrick, L., Powe, N. R, Jenckes, M. W., Gonzales, J. J., Levine, D. M., & Ford, D. E. (1997). Identification of patient attitudes and preferences regarding treatment of depression. *Journal of General Internal Medicine 12*, 431.

Corrigan, P. (2003). Beat the stigma: Come out of the closet. *Psychiatric Services, 54*, 1313.

Corrigan, P. (2004). How stigma interferes with mental health care. *American Psychologist 59*, 614–625.

Corrigan, P. W. (2002). Empowerment and serious mental illness: treatment partnerships and community opportunities. *Psychiatric Quarterly 73*, 217–228.

Corrigan, P. W., Green, A., Lundin, R., Kubiak, M. A., & Penn, D. L. (2001). Familiarity with and social distance from people who have serious mental illness. *Psychiatric Services, 52*, 953–958.

Corrigan, P. W., River, L. P., Lundin, R. K., Penn, D. L., Uphoff-Wasowski, K., Campion, J., Mathisen, J., Gagnon, C., Bergman, M., Goldstein, H., & Kubiak, M. A. (2001). Three strategies for changing attributions about severe mental illness. *Schizophrenia Bulletin 27*, 187–195.

Corrigan, P. W., Watson, A. C., Warpinski, A. C., & Gracia, G. (2004). Implications of educating the public on mental illness, violence, and stigma. *Psychiatric Services, 55*, 577–580.

Cummings, S. M., Neff, J. A., & Husaini, B. A. (2003). Functional impairment as a predictor of depressive symptomatology: The role of race, religiosity, and social support. *Health and Social Work 28*(1), 23–32.

Dain, N. (1994). Reflections on antipsychiatry and stigma in the history of American psychiatry. *Hospital and Community Psychiatry 45*(10), 1010–1015.

Desforges, D. M., Lord, C. G., Ramsey, S. L., Mason, J. A., Van Leeuwen, M. D., West, S. C., & Lepper, M. R. (1991). Effects of structured cooperative contact on changing negative attitudes toward stigmatized social groups. *Journal of Personality and Social Psychology 60*, 531–544.

Diala, C. C., Muntaner, C., Walrath, C., Nickerson, K., LaVeist, T., & Leaf, P. (2001). Racial/ethnic differences in attitudes toward seeking professional mental health services. *American Journal of Public Health 91*, 805.

Dietrich, S., Beck, M., Bujantugs, B., Kenzine, D., Matschinger, H., & Angermeyer, M. C. (2004). The relationship between public causal beliefs and social distance toward mentally ill people. *Australian and New Zealand Journal of Psychiatry 38*, 348–54; discussion 355–357.

Dietrich, S., Heider, D., Matschinger, H., & Angermeyer, M. C. (2006). Influence of newspaper reporting on adolescents' attitudes toward people with mental illness. *Social Psychiatry and Psychiatric Epidemiology 41*, 318–322.

Dietrich, S., Matschinger, H., & Angermeyer, M. C. (2006). The relationship between biogenetic causal explanations and social distance toward people with mental disorders: Results from a population survey in Germany. *International Journal of Social Psychiatry 52*, 166–174.

Dwight-Johnson, M., Sherbourne, C. D., Liao, D., & Wells, K. B. (2000). Treatment preferences among depressed primary care patients. *Journal of General Internal Medicine 15*, 527.

Eisenberg, L. (1992). Treating depression and anxiety in primary care: Closing the gap between knowledge and practice. *New England Journal of Medicine 326*(16), 1080–1084.

Ellison, C. G. (1995). Race, religious involvement and depressive symptomatology in a southeastern U.S. community. *Social Science Medicine 40*, 1561.

Fink, P. (1986). Dealing with psychiatry's stigma. *Hospital and Community Psychiatry 37*(8), 814–818.

Fink, P. (1983). Enigma of stigma and its relation to psychiatric education. *Psychiatric Annals 13,* 669–690.

Gary, F. A. (2005). Stigma: Barrier to mental health care among ethnic minorities. *Issues in Mental Health Nursing 26*, 979.

Givens, J. L., Houston, T. K., Van Voorhees, B.W., Ford, D. E., Cooper, L. A. (2007). Ethnicity and preferences for depression treatment. *General Hospital Psychiatry, 29*, 182–191.

Hazlett-Stevens, H., Craske, M. G., Roy-Byrne, P. P., Sherbourne, C. D., Stein, M. B., & Bystritsky, A. (2002). Predictors of willingness to consider medication and psychosocial treatment for panic disorder in primary care patients. *General Hospital Psychiatry 24*, 316.

Huang, F. Y., Chung, H., Kroenke, K., & Spitzer, R. L. (2006). Racial and ethnic differences in the relationship between depression severity and functional status. *Psychiatric Services, 57*, 498.

Husaini, B. A. (1999). Does public and private religiosity have a moderating effect on depression? A bi-racial study of elders in the American South. *International Journal of Aging and Human Development 48*, 63–72.

Kroenke, K., Spitzer, R. L., & Williams, J. B. (2001). The PHQ-9: Validity of a brief depression severity measure. *Journal of General Internal Medicine 16*, 606–613.

Lefley, H. P. (1989). Family burden and family stigma in major mental illness. *American Psychology, 44*(3), 556–560.

Lesser, I. M., Castro, D. B., Gaynes, B. N., Gonzalcz, J., Rush, A. J., Alpert, J. E., Trivedi, M., Luther, J. F., & Wisniewski, S. R. (2007). Ethnicity/race and outcome in the treatment of depression: Results from STAR*D. *Medical Care 45*, 1043–1051.

Link, B. G., Phelan, J. C., Bresnahan, M., Stueve, A., & Pescosolido, B. A. (1999). Public conceptions of mental illness: Labels, causes, dangerousness, and social distance. *American Journal of Public Health 89*, 1328.

Link, B. G., Struening, E. L., Neese-Todd, S., Asmussen, S., & Phelan, J. C. (2001). Stigma as a barrier to recovery: The consequences of stigma for the self-esteem of people with mental illnesses. *Psychiatric Services, 52*, 1621.

Link, B. G., Yang, L. H., Phelan, J. C., & Collins, P. Y. (2004). Measuring mental illness stigma. *Schizophrenia Bulletin 30*, 511

Masand, P., Satcher, D., Culpepper, L. (2005). *A surgeon general's report on the stigma of mental illness: Have we made progress?* Retrieved November 1, 2008, from http://www.medscape.com/viewprogram/3786_pnt

McMahon, F. J., Buervenich, S., Charney, D., Lipsky, R., Rush, A. J., Wilson, A. F., Sorant, A. J. M., Papanicolaou, G. J., Laje, G., Fava, M., Trivedi, M. H., Wisniewski, S. R., & Manji, H. (2006). Variation in the gene encoding the serotonin 2A receptor is associated with outcome of antidepressant treatment. *American Journal of Human Genetics 78*, 804.

Millet, P. E., Sullivan, B. F., Schwebel, A. I., & Myers, L. J. (1996). Black Americans' and White Americans' views of the etiology and treatment of mental health problems. *Community Mental Health Journal 32*, 235–242.

Neighbors, H. W., Musick, M. A., & Williams, D. R. (1998). The African American minister as a source of help for serious personal crises: Bridge or barrier to mental health care? *Health, Education and Behavior 25*(6), 759–777.

Primm, A. B., Cabot, D., Pettis, J., Vu, H. T., Cooper, L. A. (2002). The acceptability of a culturally-tailored depression education videotape to African Americans. *Journal of the National Medical Association 94*(11), 1007–1016.

Rüsch, N., Angermeyer, M. C., & Corrigan, P. W. (2005). Mental illness stigma: Concepts, consequences, and initiatives to reduce stigma. *European Psychiatry 20*, 529–539.

Schraufnagel, T. J., Wagner, A. W., Miranda, J., & Roy-Byrne, P. P. (2006). Treating minority patients with depression and anxiety: What does the evidence tell us? *General Hospital Psychiatry 28*, 27.

Sher, I., McGinn, L., Sirey, J. A., & Meyers, B. (2005). Effects of caregivers' perceived stigma and causal beliefs on patients' adherence to antidepressant treatment. *Psychiatric Services 56*, 564–569.

Snowden, L. R. (2001). Barriers to effective mental health services. *Mental Health Services Research 3*(4), 181–187.

U.S. Department of Health and Human Services (US DHHS). (1999). *Mental health: A report of the Surgeon General.* Rockville, MD: Author.

U.S. Department of Health and Human Services (US DHHS). (2001). *Mental health: Culture, race and ethnicity, A supplement to Mental health: A report of the surgeon general.* Rockville, MD: Author.

Van Hook, M. P. (1999). Women's help-seeking patterns for depression. *Social Work in Health Care 29*, 15.

Wahl, O. F. (1999). Mental health consumers' experience of stigma. *Schizophrenia Bulletin 25*, 467–78.

Wahl, O. F., & Harman, C. R. (1989). Family views of stigma. *Schizophrenia Bulletin 15*, 131–139.

Williams, J., Rost, K., Dietrich, A., Ciotti, M., Zyzanski, S., Cornell, J. (1999). Primary care physicians' approach to depressive disorders. *Archives of Family Medicine 8*(1), 58–67.

Wilson, C., Nairn, R., Coverdale, J., & Panapa, A. (2000). How mental illness is portrayed in children's television: A prospective study. *British Journal of Psychiatry 176*, 440–443.

Young, J. L., Griffith, E. E. H., & Williams, D. R. (2003). The integral role of pastoral counseling by African-American clergy in community mental health. *Psychiatric Services 54*, 688–692.

CHAPTER

8

HOMICIDE AND VIOLENCE AMONG AFRICAN AMERICAN YOUTH: FROM EPIDEMIC TO ENDEMIC?

EMILIE PHILLIPS SMITH
JOSEPH RICHARDSON
RHONDA BELUE

Youth violence is a problem that continues to affect the fabric of the United States. Violence seriously affects both youth and young adult populations. Homicide is an important public health issue, as the second leading cause of death for *all* U.S. youth between the ages of 15 and 24 years (National Center for Injury Prevention and Control, Centers for Disease Control and Prevention, 2008). For African American youth, homicide is *the leading cause of death*, followed by unintentional injury and suicide. Homicide is among the top three causes of death for people up to 34 years of age, claiming far too many lives in the African American community.

Unfortunately, these lives are most often taken by perpetrators known to the victims. Considering only murders for which the offender is known in 2002, 5 percent of victims ages 15–17 years were killed by parents, 5 percent by other family members, 32 percent by strangers, and 58 percent by acquaintances (Snyder & Sickmund, 2006).

According to Snyder and Sickmund (2006), juvenile offenders, who account for 25 percent of the population, participated in one of every four juvenile homicides.

Homicide and violence also contribute to health disparities between African Americans and whites. According to a recent study (Centers for Disease Control and Prevention [CDC], 2001), whites live 6.2 years longer than African Americans. In the later years of life, HIV, heart disease, and diabetes contribute to disparate years of life, but for youth, violence and homicide makes the largest contribution to health disparities between African American and whites. Homicide disproportionately influences life expectancy because it affects persons in the first few decades of life, whereas death from heart disease and cancer—the number one and number two leading contributors to the life expectancy gap—primarily affects persons in their fifth and sixth decades of life (CDC, 2001; Smith & Hasbrouck, 2006). Death rates from homicide have historically been six- to eight-fold greater for African Americans than for whites. Though violence affects the entire U.S. population, its effects are particularly endemic to the African American community, resulting in disproportionate years of youthful lives lost.

THE COSTS OF VIOLENCE AND HOMICIDE AMONG YOUTH

The economic cost of violence manifests in numerous ways, including both direct and indirect costs. Violent acts have been estimated to cost the United States more than 3 percent of the Gross Domestic Product (Waters, Hyder, Rajkotia, Basu, & Butchart, 2005). Direct costs include expenses such as the costs to the criminal justice system for processing violent crimes, the costs of police force time, adjudication and incarceration, medical expenses, lost wages due to missed days of work, and the cost of stolen property (Rutherford et al., 2007; Foster, Jones, & Conduct Problems Prevention Research Group, 2006). For example, gun and weapon crime costs society over $2 billion annually in legal processing. Furthermore, costs are also incurred in the form of imposing safety measures such as metal detectors and extra security in schools (Cook & Ludwig, 2002).

However, prevention can offset the costs of eliminating existing violence. A study conducted by the Washington State Institute for Public Policy evaluated the cost versus benefit of a variety of violence prevention strategies (Aos, Lieb, Mayfield, Miller, & Pennucci, 2004). This study found that some prevention programs, such as dialectic behavior therapy, are highly cost effective, costing $843 per youth, yet yielding benefits approximated at $32,078 per youth. In contrast, parole-based programs cost approximately $1,400 to $2,100 per child but produce $0 to -$11,000 in benefits. In this study, benefit is measured in terms of monetary values from reductions in crime, substance abuse, child abuse, and increases in educational attainment. Cost represents the amount of taxpayer dollars needed to deliver the program. However, further studies are needed to understand whether these violence prevention strategies are equally effective for families and youth of diverse racial-ethnic backgrounds. Some of these violence prevention strategies have been explicitly tested and found to be quite beneficial to African American youth and families (Henggeler, Melton, Brondino, Scherer, &

Hanley, 1997; Henggeler, Pickrel, & Brondino, 1999; Olds, 2002; Webster-Stratton, 1998; Webster-Stratton & Hammond, 1997).

Violence also results in indirect or nonmonetary costs such as increase in psychological distress for life, physical disability, loss of productivity (Rutherford et al., 2007; Foster et al., 2006), and reduced social value and life years lost for youth who are exposed to violence. Children and families exposed to violence experience a lower quality of life compared to children who are not regularly exposed to violence (Cook & Ludwig, 2002). For example, it has been estimated that in the United States, on average, starting from birth, violence reduces the average life expectancy by approximately one-third of a year for every year of exposure (Soares, 2006).

Given that violence disproportionately affects African American youth, the cost of violence also disproportionately affects African American youth. Longitudinal research has found that African American youth are more likely to continue violent and delinquent behavior into early adulthood. Moving into viable adult roles, including gainful employment, marriage, and connectedness to conventional family and friends, emerges as related to cessation of violence and delinquency in adulthood (Elliott et al., 2006). Unfortunately, these are aspects of development in emerging adulthood which African American males are less able to access, as demonstrated by higher unemployment rates and lower marriage rates (which in fact may be interrelated). Furthermore, research by Sampson has shown that levels of male unemployment are related to *both* levels of rates of marriage and levels of two-parent family structure, which in turn are related to *reduced* levels of crime and delinquency (Sampson, 1995).

In sum, violence has costs to both the individual and society in both real dollars and lost human potential. In the following sections, we present definitions of violence and describe our conceptual approach to understanding the various multilevel factors found to be related to violence and homicide among youth, with special attention to African Americans.

DEFINITIONS OF HOMICIDE AND VIOLENCE

Violence can be assessed by either official or self-report. Official reports of violence include four types of violent crime:

1. criminal homicide (the willful, non-negligent killing of one human being by another);

2. robbery (taking or attempting to take anything of value by force or threat of force);

3. aggravated assault (attack by one person on another using or threatening to use a weapon, where the victim suffers bodily injury); and

4. forcible rape (carnal knowledge of a person forcibly or against that person's will, or where the victim is incapable of giving consent) (U.S. Department of Health and Human Services [U.S. DHHS], 2001; U.S. Department of Justice, Federal Bureau of Investigation, 2000).

Though official statistics allow us to monitor the prevalence and types of violent crime reported to the police, confidential surveys of young people about their behavior can also be helpful (U.S. DHHS, 2001). There are several longitudinal studies of youth violence and delinquency that help to add understanding of important risk and protective processes related to youth-reported involvement in violence and delinquency across the life span (see, for example, longitudinal work in Thornberry and Krohn's [2003] special volume, including Hawkins et al., 2003; Huizinga, Weiher, Espiritu, & Esbensen, 2003; and Loeber et al., 2003). These important longitudinal studies add much to our knowledge of the ways in which multiple-level factors can act and interact to influence violence and delinquency across the lifespan. In the following section, we will describe our conceptual framework and multilevel risk and protective processes in violence and delinquency.

CONCEPTUAL APPROACH: AN ECO-DEVELOPMENTAL FRAMEWORK OF YOUTH VIOLENCE

Substantial attention is currently given to the multiplicity of factors likely involved in youth homicide and violence. A developmental-ecological model (O'Donnell et al., 1995; Tolan, Gorman-Smith, & Henry, 2003) recognizes that individual, family, school, and larger community factors all contribute to violence and delinquency among youth. An ecological model acknowledges that individual factors such as temperament and self-control can contribute to violence and delinquency, as can factors such as the family environment in which one is reared, peer networks, and the neighborhood and communities in which one resides and interacts. Furthermore, a developmental perspective acknowledges that some of these influences, like the family, may have primary and enduring influences on youth behavior whereas others (peer and neighborhood/community context) may become increasingly important to youth as they grow, develop, and begin to navigate their peer networks and communities more autonomously. Importantly, an eco-developmental model also considers the overarching role of sociocultural beliefs and practices, public policy, the media, racism, and discrimination (Ogbu, 1981; Coll et al., 1996). Thus, we think it is important to explore not only family and peer factors in violence and delinquency, but also the role of the larger community and societal contexts in youth violence and aggression (Figure 8.1). The following sections consider multilevel influences on youth violence and homicide at the individual, family, peer, school, neighborhood, and macrolevels, taking into account the economic environment, the media, public policy, racism, and discrimination in addition to the role of sociocultural beliefs and practices.

Individual Factors

The relevant data demonstrate fairly clearly that males are more likely than females to be involved in violent and delinquent behavior (CDC, 2004). Eighty-two percent of persons arrested for violent crime and 66.6 percent of persons arrested for property crime were male. However, given that the reasons and processes for this are not a

FIGURE 8.1 *A Sociocultural-Developmental Model.*

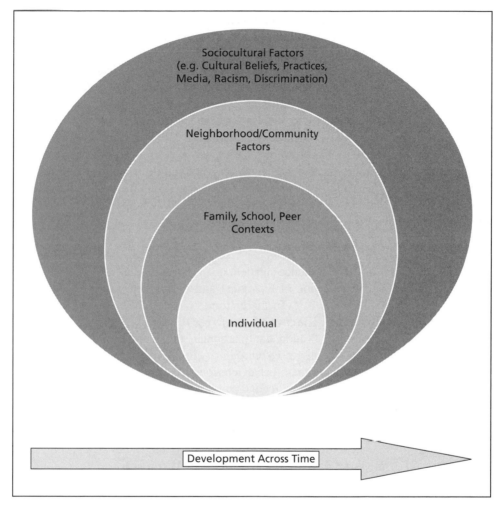

malleable, throughout these sections we will attend to the role of gender in ways that are potentially helpful in terms of directions for prevention and intervention.

Race and ethnicity have also been implicated in youth violence and delinquency. However, official reports of arrest data demonstrate that in 2007, the majority (69.7%) of persons arrested were white. Whites accounted for 58.9 percent and 67.9 percent of persons arrested for violent crimes and property crimes, respectively. Yet, among youth, African Americans are disproportionately represented, accounting for 50.7 percent of *juveniles* arrested for violent crime (U.S. Department of Justice, Federal Bureau of Investigation, 2007).

However, it is the perspective here that it is difficult to disentangle to what degree race and ethnicity are inextricably intertwined with other factors such as poverty, socioeconomic status, and neighborhood violence—factors that are relatively powerful predictors of violence and homicide. We discuss the role of family structure and socioeconomic status, particularly the gross disparities in family structure and income under family factors. Disentangling the contribution of individual factors from environmental and social factors is a complex research task.

Other important individual factors have been found to impact involvement in violent and delinquent behavior. Exposure to television and media violence have an impact and African American children watch more television (Paik & Comstock, 1994). An individual's exposure to chronic violence also has an impact in multiple ways: by increasing stress that inhibits the ability to respond calmly and thoughtfully and also by decreasing the brain functioning that allows one to adequately process multiple possible responses cognitively (Raine et al., 2001). Thus, children who have grown up with chronic exposure to violence are affected in both biological and social ways. Research shows that effective prevention programs can not only reduce the violent and aggressive behavior of the participating youth, but also can increase self-regulation and executive function exhibited by children at risk of violence and delinquency (Raine et al., 2001). By including consideration of the interaction of biological and social factors, we may actually point out that some youth benefit even more from strategies that increase individual functioning and family support. The caveat is not to use research on biological processes to label youth in a deterministic fashion, but to articulate the role of prevention activities in efforts to enhance protective processes *particularly* in instances in which exposure to violence and traumatic events may have had deleterious effects (Beauchaine et al., 2008). Supportive family environments and effective parenting practices are very important in reducing involvement in violence and delinquency and promoting positive development and achievement (Edlynn, Gaylord-Harden, Richards, & Miller, 2008; Proctor, 2006).

The Role of Family and Parenting Practices in Violence and Delinquency

Substantial research documents the important role of family in violence and delinquency. The role of family is derived by a combination of shared temperament and personality factors, by parental socialization practices, and/or by shared social situations (Moffitt, 1987).

It is well recognized that though ethnic minority youth are more likely to be involved in violent and delinquent behavior, they are also more likely to be impoverished and living in female-headed households. Seventy-six percent of white youth live in two-parent households, whereas only 38 percent of African American youth live in two-parent households (U.S. Census Bureau, 2008). Interestingly, it has been found that in minority communities, communities with higher proportions of males also have higher percentage of two-parent families *and* reduced crime and violence (Sampson, 1995). Large numbers of incarcerated men limit the number of male partners in the marriageable pool within poor African American neighborhoods, which severely affects family structure (Wilson, 1987).

Living in female-headed households is related to poverty. Thirty-seven percent of children in African American female-headed households live in poverty, compared to a 20 percent poverty rate among white children living in single-mother families (U.S. Census Bureau, 2001). These rates are even more disparate when considering that the majority of white children are reared in two-parent households with a poverty rate of 10 percent. Earnings further contribute to the disparity. Darity and Nicholson (2005) report a median income for white American families of $53,714 in contrast to a median income of $34,001 for African American families. Even at similar income and educational levels, considerable economic gaps exist, with African Americans evidencing only 9.7 percent of the net worth of white Americans ($4,418 versus $45,740), and with a home ownership rate of 46 percent compared to that of 70 percent among whites (Darity & Nicholson, 2005; Shapiro, 2001). Ethnic minority youth are more likely to live in poor, single-parent families in communities with higher levels of decay, unemployment, crime, and violence (Wilson, 1987; Williams & Guerra, 2006). However, it must be recognized that the majority of African American children are *not* involved in violence and delinquency, and that parenting may play an important role in helping to foster the success of children (Edlynn et al., 2008; Proctor, 2006).

It is now fairly well validated that parental disciplinary practices with clear standards, rewards, and consequences are superior to inconsistent, coercive, and unresponsive discipline (Lutzker, Touchette, & Campbell, 1988; Maccoby & Martin, 1983; Snyder & Huntley, 1990). Inconsistent parenting fails to establish clear limits that are rewarded or sanctioned with regularity. In coercive parenting, the parent(s) give in to nagging misbehavior or child noncompliance, unwittingly encouraging youth to continue this behavioral pattern (Chamberlain & Patterson, 1995; Martinez & Forgatch, 2001; Reid, Patterson, & Snyder, 2002). On the other hand, harsh punishment involving intense physical punishment and caustically verbal abuse is damaging emotionally for children and does not model nor teach children positive ways to behave (Lochman & van den Steenhoven, 2002).

As we consider the contexts of parenting for African American children, disproportionate numbers of children are reared in poor, female-headed households. With this in mind, the ways in which these contexts interact with parenting approaches is worth consideration. Parenting is a tough job for two parents, let alone one. Rearing children in poor, single-parent households is related to more family stress, lower income, and household and family responsibilities that hamper the ability to parent effectively (Cairney et al., 2003; Jackson et al., 2000; McLoyd, 1998). Family status variables including poverty, life stressors, family isolation, and dangerous neighborhoods are found to be related to disrupted family processes such as the family's ability to provide emotional support and discipline, processes that in turn are related to externalizing (more aggressive) and internalizing (more anxious and depressed) behavior among youth (Ceballo & McLoyd, 2002; Stern, Smith, & Jang, 1999). Thus, the circumstances of fewer resources and more responsibility make it more difficult for single parents to perform their role consistently and effectively.

This raises the issue of whether parenting programs that focus on increasing knowledge can be effective, in that helping single parents to be better parents may be not only an issue of *knowledge* of effective practices but also the wherewithal to manage their lives and *act* in accordance with that knowledge. Indeed, several important comprehensive, multifaceted prevention approaches report that it is extremely difficult to deliver prevention and intervention programming to families in the most dangerous and economically challenging circumstances (Conduct Problems Prevention Research Group, 1999, 2002; Huessman et al., 1996). It is a daunting task and the degree to which this task should include parenting knowledge *plus* community advocacy and support may be critical. Some of the more cost-effective models of intervention with African American families include both services and advocacy that helps families to procure necessary resources to leave them more time and availability to parent effectively (Henggeler et al., 1997; Henggeler et al., 1999; Olds, 2002).

Though there is a fair amount of consensus on the role of consistent and involved parenting, there is some debate concerning the role of physical punishment. Some researchers report finding a positive relationship between physical punishment and externalizing behavior among young children, regardless of race-ethnicity, for African American, European American, and Latino populations (McLoyd & Smith, 2002). Yet, other research has found physical punishment is related to increased problem behavior among whites but not among African American boys (Deater-Deckard, Dodge, Bates, & Pettit, 1996). Interestingly, McLoyd and Smith (2002) argue that physical punishment has deleterious effects on behavior across race, but this relationship does not occur when it is moderated by warm, supportive parenting. The authors purport that potentially, in the context of a warm communicative relationship, physical punishment is interpreted by children as a strategy to help and not harm them. Researchers argue that parents of African American children report being hypervigilant and more likely to use more parental control and authority when rearing children in either dangerous poor communities or in middle-income integrated communities in which they feel more pressure to have their children comply in order to avoid problems and succeed (Armistead, Forehand, Brody, & Maguen, 2002; Gonzales, Cauce, Friedman, & Mason, 1996). Particularly when examining the nature of violent and delinquent behavior, research has shown that the nature of the factors shown to be most potent in predicting violence and delinquency change over time as suggested by a developmental-ecological model (Loeber et al., 2000). Physical punishment decreases as a predictor of delinquency while poor supervision and the lack of positive parenting increase in significance.

Parenting strategies that express care, concern, and warmth, in which parents communicate with their young by listening and helping them to think about the consequences of their actions promotes children's moral development and good decision-making (Brody & Shaffer, 1982; Brody et al., 2001) and helps to build closeness in the family relationship (Rodick, Henggeler, & Hanson, 1986). Further, parents who communicate effectively with their children are more aware of *who* youth are with, *what* they are doing, and *where* they are, and are less likely to have children and youth involved in deviant peer groups or delinquent activities (Dishion, Patterson, Stoolmiller, & Skinner, 1991). In terms of family predictors of violence and delinquency, in their longitudinal research in Pittsburgh, Loeber et al. (1998) found that poor parental supervision is the best explanatory variable for delinquency, followed by poor parent-child communication. In light of this information, it seems that prevention efforts focused on African American families would benefit by focused approaches fostering positive parenting, which includes avoiding permissive and coercive patterns, and encouraging warmth and supervision with less attention to physical punishment which is less likely to have an effect in the context of warm relationships and decreases both in frequency and in prediction of violent behavior. However, there is some consensus upon important dimensions of parenting which should be the focus of efforts with African American families, along with community advocacy efforts that help the families to manage their lives and be more available to be effective parents.

Parenting to prevent violence and delinquency is important but not the only driving concern for African American parents. They also want to prepare their youth to succeed in a society in which they may experience racism and discrimination (Coll et al., 1996; Hughes et al., 2006). Indeed, criminologists discuss the extent to which African Americans might be more likely to experience police surveillance, disparate arrest rates, harsher sentencing, and disproportionate rates of incarceration due to their race (Free, 2003; Russell, 1999). Ogbu (1981) posits that shared historical, social, and cultural experiences might also inform parental perceptions of what is necessary for success within certain contexts. Perceptions of the competencies necessary for success within a particular context (avoiding bullying and violence) may vary. For example, in work with African American fathers in blighted urban neighborhoods, many fathers have been found to endorse defensive or protective violence by their sons (Caldwell et al., 2004; Caldwell, 2008). These fathers voiced a concern that their children not be the victims of violence and bullying and thought that self-defense was the most effective way to accomplish that in their children's social context. It is important to understand the sociocultural norms for dealing with provoked and unprovoked violence (Henry, Cartland, Ruch-Ross, & Monahan, 2004) that may emerge in certain contexts and to consider these norms in approaches to violence and delinquency with African American populations.

Peer Factors

As youth develop, not only is family important, but peer influences as well. The earliest notions of delinquent behavior suggested that families who permit disruptive, aggressive, and antisocial behavior from children unwittingly encourage it, resulting in children's rejection from normative peer groups and their bonding with other antisocial peers (Keenan, Loeber, Zhang, Stouthamer-Loeber, & Van Kammen, 1995). This bonding to antisocial peers could potentially lead to involvement in violent gangs, responsible for a large amount of violence. Thornberry (1998), with results from the Rochester longitudinal study of delinquency, reports that 86 percent of serious delinquency is committed by gang members, who are also responsible for 68 percent of violent delinquency and 70 percent of drug sales. Gang members are also more likely to own and carry guns. Snyder and Sickmund (2006) report that firearms were used in 78 percent of the murders of juveniles ages 12–17 years. A greater percentage of African American versus white juvenile murder victims were killed with a firearm (54% vs. 44%). Between 1984 and 1994, the number of juveniles who committed murder with a firearm increased about 320 percent, whereas murders committed without a firearm increased about 40 percent. Interestingly, only about 3 to 7 percent of non-gun owners or sport owners were involved in drug sales (Huizinga et al., 1995).

Gang membership seems to be more predominant among ethnic minority youth members, as reported by heads of law enforcement agencies who indicate that 47 percent of Latino, 31 percent of African American, 13 percent of non-Hispanic white, and 7 percent of Asian youths are gang affiliated (as cited in U.S. DHHS, 2001, p. 33). Importantly, youth involved in gangs seem to do so later in their adolescent development, resulting in more dysfunctional results including school dropout, out-of-wedlock parenthood, and unstable employment.

Attention has been given to the degree to which violent acts for youth occur as a result of gang affiliation and drug trafficking. The National Youth Gang Survey estimates that 46 percent of youth gang members are involved in street drug sales (Egley & Major, 2004). Though Blumstein and Wallman (2000) argue that multiple complex factors were involved in the decreasing trends in homicide, they surmise that drops in trafficking of crack cocaine (a cheaper, inexpensive version of cocaine favored by African Americans) also contributed to the lower trends.

However, it is important to note that minority youth, who are disproportionately involved in homicide and violence, evidence lower rates of substance use. According to data from the Monitoring the Future Study (Johnston, O'Malley, Bachman, & Schulenberg, 2004), in 2003, 10 percent of African American high school seniors said they had smoked cigarettes in the past 30 days, compared with 29 percent of whites. Fewer than one-third of African American seniors reported alcohol use in the past 30 days, compared with more than one-half of white. Of youth ages 12–14 who reported alcohol use (11% of youth in this age group), 27 percent said they used marijuana and 17 percent reported selling drugs, demonstrating a small amount of comorbidity between drug use and trafficking.

Contextual Factors and Violence

Understanding the contextual factors affecting violence is important to determining future directions for stemming the tide of homicide and violence among youth. It has become common knowledge that in contrast to adult crimes, which increase hourly between morning and evening hours, juvenile crimes peak between 3 and 4 p.m., fall to a lower level in the early evening hours, and decline substantially after 9 p.m. (Gottfredson et al., 2004; Snyder & Sickmund, 2006). Further, youth are 140 percent more likely to be victimized on school days than on non-school days (weekends and summer months). Interestingly, juvenile crimes are more likely to occur in a residence (64%), with only 19 percent occuring outdoors, 10 percent in commercial areas, and 6 percent in a school. This evidence suggests that prevention programming targeted at offering supervision during out-of-school time could potentially stem the tide of youth problem behavior and offer opportunities for positive youth development (Smith, 2007).

Neighborhood/Community Factors, and Violence Among African American Youth

Community characteristics such as concentrated poverty, unemployment, educational attainment level, vacant housing, and racial/ethnic heterogeneity are risk factors for violence, including homicide, injury, and physical abuse (Peeples & Loeber, 1994; Sampson, 2003). Interestingly, African American boys who do not live in underclass neighborhoods have similar rates of delinquent behavior as white boys once poverty and single-parent family structure are accounted for (Peeples & Loeber, 1994).

Several physical community characteristics are known correlates of violence. African Americans adolescents are more likely to live in communities characterized with concentrated poverty, vacant housing, and low educational attainment (Sampson, 2003), compared to whites. These characteristics may co-act to facilitate an environment conducive to violence. Communities with high concentrated poverty and low levels of educational attainment are known to be subject to a higher prevalence of violent events among African American adolescents. Presumably, these citizens may feel less empowered to influence their communities. Yet, with higher levels of collective efficacy, even poorer neighborhoods can exhibit reduced violence and delinquency (Sampson, Raudenbush, & Earls, 1997). On the other hand, neighborhoods with high rates of vacancy are thought to provide unoccupied space for violent crimes or activities which lead to violent crime. Furthermore, vacant housing decreases the property value of other houses in the neighborhood and, as a result, contributes to the cycle of neighborhood poverty. Adolescents who reside in neighborhoods characterized by high racial and ethnic heterogeneity are more likely to observe, participate in, or be victims of violence.

Exploring the relationship between adolescent development, social context, and youth violence has been of interest to social scientists for nearly a century (Burton, Obeidallah, & Allison, 1996). Of particular interest has been the influence of social context on the youth outcomes of poor inner-city African American adolescents (Anderson, 1999). For those African American adolescents living in communities marked by social marginalization, social disorganization, lack of informal social control, few conventional role models, and limited connections to mainstream opportunities, the creation of an "oppositional culture" is spawned with its own "code." As a result of persistent alienation, hopelessness, dislocation from the labor market, institutional racism, and structural inequality, the oppositional culture gives rise to a "street culture," which governs interpersonal relations on the street. This street culture and street-oriented environment produces a set of informal rules known as "the code of the street." Regardless of an individual's social orientation or status in the community, African American adolescents in poor urban communities are expected to know the code and the appropriate behavior for negotiating the code in public spaces. In fact, many African American parents socialize adolescents to become familiar with the code as an essential and necessary strategy to negotiate the inner-city environment.

At the heart of the code is the campaign for respect, a highly valued commodity on the streets of urban America. Anderson notes "respect is hard won but easily lost" (Anderson, 1999). For African American adolescents, particularly young African American males, this campaign for respect may place them in physical danger if they experience public disgrace or disrespect. Anderson postulates that for those invested in the code, even the most minor violations of the code (i.e., staring at an individual too long, stepping on an individual's sneaker without apology) may lead to fatal violence. Violence is often exacerbated by easy accessibility to firearms and may be significantly correlated to homicide as the leading cause of death for African American males ages 15–24 years.

For many poor urban African American male adolescents, incarceration or spending time detained in jail or prison may also result in increased social status and respect in the street-oriented culture. Yet exposure to the criminal justice system often results in increased violence and aggression (Petrosino, Turpin-Petrosino, & Buehler, 2003; Petrosino, Turpin-Petrosino, & Finckenauer, 2000). In a study of African American male youth recently released from a juvenile detention facility in Chicago, Teplin et al. (2005) found the rates of early violent death to be four times higher than for the general population of youth. Furthermore, more than 90 percent of all homicides among this population were firearm-related (Teplin et al., 2005).

In spite of the oppositional culture and code of the street that thrives in many inner-city communities, young African American males and parents familiar with the code often utilize a variety of social resources and parenting to move their children out of poverty and away from engaging in youth violence. Key to this discussion is the role of social capital in the analysis of violence among young African American males.

SOCIAL CAPITAL: AN INNOVATIVE AND INTEGRATIVE APPROACH TO YOUTH VIOLENCE

How social structures and cultures interact with individuals' psycho-social development to influence violent behavior is now a research priority for criminologists, especially those concerned with violence and its effects on children's social development (Reiss & Roth, 1993). The theoretical concept of social capital is a valuable and innovative tool for examining violent youth behavior because it integrates both individual and community-level modes of analysis. Social capital is a multi-dimensional theoretical tool that examines informal social controls, network ties (familial, extended "fictive" kinship, friendships, and extra-local power), and mutually trusting relationships among individuals and their potential buffering role in regard to youth violence (Sampson, 1992). Thus, social capital is an important concept because it is lodged not only in individuals but also in the social structures and organization of communities as well.

Furstenberg (1993) suggests that community social cohesion has indirect contextual effects on the control of delinquency and youth violence by facilitating social capital available to families, particularly the establishment of effective monitoring and supervision through parent-child and adult-peer social networks. Because few studies on youth violence among young African American males have effectively managed to integrate both community- and individual-level analysis of the factors that may foster or mitigate delinquent behavior, social capital is a theoretical tool ripe for this task. Social capital also resides in the form of social organizations and social structures that produce something of value for the individuals involved (Furstenberg, 1993).

Following up on the work conducted by prominent social capital and capitalization theorists (Coleman, 1988; Hagan, 2002; and Furstenberg, 1993), the contextual analysis of social capital and its relationship to youth violence will primarily focus on the individuals' connection to social networks composed of family and extended fictive kinship networks (Stack, 1974; Jarrett, 1995, 1997). Family members are connected to other families within communities through friendships and associations of parents and children, and these contacts extend the social capital of the family out into the community through schools, clubs, recreational sport organizations, and other voluntary groups. This implies that social capital is not simply a property of individuals, but of collectivities as well. Sampson and Laub (2005) concluded that parents who are well situated within secure and supportive social networks usually are inclined or driven by their capital positions to endow their children with forms of social, human, and cultural capital that increase their likelihood of success in school and later in life. However, in less advantaged community and family settings, parents who lack abundant social and cultural capital are less able to endow or transmit opportunities to their children and must continually adapt to diminished circumstances and opportunities they encounter (Hagan, 2002). Social capital potentially unites individuals within a neighborhood, thereby initiating and enhancing a sense of collectivity (Rose & Clear, 1998). In communities with large supplies of social capital, adolescents are encouraged to complete their education, discouraged from delinquency and violence, and sanctioned appropriately in informal and intimate relationships (Rose & Clear, 1998; Hagan, 2002).

It is important to highlight that the "involvement in delinquency or antisocial behavior during adolescence is relatively common among young males but does not generally lead to a life of serious crime. Not every troubled child becomes a delinquent; not every juvenile who commits an illegal offense becomes a habitual and chronic offender; and not every juvenile offender becomes a career criminal" (Sullivan, 1989). Furstenberg and colleagues (1999) note that the presence or absence of social capital in a community may be an important link between the structure of communities, families, and the development of children. Bonds to families, schools, communities, and other prosocial contexts can protect youth against the elaboration and extension of problem behaviors, particularly participation in youth violence.

The Interaction of Neighborhood Effects, Social Capital, and Youth Violence

At the most general level, community social organization may be conceptualized as the ability of a community structure to realize the common values of its residents and maintain effective social controls (Kornhauser, 1978; Bursik, 1988; Sampson & Groves, 1989). Some of the more central and salient goals among inner-city residents and families are the collective desires to live in a safe and orderly environment free of predatory crime, and to have adequate housing, effective schools, and a healthy living environment for their children. In order to achieve these common and shared goals, informal role relationships are established to achieve social regulation (Kornhauser, 1978).

This social control approach to community is grounded in what social control theorists Kasarda and Janowitz (1974) coined the "systemic model," where community is viewed as a complex system of friendships and kinship networks, and formal and informal associational ties rooted in family life, ongoing socialization processes, and local institutions. Sampson and colleagues (1999) argue that this systemic approach to social control is theoretically compatible with more recent formulations in the recent social science literature of what has been termed *social capital*. Putnam (1995) similarly defines social capital as "features of social organization such as networks, norms, and trust that facilitate coordination and cooperation by community members for mutual benefit."

In contrast, Sampson and Wilson (1995) argue that the loss of stable employment among families living in distressed urban areas has undermined the collective socialization of youth, consequently decreasing social capital for youth and families. Decreased social capital is reflected in the forms of less neighborhood monitoring practices, institutional resources (i.e., inadequate and failing schools, and fewer recreational activities), and fewer adult role models or "oldheads" (Anderson, 1999). The result of a decreased pool of social capital (i.e., stable families and employed adult African American males) within poor inner-city African American neighborhoods plays a crucial role in weakening informal social controls and also weakens links of local youth to wider social institutions and fostering of desired principles and values (Kornhauser, 1978). Consequently, more unsupervised youth groups "hang out," providing the opportunity for more serious crime and violence.

However, few research efforts have examined the effects of social capital and family disruptions on inner-city variations in serious youth crime, and none of these focused on racially disaggregated rates of African American male youth violence. This despite research having consistently demonstrated the importance of community family structure in predicting offending and victimization rates among African American youth (Sampson, 1997).

A theoretical framework for integrating social disorganization theory with the concept of social capital aids in our understanding of the effects of community and family structure on crime. Furstenberg and colleagues (1999) note that "families provide a crucial link between community and the successful development of at-risk youth." Particular emphasis is placed on the family experience in creating social capital and "community-bridging strategies" for their children (Jarrett, 1995). Emerging research examining the linkages between family and community has found that families who feel closer to their communities are more efficacious in their parenting, which results in youth who are less prone to negative peer affiliation (Simons, Simons, Burt, Brody, Cutrona, 2005). There are numerous examples of the strategies devised by families that create positive social networks across family, school, church, and community. Within extended familial networks a great deal of male role modeling may occur (Richardson, 2009). Poor urban families often create their own strategies for the successful development of young African American males through the use of local basketball leagues with male mentoring programs, the Boy Scouts, or by simply utilizing the positive male role models within their families and extended social networks such as uncles, older brothers, older cousins, family friends, etc. These men often serve as surrogate parents to young African American men (Richardson, 2009). Furthermore, structured and regular mentoring experiences, such as implemented by the Big Brothers/Big Sisters Program, have been found to be effective in improving youth achievement and reducing problem behavior (Grossman & Tierney, 1998).

These are merely a few of the examples that have been particularly useful in helping to understand the microlevel differences in social context that contribute to explaining how these young men and their families manage to " make it" (Furstenberg et al., 1999), a term used to imply successful adolescent development in high-risk settings over the life course in school and the community. How families, particularly parents, manage social capital and are able to "work informal and formal systems" to access and activate social resources for the social benefit of their children may be critical to the level of engagement in serious youth violence.

Moreover, the effect of incarceration has disproportionately affected the social capital of poor African American communities and families, severely weakening community structures and families, and their ability to self-regulate neighborhoods and youth. In 2004, one out of three African American males aged 16 to 34 years, living in metropolitan areas and contiguous counties, was admitted to prison. According to the Pew Center on the States Report (Warren, 2008) entitled "One in 100: Behind Bars in America 2008," one in every fifteen black males age 18 or older is in jail or prison. Furthermore, the lifetime probability of an African American male going to state or federal prison is 29 percent. Consequently, the impact of incarceration on African American communities has severely depleted the supplies of social capital in poor urban areas already suffering from extreme social disorganization. Rose and Clear (1998) argue that the impact of incarcerating African American males drains African American communities and families of critical social resources. Men who leave their communities for lengthy prison terms potentially "take with them the support they have been providing to networks that sustain private and parochial controls" in poor urban communities (p. 452). A lack of support and employment inhibits the ability of many African American men to contribute both socially and economically (Wilson, 1987). Alternatively, Sullivan's (1989) ethnographic study of young offenders found that many of these young men contributed financially and socially to the welfare of their neighborhoods, families, and children. Other ethnographies also show that young male offenders live within close associational networks of families and children, and act as resources to those networks (Rose & Clear, 1998). The caution here is that parental incarceration is considered an environmental risk factor (not a predestinating or biological one) for future violence and delinquency (Moffitt, 1987). At any rate, the depletion of African American men via incarceration disrupts the potential for social capital and individual networks used by young at-risk African American males, which in turn disrupts community networks. This process compounds a community's inability to provide informal social control over its youth. The literature review on neighborhood effects and families and youth violence has documented that, at the basic level, the absence of males limits the number of available men to supervise young people in the community. Sampson and Groves (1989) have documented that the presence of large numbers of unsupervised youth is predictive of serious crime and violence at the neighborhood level.

Although we can hypothesize about the implications of these patterns, ironically, not much is known about the social networks so fundamental to social capital and social control among poor African American communities, families, and adolescent males (Rose & Clear, 1998). Bourdieu (1986) suggests that "how the social networks are used may be as valuable (or even more so) than social networks themselves." Even though we can assume that social capital enhances the neighborhood and families' ability to self-regulate and self-control, within criminology not much work has focused on the nature of networks and their impact on children, families, and communities in regard to serious youth violence, specifically among at-risk young African American males. The potential contribution of social capital to youth behavior is a ripe uncharted area of scientific inquiry.

APPROACHES TO ADDRESSING YOUTH VIOLENCE AND HOMICIDE: IMPLICATIONS FOR PREVENTION AND INTERVENTION

Addressing the multilevel complexities of violence among African American youth requires a culturally appropriate approach that takes into consideration the influence of individual, family, and community characteristics which co-act to produce the epidemic of violence. Furthermore, if we are to be successful in reducing and eventually eliminating violence, we must consider the elimination of deleterious risk factors, but must also promote healthy protective factors. The PEN-3 Model (Airhihenbuwa, 1993), recognizing the role of the Person/Individual, Extended Family, and Neighborhood in public health problems such as youth violence, is specifically designed to facilitate intervention and policy planning across multiple contexts while considering cultural aspects of the target populations of African descent.

Qualitative research has been helpful in identifying successful parenting strategies. One of the successful strategies identified in qualitative studies of parenting in high-risk communities is the family protection strategy (Jarrett, 1997). Family protection strategies include avoidance of dangerous areas, temporal use of the neighborhood, restrictions on neighboring relations, and ideological support of mainstream orientations. Other successful parenting strategies identified were protective monitoring strategies and parental resource-seeking strategies (Jarrett, 1997; Furstenberg, 2000). Protective monitoring strategies include chaperonage, intensive collective supervision by adults, and community-bridging. Parental resource-seeking strategies encompass parents who allocate a significant portion of their time and energy seeking out local and extra-local resources and opportunities for the social benefit of their children. Despite limited resources in poor African American communities, parents are able to locate, access, and acquire social resources that buffer children from engaging in high-risk behaviors. Resources within and outside the community are frequently accessed through social relationships such as kinship ties, labor market connections, and relationships with neighbors and community institutions.

Empirical research has helped to validate some of these strategies uncovered by ethnographic approaches. Substantial research has demonstrated the usefulness of programs for parents that are designed to help promote effective disciplinary practices, monitoring, supervision, and warm family relationships (Conduct Problems Prevention Research Group, 1999, 2002; Henggeler et al., 1997, 1999; Olds, 2002; Smith et al., 2004; Webster-Stratton, 1998). More recently, there are approaches that draw on the cultural traditions and strengths of African American families in fostering positive parenting and youth development (Murry et al., 2007).

As described above, there are additional strategies that have yet to be researched extensively, including involving social fathers and fictive kin. The closest approach approximating this strategy is the use of mentors, though these mentors are diverse in terms of racial-ethnic background and socioeconomic status, with most being upwardly mobile professionals (Grossman & Tierney, 1998). Research rarely examines the affective roles and functions of men in African American families. Men in extended familial networks, such as uncles, play a significant role in the lives of African American male youth as social fathers in the absence of the biological father. These men are valuable forms of family-based social capital and social support in the lives of at-risk youth. They often provide adult supervision, monitoring, and chaperonage (Jarrett, 1997).

Parental resource-seeking strategies that provide community bridges to social resources and cultural activities, extending beyond the local community, are also successful parenting practices. Community-bridging parenting strategies provide the opportunity for parents to connect at-risk African American youth to human, social, and cultural capital outside of the local community. This strategy exposes African American male youth imprisoned by a world of poverty to mainstream educational, social, and cultural opportunities. Examples of these educational, social, and cultural opportunities are programs such as the Fresh Air Fund, A Better Chance, AAU Basketball Leagues, etc. Exposing at-risk African American male youth to social worlds that extend beyond the local community provides an alternate reality not limited to daily survival, the code of the street, violence, and poverty.

Similarly, empirical work is beginning to examine approaches aimed at strategies that combine approaches designed to enhance both family processes and linkages to helpful community resources (Huston et al., 2001, 2005). The New Hope Project provides child care and structured community offerings in addition to helping to support parents in rearing their young. Children engaged in the project are found to spend more time in supervised engaging offerings in the afternoon than nonparticipating children.

The project has been found to exhibit benefits to both families and to their children in terms of their academic achievement and reductions in problem behavior.

With this idea of connecting families to community resources, more work is being conducted in community-based out-of-school learning opportunities and after-school programs as a mechanism for fostering youth positive engagement in the community and social capital. Though few rigorous trials exist, preliminary evidence suggests that after-school settings can be helpful in reducing problem behavior and promoting positive youth development (Durlak & Weissberg, 2007; Gottfredson et al., 2004).

In sum, for interventions and policies to be effective in reversing the epidemic of violence, they must account for the African American youth within multiple contexts, positive and negative influences from multiple sources, and most importantly, how sociocultural factors shape the contexts of African American youth.

REFERENCES

Airhihenbuwa, C. (1993). Health promotion for child survival in Africa: Implications for cultural appropriateness. *Hygiene, 12*(3), 10–15.

Anderson, E. (1999). *Code of the street: Decency, violence and the moral life of the inner-city*. New York: W. W. Norton & Company.

Aos, S., Lieb, R., Mayfield, J., Miller, M., & Pennucci, A. (2004). *Benefits and costs of prevention and early intervention programs for youth*. Olympia, WA: Washington State Institute for Public Policy.

Armistead, L., Forehand, R., Brody, G., & Maguen, S. (2002). Parenting and child psychosocial adjustment in single-parent African American families: Is community context important? *Behavior Therapy, 33*, 361–375.

Beauchaine, T. P., Neuhaus, E., Brenner, S. L., & Gatzke-Kopp, L. (2008). Ten good reasons to consider biological processes in prevention and intervention research. *Development and Psychopathology. Special Issue: Integrating biological measures into the design and evaluation of preventive interventions, 20*(3), 745–774.

Blumstein, A., & Wallman, J. (Eds.). (2000). *The crime drop in America*. New York: Cambridge University Press.

Bourdieu, P. (1986). *The forms of capital: Handbook of theory and research for the sociology of education*. New York: Greenwood Publishing Group.

Brody, G. H., Ge, X., Conger, R. D., Gibbons, F. X., Murry, V. B., Gerrard, M., et al. (2001). The influence of neighborhood disadvantage, collective socialization, and parenting on African American children's affiliation with deviant peers. *Child Development, 72*, 1231–1246.

Brody, G. H., & Shaffer, J. N. (1982). Contributions of parents and peers to children's moral socialization. *Developmental View 2*(1), 31–75.

Bursik, R. J., Jr. (1988). Social disorganization and theories of crime and deliquency: Problems and prospects. *Criminology, 26*, 519–552.

Burton, L. M., Obeidallah, D. A., & Allison, K. (1996). Ethnographic perspectives on social context and adolescent development among inner-city African-American teens. In D. Jessor, A. Colby, & R. Shweder (Eds.), *Ethnography and human development: Context and meaning in social inquiry* (pp. 395–418). Chicago: University of Chicago Press.

Cairney, J., Boyle, M., Offord, D. R., & Racine, Y. (2003). Stress, social support and depression in single and married mothers. *Social Psychiatry and Psychiatric Epidemiology, 38*, 442–449.

Caldwell, C. (2008). *Pathways to prevention: Influencing the parenting attitudes and behaviors of non-resident African American fathers as protection against adolescent risk behaviors*. Invited presentation for the Center for Family Research in Diverse Contexts and the Child Study Center, The Pennsylvania State University, University Park, PA.

Caldwell, C. H., Wright, J. C., Zimmerman, M. A., Walsemann, K. M., Williams, D., & Isichei, P. A. C. (2004). Enhancing adolescent health behaviors through strengthening non-resident father-son relationships: A model for intervention with African-American families. *Health Education Research, 19*(6), 644–656.

Ceballo, R., & McLoyd, V. C. (2002). Social support and parenting in poor, dangerous neighborhoods. *Child Development, 73*(4), 1310–1321.

Centers for Disease Control and Prevention. (2001). *Morbidity and mortality weekly report, 50,* 780–783.

Centers for Disease Control and Prevention. (2004). Youth risk behavior surveillance—United States, 2003. *Morbidity and Mortality Weekly Report, 53*(SS–2).

Chamberlain, P., & Patterson, G. R. (1995). Discipline and child compliance in parenting. In M. H. Bornstein (Ed.), *Handbook of parenting*: Vol. 4 (pp. 204–225). Hillsdale, NJ: Erlbaum.

Coleman, J. S. (1988). Social capital in the creation of human capital. *American Journal of Sociology 94*: S95–S120.

Coll, C. G., Crnic, K., Lamberty, G., Wasik, B. J., Jenkins, R., Garcia, H.V., & McAdoo, H. P. (1996). An integerative model for the study of developmental competencies in minority children. *Child Development, 67,* 1891–1914.

Conduct Problems Prevention Research Group. (1999). Initial impact of the fast track prevention trial for conduct problems: I. The high-risk sample. *Journal of Consulting and Clinical Psychology, 60,* 783–792.

Conduct Problems Prevention Research Group. (2002). Evaluation of the first three years of the fast track prevention trial with children at high risk for adolescent conduct problems. *Journal of Abnormal Child Psychology, 30*(2), 19–35.

Cook, P. J., & Ludwig, J. (2002). The costs of gun violence against children. *The Future of Children, 12*(2), 87–100.

Darity, W., Jr., & Nicholson, M. J. (2005). Racial wealth inequality and the black family. In V. C. McLoyd, N. E. Hill, & K. A. Dodge (Eds.), *African American family life: Ecological and cultural diversity* (pp. 78–85). New York: Guilford Press.

Deater-Deckard, K., Dodge, K. A., Bates, J. E., & Pettit, G. S. (1996). Physical discipline among African American and European American mothers: Links to children's externalizing behaviors. *Developmental Psychology, 32*(6), 1065–1072.

Dishion, T. J., Patterson, G. R., Stoolmiller, M., & Skinner, M. L. (1991). Family, school, and behavioral antecedents to early adolescent involvement with antisocial peers. *Developmental Psychology, 27,* 172–180.

Durlak, J. A., & Weissberg, R. P. (2007). *The impact of after-school programs that promote personal and social skills.* Chicago: The University of Illinois at Chicago.

Edlynn, E. S., Gaylord-Harden, N. K, Richards, M. H., & Miller, S. A. (2008). African American inner-city youth exposed to violence: Coping skills as a moderator for anxiety. *American Journal of Orthopsychiatry, 78*(2), 249–258.

Egley, A., & Major, A. (2004). Highlights of the 2002 National Youth Gang Survey. *OJJDP Fact Sheet* (#01). Washington, DC: U.S. Department of Justice, Office of Justice Programs, Office of Juvenile Justice and Delinquency Prevention.

Elliott, D. S., Menard, S., Rankin, B., Elliott, A., Wilson, W. J., & Huizinga, D. (2006). *Good kids from bad neighborhoods: Successful development in social context.* New York: Cambridge University Press.

Foster, E. M., Jones, D., & Conduct Problems Prevention Research Group. (2006). Can a costly intervention be cost-effective? An analysis of violence prevention. *Archives of General Psychiatry, 63,* 1284–1291.

Free, M. D. (2003). Race and presentencing decisions: The cost of being African American. In M. D. Free (Ed.), *Racial issues in criminal justice: The case of African Americans* (pp. 137–157). Westport, CT: Praeger.

Furstenberg, F. (1993). How families manage risk and opportunity in dangerous neighborhoods. In W. J. Wilson (Ed.), *Sociology and the public agenda* (pp. 231–258). Newbury Park, CA: Sage.

Furstenberg, F. (2000). The sociology of adolescence and youth in the 1990s: A critical commentary. *Journal of Marriage and the Family, 62,* 896–910.

Furstenberg, F., Cook, T., Eccles, J., Elder, G., & Sameroff, A. (1999). *Managing to make it: Urban families and adolescent success.* Chicago: University of Chicago Press.

Gonzales, N. A., Cauce, A. M., Friedman, R. J., & Mason, C. A. (1996). Family, peer, and neighborhood influence on academic achievement among African American adolescents: One year prospective effects. *American Journal of Community Psychology, 24,* 365–387.

Gottfredson, D. C., Gerstenblith, S. A., Soule, D. A., Womer, S. C., & Lu, S. (2004). Do after school programs reduce delinquency? *Prevention Science, 5*(4), 253–266.

Grossman, J. B., & Tierney, J. P. (1998). Does mentoring work? An impact study of the Big Brothers Big Sisters Program. *Evaluation Review, 22*(3), 403–426.

Hagan, J. (2002). In and out of harm's way: Violent victimization and the social capital of fictive street families. *Criminology, 40,* 831–866.

Hawkins, J. D., Smith, B. H., Hill, K. G., Kosterman, R., Catalano, R. F., & Abbott, R. D. (2003). Understanding and Preventing Crime and Violence. In T. Thornberry and M. D. Krohn (Eds.). *Taking stock of delinquency: An overview of findings from contemporary longitudinal studies* (pp. 255–312). New York: Kluwer Academics.

Henggeler, S. W., Melton, G. B., Brondino, M. J., Scherer, D. G., & Hanley, J. H. (1997). Multisystemic therapy with violent and chronic juvenile offenders and their families: The role of treatment fidelity in successful dissemination. *Journal of Consulting and Clinical Psychology, 65*, 821–833.

Henggeler, S. W., Pickrel, S. G., & Brondino, M. J. (1999). Multisystemic treatment of substance abusing and dependent delinquents: Outcomes, treatment fidelity, and transportability. *Mental Health Services Research, 1*, 171–184.

Henry, D. B., Cartland, J., Ruch-Ross, H., & Monahan, K. (2004). A return potential model of setting norms for aggression. *American Journal of Community Psychology, 33*, 131–149.

Huesmann, L. R., Maxwell, C. D., Eron, L., Dalhberg, L., Guerra, N. G., Tolan, P. H., VanAcker, R., & Henry, D. (1996). Evaluating a cognitive/ecological program for the prevention of aggression among urban children. *American Journal of Preventive Medicine, 12*(5, Suppl), 120–128.

Hughes, D., Rodriguez, J., Smith, E. P., Johnson, D. J., Stevenson, H. C., & Spicer, P. (2006). Parents' ethnic-racial socialization practices: A review of the research and directions for future study. *Developmental Psychology, 42*, 747–770.

Huizinga, D., Loeber, R., & Thornberry, T. P. (1995). Recent findings from the program of research on the causes and correlates of delinquency. Washington, DC: U.S. Department of Justice, Office of Justice Programs, Office of Juvenile Justice and Delinquency Prevention, NCJ 1599042.

Huizinga, D., Weiher, A. W., Espiritu, R., & Esbensen, F. (2003). Delinquency and crime: Some highlights from the Denver Youth Survey. In T. Thornberry and M. D. Krohn (Eds.) *Taking stock of delinquency: An overview of findings from contemporary longitudinal studies* (pp. 47–91). New York: Kluwer Academics.

Huston, A., Duncan, G., Granger, R.T., Bos, J., McLoyd, L., Mistry, R., Crosby, D., Gibson, C., Magnuson, K., Romich, J., & Ventura, A. (2001). Work-based antipoverty programs for parents can enhance the school performance and social behavior of children. *Child development, 72*(1), 318–336.

Huston, A., Duncan, G., McLoyd, V., Crosby, D., Ripke, M., Weisner, T., & Eldred, C. (2005). Impacts on children of a policy to promote employment and reduce poverty for low-income parents: New hope after 5 years. *Developmental Psychology, 41*(6), 902–918.

Jackson, A. P., Brooks-Gunn, J., Huang, C. C., & Glassman, M. (2000). Single mothers in low-wage jobs: Financial strain, parenting, and preschoolers' outcomes. *Child Development, 71*(5), 1409–1423.

Jarrett, R. (1997). African-American family and parenting strategies in impoverished neighborhoods. *Qualitative Sociology, 20*, 275–288.

Jarrett, R. (1995). Growing up poor: The family experiences of socially mobile youth in low-income African-American neighborhoods. *Journal of Adolescent Research, 10*, 111–135.

Johnston, L., O'Malley, P., Bachman, J., & Schulenberg, J. (2004). Demographic subgroup trends for various licit and illicit drugs, 1975–2003. *Monitoring the Future Occasional Paper* (No. 60). Ann Arbor, MI: Institute for Social Research.

Kasarda, J., & Janowitz, M. (1974). Community attachment in mass society. *American Sociological Review, 39*, 328–339.

Keenan, K., Loeber, R., Zhang, Q., Stouthamer-Loeber, M., & Van Kammen, W. B. (1995). The influence of deviant peers on the development of boys' disruptive and delinquent behavior: A temporal analysis. *Development & Psychopathology, 7*, 715–726.

Kornhauser, R. (1978). *Sources of delinquency*. Chicago: University of Chicago Press.

Lochman, J. E., & van den Steenhoven, A. (2002). Family-based approaches to substance abuse prevention. *Journal of Primary Prevention, 23*(1), 49–114.

Loeber, R., Drinkwater, M., Yin, Y., Anderson, S. J., Schmidt, L. C., & Crawford, A. (2000). Stability of family interactions from ages 6 to 18. *Journal of Abnormal Child Psychology, 28*, 353–369.

Loeber, R., Farrington, D. P., Stouthamer-Loeber, M., Moffitt, T. Caspi, A., White, H. R., Wei, E., & Beyers, J., (2003). The development of male offending: Key findings from fourteen years of the Pittsburgh Youth Study. In T. Thornberry and M. D. Krohn (Eds.), *Taking stock of delinquency: An overview of findings from contemporary longitudinal studies* (pp. 93–136). New York:Kluwer Academics.

Loeber, R., Farrington, D. P., Stouthamer-Loeber, M., & Van Kammen, W. B. H. (1998). *Antisocial behavior and mental health problems: Explanatory factors in childhood and adolescence*. Mahwah, NJ: Lawrence Erlbaum.

Lutzker, J. R., Touchette, P. E., & Campbell, R. V. (1988). Parental positive reinforcement might make a difference: A rejoinder to Forehand. *Child and Family Behavior Therapy, 10*(4), 2–33.

Maccoby, E. A., & Martin, J. A. (1983). Socialization in the context of the family: Parent-child interaction. In P. H. Mussen (Ed.), *Handbook of child psychology*: Vol. IV (4th ed., pp. 1–101). New York: Wiley.

Martinez, C. R., & Forgatch, M. S. (2001). Preventing problems with boys' noncompliance: Effect of a parent training intervention for divorcing mothers. *Journal of Consulting and Clinical Psychology, 69*(3), 416–428.

McLoyd, V. C. (1998). Socioeconomic disadvantage and child development. *American Psychologist, 53*(2), 185–204.

McLoyd, V. C., & Smith, J. (2002). Physical discipline and behavior problems in African American, European American, and Latino children: Emotional support as a moderator. *Journal of Marriage and the Family, 64*, 40–53.

Moffitt, T E. (1987). Parental mental disorder and off-spring criminal behavior: An adoption study. *Psychiatry, 50*, 346–360.

Murry, V., Berkel, C. Brody, G., Gibbons, M., & Gibbons, F. (2007). The strong African American families program: Longitudinal pathways to sexual risk reduction. *Journal of Adolescent Health, 41*(4), 333–342.

National Center for Injury Prevention and Control, Centers for Disease Control and Prevention. *The National Violent Death Reporting System.* Retrieved December 4, 2008, from http://www.cdc.gov/ViolencePrevention/NVDRS/index.html

O'Donnell, J., Hawkins, J. D., Catalano, R. F., Abbott, R. D., & Day, L. E. (1995). Preventing school failure, drug use, and delinquency among low-income children: Long-term intervention in elementary schools. *American Journal of Orthopsychiatry, 65*, 87–100.

Ogbu, J. J. (1981). Origins of human competence: A cultural-ecological perspective. *Child Development, 52*, 413–429.

Olds, D. L. (2002). Prenatal and infancy home visiting by nurses: From randomized trials to community replication. *Prevention-Science, 3*(3), 153–172.

Paik, H. & Comstock, G. (1994). The effects of television violence on antisocial behavior: A meta-analysis. *Communication Research, 21*, 516–546.

Peeples, F., & Loeber, R. (1994). Do individual factors and neighborhood context explain ethnic differences in juvenile delinquency? *Journal of Quantitative Criminology, 10*, 141–157.

Petrosino, A., Turpin-Petrosino, C., & Buehler, J. (2003). Scared straight and other juvenile awareness programs for preventing juvenile delinquency: A systematic review of the randomized experimental evidence. *The Annals of the American Academy of Political and Social Science, 589*, 41–62.

Petrosino, A., Turpin-Petrosino, C., & Finckenauer, J. (2000). Well meaning programs can have harmful effects! Lessons from experiments of programs such as Scared Straight. *Crime and Delinquency, 46*, 354–379.

Proctor, L. J. (2006). Children growing up in a violent community: The role of the family. *Aggression and Violent Behavior, 11*, 558–576.

Putnam, R. (1995). Bowling alone: America's declining social capital. *Journal of Democracy, 6*, 65–78.

Raine, A., Venables, P., Dalais, C., Mellingen, K., Reynolds, C., & Mednick, S. (2001). Early educational and health enrichment at age 3–5 years is associated with increased autonomic and central nervous system arousal and orienting at age 11 years: Evidence from the Mauritius Child Health Project. *Psychophysiology, 38*, 254–266.

Reid, J. B., Patterson, G. R., & Snyder, J. (2002). *Antisocial behavior in children and adolescents: A developmental analysis and model for intervention.* Washington, DC: American Psychological Association.

Reiss, A. J., & Roth, J. A. (1993). *Understanding and preventing violence.* Washington, DC: National Academies Press.

Richardson, J. (2009). Men do matter: Ethnographic insights on the socially supportive role of the African American uncle in the lives of inner-city African American male youth. *Journal of Family Issues, 30*, 1041–1069.

Rodick, J. D., Henggeler, S. W., & Hanson, C. L. (1986). An evaluation of the Family Adaptability and Cohesion Evaluation Scales and the Circumplex Model. *Journal of Abnormal Child Psychology, 14*(1), 77–87.

Rose, D., & Clear, T. (1998). Incarceration, social capital and crime: Implications for social disorganization theory. *Criminology, 36*, 441–479.

Russell, K. K. (1999). Driving while black: Corollary phenomena and collateral consequences. *Boston Law Review, 40*, 717–731.

Rutherford, A., Zwi, A. B., Grove, N. J., & Butchart, A. (2007). Violence: A priority for public health? (part 2). *Journal of Epidemiology and Community Health, 61*(9), 764–770.

Sampson, R. J., & Groves, W. B. (1989). Community structure and crime: Testing social disorganization theory. *American Journal of Sociology, 94*, 774.

Sampson, R. J. (1997). The embeddedness of child and adolescent development: A community-level perspective on urban violence. In J. McCord (Ed.), *Childhood and violence in the inner city* (pp. 31–77). New York: Cambridge University Press.

Sampson, R. J. (1992). Family management and child development: Insights from social disorganization theory. In J. McCord (Ed.), *Advances in criminal theory* (pp. 63–93). New Brunswick, NJ: Transaction Books.

Sampson, R. J. (2003). The neighborhood context of well-being. *Perspectives in Biology and Medicine, 46*(3 Supp. Summer 2003), S53–S64.

Sampson, R. J. (1995). Unemployment and imbalanced sex ratios: Race-specific consequences for family structure and crime. In M. B. Tucker & C. Mitchell-Kernan (Eds.), *The decline in marriage among African Americans* (pp. 229–260). New York: Russell Sage.

Sampson, R. J., & Laub, J. (2005). A life-course view of the development of crime. *The Annals of the American Academy of Political and Social Science, 602*, 12–45.

Sampson, R. J., Morenoff, J., & Earls, F. (1999). Beyond social capital: Spatial dynamics of collective efficacy for children. *American Sociological Review*, 64, 633–660.

Sampson, R. J., Raudenbush, S. W., & Earls, F. (1997). Neighborhoods and violent crime: A multilevel study of collective efficacy. *Science, 277*(5328), 918–924.

Sampson, R. J., & Wilson, W. J. (1995). Toward a theory of race, crime, and urban inequality. In J. Hagan & R. Peterson (Eds.), *Crime and inequality* (pp. 37–56). Stanford, CA: Stanford University Press.

Shapiro, T. (2001). The importance of assets: The benefits of spreading asset ownership. In T. N. Shapiro & E. Wolff (Eds.), *Assets for the poor: The benefits of spreading asset ownership* (pp. 11–333). New York: Russell Sage Foundation.

Simons, R., Simons, L., Burt, C., Brody, G., Cutrona, C. (2005). Collective efficacy, authoritative parenting and delinquency: A longitudinal test of a model integrating community - and family-level processes. *Criminology: An Interdisciplinary Journal, 43*(4), 989–1029.

Smith, E. P. (2007). The role of afterschool settings in positive youth development. *Journal of Adolescent Health, 41*(3), 219–220.

Smith, E. P., Gorman-Smith, D. Quinn, W., Rabiner, D., Winn, D., & the Multi-site Violence Prevention Project. (2004). Community-based multiple family groups to prevent and reduce violent and aggressive behavior: The G.R.E.A.T. Families Program. *American Journal of Preventive Medicine, 26*(1S), 39–47.

Smith, E. P., & Hasbrouck, L. M. (2006). Preventing youth violence among African American youth: The sociocultural context of risk and protective factors. In N. G. Guerra & E. P. Smith (Eds.), *Preventing youth violence in a multicultural society* (pp. 17–46). Washington, DC: American Psychological Association.

Snyder, H. N., & Sickmund, M. (2006). *Juvenile offenders and victims: 2006 national report*. Washington, DC: U.S. Department of Justice, Office of Justice Programs, Office of Juvenile Justice and Delinquency Prevention.

Snyder, J. J., & Huntley, D. (1990). Troubled families and troubled youth: The development of antisocial behavior and depression in children. In P. E. Leone (Ed.), *Understanding troubled and troubling youth* (pp. 194–225). Newbury Park, CA: Sage.

Soares, R. R. (2006, September). The welfare cost of violence across countries. *Journal of Health Economics 25*(5),821–846.

Stack, C. (1974). *All our kin*. New York: Basic Books.

Stern, S. B., Smith, C.A., & Jang, S. J. (1999). Urban families and adolescent mental health. *Social Work Research, 23*, 15–27.

Sullivan, M. (1989). *Getting paid: Youth crime and work in the inner-city*. Ithaca, NY: Cornell University Press.

Teplin, L., McClelland, G., Abram, K., & Milusenic, D. (2005). Early violent deaths among delinquent youth: A prospective longitudinal study. *Pediatrics, 115*, 1586–1593.

Thornberry, T. P. (1998). Membership in youth gangs and involvement in serious and violent offending. In R. Loeber & D. P. Farrington (Eds.), *Serious and violent juvenile offenders: Risk factors and successful interventions* (pp. 147–166). Thousand Oaks, CA: Sage.

Thornberry, T. P., & Krohn, M. D. (2003). *Taking stock of delinquency: An overview of findings from contemporary longitudinal studies*. New York: Kluwer Academics.

Tolan, P., Gorman-Smith, D., & Henry, D. B. (2003). The developmental ecology of urban males' youth violence. *Developmental Psychology. Special Issue: Violent children, 39*(2), 274–291.

U.S. Census Bureau. (2001). Historical Tables. Retrieved from http://www.census.gov/hhes/www/poverty/histpov/hstpov2.html; and Poverty in the United States, 2001. Retrieved from http:// www.census.gov/hhes/www/poverty/histpov/famindex.html

U.S. Census Bureau. (2008). America's families and living arrangements: 2008. In *Current population survey, 2008 annual social and economic supplement* (Table C9). Retrieved August 31, 2009, from http://www.census.gov/population/www/socdemo/hh-fam.html

U.S. Department of Health and Human Services. (2001). *Youth violence: A report of the Surgeon General*. Rockville, MD: Author.

U.S. Department of Justice, Federal Bureau of Investigation. (2000). *Crime in the United States, 1999*. Washington, DC: U.S. Government Printing Office.

U.S. Department of Justice, Federal Bureau of Investigation. (2007). *Crime in the United States*. Washington, DC: U.S. Government Printing Office. Retrieved December 11, 2008, from http://www.fbi.gov/ucr/cius2007/arrests/index.html

Warren, J. (2008). *One in 100: Behind bars in America 2008*. Philadelphia: Pew Center on the States.

Waters, H., Hyder, A., Rajkotia, Y., Basu, S., & Butchart, A. (2005). The costs of interpersonal violence: An international review. *Health Policy, 73*, 303–315.

Webster-Stratton, C. (1998). Preventing conduct problems in Head Start children: Strengthening parenting competencies. *Journal of Consulting and Clinical Psychology, 66*, 715–730.

Webster-Stratton, C., & Hammond, M. (1997). Treating children with early-onset conduct problems: A comparison of child and parent training interventions. *Journal of Consulting and Clinical Psychology, 65*, 93–109.

Williams, K. R., & Guerra, N. G. (2006). Ethnicity, youth violence, and the ecology of development. In N. G. Guerra & E. P. Smith (Eds.), *Preventing youth violence in a multicultural society* (pp. 17–46). Washington, DC: American Psychological Association.

Wilson, W. (1987). *The truly disadvantaged: The inner city, the underclass, and public policy*. Chicago: University of Chicago Press.

CHAPTER

9

NARROWING THE GAP BETWEEN SUPPLY AND DEMAND OF ORGANS FOR TRANSPLANTATION

Current Issues for African Americans

KIMBERLY JACOB ARRIOLA
DANA H. Z. ROBINSON
L. EBONY BOULWARE

Organ and tissue transplantation has extended and saved lives, improved quality of life, decreased overall mortality from certain diseases and conditions, and is the preferred therapy for many types of end-organ failure. However, the gap between the number of transplants needed and the number of organs available for transplant continues to increase. Viable organs for transplantation are a scarce resource, particularly for African Americans, and a disproportionate number of African Americans suffer from diseases that cause end-stage organ failure (U.S. Department of Health and Human Services [DHHS], 2008). At the same time, rates of organ donation on the part of African Americans do not match the greater need for organs. The task of narrowing the disparity in supply and demand is a difficult one.

In this chapter, we will describe the gap between the demand for transplants and the supply of organs for African Americans, and we will explore the factors that serve to increase demand and limit supply. We will also explore current strategies to reduce the gap between supply and demand, and in doing so raise several ethical concerns currently being debated in the field. We conclude with a discussion of the mechanisms through which new policies could work to narrow the gap.

THE NEED FOR TRANSPLANTATION AMONG MINORITIES

Ethnic/racial minorities comprise approximately 33 percent of the U.S. population but account for more than 53 percent of the 100,300 persons on the national transplant waiting list (Organ Procurement and Transplantation Network [OPTN], 2008a). Trends among ethnic/minorities are particularly dramatic among African Americans. Over the past decade, African Americans have consistently suffered disproportionately greater rates of organ failure than whites. When compared to their white counterparts, African Americans are up to four times more likely to develop end-stage kidney disease (United States Renal Data System [USRDS], 2008), up to four times more likely to develop heart failure (Loehr, Rosamond, Chang, Folsom, & Chambless, 2008), and more than twice as likely to develop diseases leading to liver failure (Nguyen, Segev, & Thuluvath, 2007).

Relative to the need for transplants, rates of organ and tissue donation among African Americans are comparatively low. Although African Americans donate at population parity, accounting for approximately 14 percent of living and deceased donations in 2008 (see Figure 9.1; OPTN, 2008a), they comprised approximately 30

FIGURE 9.1 *Living/Deceased Donors Recovered in the U.S. by Ethnicity.*

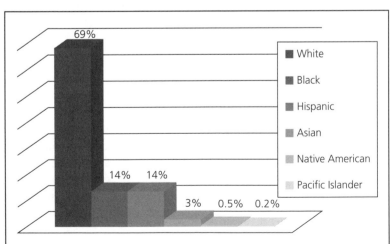

percent of those on the waiting list to receive a life-saving organ in 2008 (see Figure 9.2; OPTN, 2008b). Moreover, over 90 percent of African Americans on the national transplant waiting list are in need of a kidney (OPTN, 2008b). Although cross-race transplantation is the norm, transplantation is often most successful when donated organs are matched to others who are genetically similar. The kidney matching process is heavily dependent on the similarity of the protein complex HLA (human lymphocyte antigens), which is found abundantly in the immune system. Persons of the same racial/ethnic group tend to have a better HLA match than persons across different races (U.S. DHHS, 2008). Although recent improvements in immunosuppressant regimens have helped to overcome some issues related to immunologic incompatibility between donors and recipients, African Americans are among those most impacted by the donor shortage. They spend more than twice the amount of time on the national transplant waiting list and generally have less access to transplantation as compared to whites (Louis, Sankar, & Ubel, 1997; Rozon-Solomon & Burrows, 1999; Danovitch et al., 2005; Young & Gaston, 2003; USRDS, 2008).

EXAMINING THE FORCES OF DEMAND FOR TRANSPLANTS AND SUPPLY OF ORGANS

Forces at several levels (individual, interpersonal, organizational, and systemic) drive both demand for transplants and supply of organs (see Figure 9.3). Forces influencing the demand for transplants include patient knowledge, preferences, communication

FIGURE 9.2 *Waiting List Candidates by Ethnicity.*

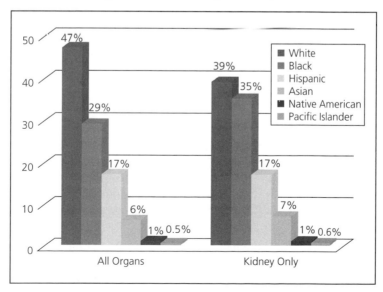

FIGURE 9.3 *Patient, Physician, and System Level Factors Affecting Demand and Supply for Organ Transplants.*

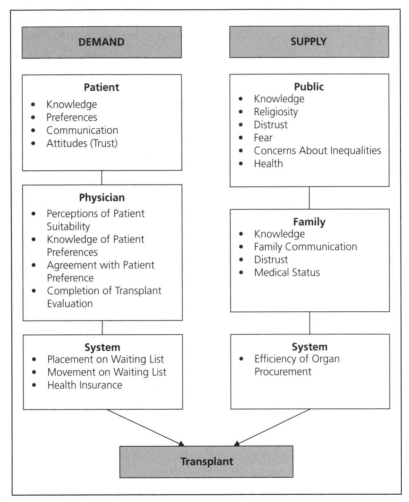

patterns, and attitudes that affect the desire for transplantation at the patient level; physician perceptions, knowledge, and attitudes that affect their ability to help patients achieve transplantation at the provider level; and system factors that affect rates at which patients are placed on waiting lists or advance up waiting lists toward transplants. Forces influencing the supply of organs for transplant include the general public's knowledge of the need for transplantation, religiosity, attitudes (such as fear or distrust), and concerns that affect rates at which people are willing to become deceased organ and tissue donors. In the case of living organ donation, families are often the donors. Therefore family knowledge, communication, attitudes, and medical status play a role in the rates at which living donation occurs. Finally, the efficiency of organ procurement at the time of potential donors' deaths and efficiencies in the organ allocation system both affect the rates at which organs are appropriately harvested and distributed for transplantation. In the following sections, we will discuss these forces in more depth.

Factors Influencing Demand for Transplants

The demand for transplants is driven by patient factors (including patients' knowledge about transplant as a treatment option, their desire to receive a transplant, their communication of their preferences for transplant, and attitudes they may have such as trust), physician factors (including their perceptions of patients' suitability for transplant, their knowledge of patients' preferences, communication, and agreement with patients regarding patients' preferences for transplant), and system factors (including patients' completion of clinical evaluations needed to receive transplants, placement on transplant waiting lists, and movement up the waiting list). Barriers to African Americans' receipt of organ transplants have been demonstrated to exist at several points in this scheme.

African American patients' knowledge, preference, communication, and attitudes have been demonstrated to be associated with their willingness to pursue transplantation as a treatment option. Two large multi-state studies of patients receiving dialysis for kidney failure have revealed that African Americans were significantly less likely than their white counterparts to report they were definitely interested in seeking a transplant (Alexander & Sehgal, 1998; Ayanian, Cleary, Weissman, & Epstein, 1999). However, one of these studies indicated that few patients learned about transplantation as a treatment option before they developed kidney failure, with lowest rates of knowledge among African American men and women (Ayanian et al., 1999). Other studies have suggested that African American patients may be less likely than their white counterparts to admit they need a transplant (Lunsford, Simpson, Chavin, Hildebrand, et al., 2006), and may be hesitant to discuss their desires for a transplant with family because of fears that potential family members (who could serve as living donors for some transplants) might be at risk with living kidney donation (Lunsford, Simpson, Chavin, Hildebrand, et al., 2006; Shilling et al., 2006; Waterman, Stanley, Covelli, et al., 2006). Patient and family communication may play a role in the manner in which patients seek both deceased and living transplantation. A recent study of African American patients with kidney failure and their families indicated that although a majority of patients with kidney failure reported they desired a kidney transplant, less than half reported they had discussed their desires for a transplant with their spouses and children. In this same study, patients and their family members often reported they had not discussed transplantation as a treatment option with patients' physicians, suggesting that a lack of discussion between patients and physicians as well as among families may be a significant obstacle for African Americans (Boulware et al., 2005). Studies also indicate that African American patients' fear of surgery and distrust of the medical community may pose a significant barrier to seeking transplant therapy (Shilling et al., 2006).

Practice patterns of physicians caring for patients with organ failure—the doctors responsible for determining patients' eligibility to receive transplants and for referring patients for testing needed as part of the process for placing patients on transplant waiting lists—have also been demonstrated to pose a barrier to the receipt of transplants for African Americans. A large study of physicians and their patients with kidney failure from five U.S. states indicated that, compared to their white counterparts, African American patients who were considered (by independent clinical experts) to be appropriate for receiving transplants were less likely than whites to be referred to transplant centers for further evaluation and testing. This same study demonstrated that whites deemed to be ineligible to receive a transplant were more likely than their African American counterparts to be inappropriately referred to transplant centers for further evaluation and testing, providing evidence of racial bias in physician practice patterns (Epstein et al., 2000). A separate study performed in three U.S. states revealed that African Americans receiving dialysis for kidney failure were less likely than their white counterparts to have completed the testing and clinical evaluation needed to get them placed on the kidney transplant waiting list (Alexander & Sehgal, 1998).

System factors, including health insurance and patients' placement and movement on the waiting list, have been demonstrated to play a role in access to organ transplants. For kidney transplantation, studies have demonstrated that even when patients have received all the testing needed to place them on the waiting list, rates of placement on the list and rates of movement up the list are significantly less for African Americans than for whites (Alexander & Sehgal, 1998, 2001). Several studies have identified suboptimal access to private health insurance as a major barrier to placement on transplant waiting lists. In a national study, both ethnic/racial minorities and whites with government health insurance were significantly less likely than their counterparts with private insurance to be placed on the waiting list for a transplant before dialysis. Rates of placement on the waiting list were the lowest for minorities with government health insurance (Keith, Ashby, Port, & Leichtman, 2008). Similarly, other studies have identified being of the African American race and lacking private health insurance as barriers to receiving heart transplants (Coughlin, Halabi, & Metayer, 1998). Although a majority of patients with kidney failure receive either state or federal government insurance, this benefit does not exist for patients with other forms of organ failure, exacerbating racial differences in access to transplants for these organs (USRDS, 2008; King et al., 2005).

Factors Influencing Supply of Organs for Transplant

The supply of viable organs and tissues for transplant is influenced by factors related to the public (including knowledge, religious views, distrust, fear, and concern about social inequalities), family (including knowledge, family communication, distrust, and health status), and system. All of these factors can potentially facilitate conversion of a potential donor into an actual donor (see Figure 9.3). In the case of deceased donation, most donated organs come from patients who are declared brain dead, most often as a result of injury (e.g., brain hemorrhage and injuries such as motor vehicle crashes, asphyxiation, and stabbing or gunshot wounds) or disease (OPTN, 2008c). Thus, in this situation, donation is contingent on the potential donor's prior decision to become a donor and the expression of this wish either verbally (by sharing one's views with family) or in written form (via a donor card or registering on the state donor registry via one's driver's license). In the case of living donation, the potential donor must be aware of living donation as an option, willing to donate, and able both physically and mentally to serve as a donor. Considerable research literature suggests that multiple barriers to expressing donation intentions, relevant to both living and deceased donation, exist, particularly among African Americans.

Although there is some evidence for African Americans' support for donation (Arriola, Perryman, & Doldren, 2005), research consistently finds that, compared to people of other racial/ethnic groups, African Americans are less willing to engage in both living and deceased donation (Boulware, et al., 2002; Morgan, Miller, & Arasaratnam, 2003; Lunsford, Simpson, Chavin, Menching, et al., 2006). The underlying reasons for this finding are complex, but five general areas have been explored in the research literature:

1. lack of knowledge of renal disease and the magnitude of the need for transplantation within the African American community (Arriola, Robinson, Perryman, & Thompson, 2008b; Callender, Miles, & Hall, 2002);

2. religious myths, misperceptions, and superstitions that promote a desire to remain whole when entering heaven (Arriola, Perryman, Doldren, Warren, & Robinson, 2007; Callender, Miles, Hall, & Gordon, 2002; Callender & Washington, 1997; Durand, Decker, & Bruder, 2002; Hall et al., 1991; Thompson, 1993);

3. lack of trust in the health care system in general and the organ allocation system specifically due in part to the legacy of the Tuskegee Syphyllis Study (Boulware, Troll, Wang, & Powe, 2007; Callendar, Miles, Hall, & Gordon, 2002; Callender, Hall, & Branch, 2001; Callender & Washington, 1997);

4. fear that signing an organ donor card might change the emphasis from life-saving to organ donor priority in the event of an emergency, not realizing that the medical team is separate from the requesting and transplantation teams; and

5. fear that racism would cause organs donated by African Americans to go to white patients (Callender, Miles, Hall, & Gordon, 2002; Callender, Miles, & Hall, 2002; Schutte & Kappel, 1997).

Patients may grapple with these concerns in advance of potentially becoming a deceased donor, but the family of the deceased patient could also face these same concerns at the time of consent for donation. These views can influence their decision of whether to consent to donation of their family member's organs, especially if the patient has not made his/her wishes known.

In the case of living donation, the family dynamics around consent are quite different. A family member has to personally consent to serve as a living donor. This cannot happen unless the patient and/or family member is aware that living donation is a viable option. It also requires that there be enough open family communication for the patient to be willing to approach a loved one and accept his or her offer of an organ (Rodrigue, Cornell, Kaplan, & Howard, 2008a; Waterman, Stanley, Covelli, et al., 2006; Shilling et al., 2006). One study found that of 115 dialysis clinic patients, 60 percent never talked with anyone about the possibility of living donation, and 80 percent actually refused to consider the possibility of receiving an organ from a family member (Murray, Conrad, & Zarifian, 1999). Other studies have similarly found that many patients refuse to have potential matching donors evaluated and are not willing to actively pursue living donation as a treatment option (Gordon, 2001; Waterman, Stanley, Barrett, et al., 2006; Kranenburg et al., 2005). A study of African American patients with kidney failure and their families revealed that, despite high levels of desire on the part of patients to seek a transplant, rates of family discussion about living kidney transplantation were low, and family members often did not agree on whether a discussion about transplantation or donation had occurred (Boulware et al., 2005).

Numerous patients choose to stay on dialysis due to concerns about harming the potential donor, possible resentment after donation, graft rejection, and feelings of indebtedness to the donor (Rodrigue et al., 2008a; Gordon, 2001; Waterman, Stanley, Covelli, et al., 2006; Kranenburg et al., 2005). All of these feelings exist within a context of distrust that the health care establishment will provide all the needed care for the loved one serving as a living donor. Even when these barriers are overcome and the decision is made for a family member to undergo evaluation as a potential living donor, the actual living donation is thwarted for many African Americans by the presence of conditions such as hypertension, heart disease, diabetes, kidney dysfunction, hepatitis, high body mass indexes, and pancreas, bladder, and liver problems, all of which may render potential living donors unsuitable (Lunsford, Simpson, Chavin, Menching, et al., 2006; Reeves-Daniel et al., 2008; Shilling et al., 2006).

The final issue related to supply concerns the rate at which potential donors are converted to actual donors. In the case of deceased donation, this is a function of the requesting process, and research suggests that the families of African American patients are less likely to be approached for donation (Guadagnoli et al., 1999; Siminoff, Lawrence, & Arnold, 2003), have more negative attitudes toward donation (Siminoff et al., 2003), and are less likely to agree to donation than are white patients (Rodrigue, Cornell, & Howard, 2006; Siminoff et al., 2003). Certainly, many of the previously discussed patient-level concerns are relevant to the families of African American patients having more negative attitudes toward donation than the families of white patients (e.g., religiosity, distrust of the health care system, fear, and concerns about inequalities), but characteristics of the requesting process that contribute to conversion also deserve attention. One characteristic that has garnered some research attention is race/ethnicity of the procurer. One study found that same-race procurers are more effective at obtaining consent to donation among families of African American patients than those of a different race (Gentry, Brown-Holbert, & Andrews, 1997), although much more research is needed in this area.

APPROACHES TO CREATING A STATE OF EQUILIBRIUM

Enhancing Access to Transplantation

Efforts to address barriers to the demand for organ and tissue transplantation have focused primarily on enhancing potential organ recipients' access to organ transplants through interventions addressing the need for greater patient education about transplantation as well as interventions focusing on provider and system-level contributions to disparities in access. Though the intensity of efforts to improve access to transplants have varied (originating from both public and private sources), few efforts have specifically targeted minorities.

One notable exception is the Minority Organ/Tissue Transplant Education Program (MOTTEP), a National Institutes of Health–funded program that initially targeted only African Americans and expanded to include Hispanic Americans, Asian Americans, Pacific Islanders, Alaska Natives, and Native Americans. MOTTEP is a demonstration research program with primary goals of

1. educating minority communities about organ and tissue transplantation,

2. empowering minority communities to develop transplant education programs,

3. increasing minority participation in organ and tissue transplant endeavors,

4. encouraging and increasing family discussions about organ and tissue donation,

5. increasing the number of minority individuals who donate organs and tissues, and

6. promoting healthy lifestyle choices to prevent the need for transplantation.

MOTTEP employs a variety of efforts to achieve its multifaceted goals, including program marketing and public relations, dissemination of health messages and disease prevention materials, and collaboration with other patient advocacy and policy organizations to address disparities in organ donation and transplantation. The program has been successful at establishing community-based networks through which health education related to minority organ and tissue donation as well as transplantation is disseminated. MOTTEP has successfully demonstrated effectiveness in affecting public attitudes regarding health behaviors that contribute to the need for transplants (Callender, Miles, & Hall, 2002).

Beyond MOTTEP, few interventions have been designed to specifically enhance rates at which minorities consider transplants. In a single study of a culturally sensitive educational program (targeted toward both minorities and nonminorities) in which potential kidney transplant recipients and their families met with transplant professionals in their homes to discuss transplantation, investigators reported an increase in rates of pursuit of living kidney donation among all families, with a greater increase among African Americans relative to whites (Rodrigue et al., 2008b). Few additional interventions have been specifically designed to enhance minority patient and family decision making regarding transplantation and to enhance access to transplantation through education. Two such ongoing studies offer promise of their ability to potentially identify interventions that can increase rates of living kidney transplantation among African Americans.

The Talking about Living Kidney Donation (TALK) Study is an ongoing Health Resources and Services Administration–sponsored program that has developed a culturally targeted intervention to enhance minority and nonminority rates of consideration for living kidney transplant as a treatment option. This study is designed to assess the effectiveness of an educational video and written educational materials to narrow ethnic/racial disparities in access to live kidney transplantation by providing potential transplant recipients knowledge about transplantation as a treatment option for kidney failure and by enhancing family discussion of living transplantation as a treatment option. The Providing Resources to Enhance PAtients' REadiness to make Decisions about kidney disease (PREPARED) Study is a recently funded NIH-sponsored program that will assess the effectiveness of a culturally targeted educational intervention to improve African Americans' ability to make informed decisions about transplantation as a treatment option for kidney failure. Both the TALK and PREPARED studies will contribute needed evidence regarding steps that are needed to address patient-level barriers to the receipt of kidney transplants. These study findings may also translate to other forms of transplantation as well.

Efforts aimed at addressing physician-level barriers to transplant have been limited to date, and have primarily focused on health policies addressing the need for physicians to educate patients regarding transplant in a more frequent and comprehensive fashion. The Medicare Improvements for Patients and Providers Act of 2008 (H.R. 6331), enacted in July 2008, expands Medicare payments to physicians caring for patients with kidney disease to provide reimbursement for up to six sessions of education about all treatment options (including transplantation) for kidney failure, with an emphasis of helping patients actively participate in their choice of a therapy (Medicare Improvements, 2008). Though this legislation does not specifically target ethnic minorities, it does specify that educational efforts should be tailored to individual patients' needs. Similar policy interventions for other types of transplants have not been enacted.

Enhancing Rates of Organ Donation

Approaches to increasing the supply of available organs and tissues are broad and exist at multiple levels. National and state legislation and policies, programs within transplant centers, and national, state, and community-based public education interventions all have the goal of increasing the number of living and deceased donors. The extent to which the effectiveness of these approaches has been scientifically evaluated varies greatly, and certainly more work is needed in this area. Nevertheless, we provide examples of how each of these approaches has been applied and discuss the relevance to African Americans where appropriate.

First-person consent legislation, which is acknowledged in forty-eight of fifty states (excluding Mississippi and New York) (United Network for Organ Sharing [UNOS], 2008a), is perhaps impacting the largest number of people. This law allows a potential donor to be designated as such on a legally binding document such as a driver's license or an official signed donor document. It also gives hospitals legal authority to proceed with organ procurement and removes the burden of the donation decision from the family and legal next-of-kin (UNOS, 2008a). This legislation has important implications for African Americans, who tend to be characterized by strong extended family networks. In situations in which there is disagreement among family members about whether to consent to deceased donation (even though the decision technically rests with the legal next-of-kin) it might ameliorate the situation to remove the burden of the donation decision from the family when written documentation exists.

There has also been national and state legislation to support living donors. The Organ Donation and Recovery Act is one of the most important federal laws with respect to donation incentives. It has authorized $25 million in program development, grants, reporting authority, and direct funding. One of the key provisions of the legislation is the development of a federal grant program that provides supplementary assistance to potential living donors for travel and incidental nonmedical-related expenses incurred during the process and as a result of individuals making a living donation (Library of Congress, n.d). The goal of this program is to ease the donation burden so economics do not impact the final choice of whether or not to donate. These types of programs are particularly relevant to African American patients, many of whom see financial barriers as significant deterrents to living donation for their family members.

As of January 1, 2006, twenty-seven states enacted legislation to provide support for living donors. Of these, twenty-two states enacted legislation mandating paid leave for donors, whereas only nine and three states enacted legislation mandating tax benefits and unpaid leave, respectively (Boulware, Troll, Plantinga, & Powe, 2008; UNOS, 2008b). It is hoped legislation would enhance rates of donation by supporting donor concerns, but recent studies reveal there has been no association between the enactment of legislation and living related donation rates over the past sixteen years (Boulware et al., 2008). The effect of legislation specifically on minority donation rates is currently unknown.

Other mechanisms for financial support include the National Living Donor Assistance Program, funded by the Division of Transplantation, which receives support per the Organ Donation and Recovery Improvement Act. This program, similar to the legislation previously described, provides for travel, subsistence expenses, and other nonmedical expenses to reduce financial disincentives to living donation (National Living Donor Assistance Center, 2007). Similar programs that offer financial support to living donors (e.g., employment insurance, short-term disability, tax credit for medical expenses, paid leave, travel, accommodations) exist in Canada, France, and the United Kingdom (Klarenbach & Garg, 2006).

Whereas living donor support is widely accepted, much ethical debate has centered around actual compensation for living donors and/or the families of deceased donors. The National Organ Transplant Act (NOTA) of 1984 implicitly prohibits "any person knowingly to acquire, receive or otherwise transfer any human organ for valuable consideration for use in a human transplantation if the transfer affects interstate commerce" (Organ Procurement and Transplantation Network [OPTN], 1984, p. 8).

The purpose of this legislation was to protect the poor and disenfranchised from potential exploitation (Monaco, 2006; Siminoff & Mercer, 2001) and since its inception several countries and the World Health Organization have implemented similar regulations (World Health Organization [WHO], 1991, 2004). Whereas proponents of such legislation argue that incentives are coercive to the poor and dehumanizing, opponents disagree and think that individuals should be allowed to act autonomously, consistent with their self-interests (Bryce et al., 2005; Matas, Hippen, & Satel, 2008).

In a national survey of attitudes regarding rewards for living donation, African Americans were more likely than whites to be in favor of monetary incentives (e.g., tax breaks or credits, direct payment from the government, and financial compensation from living donors' employers) (Boulware, Troll, Wang, & Powe, 2006). With respect to deceased donation, the question concerns whether offering financial incentives, benefits, or reimbursements will actually increase donation rates. According to a study conducted by Siminoff and colleagues (2001), only 20 percent of families would appreciate a financial incentive and 92.5 percent of families that previously refused donation would not be encouraged to donate if such an offer were made. The 2005 Gallup study of 2,500 individuals found similar results such that the majority of individuals would be unaffected by financial incentives to donate their own organs (74.2%) as well as those of family members (72.4%) (Gallup Organization, 2005). In a national study of attitudes toward financial rewards for deceased organ donation, fewer than 20 percent of all respondents were in favor of family members of organ donors receiving cash incentives, although African Americans were somewhat more likely than their white counterparts to favor this idea (Boulware et al., 2006).

At the center of many ethical debates is the use of expanded donor criteria (EDC) for both living and deceased donor candidates (Merion, 2005; Schold et al., 2006; Spital, 1997). Implemented in October 2002, the intent of this policy is to increase the recovery and utilization of viable kidneys by expanding the higher-risk deceased donor pool, thereby increasing the likelihood of transplantation, while improving the efficiency of the allocation process (Schold et al., 2006). In general, the EDC policy identifies higher-risk organs from deceased persons who have a prior history of hypertension, diabetes, stroke, and Hepatitis B or C. This is particularly relevant to African Americans because they suffer from many of these comorbidities, thereby preventing them from being able to serve as donors. A deceased donor of older age (i.e., greater than 60) is also identified as being of higher risk per the EDC policy. According to EDC policy, transplant recipient candidates are informed of the risks involved with consent to accept an EDC transplant. By consenting to receive an EDC kidney, candidate wait time is potentially reduced in exchange for receiving an organ that is potentially of a lower quality.

There is also public education at the national, state, and local levels targeting African Americans. For example, MOTTEP, which was previously described, represents the first national education campaign in the United States to systematically target minorities with education relative to organ and tissue transplantation. Project ACTS:

About Choices in Transplantation and Sharing is another example. This National Institutes of Health–funded culturally sensitive family-focused self-education intervention was developed to increase readiness for organ and tissue donation among African American adults. Developed for delivery in a community setting, the Project ACTS intervention package consists of a DVD or VHS, an educational pamphlet, a donor card, a National Donor Sabbath pendant, and several additional items embossed with the project name and logo (e.g., pen, notepad, refrigerator magnet, and bookmark). The DVD/VHS is hosted by gospel singing group Trin-i-tee 5:7, and features excerpts from individual and family conversations about beliefs, attitudes, myths, misconceptions, and fears about the organ donation/transplantation process. Interspersed throughout the video are biblical and spiritual themes to encourage organ donation (e.g., an excerpt from the biblical Book of Acts 20:35, "It is more blessed to give than to receive"). Additionally, the DVD/VHS seeks to motivate viewers by including heartfelt personal stories from individual organ recipients, donor family members, those on the waiting list to receive an organ, and living donors. The Project ACTS educational booklet contains statistical information on the overrepresentation of African Americans on the waiting list, information on how the allocation system works, resources for additional information, and a donor card.

To evaluate the effectiveness of the intervention, nine churches (N=425 participants) were randomly assigned to receive donation education materials currently available to consumers (control group) or Project ACTS educational materials (intervention group). The primary outcomes assessed at one-year follow-up were readiness to express donation intentions via one's driver's license, donor card, and discussion with family. Results indicate a significant increase in readiness to discuss donation intentions with family among participants in the intervention group as compared to the control group ($p < .05$). Additionally, all participants significantly increased in their readiness to sign a donor card at follow-up, regardless of condition ($p < .01$). However, there were no significant changes in readiness to express donation intentions via one's driver's license. Project ACTS may be an effective tool for stimulating family discussion of donation intentions among African Americans, although additional research is needed to explore how to more effectively impact written intentions (Arriola et al., 2008a).

At the transplant center level there are donor matching programs and paired exchange programs (Mahendran & Veitch, 2007; Marshall, 2008). In many circumstances a would-be living donor is medically incompatible with the intended recipient due to a mismatch of ABO blood group or HLAs, which are essential in the matching process for most organs. As a result, multiple living donation paired exchange programs have been developed to create a mechanism for two live donors who are otherwise incompatible with their intended recipients to essentially "swap" organs so that appropriately matched recipients receive the needed organ. However, the ethics of these and similar unrelated living donation programs are often debated because they are viewed by some as creating a mechanism for commercial interests to be served (Spital, 1997; Stephan, Barbari, & Younan, 2007).

POLICY IMPLICATIONS, RECOMMENDATIONS FOR CLOSING THE GAP, AND CONCLUSIONS

The broad array of issues encompassed by the tension between demand and supply of organs for transplantation leaves tremendous opportunities for policy interventions to significantly impact rates of transplant, particularly for racial/ethnic minorities. Although many of the ethical dilemmas facing policymakers may not be easily addressed, there are several aspects of the supply/demand gap that might be more easily addressed and could still have a significant impact in enhancing rates of transplantation for minorities.

Policies to enhance access to transplantation should address:

1. minority patients' access to information about transplantation as a treatment option,

2. physician barriers to transplants, and

3. gaps in health insurance that limit access to life-saving transplant therapy.

Although Medicare has already mandated improved education for persons with kidney failure, the content of newly mandated educational programs has yet to be established. Efforts to ensure that educational programs provide balanced perspectives of all treatment options, with equal attention paid to benefits and risks of transplant therapy, will provide patients greater opportunity to choose treatments based on their preferences for length and quality of life. Similar legislation is needed to ensure patients suffering from other forms of organ failure also have equal access to education regarding transplant therapies. Policies designed to enhance education should focus attention on addressing health literacy issues documented among minorities (Georges, Bolton, & Bennett, 2004; Osborn et al., 2007). Policies to improve physician practice patterns regarding improved access to transplantation should focus on enhancing physician education and training, with emphasis on educating physicians regarding clinical criteria for transplant eligibility, helping physicians assess patients' preferences for care, and guiding physicians on the optimal methods through which transplantation can be discussed with patients and their families.

The development and implementation of approaches to enhance patient education should be guided by rigorously tested interventions. Although Medicare provides coverage for dialysis and transplantation for patients with kidney failure, similar coverage for other organ transplants does not exist, creating large inequities in access to care based on access to private health insurance as well as private insurers' coverage policies. Efforts should be made to broaden coverage for all persons with organ failure, as well as to enhance coverage for persons receiving kidney transplants. For instance, three years after a successful kidney transplant, Medicare coverage ceases. This has been demonstrated to affect rates of transplant graft failure, with a possibly disproportionate effect on minorities (Butkus, Meydrech, & Raju, 1992; Centers for Medicare & Medicaid Services [CMMS], 2008). Efforts to address deficiencies in existing legislation could therefore not only improve access to transplant but also improve long-term clinical outcomes.

Policies to enhance the supply of organs should

1. address public knowledge of the need for organ donation and encourage family discussion of donation plans,

2. enhance transparency of organ allocation systems and current policies protecting donors, and

3. address inequities in health care that contribute to the lack of trust strongly associated with poor donation rates in minority communities.

Current efforts to enhance donation rates are focused on enhancing public knowledge and encouraging donation plans, but likely need greater penetration among ethnic minority communities. Efforts should be made to enhance minorities' knowledge about the greater need for transplants among ethnic minorities and the benefits of donation, with special attention paid to the optimal venues/settings (e.g., religious settings) in which such messages should be delivered. Greater clarification of the various allocation systems for organs is needed, and will likely enhance rates at which public trust, and in particular the trust of minorities, can be enhanced. Additional ongoing efforts on the part of local, state, and federal agencies to address past failures of the U.S. public health system to act in the best interest of minorities are needed to enhance overall rates of trust and willingness on the part of ethnic minorities to engage in organ donation. Such efforts should simultaneously address issues of historic and current racism and discrimination in health care that contribute to poorer health of minorities compared to nonminorities.

In conclusion, a broad variety of factors contribute to the widening gap between the number of viable organs for transplant and the need for transplantation among African American patients with end-stage organ failure. There is a need for scientifically rigorous, theoretically driven, population-based multilevel research that continues to develop knowledge in this area in order to inform the development of behavioral and policy interventions. The possibility exists for reducing this current gap in supply and demand, which disproportionately impacts African Americans, while restoring African Americans' trust in the transplantation system and ultimately improving the health of all.

Acknowledgments

This work was supported in part by the National Institute of Diabetes & Digestive and Kidney Diseases (Grant numbers 5R01DK079713-02 and 5R01DK079682-02). Also, we thank Katelyn Upcraft for her assistance in the preparation of this chapter.

REFERENCES

Alexander, G. C., & Sehgal, A. R. (1998). Barriers to cadaveric renal transplantation among blacks, women, and the poor. *JAMA, 280*(13), 1148–1152.

Alexander, G. C., & Sehgal, A. R. (2001). Why hemodialysis patients fail to complete the transplantation process. *American Journal of Kidney Disease, 37*(2), 321–328.

Arriola, K. R. J., Perryman, J., & Doldren, M. (2005). Moving beyond attitudinal barriers: Understanding African Americans' support for organ and tissue donation. *Journal of the National Medical Association, 97*, 339–350.

Arriola, K. R. J., Perryman, J. P., Doldren, M., Warren, C. M., & Robinson, D. H. Z. (2007). Understanding the role of clergy in African American organ and tissue donation decision making. *Ethnicity and Health, 12*(5), 465–482.

Arriola, K. R. J., Robinson, D. H. Z., Perryman, J. P., & Thompson, N. (2008a). Project ACTS: An intervention to increase organ and tissue donation intentions among African Americans. Manuscript submitted for publication.

Arriola, K. R. J., Robinson, D. H. Z., Perryman, J. P., & Thompson, N. (2008b). Understanding the relationship between knowledge and African American's donation decision-making. *Patient Education and Counseling, 70*, 242–250.

Ayanian, J. Z., Cleary, P. D., Weissman, J. S., & Epstein, A. M. (1999). The effect of patients' preferences on racial differences in access to renal transplantation. *New England Journal of Medicine, 341*(22), 1661–1669.

Boulware, L. E., Meoni, L. A., Fink, N. E., Parekh, K. S., Kao, W. H., Klag, M. J., & Powe, N. R. (2005). Preferences, knowledge, communication and patient-physician discussion of living kidney transplantation in African American families. *American Journal of Transplantation, 5*(6), 1503–1512.

Boulware, L. E., Ratner, L. E., Cooper, L. A., Sosa, J. A., LaVeist, T. A., & Powe, N. R. (2002). Understanding disparities in donor behavior: Race and gender differences in willingness to donate blood and cadaveric organs. *Medical Care, 40*(2), 85–95.

Boulware, L. E., Troll, M. U. Plantinga, L. C., & Powe, N. R. (2008). The Association of State and National Legislation with living kidney donation rates in the United States: A national study. *American Journal of Transplantation, 8,* 1–20.

Boulware, L. E., Troll, M. U., Wang, N. Y., & Powe, N. R. (2006). Public attitudes toward incentives for organ donation: A national study of different racial/ethnic and income groups. *American Journal of Transplantation, 6*(11), 2774–2785.

Boulware, L. E., Troll, M. U., Wang, N. Y., & Powe, N. R. (2007). Perceived transparency and fairness of the organ allocation system and willingness to donate organs: A national study. *American Journal of Transplantation, 7*, 1778–1787.

Bryce, C. L., Siminoff, L. A., Ubel, P. A., Nathan, H., Caplan, A., & Arnold, R. M. (2005). Do incentives matter? Providing benefits to families of organ donors. *American Journal of Transplantation, 5*, 2999–3008.

Butkus, D. E., Meydrech, E. F., & Raju, S. S. (1992). Racial differences in the survival of cadaveric renal allografts. Overriding effects of HLA matching and socioeconomic factors. *New England Journal of Medicine, 327*(12), 840–845.

Callender, C. O., Hall, M. B., & Branch, D. (2001). An assessment of the effectiveness of the MOTTEP Model for increasing donation rates and preventing the need for transplantation-adult findings: Program years 1998 and 1999. *Seminars in Nephrology, 21*(4), 419–428.

Callender, C. O., Miles, P. V., & Hall, M. B. (2002) National MOTTEP: Educating to prevent the need for transplantation. *Ethnicity and Disease, 12*, S1–34–S1–37.

Callender, C. O., Miles, P. V., Hall, M. B., & Gordon, S. (2002). Blacks and whites and kidney transplantation: A disparity! But why and why won't it go away?. *Transplantation Reviews, 16*, 163–176.

Callender, C. O., & Washington, A. W. (1997). Organ/tissue donation the problem! Education the solution: A review. *Journal of the National Medical Association, 89*(10), 689–693.

Centers for Medicare & Medicaid Services (2008, May). Medicare coverage of kidney dialysis and kidney transplant services. Retrieved from http://www.medicare.gov/Publications/Pubs/pdf/esrdcoverage.pdf.

Coughlin, S. S., Halabi, S., & Metayer, C. (1998). Barriers to cardiac transplantation in idiopathic dilated cardiomyopathy: The Washington, DC, Dilated Cardiomyopathy Study. *Journal of the National Medical Association, 90*, 342–348.

Danovitch, G. M., Cohen, D. J., Weir, M. R., Stock, P. G., Bennett, W. M., Christensen, L. L., & Sung, R. S. (2005). Current status of kidney and pancreas transplantation in the United States, 1994–2003. *American Journal of Transplantation, 5*(Part 2), 904–915.

Durand, R., Decker, P. J., & Bruder, P. (2002). Organ donation among African Americans: Opportunities for increasing donor rates. *Hospital Topics, 80*(3), 34–37.

Epstein, A. M., Ayanian, J. Z., Keogh, J. H., Noonan, S. J., Armistead, N., Cleary, P. D., Weissman, J. S., David-Kasdan, J., Carlson, D., Fuller, J., Marsh, D., & Conti, R. M. (2000). Racial disparities in access to renal transplantation—clinically appropriate or due to underuse or overuse? *New England Journal of Medicine, 343,* 1537–1545.

Gallup Organization (2005). 2005 National Survey of Organ and Tissue Donation Attitudes and Behaviors. Retrieved October 29, 2008, from http://www.organdonor.gov/survey2005/financial_issues.shtm.

Gentry, D. G., Brown-Holbert, J., & Andrews, C. (1997). Racial impact: Increasing minority consent rate by altering the racial mix of an organ procurement organization. *Transplantation Proceedings, 29,* 3758–3759.

Georges, C. A., Bolton, L. B., & Bennett, C. (2004). Functional health literacy: An issue in African-American and other ethnic and racial communities. *Journal of the National Black Nurses Association, 15*(1), 1–4.

Gordon, E. J. (2001). Patients' decisions for treatment of end-stage renal disease and their implications for access to transplantation. *Social Science & Medicine, 53,* 971–987.

Guadagnoli, E., McNamara, M. J., Evanisko, C., Beasley, C. O., Callender, C., & Poretsky, A. (1999). The influence of race on approaching families for organ donation and their decision to donate. *American Journal of Public Health, 89,* 244–247.

Hall, L., Callender, C. O., Yeager, C. L., Barber, J. B., Dunston, G. M., & Pinn-Wiggins, V. W. (1991). Organ donation and blacks: The next frontier. *Transplant Proceedings, 23*(5), 2500–2504.

Keith, D., Ashby, V. B., Port, F. K., & Leichtman, A. B. (2008). Insurance type and minority status associated with large disparities in prelisting dialysis among candidates for kidney transplantation. *Clinical Journal of the American Society of Nephrology, 3*(2), 463–470.

King, L. P., Siminoff, L. A., Meyer, D. M., Yancy, C. W., Ring, W. S., Mayo, T. W., & Drazner, M. H. (2005). Health insurance and cardiac transplantation: A call for reform. *Journal of the American College of Cardiology, 45*(9), 1388–1391.

Klarenbach, S., & Garg, A. X. (2006). Living organ donors face financial barriers: A national reimbursement policy is needed. *Canadian Medical Association Journal, 174*(6), 797–798.

Kranenburg, L., Zuidema, W., Weimar, W., Ijzermans, J., Passchier, J., Hilhorst, M., & Busschbach, J. (2005). Postmortal or living related donor: Preferences of kidney patients. *Transplant International,18,* 519–523.

Library of Congress. (n.d.) Organ Donation and Recovery Improvement Act (S. 1949). Retrieved October 29, 2008, from http://thomas.loc.gov/home/bills_res.html

Loehr, L. R., Rosamond, W. D., Chang, P. P., Folsom, A. R., & Chambless, L. E. (2008). Heart failure incidence and survival (from the Atherosclerosis Risk in Communities study). *American Journal of Cardiology, 101*(7), 1016–1022.

Louis, O. N., Sankar, P., & Ubel, P. A. (1997). Kidney transplant candidates' views of the transplant allocation system. *Journal of General Internal Medicine, 12*(8), 478–484.

Lunsford, S. L., Simpson, K. S., Chavin, K. D., Hildebrand, L. G., Miles, L. G., Shilling, L. M., Smalls, G. R., & Baliga, P. K. (2006). Racial differences in coping with the need for kidney transplantation and willingness to ask for live organ donation. *American Journal of Kidney Diseases, 47*(2), 324–331.

Lunsford, S. L., Simpson, K. S., Chavin, K. D., Menching, K. J., Miles, L. G., Shilling, L. M., Smalls, G. R., & Baliga, P. K. (2006). Racial disparities in living kidney donation: Is there a lack of willing donors or an excess of medically unsuitable candidates? *Transplantation, 82*(7), 876–881.

Mahendran, A. O., & Veitch, P. S. (2007). Paired exchange programmes can expand the live kidney donor pool. *British Journal of Surgery, 94,* 657–664.

Marshall, K. C. (2008, March 28). Re: Legality of Alternative Organ Donation Practices Under 42 U.S.C. § 247e, Memorandum for Daniel Meron, General Counsel, Department of Health and Human Services. Office of the Deputy Assistant Attorney General. Retrieved August 4, 2008, from http://www.usdoj.gov/olc/2007/organtransplant.pdf

Matas, A. J., Hippen, B., & Satel, S. (2008). In defense of a regulated system of compensation for living donation. *Current Opinion in Organ Transplantation, 13*(4), 379–385.

Medicare Improvements for Patients and Providers Act of 2008, H.R. 6331 (2008).

Merion, R. M. (2005). Expanded criteria donors for kidney transplantation. *Transplantation Proceedings, 37,* 3655–3657.

Monaco, A. P. (2006). Rewards for organ donation: The time has come. *Kidney International, 69,* 955–957.

Morgan, S. E., Miller, J. K., & Arasaratnam, L. A. (2003). Similarities and differences between African Americans' and European Americans' attitudes, knowledge, and willingness to communicate about organ donation. *Journal of Applied Social Psychology, 33*(4). 693–715.

Murray, L. R., Conrad, N. E., & Zarifian, A. (1999). Perceptions of kidney transplant by persons with end stage renal disease. *ANNA Journal, 26*(5), 479–500.

National Living Donor Assistance Center (2007). National Living Donor Assistance Program. Retrieved October 29, 2008, from http://www.livingdonorassistance.org/theprogram/background.aspx.

Nguyen, G. C., Segev, D. L., & Thuluvath, P. J. (2007). Racial disparities in the management of hospitalized patients with cirrhosis and complications of portal hypertension: A national study. *Hepatology, 45*(5), 1282–1289.

Organ Procurement and Transplantation Network. (1984). National Organ Transplant Act, 3 USC § 9401 (1984). Retrieved October 28, 2008, from http://optn.transplant.hrsa.gov/policiesAndBylaws/nota.asp

Organ Procurement and Transplantation Network. (2008a). Data: View data reports, waiting list candidates by ethnicity, 1988–2008. Retrieved October 29, 2008 from http://www.optn.org/latestData/viewDataReports.asp

Organ Procurement and Transplantation Network. (2008b). Data: View data reports, deceased and living donors by ethnicity, 1988–2008. Retrieved October 29, 2008, from http://www.optn.org/latestData/viewDataReports.asp.

Organ Procurement and Transplantation Network. (2008c). Data: View data reports, deceased donors recovered in the U.S. by cause of death, 1988–2008. Retrieved October 29, 2008, from http://optn.transplant.hrsa.gov/latestData/viewDataReports.asp

Osborn, C. Y., Paasche-Orlow, M. K., Davis, T. C., & Wolf, M. S. (2007). Health literacy: An overlooked factor in understanding HIV health disparities. *American Journal of Preventive Medicine, 33*(5), 374–378.

Reeves-Daniel, A., Adams, P. L., Daniel, K., Assimos, D., Westcott, C., Alcorn, S. G., Rogers, J., Farney, A. C., Stratta, R. J., & Hartmann, E. L. (2008). Impact of race and gender on live kidney donation. *Clinical Transplant, 23*(1), 39–46.

Rodrigue, J. R., Cornell, D. L., & Howard, R. J. (2006). Organ donation decision: Comparison of donor and nondonor families. *American Journal of Transplantation, 6*(1), 190–198.

Rodrigue, J. R., Cornell, D. L., Kaplan, B., & Howard, R. J. (2008a). Patients' willingness to talk to others about living kidney donation. *Progress in Transplantation, 18*, 25–31.

Rodrigue, J. R., Cornell, D. L., Kaplan, B., & Howard, R. J. (2008b). A randomized trial of a home-based educational approach to increase live donor kidney transplantation: Effects in blacks and whites. *American Journal of Kidney Disease, 51*(4), 663–670.

Rozon-Solomon, M., & Burrows, L. (1999). Tis better to receive than to give: The relative failure of the African American community to provide organs for transplantation. *Mt Sinai Journal of Medicine, 66*, 273–276.

Schold, J. D., Howard, R. J., Scicchitano, M. J., & Meier-Kreische, H. U. (2006). The Expanded Criteria Donor Policy: An evaluation of program objectives and indirect ramifications. *American Journal of Transplantation, 6*, 1689–1695.

Schutte, L. K., & Kappel, D. (1997). Barriers to donation in minority, low-income, and rural populations. *Transplantation Proceedings, 29*(8), 3746–3747.

Shilling, L. M., Norman, M. L., Chavin, K. D., Hildebrand, L. G., Lunsford, S. L., & Martin, M. S. (2006). Healthcare professionals' perceptions of the barriers to living donor kidney transplantation among African Americans. *Journal of the National Medical Association, 98*, 834–840.

Siminoff, L. A., Lawrence, R. H., & Arnold, R. M. (2003). Comparison of black and white family experiences and perceptions regarding organ donation requests. *Critical Care Medicine, 31*, 146–151.

Siminoff, L. A., & Mercer, M. B. (2001). Public policy, public opinion, and consent for organ donation. *Cambridge Quarterly of Healthcare Ethics, 10*, 377–386.

Spital, A. (1997). Ethical and policy issues in altruistic living and cadaveric organ donation. *Clinical Transplant, 11*(2), 77–87.

Stephan, A., Barbari, A., & Younan, F. (2007). Ethical aspects of organ donation activities. *Experimental and Clinical Transplantation, 2*, 633–637.

Thompson, V. L. S. (1993). Educating the African-American community on organ donation. *Journal of the National Medical Association, 85*, 17–19.

United Network for Organ Sharing. (2008a). Donor designation (first person consent) status by state. Retrieved October 29, 2008, from http://www.unos.org/inTheNews/factsheets.asp?fs=6.

United Network for Organ Sharing. (2008b). Transplant Living: Federal Legislation. Retrieved October 29, 2008, from http://www.transplantliving.org/livingdonation/financialaspects/legislation.aspx.

U. S. Department of Health and Human Services, Office of Minority Health (2008). Organ and Tissue Donation 101. Retrieved October 29, 2008, from http://www.omhrc.gov

United States Renal Data System. (2008). *USRDS 2008 annual data report: Atlas of chronic kidney disease and end stage renal disease in the United States.* Bethesda, MD: National Institutes of Health, National Institute of Diabetes and Digestive and Kidney Diseases.

Waterman, A. D., Stanley, S. L., Barrett, A. C., Waterman, B. M., Shenoy, S., & Brennan, D. C. (2006). Refusing living donors?: Renal patient predictors of not having living donors evaluated. World Transplant Congress 2006.

Waterman, A. D., Stanley, S. L., Covelli, T., Hazel, E., Hong, B. A., & Brennan, D. C. (2006). Living donation decision making: Recipients' concerns and educational needs. *Progress in Transplant, 16*(1), 17–23.

World Health Organization. (1991). Guiding principles on human organ transplantation. *Lancet, 337*(8755), 1470.

World Health Organization. (2004). Ethics, access and safety in tissue and organ transplantation: Issues of global concern. Retrieved August 14, 2009, from http://www.who.int/ethics/Tissue%20and%20Organ%20Transplantation.pdf

Young, C. J., & Gaston, R. S. (2003). African Americans and renal transplantation: Disproportionate need, limited access, and impaired outcomes. *American Journal of Medical Science, 323*(2), 94–99.

CHAPTER

10

AFRICAN AMERICANS ON THE FRONT LINE OF ENVIRONMENTAL ASSAULT

ROBERT D. BULLARD
GLENN S. JOHNSON
ANGEL O. TORRES

Despite significant improvements in environmental protection over the past several decades, millions of African Americans continue to live in unsafe and unhealthy physical environments. Many economically impoverished communities and their inhabitants are exposed to greater health hazards in their homes, on the jobs, and in their neighborhoods than are their more affluent counterparts (Bullard, 1994a; Bryant & Mohai, 1992). Hardly a day passes without the media discovering some community or neighborhood fighting a landfill, incinerator, chemical plant, or some other polluting industry. This was not always the case.

This chapter attempts to lay the historical foundations and social context of the environmental justice movement (EJM) in the United States. It provides a critique and analysis of government policies and industry practices that endanger the health and safety of African Americans in their neighborhoods, workplaces, and playgrounds. Our discussion also examines the role of grassroots groups, community-based organizations, and black institutions in dismantling the legacy of environmental racism (ER).

HISTORICAL BACKDROP

Just three decades ago, the concept of environmental justice (EJ) had not registered on the radar screens of environmental, civil rights, or social justice groups (Bullard, 1994b). Nevertheless, it should not be forgotten that Dr. Martin Luther King Jr. went to Memphis in 1968 on an environmental and economic justice mission for the striking black garbage workers. The strikers were demanding equal pay and better work conditions. Of course, Dr. King was assassinated before he could complete his mission.

Another landmark garbage dispute took place a decade later in Houston, when African American homeowners began a bitter fight to keep a sanitary landfill out of their suburban middle-income neighborhood (Bullard, 1983). Residents formed the Northeast Community Action Group or NECAG. NECAG and their attorney, Linda McKeever Bullard, filed a class action lawsuit to block the facility from being built. The 1979 lawsuit, *Bean v. Southwestern Waste Management, Inc.*, was the first of its kind to challenge the siting of a waste facility under civil rights law. The landmark Houston case occurred three years before the environmental justice movement was catapulted into the national limelight in rural and mostly African American Warren County, North Carolina.

The environmental justice movement has come a long way since its humble beginning in Warren County, North Carolina, where a PCB landfill ignited protests and over five hundred arrests. The Warren County protests provided the impetus for a U.S. General Accounting Office (1983) study, *Siting of Hazardous Waste Landfills and Their Correlation with Racial and Economic Status of Surrounding Communities*. That study revealed that three out of four of the off-site, commercial hazardous waste landfills in Region Four (which includes Alabama, Florida, Georgia, Kentucky, Mississippi, North Carolina, South Carolina, and Tennessee) happened to be located in predominantly African American communities, although African Americans made up only 20 percent of the region's population. The protests in North Carolina put "environmental racism" on the map.

The protests also led the Commission for Racial Justice (1987) to produce *Toxic Wastes and Race*, the first national study to correlate waste facility sites and demographic characteristics. Race was found to be the most potent variable in predicting where these facilities were located—more powerful than poverty, land values, and home ownership. The *Toxic Wastes and Race at Twenty 1987–2007* report concludes that significant racial and socioeconomic disparities persist in the distribution of the nation's commercial hazardous waste facilities. The current assessment uses newer methods that better match where people and hazardous waste facilities are located, and in fact, people of color are found to be more concentrated around hazardous waste facilities than previously shown (Bullard 2007a). In 1990, *Dumping in Dixie: Race, Class, and Environmental Quality* chronicled the convergence of two social movements—social justice and environmental movements—into the environmental justice movement (Bullard, 1994a). This book highlighted African American environmental activism in the South, the same region that gave birth to the modern civil rights movement. What started out as local and often isolated community-based struggles against toxics and facility siting blossomed into a multi-issue, multi-ethnic, and multi-regional movement.

The 1991 First National People of Color Environmental Leadership Summit was the most important single event in the environmental justice movement's history. The Summit broadened the movement beyond its somewhat narrow anti-toxics focus to include issues of public health, worker safety, land use, transportation, housing, resource allocation, and community empowerment (Lang Lee, 1992). The meeting also demonstrated that it is possible to build a multi-racial grassroots movement around environmental and economic justice (Alston, 1992).

Held in Washington, D.C., the four-day Summit was attended by over 650 grassroots and national leaders from around the world. Delegates came from all fifty states, Puerto Rico, Chile, Mexico, and as far away as the Marshall Islands. People attended the Summit to share their action strategies, redefine the environmental movement, and develop common plans for addressing environmental problems affecting people of color in the United States and around the world.

On September 27, 1991, Summit delegates adopted 17 "Principles of Environmental Justice." These principles were developed as a guide for organizing, networking, and relating to government nongovernmental organizations (NGOs). By June 1992, Spanish and Portuguese translations of the Principles were being used and circulated by NGOs and environmental justice groups at the Earth Summit in Rio de Janeiro.

The publication of the *People of Color Environmental Groups Directory* in 1992, 1994, and 2000 further illustrates that environmental justice organizations are found in the United States from coast to coast, in Puerto Rico, in Mexico, and in Canada. Groups have come to embrace a wide range of issues, including public health, children's health, pollution prevention, facility siting, housing, brownfields, community reinvestment, air pollution, urban sprawl, land use, worker safety, public participation, transportation discrimination, smart growth, and regional equity (Bullard, 2000).

Warren County PCB Landfill Detoxification

In December 2003, after waiting more than two decades, an environmental justice victory finally came to the residents of predominantly black Warren County, North Carolina. Since 1982, county residents had lived with the legacy of a 142-acre toxic-waste dump. The toxic-waste dump was forced on the tiny Afton community—more than 84 percent of which was black in 1982—helping trigger the national EJM. While the "midnight dumpers" were fined and jailed, the innocent Afton community was handed a twenty-year sentence of living in a toxic-waste prison.

The PCB landfill became the most recognized symbol in the county. Despite the stigma, Warren County also became a symbol of the EJM. Warren County residents pleaded for a more permanent solution, rather than a cheap "quick fix" that would eventually end up with the PCBs leaking into the groundwater and wells. Their voices fell on deaf ears. State and federal officials chose to build a landfill, the cheap way out. By 1993, the landfill was failing, and for a decade community leaders pressed the state to decontaminate the site.

Detoxification work finally began on the dump in June 2001 and the last clean-up work ended in December 2003. State and federal sources spent $18 million to detoxify or neutralize contaminated soil stored at the Warren County PCB landfill (Rawlins, 2003). A private contractor hired by the state dug up and burned 81,500 tons of oil-laced soil in a kiln that reached more than 800 degrees Fahrenheit to remove the PCBs (polychlorinated biphenyls). The soil was put back in a football-field-size pit, re-covered to form a mound, graded, and seeded with grass.

This was no small win given state deficits, budget cuts, and past broken promises, but residents and officials still must grapple with what to do with the site. Even after detoxification, some Warren County residents still question the completeness of the clean-up, especially contamination that may have migrated beyond the three-acre landfill site—into the 137-acre buffer zone that surrounds the landfill and the nearby creek and outlet basin. PCBs are persistent, bioaccumulative, and toxic pollutants (PBTs). That is, they are highly toxic, long-lasting substances that can build up in the food chain to levels that are harmful to human and ecosystem health. PCBs are not something most Americans would want as a next-door neighbor. PCBs are probable human carcinogens. They also cause developmental effects such as low birth weight, and they disrupt hormone function.

Warren County is located in eastern North Carolina. The twenty-nine counties located "Down East" are noticeably different from the rest of North Carolina (Ricketts & Pope, 2002). According to the 2000 census, whites comprised 62 percent of the population in eastern North Carolina and 72 percent statewide. Blacks are concentrated in the northeastern and the central parts of the region. Warren County is one of six counties in the region where blacks comprised a majority of the population in 2000: Bertie County (62.3%), Hertford (59.6%), Northhampton (59.4%), Edgecombe (57.5%), Warren (54.5%), and Halifax (52.6%). Eastern North Carolina is also significantly poorer than the rest of the state (McLaughlin, n.d.). In 1999, per capita income in North Carolina was $26,463, but in the eastern region it was only $18,550 (Ricketts & Pope, 2002).

Warren County is vulnerable to a "quadruple whammy" of being mostly black, poor, rural, and politically powerless. In 1980, not long before the toxic-waste dump was established, the county had a population of 16,232. Blacks comprised 63.7 percent of the county population and 24.2 percent of the state population. The county continues to be economically worse off than the state as a whole on all major social indicators. Per capita income for Warren County residents was $6,984 in 1982 compared with $9,283 for the state. Warren County residents earned about 75 percent of the average state per capita income. Infrastructure development in this part of North Carolina diverted traffic and economic development away from Warren County. Generally, development often follows along major highways, but economic development bypassed much of the county. Over 19.4 percent of Warren County residents (compared with 12.3% of state residents) lived below the poverty level in 1999. Warren County has failed to attract new business.

It is important that the state finally detoxified the Warren County PCB landfill—a problem it created for local residents. This is a major victory for local residents and the EJM. However, it is also important that the surrounding land area and local community be made environmentally whole. Detoxifying the landfill does not bring the community back to its pre-1982 PCB-free environmental condition. Soil still containing low PCB levels is buried at least fifteen feet below the surface in the dump. Government officials claim the site is safe and suitable for reuse. However none of them live next door to the dump. There remain questions about suitable reuse of the site, and there is no evidence that the land has been brought back to its pre-1982 condition— where homes with deep basements could have been built and occupied and backyard vegetable gardens grown with little worry about toxic contamination or safety.

The placement of the PCB landfill in Afton is a textbook case of environmental racism. Around the world, environmental racism is defined as a human rights violation. Strong and persuasive arguments have been made for reparations as a remedy for serious human rights abuse. Under traditional human rights law and policy, we expect governments that practice or tolerate racial discrimination to acknowledge and end this human rights violation and compensate the victims. Environmental remediation is not reparations. Justice will not be complete until the 20,000 Warren County residents receive a public apology and some form of financial reparations for the two decades of economic loss, psychological damage, and mental anguish they have suffered. How much reparations should be paid is problematic because it is difficult for anyone to put a price tag on peace of mind. At minimum, Warren County residents should be paid reparations equal to the cost of detoxifying the landfill site, or $18 million. Another reparations formula might include payment of a minimum of $1 million a year for every year the mostly black Afton community hosted the PCB landfill, totaling $21 million.

Until the impacted community is made whole, the PCB-landfill detoxification victory won by the tenacity and perseverance of local Warren County residents will remain incomplete.

THE ENVIRONMENTAL JUSTICE PARADIGM

Despite significant improvements in environmental protection over the past several decades, millions of Americans continue to live in unsafe and unhealthy physical environments. As we stated earlier, many economically impoverished communities and their inhabitants are exposed to greater health hazards in their homes, on the jobs, and in their neighborhoods when compared to their more affluent counterparts (Bullard, 1994a, 1994b; U.S. EPA, 1992; Bryant & Mohai, 1992; Bryant, 1995; Calloway & Decker, 1997; Collin & Morris: Collin & Morris Collin, 1998). When it comes to enforcing the rights of poor people and people of color in the United States, government officials often look the other way. Unequal enforcement has left a gaping environmental protection hole in many poor communities and communities of color. Waiting for government to act is a recipe for disaster.

From New York to Los Angeles, grassroots community resistance has emerged in response to practices, policies, and conditions that residents have judged to be unjust, unfair, and illegal. Some of these conditions include:

1. unequal enforcement of environmental, civil rights, and public health laws;

2. differential exposure of some populations to harmful chemicals, pesticides, and other toxins in the home, school, neighborhood, and workplace;

3. faulty assumptions in calculating, assessing, and managing risks;

4. discriminatory zoning and land-use practices; and

5. exclusionary practices that limit some individuals and groups from participation in decision making (Lee, 1992; Bullard, 1993c).

Environmental justice is defined as the fair treatment and meaningful involvement of all people regardless of race, color, national origin, or income with respect to the development, implementation, and enforcement of environmental laws, regulations, and policies. Fair treatment means that no group of people, including racial, ethnic, or socioeconomic groups, should bear a disproportionate share of the negative environmental consequences resulting from industrial, municipal, and commercial operations or the execution of federal, state, local, and tribal programs and policies (U.S. EPA, 1998). Yet a growing body of evidence reveals that people of color and low-income persons have borne greater environmental and health risks than the society at large in their neighborhoods, workplaces, and playgrounds (Johnson, et al. 1992; National Institute for Environmental Health Sciences, 1995).

During its forty-year history, the U.S. Environmental Protection Agency (EPA) has not always recognized that many government and industry practices have adverse impact (whether intended or unintended) on poor people and people of color. Growing grassroots community resistance emerged in response to practices, policies, and conditions that residents judged to be unjust, unfair, and illegal. The EPA is mandated to enforce the nation's environmental laws and regulations equally across the board. It is required to protect all Americans, not just individuals or groups who can afford lawyers, lobbyists, and experts. Environmental protection is not a privilege reserved for a few who can "vote with their feet" and escape or fend off environmental stressors.

The current environmental protection apparatus manages, regulates, and distributes risks (Bullard, 1996). The dominant environmental protection paradigm institutionalizes unequal enforcement; trades human health for profit; places the burden of proof on the "victims" and not the polluting industry; legitimates human exposure to harmful chemicals, pesticides, and hazardous substances; promotes "risky" technologies; exploits the vulnerability of economically and politically disenfranchised communities; subsidizes ecological destruction; creates an industry around risk assessment and risk management; delays clean-up actions; and fails to develop pollution prevention as the overarching and dominant strategy (Bullard, 1993a, 1993b).

On the other hand, the environmental justice paradigm embraces a holistic approach to formulating environmental health policies and regulations, developing risk reduction strategies for multiple, cumulative, and synergistic risks, ensuring public health, enhancing public participation in environmental decision making, building infrastructure for achieving environmental justice and sustainable communities, ensuring interagency cooperation and coordination, developing innovative public/private partnerships and collaboratives, enhancing community-based pollution prevention strategies, ensuring community-based sustainable economic development, and developing geographically oriented community-wide programming.

The question of EJ is not anchored in a debate about whether or not decision makers should tinker with risk assessment and risk management. The environmental justice framework (EJF) rests on developing tools and strategies to eliminate unfair, unjust, and inequitable conditions and decisions (Bullard, 1996). The framework also attempts to uncover the underlying assumptions that may contribute to and produce differential exposure and unequal protection. It brings to the surface the ethical and political questions of "who gets what, when, why, and how much." Some general characteristics of this framework include

- adopting a public health model of prevention (i.e., elimination of the threat before harm occurs) as the preferred strategy.

- shifting the burden of proof to polluters/dischargers who do harm, who discriminate, or who do not give equal protection to people of color, low-income persons, and other "protected" classes.

- allowing disparate impact and statistical weight or an "effect" test, as opposed to "intent," to infer discrimination.

- redressing disproportionate impact through "targeted" action and resources. In general, this strategy would target resources where environmental and health problems are greatest (as determined by some ranking scheme but not limited to risk assessment).

In response to growing public concern and mounting scientific evidence, President Clinton on February 11, 1994 (the second day of the national health symposium) issued Executive Order 12898, "Federal Actions to Address Environmental Justice in Minority Populations and Low-Income Populations." This Order attempts to address environmental injustice within existing federal laws and regulations.

Executive Order 12898 reinforces the thirty-five-year-old Civil Rights Act of 1964, Title VI, which prohibits discriminatory practices in programs receiving federal funds. The Order also focuses the spotlight back on the National Environmental Policy Act (NEPA), a twenty-five-year-old law that set policy goals for the protection, maintenance, and enhancement of the environment. NEPA's goal is to ensure for all Americans a safe, healthful, productive, and aesthetically and culturally pleasing environment. NEPA requires federal agencies to prepare a detailed statement on the environmental effects of proposed federal actions that significantly affect the quality of human health (Council on Environmental Quality, 1997).

The Executive Order encourages participation of the impacted populations in the various phases of assessing impacts, including scoping, data gathering, alternatives, analysis, mitigation, and monitoring. It also calls for improved methodologies for assessing and mitigating impacts, assessing health effects from multiple and cumulative exposure, collection of data on low-income and minority populations who may be disproportionately at risk, and impacts on subsistence fishers and wildlife consumers. There are many people who are subsistence fishers, who fish for protein, while subsidizing their budgets and their diets by fishing from rivers, streams, and lakes that are polluted. These subpopulations may be underprotected when basic assumptions are made using the dominant risk paradigm.

DEADLY DUMPING GROUNDS AT THE FENCELINE

Clearly, African American communities continue to be disproportionately and adversely impacted by environmental toxins. African American residents in fenceline communities comprise a special needs population that deserves special attention. A 2005 study from the Associated Press reported African Americans are 79 percent more likely than whites to live in neighborhoods where industrial pollution is suspected of posing the greatest health danger (Pace, 2005).

Using EPA's own data and government scientists, the AP analyzed the health risk posed by industrial air pollution using toxic chemical air releases reported by factories to calculate a health risk score for each square kilometer of the United States. The scores can be used to compare risks from long-term exposure to factory pollution from one area to another. Analysis revealed that in nineteen states, blacks were more than twice as likely as whites to live in neighborhoods where air pollution seems to pose the greatest health danger.

Toxic chemical assaults are not new for many Americans who are forced to live adjacent to and often on the fenceline with chemical industries that spew their poisons into the air, water, and ground (Bullard, 2005b). When chemical accidents inevitably occur, government and industry officials often instruct the fenceline community residents to "shelter in place." In reality, locked doors and closed windows do not block the chemical assault on the nearby communities, nor do they remove the cause of the anxiety and fear of the unknown health problems that may not show up for decades.

High-Tech Weapons Contamination in Tallevast, Florida

Tallevast is a historically African American community tucked between Brandenton and Sarasota in Manatee County in southwest Florida. It dates back to the late 1800s, when freed slaves settled in the area looking for work tapping sap from the local pine trees (Weisenmiller, 2007). Many of the more than three hundred residents are descendants of the original settlers, occupying about eighty homes (Fischbein, 2005c).

The private wells in the community are poisoned with cancer-causing chemicals that leaked from an old beryllium plant that moved into the area in 1948. Beryllium, a known carcinogen, is a chemical element known for its strength and light weight. In 1961, the plant was purchased by the American Beryllium Company (ABC), which worked under contract with the U.S. Department of Defense and the U.S. Department of Energy to make parts for nuclear reactors and weapons.

In 1996, Lockheed Martin purchased American Beryllium's parent, Loral Corporation (Lerner, 2008), and the plant ceased operations. With $42 billion in annual revenue, Lockheed Martin is the nation's largest military contractor, employing about 140,000 people worldwide. In 1997, Lockheed Martin decided to sell the property.

While sampling soil around the property, engineers noticed an underground leak (Weisenmiller, 2007). Further testing revealed high levels of beryllium, chromium, tetrachloroethylene, trichloroethylene (TCE), and 1,1-dichloroethylene in the groundwater, as well as volatile organic compounds, vinyl chloride, total petroleum hydrocarbons, and other harmful compounds and metals in the soil and groundwater (Lerner 2008). In 1999, results were reexamined. The new samples near four sumps exceeded clean-up target levels for total petroleum hydrocarbons and the toxin tetrachloroethylene. Although Lockheed Martin informed Manatee County officials and the Florida Department of Environmental Protection about the contamination as early as 1999, Tallevest residents did not learn of the contamination in their backyards until late 2003, almost four years later (Fischbein, 2005b; Green, 2008).

Since July 2000, the Florida Department of Environmental Protection has overseen a voluntary clean-up by Lockheed Martin at the former American Beryllium site. In September 2001, more than 583 tons of contaminated soil were moved off-site and replaced with new soil as an interim measure (Sole, 2004). The 1.5-square-mile community is sitting on top of a two-hundred-acre toxic plume (Green, 2008). The company continued to conduct tests and hold meetings with state officials in 2002. Yet, Tallevast residents were told nothing—even in 2002, as records show the state "raised concerns about potential impacts to off-site private wells" (Green, 2008). Concentration of cancer-causing TCE was 10,000 times above state standards and five of the seven irrigation wells the state sampled showed elevated TCE above Florida drinking-water standards. Tallevast resident Laura Ward first learned of toxic chemicals beneath her community in 2003 when she looked out her window one day to see a giant rig drilling monitoring wells on her property. She asked the workers what they were doing on her property. "You don't know, but the water's contaminated here. . . . We're putting in monitoring wells in your community," was the reply Ward received (Green, 2008, p. A1). Naturally, she was startled.

In October 2003, in response to community inquiries, Lockheed Martin informed the community of the results of the site assessment and the believed extent of the contamination. Because of the proximity between the property fenceline and the community, residents grew concerned about contaminated groundwater. Several residential wells were sampled and the neighborhood was warned of an underground toxic plume twenty-five acres wide (Fischbein, 2005c). Bottled water was provided to residents who were on well water, and county hookups were provided to homes not previously linked to the public supply. A month later, a report by Lockheed Martin revealed a toxic plume believed to be 183 acres wide. Despite assurances from the company that the plume was not growing and that the increase in size should not raise concerns, by March 2005, the plume was more than two hundred acres wide (Fischbein, 2005a).

In February 2005, an informal health survey conducted by the retired nurse for the residents found fifteen out of eighty-seven households surveyed had cancer. The survey also found suspiciously high incidence of miscarriages, sterility, low birth rates, neurological disorders, and retardation (Lerner, 2008). A health study conducted by the Florida Department of Health (DOH) erroneously identified only three cancer cases in the community. In contrast, a survey by residents showed about ninety cases of cancer or beryllium-related diseases in the community. DOH officials agreed that their own numbers, based on a state database and figures from a local hospital, were "way off the mark" and that they had studied the wrong zip code (O'Donnell, 2008b).

Lockheed Martin has maintained from the beginning that the plume poses no health risk to residents and will have minimal if any impact on property values (Fischbein, 2006). Who would buy a house that sits atop a beryllium and TCE plume, and at what price? *Miami Herald* reporter Ronnie Green (2008) described the community's current condition:

> Today the village is little more than a giant environmental testing ground, where day-to-day life has stalled as more than 200 wells monitor a plume that spread from an initial estimate of five acres to more than 200. Residents' yards are cluttered with orange flags that mark soil-boring tests.

The Wards' eight-acre homestead is covered with thirteen monitoring wells and more than two dozen orange flags. The Ward family along with other community leaders filed lawsuits against Lockheed Martin and others, seeking medical testing, relocation to a community with clean air and water, and damages for lost property values.

Residents claim Manatee County officials have ignored them and that Lockheed Martin deliberately misled them. Lockheed Martin officials argue that state laws in effect at the time did not require the company or state to inform residents of the pollution problem. In 2005, local residents were instrumental in getting the Tallevast Bill passed—a change in Florida's law that requires polluters to notify communities within thirty days and survey all wells near a contamination source. Lockheed Martin officials say cleaning up the majority of the polluted groundwater in Tallevast could take thirty years, and getting it all could take a century. But some experts fear that the Tallevast pollution will never be completely cleaned up and the community made whole. In late 2008, the company temporarily relocated about thirty-five families while two buildings at the former plant are demolished (O'Donnell, 2008a). The residents' lawsuit is still pending.

Poisoned Water in DeBerry, Texas

A July 2006 *New York Times* article detailed the clear racial divide in the way government responds to toxic contamination in black and white communities, with a report on DeBerry, a small black community in East Texas (Blumenthal, 2006). The case involves Frank and Earnestene Roberson and their relatives, who live on County Road 329 in a historically African American enclave in the East Texas oilfields. The Roberson family are the descendants of an African American settler, George Adams, who bought forty acres and a mule there in 1911 for $289. In the 1920s oil was discovered in the area, and DeBerry enjoyed a brief boom.

The family suspects their wells were poisoned by Basic Energy Services' deep injection wells for saltwater wastes from drilling operations, which began around 1980. Basic Energy Services, a Midland, Texas–based oil and gas producing company, is the nation's third largest well servicing contractor. Years before the saltwater injection wells, cool water flowed from wells drilled into the ground and through the pipes inside area homes. Now, none of the seven families along County Road 329 in Panola County can drink their well water because various levels of methyl tertiary butyl ether (MTBE), benzene, petroleum hydrocarbons, arsenic, lead, barium, cadmium, mercury, fecal coliform, and E. coli have been detected in multiple samples. Their water is unsafe for domestic use (Welborn, 2005).

Because of the contamination, some families were forced to drive twenty-three miles to a Wal-Mart near Shreveport for clean water. Other family members depended on visits from the Music Mountain truck for water delivery, at a cost of $40 a month. In August 2005, free drinking water was delivered weekly in five-gallon containers to residents' homes—compliments of the Environmental Protection Agency Region Six Emergency Response, located in Dallas, and the Texas Commission of Environmental Quality (Welborn, 2005, 2006).

The Roberson family first complained about spillover from Basic Energy Services' injection well to the Texas Railroad Commission (RRC), which regulates the state's oil and gas industry, back in 1987—the same year the United Church of Christ Commission for Racial Justice (1987) published its groundbreaking *Toxic Wastes and Race in the United States* study—but to no avail. Nearly a decade later, in 1996, the railroad commission took samples and found "no contamination in the Robersons' household supply water that can be attributed to oilfield sources."

In 2003, testing by the Railroad Commission found benzene, barium, arsenic, cadmium, lead and mercury in the wells at concentrations exceeding primary drinking-water standards. In October 2003, after a second round of well testing showed high levels of hazardous chemicals, the Railroad Commission sent letters to affected residents advising them that their water contained material "that may pose adverse health effects. We do not recommend that it be used for any domestic purposes."

Still, no government clean-up actions were taken to protect the Robersons and other black families in the community. In June 2006, the Roberson family filed suit in federal court, accusing the Texas Railroad Commission of failing to enforce safety regulations and of "intentionally giving citizens false information based on their race and economic status."

The Robersons point to the slow government response to the toxic contamination in their mostly black community compared to the rapid clean-up response by the Railroad Commission in Manvel, a largely white suburb of Houston. The DeBerry site was closed only after the Panola County District Attorney discovered a pipe for runoff had been illegally drilled under the county road for piping in waste. Because the site sits on an incline, runoff naturally goes downhill to the County Road 329 community. Because of this, Rev. David Hudson, the Robersons' nephew and a retired California radio and television station manager, is waging a one-man crusade to get justice for his community.

Tests performed in April 2004 on wells on the disposal site and at Hudson's home detected levels of dichloromethane (DME), which is a colorless organic liquid often used as a paint remover, industry solvent, and cleaning agent. Residents' wells and a nearby spring have an oil sheen and odor. Ron Kitchens, executive director of the Texas Railroad Commission, agrees that the families' wells are contaminated, but he stops short of saying the contamination is from oil and gas operations. Though there is a general consensus that the residents' wells are fouled, no one is willing to finger the culprit (Sorg, 2006). Basic Energy's monitoring wells at the disposal site and the neighborhood spring register nearly identical concentrations of barium and chloride. Someone wrote 'interesting coincidence' in the margin of a CEQ document reviewing Basic Energy's test results.

According to a 2004 report by the Texas Groundwater Protection Committee, of which the RRC is a member, of the 230 closed cases of groundwater contamination related to oilfield operations in Texas since 1989, 222 were linked to commercial saltwater-disposal wells. *Shreveport Times* reporter Lisa Sorg (2006) draws distinctions regarding how saltwater disposal is handled in Louisiana and Texas:

> In Louisiana, commercial saltwater-disposal wells are considered hazardous enough that state regulations prohibit their property boundaries to be within 500 feet of a residence, church, or school. But in Texas, there are no such regulations, although local governments can pass ordinances to restrict their use. Panola County has passed no such law, and the property boundary of the Basic well is within 300 feet of the church and two homes. All the houses on CR 329 are within 700 feet of the disposal-well property.

It is cheaper for energy companies to haul their waste to East Texas where, with laxer rules, the wells are abundant. Hudson and his neighbors sought relief from the Railroad Commission, the Texas Commission of Environmental Quality, and the federal Environmental Protection Agency. In January 2005, the Railroad Commission canceled the company's permit. In April, Basic Energy plugged the wells, removed the tanks, and plugged lines with cement. A July 6, 2006, memorandum from the EPA Office of the Inspector General (2006) presented its preliminary findings on the Basic Energy site.

In September 2007, the OIG final report, *Complete Assessment Needed to Ensure Rural Texas Community Has Safe Drinking Water*, confirmed that the groundwater in the community is contaminated and should not be used for domestic purposes (U.S. EPA 2007). However, it did not determine the source of the groundwater contamination. The OIG report cost taxpayers $375,251. The cost for the RRC to drill a recent monitoring well: $45,000 (they have drilled a total of twelve so far). In comparison, the original cost to connect residents who live on County Road 329 to a public water supply system only a mile and half away was only $60,000.

In February 2007, the EPA did not link the contamination to the abandoned injection well. It determined that the private water wells of Hudson and his neighbors who brought the lawsuit only tested positive for fecal coliform and placed the blame on surface water carrying contaminants from septic systems and possible oilfield spills, not from the Basic Energy Services operations. However, the natural springs and monitoring wells were found to be contaminated with metals and radionuclides that exceed levels considered safe for drinking water. The radionuclides include materials such as barium, cadmium, and beryllium, all byproducts of oil and gas production.

In June 2008, EPA Region Six announced fresh water finally would be coming to DeBerry residents (Welborn, 2008). After the water lines are installed, families will be responsible for service lines to their homes and the water meters. Residents view the decision as a partial victory, because toxic contamination remains in their community. The elderly Robersons are counting the days until they can simply turn on the faucet and get fresh water. The family continued to bathe in the contaminated water because they had no other options given their limited means.

Hudson and his neighbors' civil lawsuit against Basic Energy Services was settled out of court in June 2006. Nevertheless, Rev. Hudson and the residents press on for environmental justice and redress for the harm unnecessarily inflicted on the community.

Incineration of VX Gas Wastewater in Port Arthur, Texas

The incineration of wastewater from the deadly nerve agent VX in Port Arthur, Texas, typifies the environmental justice challenges facing African Americans. Veolia Environmental Services of Lombard, Ill., won a $49 million contract from the U.S. Army to incinerate 1.8 million gallons of caustic VX hydrolysate wastewater near Port Arthur's Carver Terrace housing project. Residents in New Jersey and Ohio had fought off plans to incinerate the waste there. Army and city officials did not announce the project in Port Arthur until the deal was sealed. The first batch of VX hydrolysate was incinerated in Port Arthur on April 22, 2007—Earth Day.

About 60 percent of Port Arthur's population is African American, and Jim Crow segregation forced them to the west part of town. There the city built the Carver Terrace housing development for low-income blacks. Port Arthur is encircled by major refineries and chemical plants operated by such companies as Motiva, Chevron Phillips, Valero, and BASF. Residents whose homes are located at the fenceline are riddled with cancer, asthma, and liver and kidney disease that some blame on the pollution from nearby industries.

The Carver Terrace housing project abuts the Motiva oil refinery. Jefferson County, where Port Arthur is located, is home to one of the country's largest chemical-industrial complexes and is consistently ranked among the top 10 percent of America's dirtiest counties. In June 2007, the U.S. Army temporarily suspended shipments of the former nerve gas agent in the form of caustic wastewater while the federal court in Terre Haute, Ind., listened to the case (Meux 2007). A judge in late September ruled that the disposal plan didn't violate federal or state laws (Levine, 2008).

TCE Contamination in Dickson, Tennessee

There are literally dozens of locations across the nation where ER has left an ugly scar. Dickson, Tennessee, is a textbook case—the "poster child" for ER. Dickson is a town of 12,244 located about 35 miles west of Nashville. Dickson County was only 4.5

percent African American in 2000 (U.S. Census Bureau, 2000), but Dickson's mostly African American Eno Road community has been used as the dumping ground for garbage and toxic wastes dating back more than four decades (Cornwell, 2003). The Eno Road community was first used as the site of the Dickson "city dump" and subsequent city and county Class I sanitary landfills, Class III and IV construction and demolition landfills, balefills, and processing centers.

The Dickson County Landfill consists of seventy-four acres off Eno Road, 1.5 miles southwest of Dickson. Scovill-Shrader automotive company opened in Dickson, Tennessee, in 1964—the same year the U.S. Congress passed the sweeping Civil Rights Act that outlawed racial discrimination. The plant manufactured automotive tire valves and gauges. The process included metal plating, etching, rubber molding and application, polishing, degreasing, and painting, according to documents prepared by the TDEC Division of Water Supply. Such an industrial operation generates quantities of hazardous wastes that must be disposed of.

According to government records, in 1968, the same year Dr. Martin Luther King was assassinated in Memphis, Scovill-Shrader and several other local industries buried drums of industrial waste solvents at an "open dump" landfill site (Tetra Tech EM Inc., 2004). In 1972, the unlined landfill was granted a permit by the Tennessee Department of Health and Environment (TDEH). The town of Dickson operated the landfill until 1977, when it was taken over and operated by Dickson County (Tetra Tech EM Inc., 2004, p. 15). More than 1,400 people obtain their drinking water from private wells or springs within a four-mile radius of the landfill (Halliburton NUS Environmental Corporation, 1991, p.ES-1). A 1991 Halliburton report acknowledged the fact that the Harry Holt well (described later) is close to the landfill. It states, "the closest private well [Harry Holt well] is located approximately 500 feet east of the landfill" (Halliburton NUS Environmental Corporation, 1991, p. 9).

Contaminated waste material was cleaned up from other areas of this mostly white county and trucked to the landfill in the mostly black Eno Road community. For example, Ebbtide Corporation (Winner Boats) removed material from an on-site dump and transferred it to the Dickson County Landfill (Halliburton NUS Environmental Corporation, 1991, p. 17), disposing of drummed wastes every week for three to four years. Scovill-Shrader Automotive manufacturing plant buried drums of industrial waste solvents at the landfill. The company's wastes are known to have contained acetone and paint thinner (Halliburton NUS Environmental Corporation, 1991, p. 31). A 1991 EPA Site Inspection Report notes that soil containing benzene, toluene, ethylbenzene, xylenes, and petroleum hydrocarbons from underground storage tank cleanups was brought to the landfill (Halliburton NUS Environmental Corporation, 1991, p. 17).

The Dickson County Landfill has received numerous unsatisfactory operational notices. The landfill received five notices of violations (NOV) from July 18, 1988, to April 12, 1999, including inadequate daily cover, violation of Groundwater Protection Standards, cadmium detected in ground water and springs at concentrations exceeding the MCL (the maximum concentration of a chemical that is allowed in public drinking-water systems), and violation of inadequate depth cover and pooling of water on landfill cover (Tetra Tech EM Inc., p. 19).

Despite repeated violations at the Dickson County Landfill, the TDEC continued to grant permits for the site on Eno Road. TDEC permitted at least four landfills for the Eno Road site after 1988. In February 2007, Dickson County began operating a recycling center, garbage transfer station, and C&D landfill at the Eno Road site. The garbage transfer station alone handles approximately 35,000 tons annually, with 20–25 heavy-duty diesel trucks entering the sites each day and leaving behind noxious fumes, dangerous particulates, household garbage, recyclables, and demolition debris from around Middle Tennessee.

It is no accident or statistical fluke that all the permitted landfills in Dickson County are concentrated in this black community (Bullard, 2007a). When *New York Times* columnist Bob Herbert queried Dickson County attorney Eric Thornton for an October 2006 article, "Poisoned on Eno Road," about why the Eno Road community had been chosen to absorb so much of the county's garbage and hazardous waste, Thornton's reply was "it has to be at some location" (Herbert, 2006). Though this may be true, why must the "Somewhere USA" generally end up being in the communities of African Americans and other people of color?

Treatment of the African American Holt Family   The Harry Holt family, a family of black landowners that have deep roots in the Eno Road community, has been especially harmed by the toxic assaults of the city and county landfills and government inaction. The Holt family's American Dream of land ownership has become a "toxic nightmare." For more than a decade, they have experienced the terror of not knowing what health problems may lay ahead for their children and their children's children. The State of Tennessee approved the Dickson County Landfill permit on December 2, 1988, even though government test results completed on November 18, 1988 on the Harry Holt and Lavenia Holt wells showed TCE contamination. TCE is a suspected carcinogen with adverse health effects if ingested including liver disease, hypertension, speech impediment, hearing impairment, stroke, anemia and other blood disorders, diabetes, kidney disease, urinary tract disorders, and skin rashes (Agency for Toxic Substances and Disease Registry [ATSDR], 2003; Gist & Burg, 2006).

The TDHE letters to Harry Holt and Lavenia Holt on December 8, 1988 informing the family of the test results finding of contamination in their wells, stated: "Your water is of good quality for the parameters tested. It is felt that the low levels of methylene or trichloroethylene may be due to either lab or sampling error" (Letter from Mark McWhorter, 1988).

On January 28, 1990, government tests found 26 ppb (parts per billion) TCE in the Harry Holt well—five times above the established Maximum Contaminant Level (MCL) of 5 ppb set by the federal EPA. Follow-up tests in August 1990 and August 1991 found 3.9 ppb TCE and 3.7 ppb TCE in the Harry Holt well.

A January 28, 1991, EPA potential hazardous waste site inspection of the landfill was performed. And on December 3, 1991 the EPA sent Harry Holt a letter informing him of the three tests performed on his well and deemed it safe. The letter states: "Use of your well water should not result in any adverse health effects" (Letter from Wayne Aronson, 1991).

A December 17, 1991 letter from the TDEC expressed some concern about the level of TCE contamination found in the Holts' well. Tennessee Department of Health and Environment officials agreed that Mr. Holt's well should continue to be sampled. However, this was not done. The letter states: "Our program is concerned that the sampling twice with one considerably above MCL and one slightly below MCL in a karst area such as Dickson is in no way an assurance that Mr. Holt's well water will stay below MCL's. There is a considerably seasonal variation for contaminants in karst environments and 3.9 ppb TCE is only slightly under the MCL of 5 ppb" (Letter from Thomas A. Moss, 1991).

Although Tennessee state officials expressed concern about the tests, they stood by and allowed the Holt family to continue to drink contaminated well water. A January 6, 1992, letter from the TDHE continued to express concern about the level of contamination found in the Holt well (Letter from Thomas Moss, 1992).

A month later, on February 12, 1992, state officials continued to discuss the TCE contamination in the Holt family wells and the Dickson County Landfill. The letter states:

A search of our Division's files has been made concerning the allegation that a domestic well, located on the Harry and Lavenia Holt property, may have been adversely impacted by the Dickson County Landfill. No substantial evidence was found in our files to support this allegation. Attached is a 1988 memo from our Division showing that groundwater samples from the Holt well were obtained and analyzed at that time. Those sample results showed that trichloroethylene (TCE) and methylene chloride were found to be at the upper regulatory limit of the acceptable drinking water standards set by EPA. It was concluded by this Division that these detection levels may have been due to either laboratory or sample error. There is no record that any additional samples were obtained at a later date by either our Division or by the EPA (Memorandum Written by Debbie Sanders, 1992).

A March 13, 1992 letter from the TDHE sides with EPA on the Holt family well water being "safe." The letter states:

Since EPA has already completed a site investigation, has identified the pollutants involved, and has, in part, determined the extent of the leaching, I would suggest that they, EPA, continue with their chosen course of action, rather than create the added confusion of various agencies making their own agendas. I would suggest that if Mr. Holt is concerned about possible health risks in using his well water between now and June (when EPA's priority decision is made), that he should rely on bottled or city water for cooking and drinking purposes until he is convinced that his well water is safe (Sanders, 1992).

In the final analysis, the state handed the ball off to the federal government, and records show that the Harry Holt well was *not* retested or monitored as recommended by state officials. According to the 2004 EPA *Dickson County Landfill Reassessment Report*, no government tests were performed on the Harry Holt family well between August 24, 1991 and October 8, 2000—a full nine years (Tetra Tech EM Inc. 2004, p. 28). No scientific explanation has been given for this gap in government testing, even though the TDHE and the federal EPA were periodically performing tests on private wells that were within a one-mile radius of the leaky Dickson County Landfill.

An April 7, 1997, TDEC confirmation sample at DK-21, a nearby well, showed TCE at 14 parts per billion and Cis-1, 2 dichloroethene at 1.3 parts per billion. On April 18, 1997, the City of Dickson closed the DK-21 well, halting its use as a supplement to the municipal water source, after a call from the state requiring an aeration, or water filtration, system, and began using the Piney River exclusively as the municipal water source, according to the TDEC Division of Water Supply (Cornwell, 1991).

A dye-tracer study, *Summary and Results of Dye-Tracer Tests Conducted at the Dickson County Landfill, Tennessee, 1997 and 1998*, was conducted to help evaluate whether the landfill was a possible source of the contamination (Gresham Smith and Partners, 2000). One of the dye-tracer test sites was the Humane Society of Dickson County, a facility located at 410 Eno Road, only a few hundred feet from the Harry Holt homestead located at 390 Eno Road. The Harry Holt, Roy Holt, and Lavenia Holt family wells were not part of the 1997–1998 government study even though they are all within several hundred feet of the landfill.

The Harry Holt well was not retested until October 9, 2000, when it registered a whopping 120 ppb TCE. A second test on October 25, 2000, registered 145 ppb. These numbers are 24 times and 29 times higher than the MCL of 5 ppb set by the federal EPA (Tetra Tech EM Inc. 2004, p. 28). It was only after the extremely high TCE levels in 2000 that a Dickson County Landfill official visited the Holt family home, informing them that their wells were unsafe. No written reports or letters were sent to the Holt family explaining the October 9, 2000, test results.

The Holt family was placed on Dickson City water on October 20, 2000—twelve years after the first government tests found TCE in their well. The county paid the Holts' entire water bills because well water on the property tested positive for TCE. On December 2, 2003, the Harry Holt family filed a lawsuit against the City of Dickson, County of Dickson, and Scovill-Shrader, and immediately afterward, the Dickson County Commission stopped paying the family's water bills (Cornwell, 2004). Before the county landfill was sited, the Holt family wells were clean and the water was safe to drink and it was free. Now the Holt family must incur an added expense of paying the county for clean water.

The Holts received different treatment from white families as recently as November 6, 2006—when in a special called meeting, Dickson County Commissioners voted unanimously to settle lawsuits with several white families that had alleged groundwater contamination from the leaky Dickson County Landfill (Kimbro 2006). No such settlement has been reached with the Holt family. On November 28, 2007, one day before the "Take Back Black Health Toxics Tour" in Dickson, a front-page story ran in the *Dickson Herald* reporting that the Dickson County Commission had agreed to accept a $400,000 offer on its $4 million claim against a former local company that dumped toxic waste at the landfill several years ago (Burton, 2007).

Treatment of White Families in Dickson County   Government testing and monitoring of the African American Holt family's wells differed markedly in terms of testing, notification, remediation, and provision of alternative water supply—temporary (providing bottled water) and permanent (connecting to city water system)—from white families whose spring and wells were contaminated. On March 5, 1994, TCE was detected in Sullivan Spring, a water supply located one-third mile from the landfill and used by two white families. On September 1, 1994, tests were conducted on the spring to confirm it was indeed contaminated. On September 8, 1994, TDEC sent the white families a "Notification of Contaminants in Drinking Water" letter. The letter stated that the spring used to supply drinking water to them showed levels of trichloroethylenecis-1, 2-dichloroethene, and dichloroethene above the allowable levels, and to discontinue use of the water (Letter from C. Jason Repsher, 1994).

Dickson County officials even dug the white family a well to be used as an alternate water supply. The family was placed on the city tap water system after the new well was found to be contaminated. A total of nine tests were performed on the family's spring between June 25, 1994, and September 20, 2000 (Tetra Tech EM Inc. 2004, p. 27). Government tests were continued on the family's spring even after its family members were placed on the city water system. The care and precaution that the government officials initiated to protect the health of the white families was not extended to the black Holt family. White families near the site were notified within 48 hours, provided with bottled water, and placed on the city water system. The black family was allowed to drink TCE-contaminated well water for twelve years. This differential treatment resulted in the African American Holt family experiencing prolonged exposure to contaminated drinking water and subjected them to unnecessary health risks.

The Harry Holt family 2003 lawsuit was still pending in court when he died of cancer on January 9, 2007. Mr. Holt was 66 years old and had lived in the Eno Road community all of his life. Generations of Holts survived the horrors of post-slavery racism and "Jim Crow" segregation, but may not survive the toxic assault and contamination from the Dickson County Landfill (Duke, 2007; Gordy, 2007; Rysavy, 2007). The Holt family is represented by the NAACP Legal Defense and Education Fund (NAACP Legal Defense and Education Fund, 2007).

Environmental and Health Threats in Post-Katrina New Orleans

On August 29, 2005, Hurricane Katrina laid waste to New Orleans, an American city built mostly below sea level and whose coastal wetlands, which normally serve as a natural buffer against storm surge, had been destroyed by developers (Pastor et al., 2006; Colton, 2007). Katrina has been described as one of the most devastating, costly, and deadly disasters in U.S. history—a disaster that is still ongoing (Dyson, 2006; Heerden & Bryan, 2006; Horne, 2006; Mann, 2006; Brunsma et al., 2007). A September 2005 *Business Week* commentary described the handling of the untold tons of "lethal goop" as the "mother of all toxic clean-ups" (*Business Week*, 2005). However, the billion-dollar question facing New Orleans is which neighborhoods will get cleaned up, which ones will be left contaminated, and which ones will be targeted as new sites to dump storm debris and waste from flooded homes.

Cleaning Up Toxic Neighborhoods Flooding in the New Orleans metropolitan area largely resulted from breached levees and flood walls (Gabe et al., 2005). A May 2006 report from the Russell Sage Foundation, *In the Wake of the Storm: Environment, Disaster, and Race after Katrina*, found that minority groups often experience a "second disaster" after the initial storm (Pastor et al., 2006). Quite often the scale of a disaster's impact, as in the case of Hurricane Katrina, has more to do with the political economy of the country, region, and state than with the hurricane's category strength (Jackson, 2005; Hartman & Squires, 2007).

Quite often measures to prevent or contain the effects of disaster vulnerability are not equally provided to all (Bullard, 2005a). Typically, flood-control investments provide location-specific benefits, with the greatest benefits going to populations who live or own assets in the protected area. Thus, by virtue of where people live, work, or own property, they may be excluded from the benefits of government-funded flood-control investments (Boyce, 2004).

Hurricane Katrina left debris across a 90,000-square-mile disaster area in Louisiana, Mississippi, and Alabama (compared to the 16 acres of the 9/11 terrorist attack in New York) (Luther, 2006). Ten months after the storm, FEMA had spent $3.6 billion to remove 98.6 million cubic yards of debris (Jordan, 2006). This is enough trash to pile two miles high across five football fields. Still, an estimated 20 million cubic yards littered New Orleans and Mississippi waterways, with about 96 percent or 17.8 million cubic yards of remaining wreckage in Orleans, St. Bernard, St. Tammany, Washington, and Plaquemine parishes. Louisiana parishes hauled away 25 times more debris than was collected after the 9/11 terrorist attack (Shields, 2006).

EPA and LDEQ officials estimated that 140,000 to 160,000 homes in Louisiana may need to be demolished and disposed of (U.S. EPA & Louisiana Dept. of Environmental Quality, 2005). More than 110,000 of New Orleans' 180,000 homes were flooded, and half sat for days or weeks in more than six feet of water (Nossiter, 2005). Government officials estimate that as many as 30,000 to 50,000 homes city-wide may need to be demolished. An additional 350,000 automobiles had to be drained of oil and gasoline and then recycled; 60,000 boats needed to be destroyed; and 300,000 underground fuel tanks and 42,000 tons of hazardous waste had to be cleaned up and properly disposed of at licensed facilities (Varney & Moller, 2005). Government officials peg the numbers of cars lost in New Orleans alone at 145,000.

In March 2006, seven months after the storm slammed ashore, organizers of "A Safe Way Back Home" initiative, the Deep South Center for Environmental Justice at

Dillard University (DSCEJ) and the United Steel Workers (USW), undertook a proactive pilot neighborhood clean-up project, the first of its kind in New Orleans (Deep South Center for Environmental Justice, 2006). The clean-up project, located in the 8100 block of Aberdeen Road in New Orleans East, removed six inches of tainted soil from the front and back yards, replacing the soil with new sod and disposing of the contaminated dirt in a safe manner. Other residents who wish to remove the top soil from their yards—which contains sediments left by flooding—find themselves in a "Catch-22" situation with the LDEQ and EPA insisting the soil in their yards is not contaminated and the local landfill operators refusing to dispose of the soil because they expect it is contaminated. This bottleneck of what to do with the topsoil was unresolved a year and a half after the devastating flood.

Although government officials insist the dirt in residents' yards is safe, Church Hill Downs Inc., the owners of New Orleans' Fair Grounds track, felt it was not safe for its thoroughbred horses. The owners hauled off soil tainted by Hurricane Katrina's floodwaters and rebuilt a grandstand roof ripped off by the storm's wind (Martell, 2006). The Fair Grounds opened on Thanksgiving Day 2006. If tainted soil is not safe for horses, surely it is not safe for people—especially children who play and dig in the dirt.

The "A Safe Way Back Home" demonstration project serves as a catalyst for a series of activities that will attempt to reclaim the New Orleans East community following the devastation caused by Hurricane Katrina. Residents are not waiting for the government to ride in on a white horse to rescue them and clean up their neighborhoods (News from USW, 2006). The DSCEJ/USW coalition received dozens of requests and inquiries from New Orleans East homeowners associations to help clean up their neighborhoods block by block. State and federal officials labeled the voluntary clean-up efforts as "scaremongering" (Simmons, 2006).

EPA and LDEQ officials said that they tested soil samples from the neighborhood in December 2005 and that there was no immediate cause for concern. According to Tom Harris, administrator of LDEQ's environmental technology division, and state toxicologist, the government originally sampled 800 locations in New Orleans and found cause for concern in only 46 samples. Generally, the soil in New Orleans is consistent with "what we saw before Katrina," says Harris. He called the "A Safe Way Back Home" program "completely unnecessary" (Williams, 2006).

A week after the voluntary clean-up project began, an LDEQ staffer ate a spoonful of dirt scraped from the Aberdeen Road pilot project. The dirt-eating publicity stunt was clearly an attempt to disparage the proactive neighborhood clean-up initiative. LDEQ officials later apologized. Despite barriers and red tape, Katrina evacuees are moving back into New Orleans' damaged homes or setting up travel trailers in their yards. One of the main questions returning residents have is: Is this place safe? They're getting mixed signals from government agencies. In December 2005, the LDEQ announced that there was no unacceptable long-term health risk directly attributable to environmental contamination resulting from the storm. Two months later, the Natural Resources Defense Council (NRDC) test results came out with different conclusions (Solomon and Rotkin-Ellman, 2006). NRDC's analyses of soil and air quality after Hurricane

Katrina revealed dangerously high levels of diesel fuel, lead, and other contaminants in Gentilly, Bywater, Orleans Parish, and other New Orleans neighborhoods.

Although many government scientists insist the soil is safe, an April 2006 multi-agency task force press release distributed by the EPA raised some questions (EPA Office of the Inspector General, 2006). It claimed that the levels of lead and other contaminants in New Orleans soil was "similar" to soil contaminant levels in other cities, but it also cautioned residents to "keep children from playing in bare dirt. Cover bare dirt with grass, bushes or four–six inches of lead-free wood chips, mulch, soil or sand." In August 2006, nearly a year after Katrina made landfall, the federal EPA gave New Orleans and surrounding communities a clean bill of health, while pledging to monitor a handful of toxic hot spots (Brown, 2006). EPA and LDEQ officials concluded that Katrina did not cause any appreciable contamination that was not already there. Although EPA tests confirmed widespread lead in the soil—a pre-storm problem in 40 percent of New Orleans—EPA dismissed residents' calls to address this problem as outside the agency's mission.

Three years after Katrina, nearly one-third of New Orleans' residents had not made it back home (Liu & Plyer, 2008). The road home for many Katrina survivors has been a bumpy one, largely due to slow government actions to distribute the billions in federal aid to residents to rebuild. The Louisiana Road Home Program for Homeowners is distributing $10.5 billion in federal funds plus $1 billion in state funds to about 160,000 Louisiana homeowner-applicants whose homes were devastated in 2005 by Hurricanes Katrina or Rita or the subsequent flooding. Eighteen months after the Louisiana Road Home Program began, it had closed 90,000 grants, but some of those are still waiting for disputed award money and another 70,000 still have not gotten any money at all (Hammer, 2008). ICF International, the program's lead contractor, has been widely criticized for the slow pace of getting money to displaced homeowners.

Health Threats from Toxic FEMA Trailers Immediately after Katrina, FEMA purchased roughly 102,000 travel trailers for $2.6 billion or roughly $15,000 each (Spake, 2007). There were soon reports of residents becoming ill in these trailers due to the release of potentially dangerous levels of formaldehyde. In fact, formaldehyde is the industrial chemical (in glues, plastics, building materials, composite wood, plywood panels, and particle board) that was used to manufacture the travel trailers (Babington, 2007). In Mississippi, FEMA received 46 complaints of individuals who indicated that they had symptoms of formaldehyde exposure, including eye, nose and throat irritation, nausea, skin rashes, sinus infections, depression, mucus membrane irritations, asthma attacks, headaches, insomnia, intestinal problems, memory impairment, and breathing difficulties (Spake, 2007).

Even though FEMA received numerous complaints about toxic trailers, the agency only tested one occupied trailer to determine the levels of formaldehyde in it (U.S. House of Representatives Committee on Oversight and Government Reform, 2007). The test confirmed that the levels of formaldehyde were extraordinarily high and presented an immediate health risk to the occupants. Unfortunately, FEMA did not test any more occupied trailers and released a public statement discounting any risk associated with formaldehyde exposure.

FEMA deliberately neglected to investigate any reports of high levels of formaldehyde in trailers so as to bolster FEMA's litigation position just in case individuals affected by their negligence decided to sue them (Babington, 2007). More than five hundred hurricane survivors and evacuees in Louisiana are pursuing legal action against the trailer manufacturers.

In February of 2007, ATSDR released a health consultation entitled "Formaldehyde Sampling at FEMA Temporary Housing Units" in which ninety-six unoccupied trailers were tested for formaldehyde and other VOCs (ATSDR, 2007a). The study found that nonventilated trailers had readings higher than 0.3 ppm (at the time ATSDR stated 0.3 ppm as the level of concern for sensitive individuals), with levels dropping below this level for trailers that were adequately ventilated. According to the report, the air was safe to breathe and the contamination would not reach a "level of concern" as long as residents kept the windows open (ATSDR, 2007a).

In July 2007, FEMA stopped buying and selling disaster relief trailers because of the formaldehyde contamination. In August 2007, FEMA began moving families out of the toxic trailers and finding them new rental housing. Testing of FEMA travel trailers for formaldehyde and other hazards began in September 2007 (Treadway, 2007). The Centers for Disease Control and Prevention was assigned the lead agency in developing parameters for testing the travel trailers.

In October of 2007, ATSDR issued a report that replaced the health consultation released in February 2007. The newer report acknowledged that the February health consultation contained insufficient discussion of the health implications of formaldehyde exposure, and some language may have been unclear, potentially leading readers to draw incorrect or inappropriate conclusions. Analyses of formaldehyde levels by trailer type and by daily temperature were not conducted (ATSDR, 2007b). But the follow-up report also used the same 0.3 ppm standard used on the first study, although proPublica, an investigative journalism organization based in New York City, stated that ATSDR should have utilized a 0.03 ppm standard. The larger standard is only used for brief one-time exposure. For longer term, eight to twenty-four hours, the researchers should have applied the lower standard. The use of the wrong standard caused residents' exposure levels to be ten times higher than acceptable (Sapien, 2008). At levels so high, formaldehyde can cause respiratory problems and irritation within two hours of exposure. In October of 2008, the U.S. House of Representatives' Committee on Science and Technology published a report detailing their investigation into the trailer issue. The report states:

> *ATSDR's reaction was marred by scientific flaws, ineffective leadership, a sluggish response to inform trailer residents of the potential risks they faced, and a lack of urgency to actually remove them from harm's way. Most disturbingly, there was a concerted and continuing effort by the agency's leadership to both mask their own*

involvement in the formaldehyde study, and to push the blame for their fumbling of this critical public health issue down the line to others. The health consultation itself, conducted at the request of FEMA's Office of General Counsel because of expected litigation concerns, was scientifically flawed and omitted critical health information (U.S. House of Representatives, 2008).

The Congressional report also states that ATSDR failed to serve the public by not using the best science, by not taking responsive public health actions, and by not providing trusted health information to prevent harmful exposures and disease related to toxic substances (U.S. House of Representatives, 2008).

A December 2008 report by The Children's Health Fund (CHF) reviewed the medical charts of 261 children living in a FEMA village in Baton Rouge and discovered shocking health outcomes. The report found:

- 41 percent of children younger than four had iron-deficiency anemia, which causes fatigue, attention-deficit disorders, and skin problems.

- 55 percent of these displaced children exhibited learning or behavior problems.

- 42 percent developed allergic rhinitis, also called hay fever, and upper respiratory infection.

- 24 percent developed a cluster of ailments affecting the skin and upper respiratory tract, including allergies.

The report also found that for these kids, the health level has actually declined since the storm and they are worse off today (CHF, 2008).

After Katrina survivors and communities refused the trailers, more than 10,800 of them were sold to the public for 40 cents on the dollar by the General Service Administration from July 2006 to July 2007. After suspending sales, FEMA offered to buy back the toxic trailers purchased by the public and Katrina evacuees. In January 2008, more than 40,000 FEMA trailers were still being used as emergency shelter along the Gulf Coast, with the vast majority located in Louisiana (Kaufman, 2008). In December 2008, more than 9,300 families were living in temporary trailers and an additional 1,600 lived in hotel rooms throughout the Gulf Coast region (CHF, 2008).

A CALL FOR CLIMATE JUSTICE

Climate change looms as the global environmental justice issue of the twenty-first century. Climate change poses special environmental justice challenges for communities that are already overburdened with air pollution, poverty, and environmentally related illnesses (Adger et al., 2006; Roberts and Parks, 2006; Frumkin et al., 2008; Jackson & Shields, 2008). This is especially the case for African Americans.

Though the science on global climate change is clear, questions about mitigation (actions taken to minimize the effects of global warming), and adaptation (actions taken to minimize the effects of global warming) are less clear. What do we do about the harmful effects of global warming? How will the mitigation plans impact different people and the environment? How is fairness addressed? How will different populations adapt? These climate justice questions remain unanswered (Roberts & Parks, 2006; Adger et al., 2006). Climate change poses special health and environmental threats to vulnerable populations (Frumkin et al., 2008; Jackson & Shields, 2008).

Will the U.S. government response to climate change be fair? Does fairness matter? The jury is still out given the way government has handled health and environmental threats in the past and more recently its gross mismanagement of emergency preparedness and response to Hurricane Katrina and its aftermath (Pastor et al., 2006; Brunsma et al., 2007; Mann, 2006; Cooper & Block, 2006; Horne 2006; Heerden & Bryan, 2006).

A 2004 Congressional Black Caucus Foundation Inc. report, *Climate Change and African Americans: Unequal Burden*, concluded that there is a stark disparity in the United States between those who benefit and those who bear the costs of climate change. The report concludes:

> *African Americans are already disproportionately burdened by the health effects of climate change, including deaths during heat waves and from worsened air pollution. Similarly, unemployment and economic hardship associated with climate change will fall most heavily on the African American community. African Americans are less responsible for climate change than other Americans. Both historically and at present, African Americans emit less greenhouse gas. Policies intended to mitigate climate change can generate large health and economic benefits or costs for African Americans, depending on how they are structured. Unless appropriate actions are taken to mitigate its effects or adapt to them, climate change will worsen existing equity issues within the United States (Congressional Black Caucus Foundation, Inc., 2004, p. 2).*

Global warming will increase temperatures on hot summer days, potentially leading to more unhealthy "red alert" air pollution days in the coming years (Patz et al., 2004). In a study of fifty U.S. cities, Bell et al. (2007) report that future ozone concentrations and climate change could detrimentally affect air quality and thereby harm human health. The most vulnerable populations will suffer the earliest and most damaging setbacks, even though they have contributed least to the problem of global warming.

In fact, African Americans consistently experience higher rates of heat-related mortality during heat waves (Hoerner & Robinson, 2008). In the 1995 Chicago heat wave, excess mortality rates were 50 percent higher for African Americans than for non-Hispanic whites (Hoerner & Robinson 2008; Whitman et al., 1997). Another study of six northern U.S. cities found that "the increased risk of death during a heat episode was twice as large for African Americans as for non-Hispanic whites" (Hoerner & Robinson, 2008, p. 11). There have been several other studies that indicate similar patterns in St. Louis, Memphis, and Kansas City (McGeehin & Mirabelli, 2001). Equity is a very important component for our energy policy, and African Americans must be part of the climate change policy dialogue, general discussions, and decision-making meetings.

The most recent report of the Intergovernmental Panel on Climate Change (IPCC), *Climate Change 2007: Impacts, Adaptation and Vulnerability*, identified key vulnerabilities associated with climate-sensitive systems, including food supply, infrastructure, health, water resources, coastal systems, ecosystems, global biogeochemical cycles, ice sheets, and modes of oceanic and atmospheric circulation. The IPCC also predicts the impacts of future changes in climate are expected to fall disproportionately on the poor and communities in low-lying coastal and arid areas, with many who are highly dependent on farming, fishing, or forestry seeing their livelihoods severely curtailed or destroyed.

More social research is needed to better inform and provide data-based support for the response to climate change that include research on the association between climate change and public health (including mental health), scenario development to forecast health impacts and vulnerabilities, and development and testing of strategies to reduce risk. The issue of "who gets left behind before and after disaster strikes and why" is a core climate justice research and policy question. As seen in Hurricane Katrina, the effects of natural disaster fell heaviest on the poor and people of color (Brinkley 2006; Dyson 2006; Horne, 2006; Pastor et al., 2006).

The deadly pattern of climate change is also likely to fall disproportionately on the poor, African Americans, and other people of color across the United States who are concentrated in urban centers, coastal regions, and areas with substandard air quality—including ground-level ozone. Even so, in October 2007, the Bush administration made deep cuts in written testimony given to a U.S. Senate committee by Dr. Julie L. Gerberding, Centers for Disease Control and Prevention director, on health risks posed by global warming (Rivkin, 2007).

Entire sections on health-related effects of extreme weather, air-pollution-related health effects, allergic diseases, water- and food-borne infectious diseases, food and water scarcity, and the long-term impacts of chronic diseases and other health effects were edited out of the written testimony (Gerberding, 2007). The following passage on vulnerable populations was deleted entirely:

> In certain Southern coastal communities with little economic reserve, declining industry, difficulty accessing health care, and a greater underlying burden of disease, these stressors could be overwhelming. Similarly, in an urban area with increasingly frequent and severe heat waves, certain groups are expected to be more affected: the home-bound, elderly, poor, athletes, and minority and migrant populations, and populations that live in areas with less green space and with fewer centrally air-conditioned buildings are all more vulnerable to heat stress. Some populations of Americans are more vulnerable to the health effects of climate change than others.
>
> Children are at greater risk of worsening asthma, allergies, and certain infectious diseases, and the elderly are at higher risk for health effects due to heat waves, extreme weather events, and exacerbations of chronic disease.

In addition, people of lower socioeconomic status are particularly vulnerable to extreme weather events. Members of racial and ethnic minority groups suffer particularly from air pollution as well as inadequate health care access, while athletes and those who work outdoors are more at risk from air pollution, heat, and certain infectious diseases.

Given the differential burden of climate change's health effects on certain populations, public health preparedness for climate change must include vulnerability assessments that identify the most vulnerable populations with the most significant health disparities and anticipate their risks for particular exposures. At the same time, health communication targeting these vulnerable populations must be devised and tested, and early warning systems focused on vulnerable communities should be developed. With adequate notice and a vigorous response, the ill health effects of many exposures from climate change can be dampened.

Climate change poses special health risks to vulnerable populations already marginalized by limited means and their concentration in areas that fail to meet EPA ambient air quality standards and already facing environmental problems—coastal areas and low-lying areas that are prone to flooding and nonattainment regions. African Americans and Latinos are concentrated in the nation's dirtiest cities. Air pollution exacerbates asthma and other respiratory illnesses. Inner-city children have the highest rates for asthma prevalence, hospitalization, and mortality.

Asthma hits African Americans especially hard, with the highest asthma prevalence of any racial/ethnic group. In 2004, an estimated 3.5 million African Americans had asthma. The 2004 asthma prevalence rate among blacks was 36 percent higher than that for whites. African Americans make up about 12 percent of the U.S. population but accounted for 25 percent of the 4,099 deaths attributed to asthma in 2003. African Americans and Latinos are almost three times more likely than whites to die from asthma (Centers for Disease Control and Prevention, 2000, 2004).

More than 72 percent of African Americans live in counties that violate federal air pollution standards, compared to 58 percent of the white population. One of every four American children—over 27 million children under age 13—live in areas that regularly exceed the U.S. EPA's ozone standards. Half the pediatric asthma population, two million children, live in these areas. More than 61.3 percent of African American children, 69.2 percent of Hispanic children, and 67.7 percent of Asian American children live in areas that exceed the 0.080 ppm ozone standard, whereas 50.8 percent of white children live in such areas.

CONCLUSION

The environmental protection apparatus in the United States is broken. The current system fails to provide equal protection for all communities. The EJM emerged in response to environmental inequities, threats to public health, unequal protection, differential enforcement, and disparate treatment received by the poor and people of color. The movement redefined environmental protection as a basic right. It also emphasized pollution prevention, waste minimization, and cleaner production techniques as strategies to achieve EJ for all Americans without regard to race, color, national origin, or income.

The EJM set out clear goals of eliminating unequal enforcement of environmental, civil rights, and public health laws; correcting differential exposure of some populations to harmful chemicals, pesticides, and other toxins in the home, school, neighborhood, and workplace; amending faulty assumptions in calculating, assessing, and managing risks; stopping discriminatory zoning and land-use practices; and eliminating exclusionary policies and practices that limit some individuals and groups from participation in decision making. Many of these problems could be corrected if the existing environmental, health, housing, and civil rights laws were vigorously enforced in a nondiscriminatory way.

EJ leaders are demanding that no community or nation, rich or poor, urban or suburban, black or white, should be allowed to become a "sacrifice zone" or dumping grounds. They are also pressing governments to live up to their mandate of protecting public health and the environment. The legacy of environmental injustice remains a major barrier that impedes millions of African Americans from achieving healthy, livable, and sustainable communities. It is unlikely that we as a nation can achieve the goals of sustainability until we address these equity issues.

REFERENCES

Adger, W. N., Paavola, J., Huq, S., & Mace, M. J. (eds.). (2006). *Fairness in adaptation to climate change.* Cambridge: MIT Press.

Agency for Toxic Substances and Disease Registry. (2003). Managing hazardous incidents. Volume III – Medical management guidelines for acute chemical exposures: Trichloroethylene (TCE). Atlanta, GA: U.S. Department of Health and Human Services, Public Health Service.

Agency for Toxic Substances and Disease Registry. (2007a, February 1). Health consultation: Formaldehyde sampling at FEMA temporary housing units. Retrieved December 9, 2008, from http://www.atsdr.cdc.gov/HAC/PHA/fema_housing_formaldehyde/formaldehyde_report_0507.pdf

Agency for Toxic Substances and Disease Registry. (2007b, October). An update and revision of ATSDR's February 2007 health consultation: Formaldehyde sampling of FEMA temporary-housing trailers. Retrieved December 9, 2008 from http://www.atsdr.cdc.gov/substances/formaldehyde/pdfs/revised_formaldehyde_report_1007.pdf

Alston, D. (1992). Transforming a movement: People of color unite at Summit Against Environmental Racism. *Sojourner 21*(1), 30–31.

Babington, C. (2007, July 19). FEMA slow to test toxicity of trailers. *USA Today.* Retrieved December 2, 2008, from http://www.usatoday.com/news/topstories/2007-07-19-2231201740_x.htm

Bell, M. L., Goldberg, R., Hogrefe, C., Kinney, P. L., Knowlton, K., Lynn, B., Rosenthal, J., Rosenzweig, C., & Patz, J. A.. (2007). Climate change, ambient ozone, and health in 50 U.S. cities. *Climate Change, 82,* 61–76.

Blumenthal, Ralph. (2006, July 9). Texas lawsuit includes a mix of race and water. *The New York Times.*

Boyce, J. K. (2004). Green and brown? globalization and the environment. *Oxford Review of Economic Policy, 20*(1), 105–128. Retrieved from http://www.peri.umass.edu/fileadmin/pdf/working_papers/working_papers_51-100/WP78.pdf

Brinkley, D. (2006). *The great deluge: Hurricane Katrina, New Orleans, and the Mississippi Gulf Coast.* New York: HarperCollins Publishers.

Brown, M. (2006, August 19). Final EPA report deems N.O. safe. *The Times-Picayune.*

Brunsma, D. L., Overfelt, D., & Picou, J. S.. (2007). *The sociology of Katrina: Perspectives in a modern catastrophe.* New York: Rowman & Littlefield, p. xv.

Bryant, B. (1995). *Environmental justice: Issues, policies, and solutions.* Washington, DC: Island Press.

Bryant, B., & Mohai, P. (1992). *Race and the incidence of environmental hazards.* Boulder: Westview Press.

Bullard, R. D. (1983). Solid waste sites and the black Houston community. *Sociological Inquiry, 53*(Spring), 273–288.

Bullard, R. D. (1993a). *Confronting environmental racism: Voices from the grassroots.* Boston: South End Press.

Bullard, R. D. (1993b). Environmental racism and land use. *Land Use Forum: A Journal of Law, Policy & Practice, 2*(1), 6–11.

Bullard, R. D. (1993c). Race and environmental justice in the United States. *Yale Journal of International Law, 18*(1), 319–335.

Bullard, R. D. (1994a). *Dumping in dixie: Race, class and environmental quality.* Boulder, CO: Westview Press.

Bullard, R. D. (1994b). Grassroots flowering: The environmental justice movement comes of age. *The Amicus Journal, 16* (Spring), 32–37.

Bullard, R. D. (1996). *Unequal protection: Environmental justice and communities of color.* San Francisco: Sierra Club Books.

Bullard, R. D. (2000). *People of color environmental groups directory.* Flint, MI: C.S. Mott Foundation.

Bullard, R. D. (2005a, December 23). Katrina and the second disaster: A twenty-point plan to destroy black New Orleans. Atlanta: Environmental Justice Resource Center Report Series, Clark Atlanta University. Retrieved from http://www.ejrc.cau.edu/Bullard20PointPlan.html

Bullard, R. D. (2005b). *The quest for environmental justice: Human rights and the politics of pollution.* San Francisco: Sierra Club Books.

Bullard, R. D. (2007a, July/August). Dismantling toxic racism. *The crisis.* Retrieved from http://online.qmags.com/TCR0707/

Bullard, R. D. (2007b). Testimony of R. D. Bullard before the subcommittee on superfund and environmental health and public works committee regarding environmental justice. Retrieved from http://epw.senate.gov/public/index.cfm?FuseAction=Files.View&FileStore_id=4cdd3e73-8637-43e7-ad17-d75ab47c8204

Burton, T. (2007, November 28). Dickson County accepts $400,000 offer on dumping claim. *The Dickson Herald,* p. A1.

Business Week. (2005, September 26). The mother of all toxic clean-ups.

Calloway, C. A., & Decker, J. A. (1997). Environmental justice in the United States: A primer. *Michigan Bar Journal, 76,* 62–68.

Centers for Disease Control and Prevention. (1992). Asthma: United States, 1980–1990. *Morbidity and Mortality Weekly Report 39,* 733–735.

Centers for Disease Control and Prevention. (1996). Asthma mortality and hospitalization among children and young adults: United States, 1980–1993. *Morbidity and Mortality Weekly Report, 45,* 350–353.

Centers for Disease Control and Prevention. (2000). Death rates from 72 selected causes by year, age groups, race, and sex: United States 1979–98. Hyattsville, MD: National Center for Health Statistics.

Centers for Disease Control and Prevention. (2004). Asthma prevalence, health care use and mortality 2000–2001. Retrieved August 20, 2009, from http://www.cdc.gov/nchs/products/pubs/pubd/hestats/asthma/asthma.htm

Children's Health Fund (2008, November 4). Legacy of shame: The on-going public health disaster of children struggling in post-Katrina Louisiana. Retrieved December 8, 2008, from http://www.childrenshealthfund.org/sites/default/files/BR-White-Paper_Final_REV1-12-09F.pdf

Collin, R.. & Morris Collin, R. (1998). The role of communities in environmental decisions: Communities speaking for themselves. *Journal of Environmental Law and Litigation, 13,* 3789.

Colton, C. (2007). Environmental justice in a landscape of tragedy. *Technology in Society, 26,* 173–179.

Commission for Racial Justice. (1987). *Toxic wastes and race in the United States.* New York: United Church of Christ.

Congressional Black Caucus Foundation (CBCF), Inc. & Redefining Progress. (2004, July 21). African Americans and climate change: An unequal burden. Executive summary. Retrieved from http://www.usclimatenetwork.org/resource-database/CBCF-Climate%20Change%20report.pdf

Cooper, C., & Block, R. (2006). *Disaster: Hurricane Katrina and the failure of homeland security.* New York: Times Books.

Cornwell, K. (1991, January 28). Dickson County landfill reassessment report, appendix B: Chronology of events, pp. B14-B15.

Cornwell, K. (2003, October 2). Contamination problems date back almost forty years. *The Dickson Herald.*

Cornwell, K. (2004, June 9). County commission tables decision to pay families' water bills. *The Dickson Herald* (Tennessee).

Council on Environmental Quality. (1997, December 10). *Environmental justice: Guidance under the National Environmental Policy Act.* Washington, DC: CEQ.

Deep South Center for Environmental Justice at Dillard University. (2006). Project: A safe way back home. Retrieved November 30, 2008, from http://www.dscej.org/CommOutInit.html#ASWBH

Duke, L. (2007, March 20). A well of pain. *The Washington Post,* p. C1.

Dyson, M. E. (2006). *Come hell or high water: Hurricane Katrina and the color of disaster.* New York: Basic Books.

Fischbein, N. (2005a, April 16). Tallevast plume bigger than thought: Residents concerned. *Bradenton Herald.*

Fischbein, N. (2005b, September 3). Tallevast residents file lawsuit. *Bradenton Herald.*

Fischbein, N. (2005c, March 15). Waiting for updates in Tallevast. *Bradenton Herald.*

Fischbein, N. (2006, October 6). Lockheed done looking for Tallevast plume boundaries. *Bradenton Herald.*

Frumkin, H., Hess, J., Luber, G., Mallay, J., & McGeehin, M. (2008). Climate change: The public health response. *American Journal of Public Health, 98*(3), 1–11.

Gabe, T., Falk, G., Carthy, M., & Mason, V. W. (2005, November). *Hurricane Katrina: Social-demographic characteristics of impacted areas.* Washington, DC: Congressional Research Service Report RL33141.

Gerberding, J. L. (2007). Climate change and public health. Statement of Julie L. Gerberding, MD, MPH. Testimony Committee on Environment & Public Works United States Senate. Department of Health and Human Services. Retrieved August 20, 2009, from http://www.climatesciencewatch.org/file-uploads/Draft_CDC_testimony_23oct07.pdf

Gist, G. L. & Burg, J. R. (2006). Trichloroethylene: Review of the literature in view of the results of the trichloroethylene subregistry results.

Gordy, C. (2007, July). Troubled waters. *Essence Magazine, 38*(3), 146–151, 176.

Green, R. (2008, May 3). Small-town residents living on deadly ground. *The Miami Herald.*

Gresham Smith and Partners. (2000). USGS dye tracer study: Summary and results of dye-tracer tests conducted at the Dickson County Landfill, Tennessee, 1997 and 1998, Appendix B, April, p. 2.

Halliburton NUS Environmental Corporation. (1991, October 10). Final report: Site inspection Dickson County Landfill, Dickson, Dickson County, Tennessee. A report prepared for the U.S. EPA, p. ES-1.

Hammer, D. (2008, January 4). Road home promises more customer service. *The Times Picayune.* http://www.nola.com/news/index.ssf/2008/01/road_home_promises_more_custom.html

Hartman, C., & G. D. Squires. (2007). *There is no such thing as a natural disaster: Race, class, and Hurricane Katrina.* New York: Routledge, 1–9.

Heerden, I., & Bryan, M. (2006). *The storm: What went wrong during Hurricane Katrina, the inside story from one Louisiana scientist.* New York: Viking.

Herbert, B. (2006, October 2). Poisoned on Eno Road. *The New York Times.*

Hoerner, A., & Robinson, N. (2008, July). A climate of change: African Americans, global warming, and a just climate policy for the U.S. Oakland: Environmental Justice & Climate Change Initiative & Redefining Progress. Retrieved December 9, 2008, from http://www.ejcc.org/climateofchange.pdf

Horne, J. (2006). *Breach of faith: Hurricane Katrina and the near death of a great American city.* New York: Random House.

Jackson, S. (2005). Un/natural disasters, here and then. Understanding Katrina: Perspectives from the social sciences. New York: Social science research council, p.1.

Jackson, R., & Shields, K. N. (2008). Preparing the U.S. health community for climate change. *Annual Review of Public Health, 29*(25), 1–17.

Johnson, B. L., Williams, R. C., & Harris, C. M. (1992). *Proceedings of the 1990 National Minoritiy Health Conference: Focus on environmental contamination.* Princeton, NJ: Scientific Publishing Co., Inc.

Jordan, L. J. (2006, June 29). Washington extends full pickup costs of hurricane debris removal. *Associated Press,* WWLTV.com.

Kaufman, M. (2008, January 18). FEMA flip-flops again on trailers. *The Washington Post.*

Kimbro, P. L. (2006, November 7). County, city settle landfill lawsuits with families. *The Dickson Herald.*

Lang Lee, B. (1992). Environmental litigation on behalf of poor, minority children: Matthews v. Coye: A case study. Paper presented at the Annual Meeting of the Association for the Advancement of Science (February 9).

Lee, C. (1992). *Proceedings: The First National People of Color Environmental Leadership Summit.* New York: United Church of Christ Commission for Racial Justice.

Lerner, S. (2008). Tallavast, Florida: Rural residents live atop groundwater contamination by high-tech weapons company. The Collaborative on Health and the Environment. Retrieved August 20, 2009, from http://www.healthandenvironment.org/articles/homepage/3829

Letter from C. Jason Repsher, Geologist, Division of Solid Waste Management, Tennessee Department of Environment and Conservation, to Mrs. Ann Sullivan. (September 8, 1994).

Letter from Wayne Aronson, Acting Chief Drinking Water Section, Municipal Facilities Branch, U.S. EPA, to Mr. Harry Holt. (December 3, 1991).

Letter from Thomas A. Moss, Manager, Ground Water Management Section, Tennessee Division of Water Supply, Tennessee Department of Conservation, to Nathan Sykes, Drinking Water Section, Municipal Facilities Branch, U.S. EPA, Region IV. (December 17, 1991).

Letter from Thomas A. Moss, Manager, Ground Water Management Section, Tennessee Division of Water Supply, Tennessee Department of Conservation, to Nathan Sykes. Drinking Water Section, Municipal Facilities Branch, U.S. EPA, Region IV. (January 6, 1992).

Letter from Mark McWhorter, Division of Solid Waste, Tennessee Department of Health and Environment sent to Harry Holt and Lavenia Holt. (December 8, 1988).

Levine, D. (2008, October 15). America's Most Toxic Business. Portfolio.com. Retrieved December 8, 2008, from http://www.portfolio.com/news-markets/top-5/2008/10/15/The-Business-of-Destroying-Nerve-Gas#page4

Liu, A., & Plyer, A. (2008). *The New Orleans index: Tracking recovery of New Orleans and the metro area.* Washington, DC: The Brookings Institution and Greater New Orleans Community Data Center, p. 6.

Luther, L. (2006, June 16). *Disaster debris removal after Hurricane Katrina: Status and associated issues.* Washington, DC: Congressional Research Service Report to Congress, p. 1.

Mann, E. (2006). Katrina's legacy: *White racism and black reconstruction in New Orleans and the Gulf Coast.* Los Angeles: Front Press.

Martell, B. (2006, November 23). Horse racing returns to New Orleans. *Associated Press.*

McGeehin, M. J. A., & Mirabelli, M. (2001, May).The Potential Impacts of Climate Variability and Change Temperature-Related Morbidity and Mortality in the United States. *Environmental Health Perspective, 109*(Supplement 2), 185–188.

McLaughlin M. (n.d.). Center says eastern North Carolina lags the state on infrastructure, human need. North Carolina Center for Public Policy News Release. Retrieved August 20, 2009, from http://www.nccppr.org/easternnc2.html

Meux, M. (2007, June 18). Veolia to temporarily stop receiving VX wastewater. *Port Arthur News.*

NAACP Legal Defense and Education Fund. (2007, March 4). The color of environmental deception. Holt v. Scovill. Retrieved November 30, 2008, from http://www.naacpldf.org/content.aspx?article=1158

National Institute for Environmental Health Sciences. (1995). *Proceedings of the Health and Research Needs to Ensure Environmental Justice Symposium.* Research Triangle Park, NC: NIEHS.

News from USW: New Pollution data confirms concern. (2006, March 23). Retrieved August 21, 2009, from http://www.allbusiness.com/government/government-bodies-offices/5461813-1.html

Nossiter, A. (2005, October 2). Thousands of demolitions are likely in New Orleans. *The New York Times.*

O'Donnell, C. (2008a, December 1). Lockheed makes amends with Tallevast residents. *Herald-Tribune.*

O'Donnell, C. (2008b, March 31). State admits Tallevast pollution study way off mark. *Herald-Tribune.*

Pace, D. (2005, December 13). More blacks live with pollution. AP analysis of US research shows blacks more likely to live with dangerous pollution. *Associated Press.* Retrieved August 20, 2009, from http://www.blackherbals.com/more_blacks_live_with_pollution_.htm

Pastor, M., Bullard, R. D., Boyce, J., Fothergill, A., Morello-Frosch, R., & Wright, B. (2006, May). *In the wake of the storm: Environment, disaster and race after Katrina.* New York: Russell Sage Foundation.

Patz, J. A., Kinney, P. L., Bell, M. L., Goldberg, R., Hogrefe, C., Khoury, S., Knowlton, K., Rosenthal, J., Rosenzweig, C., & Ziska, L. (2004). *Heat advisory: How global warming causes more bad air days.* New York: NRDC.

Rawlins, W. (2003, November 11). Dump's days fade. *The News & Observer.*

Ricketts, T. C., & Pope, D. L. (2002). Demography and health care in Eastern North Carolina. *North Carolina Medical Journal, 62,* 20–25.

Roberts, J. T., & Parks, B. C. (2006). *A climate of injustice: Global inequality, north-south politics, and climate policy*. Cambridge: MIT Press.

Rysavy, T. F. (2007). Environmental justice for all. *Co-op America Quarterly, 73*(Fall), 14–17.

Sanders, D. (1992, March 13). Memorandum. Division of Solid Waste Management, Tennessee Department of Environment and Conservation.

Sanders, D. (1992, March 13). Memorandum. Division of Solid Waste Management, Tennessee Department of Environment and Conservation.

Sapien, J. (2008, October 4). Why CDC responded with 'lack of urgency' to formaldehyde warnings. ProPublica. Retrieved December 9, 2008, from http://www.propublica.org/feature/formaldehyde.

Shields, G. (2006). "Five parishes to receive help with debris clean-up," *The Advocate* (Baton Rouge), June 30.

Simmons, A. S. (2006, March 24). (Quoted in) New Orleans activists starting from the ground up. *The Los Angeles Times*.

Sole, M. W. (2004, June 29). Letter to Mr. Winston Smith, Director Waste Management Division, United States Environmental Protection Agency. Retrieved June 25, 2008, from http://www.dep.state.fl.us./secretary/news/2004/tal/epa_letter.pdf.

Solomon, G. M., & Rotkin-Ellman, M. (2006, February*). Contaminants in New Orleans sediments: An analysis of EPA data*. New York: NRDC.

Sorg, L. (2006, May 3). Not a drop to drink. *San Antonio Current*.

Spake, A. (2007, February 15). Dying for a home: Toxic trailers are making Katrina refugees ill. *San Antonio Current*.

Tetra Tech EM Inc. (2004, March 4). Dickson County landfill reassessment report. A report prepared for the U.S. EPA, Region IV. Atlanta.

Treadway, T. (2007, August 23). Formaldehyde testing on travel trailers to start in September, FEMA tells Hastings, Mahoney. Retrieved, August 20, 2009, from http://www.tcpalm.com/news/2007/aug/23/congressmen-question-fema-availability-travel-trai/

U.S. Census Bureau, State and County QuickFacts. (2000). Retrieved December 1, 2006, from http://quickfacts.census.gov/qfd/states/47/47043.html

U.S. Census Bureau, (2007, September 11). *Complete assessment needed to ensure rural Texas community has safe drinking water*. Dallas: Office of Inspector General, Report No. 2007-P-00034.

U.S. Environmental Protection Agency. (1992). *Environmental equity: Reducing risk to all communities*. Washington, DC: Author.

U.S. Environmental Protection Agency. (1998). Guidance for incorporating environmental justice in EPA's NEPA compliance analysis. Washington, DC: Author.

U.S. Environmental Protection Agency, Office of the Inspector General. (2006, July 6). Preliminary observations and recommendations: Panola County, TX, ground water contamination OIG complaint #2004-059.

U.S. Environmental Protection Agency. (2007, September 11). Complete assessment needed to ensure rural Texas community has safe drinking water. Dallas: Office of inspector general. Report no. 2007-P-00034.

U.S. Environmental Protection Agency and Louisiana Department of Environmental Quality. (2005, September 30). News release: Top state and federal environmental officials discuss progress and tasks ahead after Katrina, Retrieved July 2, 2006, from http://www.deq.louisiana.gov/portal/portals/0/news/pdf/administratorjohnson.pdf

U.S. General Accounting Office. (1983). Siting of hazardous waste landfills and their correlation with racial and economic status of surrounding communities. Washington, DC: Government Printing Office.

U.S. House of Representatives Committee on Oversight and Government Reform. (2007, July 19). Committee probes FEMA's response to reports of toxic trailers. Retrieved December 2, 2008 from http://oversight.house.gov/story.asp?ID=1413.

U.S. House of Representatives. (2008, September). Toxic trailers—toxic lethargy: How the Centers for Disease Control and Prevention has failed to protect the public health. Subcommittee on Investigations and Oversight, Committee on Science and Technology. Retrieved December 9, 2008, from http://science.house.gov/publications/caucus_detail.aspx?NewsID=2313.

Varney, J., & Moller, J. (2005, October 2). Huge task of cleaning up Louisiana will take at least a year. *Newhouse News Service*.

Weisenmiller, M. (2007, November 1). Environment-US: Toxins threaten to uproot entire town. IPS-Inter Press Service. Retrieved June 25, 2008, from http://ipsnews.net/news.asp?idnews=39889.

Welborn, V. (2005, September 12). Government agencies respond to East Texas residents' water woes. *Shreveport Times*.

Welborn, V. (2006, March 21). Request leads to records on contamination. *Shreveport Times*.

Welborn, V. (2008, June 17). Bethany finally getting fresh water. *Shreveport Times*.

Whitman, S., Good, G., Donoghue, E. R., Benbow, N., Shou, W., & Mou, S. (1997). Mortality in Chicago attributed to the July 1995 heat wave. *American Journal of Public Health, 87*(9), 1515–1518.

Williams, L. (2006, March 24). Groups Warn About Arsenic in Soil. *The Times-Picayune*.

CHAPTER

11

THE IMPACT OF INCARCERATION ON THE HEALTH OF AFRICAN AMERICANS

NICHOLAS FREUDENBERG
MEGHA RAMASWAMY

In the last three decades, the number of people in U.S. jails and prisons has increased five-fold (Mauer, 2006), and African Americans are more likely than whites to be stopped by the police, arrested, and incarcerated, and to serve longer sentences (Iguchi, Bell, Ramchand, & Fain, 2005). In this chapter, we consider the health consequences of these trends for African American men, women, children, families, and communities and the role that incarceration plays in maintaining or exacerbating disparities in health between whites and African Americans.

Our goals are to describe the health status of incarcerated African Americans both within various African American incarcerated populations and compared to incarcerated whites. We then seek to explore why incarcerated African Americans have worse health than incarcerated whites or non-incarcerated African Americans. Finally, we suggest policies and programs that may help to reduce the disproportionate adverse health effects of incarceration on African American populations. It should be noted that Latinos, Native Americans, and other racial/ethnic groups also experience a disproportionate health burden from incarceration, as do low-income whites compared to their better-off counterparts, but the focus here is on African Americans (Bonney, Clarke, Simmons, Rose, & Rich, 2008; Golembeski & Fullilove, 2005).

BACKGROUND TRENDS

Several trends provide the context for this analysis. First, incarceration rates have increased significantly, and African Americans have borne a disproportionate burden. In 2007, state and federal prisons (correctional facilities that detain people sentenced for one year or more) housed 2.3 million people, and the prevalence of imprisonment was highest for African Americans (Bureau of Justice Statistics, 2008). In the United States, each year about twelve million people pass through jails (facilities that hold detainees awaiting trial and those sentenced to less than a year). African Americans comprise 40 percent of the jail population (Bureau of Justice Statistics, 2006), despite totaling only 12.3 percent of the U.S. population (U.S. Census Bureau et al., 2001). In 2005, African Americans had a prison incarceration rate more than six times higher than whites (1,578 vs. 254 per 100,000 population) (Petterutti & Walsh, 2008). Between 1984 and 1997, the rate of incarceration among African American men went from 1 in 30 to 1 in 15 (Blankenship, Smoyer, Bray, & Mattocks, 2005). Based on current rates of first incarceration, an estimated 32 percent of African American males will enter state or federal prisons during their lifetime, compared to 17 percent of Latino males and 5.9 percent of white males (Bureau of Justice Statistics, 2008).

Among youth, one of every one hundred African American youth was in juvenile justice facilities in 1999, compared to one in five hundred white youth (Iguchi et al., 2005). At the current rates of incarceration, one out of four African American males can expect to spend time behind bars during his life, compared to one in twenty-three white males (Blankenship et al., 2005). An African American woman is seven times more likely than a white woman to spend time behind bars (Freudenberg, 2002). Many states now admit more young African American men to their jails and prisons than to their universities (Brotherton & Barrios, 2004; Dellums Commission, 2006).

This increase in incarceration and its burden on African Americans unfolded during a national war on drugs. Throughout the 1980s and 1990s, drug arrests fueled the increase in jail and prison populations, especially for women. Between 1996 and 2002, for example, the number of drug offenders increased by 37 percent, accounting for the largest source of jail population growth (Bureau of Justice Statistics, 2006). Figure 11.1 shows that though the number of admissions to prison for drug offenses increased for whites, Latinos, and African Americans between 1983 and 2001, after 1987 the increase became much steeper for African Americans (Iguchi et al., 2005). Between 1983 and 1998, drug-related incarcerations increased for African Americans twenty-six times, compared to a seven-fold increase for whites (Iguchi, London, Forge, Hickman, Fain, & Riehman, 2002). In 2002, the proportion of African Americans in U.S. jails for drug offenses was almost 1.7 times the proportion of whites jailed for drug offenses (30.6% vs. 18.5%) (Petterutti & Walsh, 2008).

FIGURE 11.1 *Imprisonment for Drug Offenses by Race/Ethnicity, 1983–2001.*

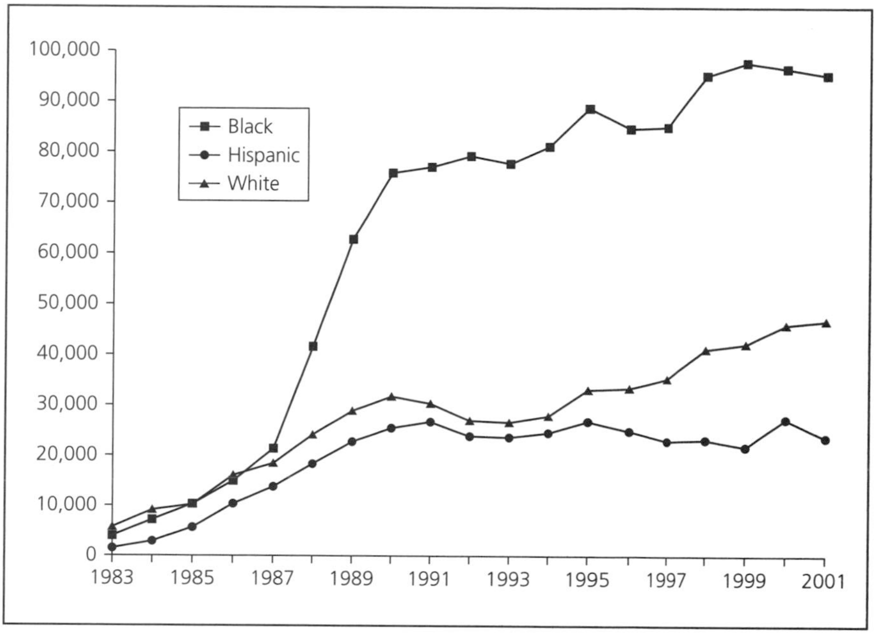

Source: Iguchi et al., 2005.

Despite the fact that African Americans use drugs less (whites are five times more likely to use marijuana and three times more likely to use cocaine), African Americans make up about 60 percent of all drug convictions in state prisons (Moore & Elkavich, 2008). Differences in prosecution for crack versus powder cocaine contribute to these disparities; penalties are often stiffer against crack sellers, 80 percent of whom are African American, compared with more predominantly white powdered cocaine sellers (Mauer, 2006). Judges sentence African Americans arrested for drug offenses about twice as often as they do whites (Blankenship et al., 2005).

A growing body of literature documents that, compared to whites, African Americans have poorer health status, higher rates of chronic and acute conditions, and shorter life spans (Braveman, 2006; King, Green, Tan-McGrory, Donahue, Kimbrough-Sugick, & Betancourt, 2008; Shavers, & Shavers, 2006). These differences in health status have been attributed to poverty, racism, exposure to higher levels of environmental hazards, and unequal access to and quality of health care.

HEALTH STATUS OF INCARCERATED AFRICAN AMERICANS

A wide variety of studies show that, in general, incarcerated populations have poorer health status than the non-incarcerated population. Within incarcerated groups, African Americans generally do worse than whites. A brief review of selected findings for various health conditions illustrates the scope and magnitude of these disparities.

Infectious Diseases

With only a few exceptions, African Americans experience higher rates of infectious and communicable diseases than do white populations (Steele, Meléndez-Morales, Campoluci, DeLuca, & Dean, 2007; Centers for Disease Control and Prevention [CDC], 2005). For example, in the general population, African Americans are seven times more likely to have chlamydia than whites and nineteen times more likely to have gonorrhea (CDC, 2006). Chlamydia and gonorrhea are the two most common sexually transmitted infections in the United States. Among women, African Americans have fifteen times the syphilis rates of whites (CDC, 2006). Rates of HIV infection are higher for African American men and women than for their white counterparts, a disparity that reflects a variety of soicodemographic and behavioral differences between these groups (Kraut-Becher, Eisenberg, Voytek, Brown, Metzger, & Aral, 2008).

This higher incidence of infectious diseases among African Americans is amplified in the correctional population both by the concentration of African Americans in this population and by criminal justice policies that select for those whose demographic and behavioral characteristics (e.g., low income, drug use, and homelessness) put them at higher risk for infectious diseases. Several studies show that incarcerated populations have higher rates of infectious diseases than non-incarcerated groups (National Commission on Correctional Health Care [NCCHC], 2002). For example, the prevalence of Hepatitis C in incarcerated populations is about nine to ten times the national prevalence (NCCHC, 2002). Moreover, a significant portion of people with infectious diseases pass through correctional facilities. One study estimated that in 1997, 20–26 percent of people living with HIV in the United States, 29–42 percent of those with Hepatitis C, and 40 percent of all those with tuberculosis passed through a correctional facility (Hammett, Harmon, & Rhodes, 2002). In that year, 48 percent of New York State inmates with AIDS were African American and 45 percent were Latino, demonstrating the racial disparities in AIDS cases (Hammett et al., 2002). A New York City study found that between 1993 and 1997, early syphilis incidence among women in jail exceeded the population rate by more than a thousand-fold (Blank, Sternberg, Neylans, Rubin, Weisfuse, & St Louis, 1999).

Within the correctional population, gender differences in infectious diseases put both genders at higher risk of some conditions. For example, women in jails and prisons are almost twice as likely as incarcerated men to be HIV-positive (Marushchak, 2004). In New York City jails, a 1998 serosurvey indicated that 18 percent of women and 21 percent of African American women were HIV-positive. As incarceration rates for women increase, the proportion of women with HIV infection in correctional facilities is also increasing (Hammett, 2006), although precise data are lacking.

Chronic Conditions

In the general population, conditions such as asthma, diabetes, hypertension, and stroke are more common among African Americans than among whites (Adler & Rehkopf, 2008) and also appear to be more prevalent in incarcerated than non-incarcerated populations. A recent analysis (Wilper et al., 2009) of federal surveys of prison and jail inmates found that inmates had a prevalence of persistent asthma of 7.7 to 8.6 percent (compared to an NHANES-based U.S. population rate of 7.5%); of diabetes mellitus of 8.1–11.1 percent (NHANES population rate 6.5%); and of hypertension of 27.9–30.8 percent (NHANES population rate 25.6%). An earlier study (NCCHC, 2002) estimated that U.S. inmates had an asthma prevalence of 8-9 percent, a diabetes rate of 5 percent, and a hypertension rate of 18 percent. Although data comparing rates by race/ethnicity within correctional facilities are scant, in a profile of the health status of Texas inmates, African American inmates had higher rates of endocrine and metabolic disorders and of circulatory and musculoskeletal systems than did whites (Baillargeon, Black, Pulvino, & Dunn, 2000). In 2002, according to the Bureau of Justice Statistics (Maruschak, 2004), 36.9 percent of U.S. jail inmates reported having any current medical problem, with arthritis (reported by 12.9%), hypertension (11.2%), asthma (9.9%), and heart problems (5.9%) leading the way. All are chronic conditions, which are the most commonly reported type of medical problems. This study did not report on prevalence by race/ethnicity.

Mental Health

Although racial/ethnic differences in the prevalence of mental health conditions vary by diagnosis, compared to whites, African Americans appear to face more barriers to care (Zuvekas & Fleishman, 2008) and to be differentially exposed to policies that contribute to mental health problems (Alegría, Peréz, & Williams, 2003).

An analysis (Wilper et al., 2009) of federal surveys of federal, state, and local inmates found that 14.8 percent of federal inmates, 25.5 percent of state inmates, and 25 percent of local jail inmates reported being diagnosed with a mental condition. According to the Bureau of Justice Statistics, 56 percent of state prison inmates, 49 percent of federal inmates, and 64.2 percent of jail inmates report having any mental health problem (James & Glaze, 2006), a prevalence several times higher than in the general population. According to the NCCHC study (2002), approximately 8 to 15 percent of people in jails had major depression, 14 to 20 percent some type of anxiety disorder, and 4 to 9 percent had post-traumatic stress disorder. Of interest and in comparison to other disease conditions, African American inmates had lower rates of mental health problems than white inmates: 54.7 percent of African American versus 62.2 percent of white state prison inmates; 45.9 percent of African American versus 49.6 percent of white federal prison inmates; and 63.4 percent of African American versus 71.2 percent of white jail inmates.

Substance Abuse

Surveys of nationally representative samples of incarcerated populations found that more than 80 percent of state prisoners and 70 percent of federal prisoners reported past drug use (Mumola, 1999). Two-thirds of jail inmates were regular drug users and more than half reported using drugs in the month before they committed the offense that led to their incarceration (Karberg & James, 2005). Inmates with mental health problems are more likely to report drug use than those without such problems (James & Glaze, 2006). Incarcerated women report higher levels of drug problems than do incarcerated men (Karberg & James, 2005).

Because criminal justice policies target drug users, it is not surprising that the prevalence of substance use is higher in correctional populations than in the general population. In addition, African American drug users are more likely to be arrested and incarcerated than white users, so they experience a disproportionate burden of incarceration. However, some evidence suggests that African American and white inmates seeking drug treatment do not differ significantly on behavioral and drug use patterns (Rounds-Bryant, Motivans & Pelissier, 2003).

Moreover, African Americans inmates are less likely to use illicit drugs than white inmates. A national survey of jail inmates in 2002 (Karberg & James, 2005) found that rates of substance dependence or abuse varied by racial or ethnic groups. White inmates had significantly higher levels of substance dependence or abuse than African American inmates (78% vs. 64% respectively). A larger proportion of white inmates than African Americans or Latinos (55% vs. 40% and 36%, respectively) were also dependent on alcohol or illicit drugs.

White inmates were also more likely than African Americans to participate in correctional treatment programs (72.5% vs. 52.9%), and among those who did get help for drug problems in jail, whites were more likely to participate in formal treatment programs than African Americans (55.5% vs. 38.9%) (Karberg & James, 2005). As with mental health services, African American drug users may encounter race-related barriers in finding treatment for their addiction (Zuvekas & Fleishman, 2008).

Injuries

A significant proportion of inmates report injuries while incarcerated. National surveys have shown that 13.4 percent of jail inmates, 32.6 percent of state inmates, and 28.2 percent of federal inmates reported an injury while confined (Maruschak, 2008). Of those seriously injured, 24.7 percent of jail inmates, 12 percent of state inmates, and 7.7 percent of federal inmates were not examined by a health provider (Wilper et al., 2009). Data are not available on differences in injury rates by race/ethnicity.

Oral Health

African Americans have poorer oral health and less access to dental care than whites (Gilbert, Duncan, & Shelton, 2003), and dental and other oral health problems are one of the most common health complaints of people in jail or prison. Few correctional facilities provide comprehensive dental care (Treadwell, Northridge, & Bethea, 2008), despite the fact that dental problems can make it more difficult for returning inmates to find and keep employment. Although little empirical data on racial/ethnic disparities in oral health status or health care among inmates is available, one study of long-term outcomes of drug users in California's Civil Addiction Program found that, compared to whites, African Americans had more missing teeth and other dental problems (Fan, Hser & Herbeck, 2006).

Mortality in Correctional Facilities and After Release

Several studies have examined mortality during and after release from incarceration. An analysis of ten years of deaths in the Cook County (Chicago, Illinois) jail system found that the mortality rates of inmates during incarceration was higher for heart diseases, infectious/inflammatory conditions, and suicide than for the general population. Most deaths were among African Americans (Kim et al., 2007). However, African American jail inmates were less likely to commit suicide in jail than whites. In U.S. jails, the suicide rate for African American inmates was 16 for every 100,000 per year compared with a rate of 96 per 100,000 per year for white inmates (Mumola, 2005).

Other studies examined mortality after release. A study in Washington state found much higher death rates in the months and years after release than among the general population (Binswanger, Stern, Deyo, Heagerty, Cheadle, Elmore, & Koepsell, 2007). Returning African American inmates had higher death rates than returning whites, but the differences between inmate and general population death rates for African Americans was smaller. Returning African Americans had a relative risk of death 2.3 times higher than African Americans in the general population, whereas returning whites has a relative risk of death 5.5 times higher than whites in the general population.

A study of deaths after release among former inmates of the North Carolina prison system found the number of deaths of African Americans from homicide and suicide, and accidents to be 1.2 and 2.7 times the expected number for the general population. Deaths from drug overdose were greater than twice that expected for the general population (Rosen, Schoenbach, & Wohl, 2008). The number of deaths from HIV infection also exceeded twice the general population number. Among African Americans, there were fewer than expected deaths from cardiovascular disease, diabetes, chronic lower respiratory diseases, "other" conditions, and most cancers, despite an excess of deaths from liver cancer.

A study of premature mortality among juveniles released from detention facilities found that the overall mortality rate was four times higher than the general population rate, and that African American youth had the highest mortality rate (Teplin, McClelland, Abram, & Mileusnic, 2005).

Gender Disparities in Health among Correctional Populations

Incarcerated women have higher rates of many health conditions compared to incarcerated men, including HIV infection and other sexually transmitted infections, mental health conditions, substance use, and histories of victimization (Lewis, 2006; Freudenberg, 2002; Henderson, 1998). In most cases, African American women fare worse than white women.

Possible explanations for gender and race differences in HIV infection rates within jails and prisons are higher rates of substance use, physical or sexual abuse, sex work, and other forms of gender and race oppression (Amaro & Raj, 2000; Bond & Salaam, 1996; O'Leary & Martins, 2000). Between 60 and 95 percent of women in the criminal justice system have reported histories of physical and sexual abuse (Fickenscher, Lapidus, Silk-Walker, & Becker, 2001; Greenfield & Snell, 1999; Kane & Dibartolo,

2002; Tsenin, 2000). Histories of abuse have been consistently associated with drug use, sex work, HIV and other sexually transmitted infections, and incarceration (Allers, Benjack, White, & Rousey, 1993; Richie & Johnsen, 1996; Widom, 2000; Wingood & DiClemente, 1997). The majority of women in all of these studies of abuse were African American.

CAUSES FOR DISPARITIES IN HEALTH AMONG AFRICAN AMERICAN AND WHITE INCARCERATED POPULATIONS

As the previous section has shown, incarcerated and returning Africans Americans suffer worse health than incarcerated and returning whites in almost every category, with only a few exceptions. In this section, we analyze some of the causes of these disparities. Our goal is to identify both upstream and downstream opportunities for intervention to mitigate or eliminate the health disparities. The factors associated with racial/ethnic health disparities among criminal justice populations operate at multiple levels of organization and through diverse pathways. Thus, it is likely that no single intervention will eradicate these inequities; rather the goal is to identify a portfolio of interventions that together will help to achieve this goal.

Disparities in Health and Health Care for African Americans in the General Population

In general, African Americans in the general population have worse health outcomes than their white counterparts for most disease conditions, including higher rates of HIV and other sexually transmitted infections, and greater mortality related to some cancers, diabetes, and heart disease (Blankenship et al., 2005; Brawley, & Jani, 2007; Harawa et al., 2004; Low, Grothe, Wofford, & Bouldin, 2007; Millett, Flores, Peterson, & Bakeman, 2007). One stark example of these differences is that, in 2003, life expectancy for U.S. African American males was 6.3 years less than that of white males, and for African American females it was 4.5 years less than for white females (Harper, Lynch, Burris, & Davey Smith, 2007).

Researchers attribute African American health disparities to a variety of factors, including poverty, education, segregation, institutional racism, health-damaging policies, behavior, and environmental exposures (Harper et al., 2007; Murray et al., 2006; Brown, 1995; Galea, & Vlahov, 2002; Geronimus & Thompson, 2004). These issues are explored in other chapters in this volume. African Americans are concentrated in some of the poorest areas of the country and in communities that often lack employment, educational, and other opportunities. Racial/ethnic disparities in health closely track disparities in educational opportunity and achievement.

Another well-studied cause of racial/ethnic disparities in health is differences in access to and quality of health care (Institute of Medicine, 2002). African Americans report less medical care and less satisfaction with medical providers than do white patients (Betancourt, Green, Carrillo, & Ananeh-Firempong 2003). For almost every health condition studied, African Americans receive poorer-quality health care than whites (Satcher & Rust, 2006).

Role of Incarceration in Health Disparities

Incarceration contributes to disparities in health for African Americans through five inter-related but distinct routes: selective recruitment of unhealthy and disproportionately African American inmates; exposure to unhealthy social and physical correctional environments; provision of inadequate medical care; failure to plan adequately for reentry; and the persistence of stigma for returning inmates. After summarizing the evidence for each of these routes, we propose a conceptual model that illustrates their connections.

Selective Recruitment of Unhealthy, Poor, and African American Inmates   Those incarcerated are overwhelmingly poor (Golembeski & Fullilove, 2005; Greenfield & Snell, 1999), and 60 percent of people in jail lack a high school diploma (Bureau of Justice Statistics, 2003). By targeting poor neighborhoods with high incidences of crime and chronic disease, criminal justice policies select for incarceration people with the demographic, socioeconomic, and behavioral factors that put people at risk of important causes of morbidity and mortality.

Drug policies, in particular, overwhelmingly target African Americans, who, as a result of their drug use, are at higher risk of Hepatitis C and HIV infection, related mental health problems, and physical and sexual abuse histories (Galca & Vlahov, 2002). Jails and prisons also house violent offenders who have experienced multiple physical and emotional traumas (Miller, 2006).

Correctional Facilities as Unhealthy Environments   Once criminal justice policies have concentrated an unhealthy, disproportionately African American population in correctional facilities, these individuals are often exposed to unhealthy physical and social conditions.

Jails and prisons are unhealthy environments for a few reasons. First, they confine many bodies in small spaces, which leads to overcrowding, transmission of communicable disease, stress, and violence. Overcrowding of jails and prisons is a direct consequence of the massive expansion of correctional populations in the last three decades (Mauer, 2006). Overcrowding can lead to unsanitary living conditions, increased transmission of communicable disease, and reduced security for inmates, leading to increased violence and more mental distress. Although a surge of prison construction in the last decade has somewhat reduced overcrowding, many municipal jail systems and several state systems, including California and Texas, continue to face overcrowding. As fiscal crises force cities and states to cut correctional spending, overcrowding may increase.

In correctional facilities, physical environmental factors that have been associated with poor health include overcrowding, lack of privacy, pests, and exposure to infectious agents (Hoge et al., 1994; Leh, 1999; Jones, Craig, Valway, Woodley, & Schaffner, 1999). Social environmental conditions associated with poor health in correctional facilities include overcrowding, exposure to physical and sexual violence, isolation from family and friends, and stigma (Hairston, 1998; Harner, 2004; Rhodes, 2005).

Though sex, drug use, and tattooing are illegal in correctional facilities, these practices flourish in men's and women's facilities. Although accurate data are scarce, researchers estimate that while incarcerated as many as two-thirds of men in prison have unprotected sex with other men (Krebs, 2002). Drug use behind bars is probably less frequent than in the free world, but most observers acknowledge that substance use does occur in correctional facilities. Paradoxically, condoms and safe injecting equipment are contraband in the majority of U.S. jails and prisons (May & Williams, 2002; US: Condoms distributed to gay inmates in LA, 2002). Countries in the European Union routinely use harm reduction approaches that make condoms and sterile injection equipment available in their correctional facilities (Gatherer, Moiler, & Hayton, 2005).

Some researchers believe that the correctional social environment may reinforce hyperaggressive masculinity, especially among African American men (Miller, 2006). Hyperaggresive masculinity may include joining official and unofficial gangs for both protection and intimidation, sexually and physically violent recruitment of members, and the victimization of weaker or marginalized inmates (Miller, 2006). This form of masculinity may also result from the need to protect one's personal space, belongings, and even food in such a stressful and confined environment. Though some of the behaviors associated with this masculinity may be protective within correctional facilities, it also puts men at risk of correctional sanctions and longer sentences and may discourage use of mental health services (Kupers, 2005). Once released, men who exhibit hyperaggresive masculine behavior may be at risk of reincarceration or perpetration of interpersonal violence.

Medical Care In 1976, the U.S. Supreme Court decided in *Estelle* v. *Gamble* (*Estelle* v. *Gamble*, 1976) that inmates had a constitutional right to health care. Although this decision is credited with improving correctional health care, many observers agree that the services provided still often fail to meet professional standards of quality and that a significant proportion of inmates fail to get the care they need (Adams & Leath, 2002; Gallagher & Dobrin, 2007; Restum, 2005; Taxman, Perdoni & Harrison, 2007; Wool, 2008). Deficits appear to be most common in areas with significant impact on community health and public safety: substance abuse, mental health, HIV care, and care for juveniles (Gallagher & Dobrin, 2007; Hammett, 2006; Taxman et al., 2007; Wells, & Bright, 2005).

Providing comprehensive primary and preventive medical care to inmates presents an opportunity for addressing the pre-existing health conditions and disparities that inmates bring to correctional facilities. A few jurisdictions demonstrate that it is possible to use correctional health services to identify and treat previously undetected health conditions and to link people with community care after release (Lincoln, Kennedy, Tuthill, Roberts, Conklin, & Hammett, 2006; Zaller, Gillani & Rich, 2007), but many correctional systems have trouble even meeting the minimal constitutional requirement not to deprive inmates of medically necessary services. This missed opportunity ensures that the incarceration experience will not reduce the health burden or the racial/ethnic disparities that inmates bring to correctional facilities.

Lack of Planning for Reentry Ninety-three percent of those who enter jails and prisons return home, most within a few months or years of incarceration. And the majority return to just a few poorly resourced urban communities (Petersilia, 2003). Inadequate reentry policies and procedures result in a precarious transition experience, and subsequently leave inmates, their partners, families, peers, and communities at public health risk. Once again, the higher proportion of African American inmates with significant health and social problems, and their concentration in a few neighborhoods, imposes higher reentry burdens on African American communities.

Though research suggests that comprehensive and intensive discharge planning and reentry services and policies can link returning inmates to substance abuse treatment, health care, mental health care, and other supportive services (Lincoln et al., 2006; Vigilante et al., 1999; Wilson & Draine, 2006; Zaller et al., 2007), correctional facilities often lack the mandate, budget, or personnel to carry out such planning for all inmates. Some evidence shows that having health care coverage (Lee et al., 2006) or continuity of health care (Sheu et al., 2002) after release is inversely related to rearrest, reincarceration, drug use, and drug sales.

Public policies often deny or restrict services (such as housing, cash assistance, food, and educational benefits) to people returning from jail (Freudenberg et al., 2006). Miller (2006) calls these "collateral civil penalties," a range of laws and policies that make successful reintegration into society much more difficult. For example, in some states public housing authorities specifically prohibit drug offenders from living in public housing or even residing with other relatives in public housing—a significant burden for inmates with children or inmates who are juvenile drug offenders (Fernandez, 2007). In addition, because landlords routinely conduct criminal background checks, ex-offenders are unofficially marginalized from regular housing (Miller, 2006). Unstable housing consistently predicts poorer health status, mental health problems, and sex and drug risk (McNiel, Binder, & Robinson, 2005; O'Leary & Martins, 2000).

State laws also prohibit some ex-offenders from receiving cash and food benefits, another significant burden for parents (Allard, 2002), who constitute almost 70 percent of people in jail and prison (Beck et al., 1993). One study (James, 2004) showed that a lack of income places a disproportionate burden on women—only one-quarter of women in jail reported previous income from wages and salary, compared to two-thirds of men. Lack of income is also related to risk for exchanging sex for drugs or money and for drug use, as well as for hunger and homelessness (Bond, Lauby, & Batson, 2005; Crepaz et al., 2006; Koblin et al., 2006; Lundgren et al., 2005; McNiel et al., 2005). Education may help to overcome some of the burdens of incarceration, but people with certain criminal justice histories are also ineligible for federal education loans (Miller, 2006).

Enduring Stigma of Criminal Justice Involvement To compound the previously described problems, people returning from correctional facilities also face the enduring stigma of incarceration. Discrimination in employment happens both officially, through restriction for certain licenses and federal jobs (Holzer, Raphael, & Stoll, 2001), and unofficially. Many employers include questions about criminal justice history on job applications, with little justification. Discrimination against the incarcerated intersects with racial discrimination. For example, Pager (2005) showed that a white man with an incarceration record was more likely to get a job than an African American man with no such record, which means that African American men face the double burden of race and incarceration.

Similarly, although there are some laws that restrict limits on housing eligibility, criminal background checks are required for most rental properties. Certain types of offenders are also prohibited from living in certain areas by law, and others are marginalized, as in the case of sex offenders, a category of conviction that has an extremely wide-ranging definition. Lack of employment and stable housing is related to both health risk and reincarceration (Bond et al., 2005; Crepaz et al., 2006; Koblin et al., 2006; Lundgren et al., 2005; McNiel et al., 2005).

Discrimination also gets passed on from family members. Ex-offenders, especially those with children, leave jail and prison eager to resume relationships with children (women in jail have on average two children under eighteen years of age) and support their families. But often these men and women return to family members or guardians of their children who are unwilling to give them a second chance (Gonnerman, 2004). Women, especially, are then forced to navigate prior relationships, often with past abusive sexual partners, to ensure housing for themselves and their young children, sometimes endangering their own safety and that of their children.

Another problem related to the reentry experience is an overwhelming feeling of alienation. Much like formerly homeless people who cannot adjust to sleeping on regular beds and prefer the floor, newly released inmates say they arrange personal living spaces in the free world to look like jail cells for emotional comfort.

Massoglia (2008) demonstrated that incarceration directly affects health as related to stress and infectious disease. He draws on theory related to primary and secondary stressors that affect health. Incarceration is viewed as a primary stressor, but factors after release, such as stigma, low income/employment, family issues, and homelessness are secondary stressors. Marmot (2005) and Marmot et al. (1984) also show that people with the lowest social status (as a result of stigma) are at greatest risk for health problems. Finally, Schnittker, & John (2007) found that any contact with the criminal justice system, rather than the length of contact, resulted in poorer health status for people released from corrections, supporting the notion that stigma creates disparities in health.

Conceptual Model

In order to illustrate how incarceration maintains or widens disparities in health, we propose a conceptual model in Figure 11.2. As shown in this model, structural factors, such as poverty, education, segregation, racism, and limited access to health care, create disparities in health for African Americans. The criminal justice system's targeting of poor, undereducated, and unhealthy people has lead to the previously described health burdens on African Americans in jails and prisons. Criminal justice facilities,

FIGURE 11.2 *Conceptual Model on the Role of Incarceration, Reentry, and Stigma in Widening Disparities in Health for African Americans.*

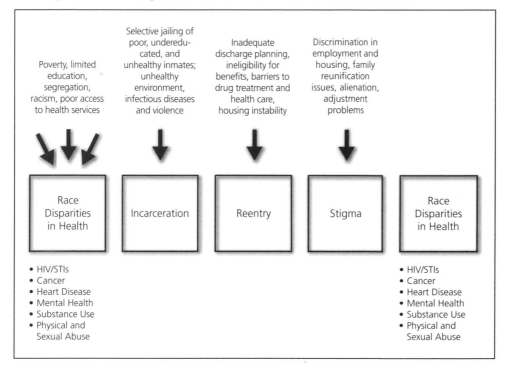

by their confined nature, provide unhealthy living environments, with potential for infectious disease transmission, exposure to social stressors, and physical and sexual violence. Poor medical care can allow diseases to worsen and/or miss the opportunities for prevention. The failure of reentry policies and programs leads to inadequate discharge planning; restriction of public benefits for income, food, housing, and education; and lower access to substance abuse treatment and health care. Finally, the additional burden of stigma related to criminal justice experience results in discrimination by multiple sectors—employment, housing, and family. We argue that the combination of these experiences maintains or widens existing disparities in health for African Americans. In the final section, we recommend policies and programs that can begin to mitigate or reverse these burdens.

RECOMMENDATIONS

The multiple determinants of poor health and health disparities among incarcerated African Americans, and the fact that these influences operate on several levels of organization, offers numerous opportunities for intervention. In this section, we use the conceptual model shown in Figure 11.2 to suggest upstream and downstream interventions that can prevent or mitigate the adverse health impact of incarceration at various points along the causal chain.

1. Reduce Income, Educational, Environmental, and Health Care Disparities in the General Population

The starting point for African American and white disparities in health is the inequitable and discriminatory living conditions and policies that are experienced by U.S. African American populations (Geronimus & Thompson, 2004). Any serious effort to reduce or eliminate these health disparities must begin with a commitment of resources and concrete actions to offer equal opportunities in education, employment, health care, and housing. These steps will in themselves begin the process of reducing the steady stream of poor people of color who fill U.S. jails and prisons. Current inequities in these areas are the fundamental causes of health disparities, and initiatives to diminish the disparate impact of criminal justice policies will succeed best if they are linked to reforms in other sectors. These issues are more fully addressed in other chapters in this volume.

2. Reduce Incarceration Rates of African Americans

Sending fewer African Americans—and other Americans—to jail and prison will bring a variety of benefits. It will reduce the number of individuals, families, and communities exposed to the adverse health and social consequences of mass incarceration. It will reduce the negative consequences of jail and prison overcrowding and allow correctional officials to focus their rehabilitative and public safety activities on a smaller and needier population. Shrinking our bloated correctional system will also free taxpayer resources for other important social goals such as employment, education, youth development, and health care—all sectors that are starved of revenues as a result of the combination of criminal justice policies and recurring fiscal crises.

In recent decades, policymakers and reformers have developed and tested a variety of innovations that can reduce incarceration rates. These include the expansion of alternatives to incarceration and violence prevention programs (Sherman, Gottfredson, MacKenzie, Eck, Reuter, & Bushway, 1997), the diversion of mentally ill inmates to mental health treatment (Loveland & Boyle, 2007) and drug users to substance abuse treatment (Belenko, 2000), the creation of community treatment programs for juvenile offenders, and the further development of "therapeutic jurisprudence" (an effort to make treatment rather than punishment a priority for certain vulnerable populations) (Wexler & Winnick, 1996). By expanding these types of programs to reach enough people and institutions to have an impact on population outcomes, it will be possible to reduce the number of people exposed to the risks of incarceration.

3. Create Health-Promoting Jails and Prisons

Though the long-term goal of U.S. criminal justice policy should be to reduce incarceration to the rates more commonly seen in the rest of the world, in the meantime, our country has the opportunity to transform jails and prisons from institutions that magnify disparities in health to ones that reduce these gaps. In Europe and elsewhere, correctional health officials and advocates have proposed the creation of health-promoting jails and prisons, facilities that seek to return inmates to their families and communities in better physical and mental health than when they entered (World Health Organization, 2006; Whitehead, 2006; Ramaswamy & Freudenberg, 2007). Among the services that could contribute to this transformation are systematic screening and treatment programs, chronic disease management, comprehensive health promotion, reproductive health care, a continuum of mental health and substance abuse treatment programs, and gender-, age-, and culture-appropriate tailoring of all health services.

4. Improve Medical Care in Jails and Prisons

Paul Farmer has advocated that, in a moral society serious about improving population health, the most vulnerable and sickest populations should receive the highest quality medical care (Farmer, 2003). In 1976, the Supreme Court ruled that depriving inmates of medical care violated their constitutional rights. By making these human and legal rights a reality, correctional facilities can contribute to achieving the national goal of reducing socioeconomic and racial/ethnic disparities in health. In the last several years, a number of organizations have promulgated standards of medical care for correctional facilities (e.g., American Public Health Association, 2003; National Commission on Correctional Health Care, 2003). For the most part, using existing medical knowledge and evidence-based protocols, it would be possible for correctional medical care to meet societal standards. No group will benefit more from improved correctional health care than African Americans.

5. Improve Reentry Policies and Procedures

Almost all inmates return home from jail or prison within days, months, or years of being incarcerated, so the process of release can have an important influence on returning individuals, their families and communities, and municipalities and states. In recent years, correctional and public health officials have developed proven or promising models of reentry services that can reduce reincarceration and drug use and improve public safety and public health (Petersilia, 2003; Taxman et al., 2003; Travis, 2005). Though further evaluation studies are needed, the priority should be on scaling up effective programs so that they can improve overall reentry outcomes. As with medical care, these changes will have a uniquely beneficial impact on African Americans returning from jail or prison. Because a disproportionate number of African American men and women encounter the criminal justice system, decreasing the risk of death or illness after release through better post-release policies and programs may decrease disparities in health outcomes in the overall population.

6. Limit the Effects of Stigma and Discrimination on African American Ex-Offenders

Finally, many African Americans encounter the triple jeopardy of stigma and discrimination based on race/ethnicity, poverty, and incarceration history. Gender, sexual orientation, substance use, and mental illness can add additional burdens of stigma. By reducing stigma for each of these categories through legislative, legal, educational, and other strategies (Thornicroft, Brohan, Kassam, & Lewis-Holmes, 2008), it will be possible to provide a post-release environment that supports rehabilitation and reintegration into society. In some jurisdictions, legislators and advocates have begun the process of dismantling the punitive and discriminatory employment, housing, and health care policies that serve as a deterrent to successful reentry.

In conclusion, current incarceration practices and policies in the United States have the unintended consequence of maintaining or exacerbating health and social disparities between whites and African Americans. By calling attention to this problem and by taking action to change the policies, programs, and attitudes that maintain or exacerbate incarceration-related disparities, health officials, health care providers, public health professionals, and advocates can make an important contribution to reducing racial and ethnic inequities in health.

REFERENCES

Adams, D. L., & Leath, B. A. (2002). Correctional health care: Implications for public health policy. *Journal of the National Medical Association, 94*(5), 294–298.

Adler, N. E., & Rehkopf, D. H. (2008). U.S. disparities in health: Descriptions, causes, and mechanisms. *Annual Review of Public Health, 29*, 235–252.

Alegría, M., Pérez, D. J., & Williams, S. (2003). The role of public policies in reducing mental health status disparities for people of color. *Health Affairs (Millwood), 22*(5), 51–64.

Allard, P. (2002). *Life sentences: Denying welfare benefits to women convicted of drug offenses.* Washington, DC: The Sentencing Project.

Allers, C., Benjack, K., White, J., & Rousey, J. (1993). HIV vulnerability and the adult survivor of childhood sexual abuse. *Child Abuse & Neglect, 17*, 291–298.

Amaro, H., & Raj, A. (2000). On the margin: Power and women's HIV risk reduction strategies. *Sex Roles, 42*(7/8), 723–749.

American Public Health Association. (2003). *Standards for Health Services in Correctional Institutions*, 3rd Ed. Washington, DC: Author.

Baillargeon, J., Black, S. A., Pulvino, J., & Dunn, K. (2000). The disease profile of Texas prison inmates. *Annals of Epidemiology, 10*(2), 74–80.

Beck, A., Gilliard, D., Greenfeld, L., Harlow, C., Hester, T., Jankowski, L., Snell, T., Stephan, J., & Morton, D. (1993). Survey of state prison inmates. Bureau of Justice Statistics, NCJ 136949.

Belenko, S. (2000). The challenges of integrating drug treatment into the criminal justice process. *Albany Law Review, 63*, 833–876.

Betancourt, J. R., Green, A. R., Carrillo, J. E., & Ananeh-Firempong, H. O. 2nd. (2003). Defining cultural competence: A practical framework for addressing racial/ethnic disparities in health and health care. *Public Health Reports, 118*, 293–302.

Binswanger, I. A., Stern, M. F., Deyo, R. A., Heagerty, P. J., Cheadle, A., Elmore, J. G., & Koepsell, T. D. (2007). Release from prison—A high risk of death for former inmates. *New England Journal of Medicine, 356*, 157–165.

Blank, S., Sternberg, M., Neylans, L. L., Rubin, S. R., Weisfuse, I. B., & St Louis, M. E. (1999). Incident syphilis among women with multiple admissions to jail in New York City. *Journal of Infectious Disease, 180*(4), 1159–1163.

Blankenship, K. M., Smoyer, A. B., Bray, S. J., & Mattocks, K. (2005). Black-white disparities in HIV/AIDS: The role of drug policy and the corrections system. *Journal of Health Care for the Poor and Underserved, 16*(4 Suppl B), 140–156.

Bond, L., Lauby, J., & Batson, H. (2005). HIV testing and the role of individual- and structural-level barriers and facilitators. *AIDS Care, 17*(2), 125–140.

Bond, L., & Salaam, S. (1996). At risk for HIV infection: Incarcerated women in a county jail in Philadelphia. *Women & Health, 24*(4), 27–45.

Bonney, L. E., Clarke, J. G., Simmons, E. M., Rose, J. S., & Rich, J. D. (2008). Racial/ethnic sexual health disparities among incarcerated women. *Journal of the National Medical Association, 100*(5), 553–558.

Braveman, P. (2006). Health disparities and health equity: Concepts and measurement. *Annual Review of Public Health, 27*, 167–194.

Brawley, O. W., & Jani, A. B. (2007). Race disparities and health. *Current Problems in Cancer, 31*(3), 114–122.

Brotherton, D. C., & Barrios, L. (2004). *The almighty Latin king and queen nation: Street politics and the transformation of a New York City gang.* New York: Columbia University Press.

Brown, P. (1995). Race, class, and environmental health: A review and systematization of the literature. *Environmental Research, 69*(1), 15–30.

Bureau of Justice Statistics. (2003). Sourcebook of criminal justice statistics, 2003. Washington, DC: Author.

Bureau of Justice Statistics. (2006). Criminal offender statistics. Washington, DC: Author.

Bureau of Justice Statistics. (2008). Prison statistics. Washington, DC: Author.

Centers for Disease Control and Prevention (CDC). (2005). Racial disparities in nationally notifiable diseases—United States, 2002. *Morbidity and Mortality Weekly Report, 54*(1), 9–11.

Centers for Disease Control and Prevention (CDC). (2006). Sexually transmitted disease surveillance, 2005. Atlanta: U.S. Department of Health and Human Services.

Crepaz, N., Lyles, C. M., Wolitski, R. J., Passin, W. F., Rama, S. M., Herbst, J. H., Purcell, D. W., Malow, R. M., & Stall, R. (2006). Do prevention interventions reduce HIV risk behaviors among people living with HIV? A meta-analytic review of controlled trials. *AIDS, 20*(2), 143–157.

Dellums Commission. (2006). A way out: Creating partners for our nation's prosperity by expanding life paths of young men of color. Washington, DC: Joint Center for Political and Economic Studies.

Estelle v. Gamble, 1976, 429 U.S. 97.

Fan, J., Hser, Y. I., & Herbeck, D. (2006). Tooth retention, tooth loss and use of dental care among long-term narcotics abusers. *Substance Abuse, 27*(1–2), 25–32.

Farmer, P. (2003). *Pathologies of power health, human rights, and the new war on the poor.* Berkeley, CA: University of California Press.

Fernandez, M. (2007, October 1). Barred from public housing, even to see family. *New York Times.*

Fickenscher, A., Lapidus, J., Silk-Walker, P., & Becker, T. (2001). Women behind bars: Health needs of inmates in a county jail. *Public Health Reports, 116*(3), 191–196.

Freudenberg, N. (2002). Adverse effects of US jail and prison policies on the health and well-being of women of color. *American Journal of Public Health, 92*(12), 1895–1899.

Freudenberg, N., Daniels, J., Crum, M., Perkins, T., & Richie, B. E. (2006). Coming home from jail: The social and health consequences of community reentry for women, male adolescents, and their families and communities. *American Journal of Public Health, 95*(1),1725–1736.

Galea, S., & Vlahov, D. (2002). Social determinants and the health of drug users: Socioeconomic status, homelessness, and incarceration. *Public Health Reports, 117*(Suppl 1), S135–S145.

Gallagher, C. A., & Dobrin, A. (2007). Can juvenile justice detention facilities meet the call of the American Academy of Pediatrics and National Commission on Correctional Health Care? A national analysis of current practices. *Pediatrics, 119*(4), 991–1001.

Gatherer, A., Moiler, L., & Hayton, P. (2005). The World Health Organization European Health in Prisons Project after 10 years: Persistent barriers and achievements. *American Journal of Public Health, 95*(10), 1696–1700.

Geronimus, A. T., & Thompson, J. P. (2004). To denigrate, ignore, or disrupt: The health impact of policy-induced breakdown of urban African American communities of support. *Du Bois Review, 1*(2), 247–279.

Gilbert, G. H., Duncan, R. P., & Shelton, B. J. (2003). Social determinants of tooth loss. *Health Services Research, 38*(6 Pt 2), 1843–1862.

Golembeski, C., & Fullilove, R. (2005). Criminal (in)justice in the city and its associated health consequences. *American Journal of Public Health, 95*(10), 1701–1706.

Gonnerman, J. (2004*). Life on the outside: The prison odyssey of Elaine Bartlett.* New York: Picador.

Greenfield, L., & Snell, T. (1999, December). Women Offenders. Bureau of Justice Statistics Special Report.

Hairston, C. F. (1998). The forgotten parent: Understanding the forces that influence incarcerated fathers' relationships with their children. *Child Welfare, 77*(5), 617–639.

Hammett, T. M. (2006). HIV/AIDS and other infectious diseases among correctional inmates: Transmission, burden, and an appropriate response. *American Journal of Public Health; 96*(6), 974–978.

Hammett, T. M., Harmon, M. P., & Rhodes, W. (2002). The burden of infectious disease among inmates of and releasees from US correctional facilities, 1997. *American Journal of Public Health, 92*(11), 1789–1794.

Harawa, N. T., Greenland, S., Bingham, T. A., Johnson, D. F., Cochran, S. D., Cunningham, W. E., Celentano, D. D., Koblin, B. A., LaLota, M., MacKellar, D. A., McFarland, W., Shehan, D., Stoyanoff, S., Thiede, H., Torian, L., & Valleroy, L. A. (2004). Associations of race/ethnicity with HIV prevalence and HIV-related behaviors among young men who have sex with men in 7 urban centers in the United States. *Journal of the Acquired Immune Deficiency Syndrome, 35*(5), 526–536.

Harner, H. M. (2004). Relationships between incarcerated women: Moving beyond stereotypes. *Journal of Psychosocial Nursing and Mental Health Services, 42*(1), 38–46.

Harper, S., Lynch, J., Burris, S., & Davey Smith, G. (2007). Trends in the black-white life expectancy gap in the United States, 1983–2003. *Journal of the American Medical Association, 297*, 1224–1232

Henderson, D. J. (1998). Drug abuse and incarcerated women. A research review. *Journal of Substance Abuse and Treatment, 15*(6), 579–587.

Hoge, C. W., Reichler, M. R., Dominguez, E. A., Bremer, J. C., Mastro, T. D., Hendricks, K. A., Musher, D. M., Elliott, J. A., Facklam, R. R., & Breiman, R. F. (1994). An epidemic of pneumococcal disease in an overcrowded, inadequately ventilated jail. *The New England Journal of Medicine, 331*(10), 643–648.

Holzer, H. J., Raphael, S., & Stoll, M. A. (2001). Will employers hire ex-offenders? Employer checks, background checks, and their determinants. Berkeley Program on Housing and Urban Policy. Working Papers: W01–005.

Iguchi, M. Y., Bell, J., Ramchand, R. N., & Fain, T. (2005). How criminal system racial disparities may translate into health disparities. *Journal of Health Care for the Poor and Underserved, 16*(4 Suppl B), 48–56.

Iguchi, M. Y., London, J. A., Forge, N. G., Hickman, L., Fain, T., & Riehman, K. (2002). Elements of well-being affected by criminalizing the drug user. *Public Health Reports, 117*(Suppl 1), S146–S150.

Institute of Medicine. (2002). Unequal treatment: What healthcare providers need to know about racial and ethnic disparities in health care. Retrieved January 8, 2009, from http://www.iom.edu/CMS/3740/4475/4175.aspx

James, D. J. (2004). Profile of jail inmates, 2002. Washington, DC: U.S. Department of Justice. Bureau of Justice Statistics special report, NCJ 201932.

James, D. J., & Glaze, L. E. (2006). Mental health problems of prison and jail inmates. Bureau of Justice Statistics Special Report NCJ 213600; 1–14.

Jones, T. F., Craig, A. S., Valway, S. E., Woodley, C. L., & Schaffner, W. (1999). Transmission of tuberculosis in a jail. *Annals of Internal Medicine, 131*(8), 557–563.

Kane, M., & DiBartolo, M. (2002). Complex physical and mental health needs of rural incarcerated women. *Issues in Mental Health Nursing, 23*, 209–229.

Karberg, J. C., & James, D. J. (2005). Substance dependence, abuse, and treatment of jail inmates, 2002 (Publication No. NCJ-209588). Washington, DC: U.S. Department of Justice, Bureau of Justice Statistics.

Kim, S., Ting, A., Puisis, M., Rodriguez, S., Benson, R., Mennella, C., & Davis, F. (2007). Deaths in the Cook County jail: 10-year report, 1995–2004. *Journal of Urban Health, 84*(1), 70–84.

King, R. K., Green, A. R., Tan-McGrory, A., Donahue, E. J., Kimbrough-Sugick, J., & Betancourt, J. R. (2008). A plan for action: Key perspectives from the racial/ethnic disparities strategy forum. *Milbank Quarterly, 86*(2), 241–272.

Koblin, B. A., Husnik, M. J., Colfax, G., Huang, Y., Madison, M., Mayer, K., Barresi, P. J., Coates, T. J., Chesney, M. A., & Buchbinder, S. (2006). Risk factors for HIV infection among men who have sex with men. *AIDS, 20*(5), 731–739.

Kraut-Becher, J., Eisenberg, M., Voytek, C., Brown, T., Metzger, D. S., & Aral, S. (2008). Examining racial disparities in HIV: Lessons from sexually transmitted infections research. *Journal of Acquired Immune Deficiency Syndrome, 47*(Suppl 1), S20–S27.

Krebs, C. P. (2002). High-risk HIV transmission behavior in prison and the prison subculture. *Prison Journal, 82*, 19–49.

Kupers, T. A. (2005). Toxic masculinity as a barrier to mental health treatment in prison. *Journal of Clinical Psychology, 61*(6), 713–724.

Lee, J., Vlahov, D., & Freudenberg, N. (2006). Primary care and health insurance among women released from New York City Jails. *Journal of Health Care for the Poor and Underserved, 17*, 200–217.

Leh, S. K. (1999). HIV infection in U.S. correctional systems: Its effect on the community. *Journal of Community Health Nursing, 16*(1), 53–63.

Lewis, C. (2006). Treating incarcerated women: Gender matters. *Psychiatric Clinical of North America, 29*(3), 773–789.

Lincoln, T., Kennedy, S., Tuthill, R., Roberts, C., Conklin, T. J., & Hammett, T. M. (2006). Facilitators and barriers to continuing healthcare after jail: A community-integrated program. *Journal of Ambulatory Care and Management, 29*(1), 2–16.

Loveland, D., & Boyle, M. (2007). Intensive case management as a jail diversion program for people with a serious mental illness: A review of the literature. *International Journal of Offender Therapy and Comparative Criminology, 51*(2), 130–150.

Low, A. K., Grothe, K. B., Wofford, T. S., & Bouldin, M. J. (2007). Addressing disparities in cardiovascular risk through community-based interventions. *Ethnicity and Disease, 17*(2 Suppl 2), S2-55-59.

Lundgren, L. M., Amodeo, M., & Chassler, D. (2005). Mental health status, drug treatment use, and needle sharing among injection drug users. *AIDS Education and Prevention, 17*(6), 525–539.

Marmot, M. (2005). Social determinants of inequalities. *Lancet, 365*, 1099–1104.

Marmot, M., Martin, S., & Gibson, R. (1984). Inequalities in death: Specific explanations of a general pattern? *Lancet, 1*, 1003–1006.

Marushchak, L. M. (2004). HIV in prisons and jails, 2002. Bureau of Justice Statistics.

Maruschak, L. M. (2008). Medical problems of jail inmates. Bureau of Justice Statistics Special Report, NCJ 210696, 1–9.

Massoglia, M. (2008). Incarceration as exposure: The prison, infectious disease, and other stress-related illnesses. *Journal of Health and Social Behavior, 49*(1), 56–71.

Mauer, M. (2006). *Race to incarcerate*. New York: The New Press.

May, J. P., & Williams, E. L. (2002). Acceptability of condom availability in a U.S. jail. *AIDS Education and Prevention, 14 (5 Suppl B)*, 85–91.

McNiel, D. E., Binder, R. L., & Robinson, J. C. (2005). Incarceration associated with homelessness, mental disorder, and co-occurring substance abuse. *Psychiatric Services, 56*, 840–846.

Miller, T. A. (2006). Incarcerated masculinities. In A. D. Mutua (Ed.), *Progressive Black Masculinities*. New York: Routledge, 155–174.

Millett, G. A., Flores, S. A., Peterson, J. L., & Bakeman, R. (2007). Explaining disparities in HIV infection among black and white men who have sex with men: A meta-analysis of HIV risk behaviors. *AIDS, 21*(15), 2083–2091.

Moore, L. D., & Elkavich, A. (2008). Who's using and who's doing time: Incarceration, the war on drugs, and public health. *American Journal of Public Health, 98*(5), 782–786.

Mumola, C. J. (1999). Substance abuse and treatment, state and federal prisoners, 1997 (Publication No. NCJ-172871). Washington, DC: Bureau of Justice Statistics.

Mumola, C. J. (2005). Suicide and homicide in state prisons and local jails. Washington, DC: Bureau of Justice Statistics; 2005. NCJ No. 210036. Retrieved January 18, 2009, from http://www.ojp.usdoj.gov/bjs/abstract/shsplj.htm

Murray, C. J., Kulkarni, S. C., Michaud, C., Tomijima, N., Bulzacchelli, M. T., Iandiorio, T. J., & Ezzati, M. (2006). Eight Americas: Investigating mortality disparities across races, counties, and race-counties in the United States. *Public Library of Science Medicine, 3*(9), e260.

National Commission on Correctional Health Care. (2002). *The health status of soon-to-be-released inmates*. A Report to Congress, 1.

National Commission on Correctional Health Care. (2003). *Standards for health services in jails*. Chicago: Author.

O'Leary, A., & Martins, P. (2000). Structural factors affecting women's HIV risk: A life-course example. *AIDS, 14*, S68–S72.

Pager, D. (2005) Double jeopardy: Race, crime, and getting a job. *Wisconsin Law Review, 2005*(2), 617–662.

Petersilia, J. (2003). *When prisoners come home: Parole and prisoner reentry*. New York: Oxford University Press.

Petteruti, A., & Walsh, N. (2008). Jailing communities: The impact of jail expansion and effective public health strategies. Washington, DC: Justice Policy Institute.

Ramaswamy, M., & Freudenberg, N. (2007). Health promotion in jails and prisons: An alternative paradigm for correctional health services. In R. Greifinger (Ed.), *Public Health Behind Bars from Prisons to Communities*. New York: Springer, 229–248.

Restum, Z. G. (2005). Public health implications of substandard correctional health care. *American Journal of Public Health, 95*(10), 1689–1691.

Rhodes, L. A. (2005). Pathological effects of the supermaximum prison. *American Journal of Public Health, 95*(10); 1692–1695.

Richie, B., & Johnsen, C. (1996). Abuse histories among newly incarcerated women in a New York City jail. *Journal of the American Medical Women's Association, 51*(3), 111–114.

Rosen, D. L., Schoenbach, V. J., & Wohl, D. A. (2008). All-cause and cause-specific mortality among men released from state prison, 1980–2005. *American Journal of Public Health, 98*(12), 2278–2284.

Rounds-Bryant, J. L., Motivans, M. A., & Pelissier, B. (2003). Comparison of background characteristics and behaviors of African American, Hispanic, and white substance abusers treated in federal prison: Results from the TRIAD Study. *Journal of Psychoactive Drugs, 35*(3), 333–341.

Satcher, D., & Rust, G. (2006). Achieving health equity in America. *Ethnicity and Disease, 16*(2 Suppl 3), S3–8-13.

Schnittker, J., & John, A. (2007). Enduring stigma: The long-term effects of incarceration on health. *Journal of Health and Social Behavior, 48*(2), 115–130.

Shavers, V. L., & Shavers, B. S. (2006). Racism and health inequity among Americans. *Journal of the National Medical Association, 98*(3), 386–396.

Sherman, L., Gottfredson, D, MacKenzie, D., Eck, J., Reuter, P., & Bushway, S. (1997). Preventing Crime: What works, what doesn't, what is promising. Washington: Report to the United States Congress prepared by the National Institute of Justice.

Sheu, M., Hogan, J., Allsworth, J., Stein, M., Vlahov, D., Schoenbaum, E. E., Schuman, P., Gardner, L., & Flanigan, T. (2002). Continuity of medical care and risk of incarceration in HIV-positive and high-risk HIV-negative women. *Journal of Womens Health, 11*(8), 743–750.

Steele, C. B., Meléndez-Morales, L., Campoluci, R., DeLuca, N., & Dean, H. D. (2007, November). Health Disparities in HIV/AIDS, Viral Hepatitis, Sexually Transmitted Diseases, and Tuberculosis: Issues, Burden, and Response, A Retrospective Review, 2000–2004. Atlanta, GA: Department of Health and Human Services, Centers for Disease Control and Prevention. Retrieved August 21, 2009, from http://www.cdc.gov/nchhstp/ healthdisparities/docs/NCHHSTP_Health%20Disparities%20Report_15-G-508.pdf

Taxman, F. S., Perdoni, M. L., & Harrison, L. D. (2007). Drug treatment services for adult offenders: The state of the state. *Journal of Substance Abuse and Treatment, 32*(3), 239–254.

Taxman, F. S., Young, D., & Byrne, J. M. (2003). *From prison safety to public safety: Best practices in offender reentry.* National Institute of Justice: Washington, DC.

Teplin, L. A., McClelland, G. M., Abram, K. M., & Mileusnic, D. (2005). Early violent death among delinquent youth: A prospective longitudinal study. *Pediatrics, 115*(6), 1586–1593.

Thornicroft, G., Brohan, E, Kassam, A., & Lewis-Holmes, E. (2008). Reducing stigma and discrimination: Candidate interventions. *International Journal of Mental Health Systems, 2*(1), 3.

Travis, J. (2005). *But they all come back: Facing the challenges of prisoner reentry.* Washington, DC: Urban Institute Press.

Treadwell, H. M., Northridge, M. E., & Bethea, T. N. (2008). Building the case for oral health care for prisoners: Presenting the evidence and calling for justice. In R. Greifinger (Ed.), *Public health behind bars from prisons to communities.* New York: Springer.

Tsenin, K. (2000, September). One judicial perspective on the sex trade. National Institute of Justice—Research on women and girls in the justice system: Plenary paper of the 1999 Conference on Criminal Justice Research and Evaluation-Enhancing Policy and Practice Through Research, 15–26.

US: Condoms distributed to gay inmates in LA. (2002). *Canadian HIV/AIDS Policy & Law Review, 6*(3), 18–19.

U.S. Census Bureau, Grieco, E. M., & Cassidy, R. C. (2001). Overview of race and Hispanic origin, 2000. Washington, DC: US Census Bureau.

Vigilante, K., Flynn, M., Affleck, P., Stunkle, J., Merriman, N., Flanigan T. P., Mitty, J., & Rich, J. (1999). Reduction in recidivism of incarcerated women through primary care, peer counseling, and discharge planning. *Journal of Women's Health, 8*(3), 409–415.

Wells, D., & Bright, L. (2005). Drug treatment and reentry for incarcerated women. *Corrections Today, 67*(7), 98–99,111.

Wexler, D., & Winnick, B. (Eds.). (1996). *Law in a therapeutic key: Developments in therapeutic jurisprudence.* Durham, NC: Carolina Academic Press.

Whitehead, D. (2006). The health promoting prison (HPP) and its imperative for nursing. *International Journal of Nursing Studies, 43*(1); 123–131.

Widom, C. (2000, September). Childhood victimization and the derailment of girls and women to the Criminal Justice System, 1999. National Institute of Justice—Research on women and girls in the justice system: Plenary paper of the 1999 Conference on Criminal Justice Research and Evaluation-Enhancing Policy and Practice Through Research, 27–36.

Wilper, A., Woolhandler, S., Boyd, W., Lasser, K. E., McCormick, D., Bor, D. H., & Himmelstein, D. (2009). The health and health care of US prisoners: A nationwide survey. *American Journal of Public Health, 99*(4): 666–72.

Wilson, A. B., &, Draine, J.(2006). Collaborations between criminal justice and mental health systems for prisoner reentry. *Psychiatric Services, 57*(6); 875–878.

Wingood, G., & DiClemente, R. (1997). Child Sexual Abuse, HIV Sexual Risk, and Gender Relation of African American Women. *American Journal of Preventive Medicine, 13*(5), 380–384.

Wool, J. (2008) Litigating for better medical care. In R. Greifinger (Ed.). *Public health behind bars from prisons to communities.* New York: Springer.

World Health Organization. (2006). Health in prisons project. Geneva: World Health Organization Regional Office for Europe. Retrieved from http://www.euro.who.int/prisons.

Zaller, N., Gillani, F. S., & Rich, J. D. (2007). A model of integrated primary care for HIV-positive patients with underlying substance use and mental illness. *AIDS Care, 19*(9), 1128–1133.

Zuvekas, S. H., & Fleishman, J. A. (2008). Self-rated mental health and racial/ethnic disparities in mental health service use. *Medical Care, 46*(9), 915–923.

PART

3

CHRONIC DISEASES

CHAPTER

12

HYPERTENSION IN AFRICAN AMERICAN COMMUNITIES

SHARON K. DAVIS
RAKALE COLLINS QUARELLS
GARY H. GIBBONS

Hypertension is one of several common, devastating, and treatable disorders that disproportionately affect African Americans. The chronic elevation of blood pressure in patients with hypertension predisposes them to cardiovascular disease complications such as stroke, myocardial infarction (heart attack), heart failure, and renal failure. These cardiovascular complications are the major contributors to racial/ethnic disparities in total mortality in the United States, and hypertension is a key driver of these conditions.

Based on the classification scheme of the National Institutes of Health Joint National Committee on High Blood Pressure, approximately 72 million people in the United States have hypertension. Although the disorder is associated with aging, there is a growing recognition that cardiovascular disease is no longer limited to economically developed nations with large elderly populations. Hypertension and its cardiovascular complications are endemic worldwide and have emerged as the leading causes of death and disability across the spectrum of rich and poor nations around the globe. There are intriguing parallels between the rapid rise in hypertension-attributable mortality observed in developing nations and the problem of cardiovascular health disparities observed in African American communities within the United States. These similarities between communities of color throughout the world are consistent with our central premise that high blood pressure is one of the consequences of the dynamic confluence of socioeconomic, psychosocial, behavioral, and biological factors associated with twenty-first-century civilization.

In this chapter we will initially describe the scope of the problem by characterizing the epidemiology of hypertension and the extent of racial disparities. We will then explore the complex interplay among biological, social, and behavioral factors that contribute to the higher prevalence of hypertension in African Americans. This multilevel analysis of the problem will conclude with a review of intervention strategies designed to prevent and/or control hypertension within African American communities.

EPIDEMIOLOGY OF HYPERTENSION

Hypertension is one of the most common risk factors for coronary heart disease and stroke. According to the latest statistics, nearly 30 percent of all Americans have hypertension (Cutler et al., 2008). Hypertension rates have increased steadily since the early 1900s. Over the past ten years, the rate of hypertension has increased by an average of 5 percent, with the overall rate increasing from 24.4 percent in 1994 to 28.9 percent in 2004. This increase has been seen across gender and racial/ethnic groups. The rates of adult hypertension range from 27.1 percent among Mexican Americans and 27.4 percent among non-Hispanic whites to 40.1 percent among non-Hispanic blacks. Among African Americans, 40.8 percent of women and 39.1 percent of men have hypertension.

Hypertension shows up earlier in African Americans than in the general population, with hypertension rates that are twice as high for young African Americans as for their peers in other racial/ethnic groups. Ten percent of African American men from 18 to 29 years old have hypertension, in comparison with 5.5 percent of white men and 3.5 percent of Mexican American men. This racial disparity is less pronounced among young women than young men. Rates of hypertension increase with age, culminating in rates of 83 percent in African American men and women age 70 years or older.

Differing hypertension rates in racial/ethnic groups appear to persist across geographic regions, although there is controversy on this topic. Recent analyses suggest that there are no differences between the rates for those living in urban versus rural areas (Howard et al., 2006). On the other hand, some studies have shown that African Americans living in the Southern region of the United States have a higher prevalence of hypertension than those in other parts of the country (Obisesan et al., 2000; Collins & Winkleby, 2002). Collins and Winkleby (2002) demonstrated that blacks living in the South had twice the rate of hypertension of African Americans living outside the South. This is consistent with the labeling of the southern region as the stroke belt, meaning that the rates of stroke are highest in this region. Interestingly, although rates of hypertension may be higher in this region, rates of awareness of and treatment for hypertension are better in this region than in the rest of the country (Howard et al.,

2006). Unfortunately, although more were under treatment for hypertension in the South, the rates of hypertension control were not comparable (Howard et al., 2006; Obisesan et al., 2000). There is also evidence that despite undergoing treatment, African Americans are more likely than members of other groups to have poor blood pressure control (Kramer, 2004).

As noted earlier, African Americans tend to have an earlier onset of hypertension than other racial/ethnic groups. The problem of hypertension has also recently become a problem among children. Din-Dzietham and colleagues (2007) have reported an increase in the prevalence of childhood hypertension since the 1980s. Currently, according to 2003–2006 NHANES data, approximately 3 percent of all youths aged 8 to 17 have hypertension, which is an increase from 2 percent in the 1988–1994 NHANES data. Non-Hispanic blacks and Mexican Americans had a higher prevalence of hypertension and prehypertension than non-Hispanic whites. In the past, hypertension in children usually was secondary to other pathologies such as renal disease. However, the rising problem of obesity has resulted in a rapidly growing incidence of primary hypertension in children (Sorof et al., 2004; Chiolero et al., 2007).

ETIOLOGY OF HYPERTENSION: THE ROLE OF BIOLOGICAL FACTORS

Blood pressure regulation involves achieving a homeostatic balance among a complex array of systems governing vascular tone and the volume of fluid within the circulatory system. Several neurohumoral systems are involved in ensuring that increases in sodium/water intake are matched by increases in sodium/water excretion such that the homeostatic balance is maintained. However, if sodium intake exceeds the kidneys' capacity to excrete the sodium load, the resultant expansion in fluid volume within the circulatory system can predispose to an elevation of blood pressure. Similarly, the activation of neurohumoral systems such as the renin-angiotensin-aldosterone or the sympathetic nervous system can promote elevations of blood pressure by increasing vascular tone or resistance. Conversely, relative deficits in neurohumoral factors that promote sodium excretion and/or vasodilation can predispose to chronic elevations of blood pressure. The maintenance of a normal level of blood pressure is so critical to the normal function of the body that dozens of redundant systems have evolved to maintain this normal state of balance. Given the complexity of these homeostatic systems, it is not surprising that pathological perturbations that predispose to hypertension may involve dozens of biological pathways and molecular mediators. Accordingly, there is no single molecular mechanism or etiology for the most common form of primary hypertension.

It is estimated that genetic factors may explain approximately 30 to 60 percent of the variance in blood pressure. Recent advances in human molecular genetics have identified a series of relatively rare diseases such as Liddle's Syndrome and Williams-Beuren Syndrome in which mutations at a single locus or gene are sufficient to cause chronic hypertension. It is noteworthy that these rare monogenic forms of human hypertension are closely aligned with the physiological principles that emphasize the central role played by sodium balance and vascular resistance as the major biological determinants of hypertension. The capacity to genetically engineer mouse models of hypertension that mimic the human condition further supports the thesis that genetic factors play an important role in predisposition for hypertension (Rossier et al., 2002).

Although substantial progress has been made in understanding these rare monogenic forms of hypertension, dissecting the genetic basis of the most common form of primary hypertension has remained elusive. It is speculated that "garden variety" hypertension reflects the cumulative impact of contributions from many different genetic variants. Moreover, the clinical manifestation of these genetic predispositions is influenced by the process of aging as well as dynamic gene-environment interactions (for example, dietary sodium intake). Therefore, a comprehensive understanding of the variance in hypertension prevalence across populations must acknowledge the potential contribution of genetic factors that render individuals more susceptible to environmental influences such as a high-sodium–low-potassium diet.

The completion of the Human Genome Project and the in-depth sequencing of individuals from a variety of different biogeographic ancestries established that there are patterns of genomic variation reflective of our population history as Homo sapiens. The prevailing "Out of Africa" hypothesis proposes that individuals of African descent constitute the oldest subgroup of Homo sapiens and therefore exhibit the greatest diversity in genomic variation. The migration of the earliest humans out of Africa populated Europe, Asia, and the Americas to yield the widely recognized biogeographic groups of today. The structure of each individual's genome reflects these patterns of population history. Moreover, each individual's genome also reflects centuries of dynamic gene-environmental interactions that may have shaped the body's metabolism and physiology over the course of multiple generations. For example, the mutations that cause sickle cell disease and glucose-6-phosphate dehydrogenase (G6PD) deficiency in African Americans reflect the genomic imprint of natural selection pressures on red blood cell metabolism as a result of exposure to endemic malaria in Sub-Saharan Africa. These adaptations are effective in improving survival from an infectious disease in the original setting of Africa but can cause devastating complications such as stroke.

Similarly, it is postulated that within environments where there is little dietary sodium, there may have been strong selection pressures to retain sodium in hot, humid climates as a means of avoiding debilitating dehydration. Indeed, there is a strong heritable component that determines an individual's capacity to excrete sodium. In accordance with this working hypothesis, these sodium-retentive genotypes would be most common among individuals of African descent. It is postulated that these "thrifty" genotypes may now be maladaptive by predisposing to hypertension in the context of Western industrialized societies where there is an overabundance of sodium in the diet (Young et al., 2005; Zhu & Cooper, 2007; Campbell & Tishkoff, 2008). It is postulated that the current differences in disease patterns by race/ethnicity may reflect in part the lingering imprint of gene-environment interactions of the ancestral population history on the genome. Ongoing research is needed to further refine our understanding of the complex interactions among genes, behavior, and environmental influences as determinants of hypertension.

ETIOLOGY OF HYPERTENSION: THE ROLE OF PSYCHOSOCIAL AND CULTURAL FACTORS

Psychosocial factors have been demonstrated to be positively associated with the incidence of hypertension in African Americans. Such factors include psychosocial stresses such as acts of racial discrimination, feelings of hostility, diet, socioeconomic status (SES), and sleep. Although each factor may be studied as an isolated contributor to the development of hypertension, it is becoming increasingly clear that there are complex interactions between these psychosocial determinants that influence health outcomes such as hypertension.

Psychosocial Stress

In the United States, people of color and individuals with lower SES experience higher rates of hypertension-related morbidity and mortality than whites and wealthier individuals (Haan, Kaplan, & Camacho, 1987; Williams & Collins 1995; Anderson & Armstead, 1995; Sorlie, Backland, & Keller, 1995; Krieger, Williams, & Moss, 1997). A growing body of research recognizes the role of "place" or environmental context as an important determinant of an individual's health. It is clear that living in areas of concentrated poverty contributes to social inequalities in health among different racial and ethnic groups in the United States (Geronimus, Bound, Waidmann, Hillemeier, & Burns, 1996; Lillie-Blanton & LaVeist, 1996; Kaplan, 1999; Diez-Roux et al., 2001). Areas of concentrated poverty are often found in urban settings and are created through processes of racial segregation and economic disinvestment (Denton & Massey, 1991). These forces can create environments where health-threatening conditions or "psychosocial stressors" are abundant, and where health-promoting or protective resources are stretched to their limits.

The identification of mechanisms linking psychosocial factors with hypertension is important in making causal inferences and therefore in designing preventive interventions. Psychosocial factors may act alone or combine in clusters (Williams et al., 1997) and may exert effects at different stages of the life course. Psychosocial factors may affect health-related behaviors such as dietary choices, alcohol consumption, or physical activity, which in turn increase the risk of hypertension. Psychosocial factors may also cause direct acute or chronic pathophysiological changes. For example, racism has been demonstrated to be a positive predictor of hypertension prevalence among African Americans (Harrel, Hall, & Taliaferro, 2003).

Diet

Evidence consistently links an increased risk of hypertension to obesity. It is believed that the greater prevalence of hypertension in African Americans may be due to the greater prevalence of obesity observed in this group, particularly among females

(Stamler, Stamler, Riedlinger, Algera, & Roberts, 1978; Chichlowska et al., 2008). Indeed, obesity has been found to be positively associated with high blood pressure in African Americans in the United States and in Africa (Hypertension Detection and Follow-up Program Cooperative Group, 1997; Seftel, Johnson, & Muller, 1980). There is a close link between food intake, metabolic rate, the activity of the sympathetic nervous system, and blood pressure. Recent evidence indicates that the expansion of adipose tissue in obese individuals generates factors that affect vascular tone and inflammatory cytokines that accelerate the progression of vascular disease. Conversely, weight loss is associated with a reduction in inflammatory biomarkers, improvements in vascular function, and a decrease in blood pressure (Mathew et al., 2007; Zhu et al., 2008). A high consumption of calorie-dense fast foods predisposes to obesity and thereby predisposes to hypertension. Individuals who live in socially deprived communities with limited access to healthful foods and a dense concentration of "fast-food" restaurants are more likely to be obese and hypertensive (Dubowitz et al., 2008). It is postulated that this confluence of factors contributes to high rates of hypertension in African American communities.

The influence of diet on blood pressure extends beyond caloric balance and fat metabolism. It has become increasingly clear that consumption of various nutrient factors in a balanced diet is an important determinant of blood pressure. The majority of research on the role of diet in hypertension has focused on four nutrients: sodium, potassium, calcium, and Vitamin D. The role of excessive sodium intake in Westernized societies remains an issue of debate (Pickering, 1981). Mechanisms underlying a sodium–blood pressure relationship have not been identified but could involve phenomena such as expansion of fluid volume, oxidative stress, decreased activity of the vasodilator nitric oxide and/or increased reactivity to vasoconstrictors (Guyton, 2002; Cowley, 2008). Although some studies have reported higher intake of dietary sodium among African Americans (Cruickshank & Beevers, 1982; Frisancho, Leonard, & Bollettino, 1984), most large-scale studies using probability samples have concluded that if racial differences in sodium intake exist, African Americans exhibit a lower, rather than a higher, intake than whites (Grim et al., 1980; Cruickshank & Beevers, 1982; Frisancho, Leonard, & Bollettino, 1984). Although African Americans may not ingest more dietary sodium than whites, African Americans appear to excrete less sodium than whites for a given amount of sodium consumed. Thus, even at low levels of sodium intake, the deleterious effects of sodium may be greater for African Americans than for whites.

Both low levels of potassium intake and a low sodium:potassium ratio (i.e., higher levels of sodium compared with potassium intake) have been linked to high blood pressure levels and adverse cardiovascular outcomes (Frisancho, Leonard, & Bollettino, 1984; Cook et al., 2009). African Americans have been found to ingest significantly less potassium and therefore to have higher dietary sodium:potassium ratios than whites (Grim et al., 1980; Frisancho, Leonard, & Bollettino, 1984). Grim et al. (1980) discovered that African American men ingest significantly less sodium than white men, with the white men eating roughly 186 mol/l per 24 hours and African American men eating 136 mol/1 per 24 hours. On the other hand, the African American men ingested significantly less potassium than white men (23 mol/l per 24 hours versus 54 mol/1). Therefore, although African American men had a lower intake of sodium, their lower potassium intake coupled with their high sodium:potassium ratio (186/23 mol/l versus 136/54 mol/l) in this group may have contributed to their higher blood pressure levels. As with sodium, the studies on potassium and hypertension among African Americans have focused primarily on racial differences to the exclusion of within-race comparisons. Similarly, there have been few multilevel analyses of the social determinants of the low sodium:potassium ratio that have addressed the interactions between access to healthy foods in the environment and cultural factors that shaped dietary choices. Future studies are needed to clarify the interplay between social and biological determinants of sodium:potassium balance and the optimal interventions for reducing the risk for hypertension and its complications.

Dietary intake of calcium has also been explored as a potential contributor to hypertension. As with potassium, low levels of calcium intake are thought to be associated with high blood pressure. The data produced by McCarron are frequently cited concerning the role of calcium in hypertension (McCarron, Morris, & Cole, 1982). Using national survey data, these investigators found that among subjects aged 20 to 70 years calcium intake was the best predictor of high blood pressure levels among the seventeen nutrients studied. Borderline hypertensives and normotensives reported similar calcium intakes, but individuals with definite hypertension (160/95 mmHg) consumed 18 percent less calcium than normotensives. The higher intake of calcium among normotensives as compared with hypertensives was evident in both African Americans and whites. African Americans have also been reported to have higher sodium:calcium ratios in their diet than whites (Lanford, Watson, & Douglas, 1980). Unfortunately, the effectiveness of calcium supplementation to lower blood pressure is an area of controversy, with some trials reporting relatively modest responses (Zemel et al., 1986; Dickinson et al., 2006).

The potential influence of dietary calcium may also be modulated by the status of Vitamin D metabolism. Deficiencies of Vitamin D have been associated with the development of hypertension (Holick, 2007). Recent surveys have documented that African Americans are prone to develop Vitamin D deficiency, with prevalence rates as high as 80 percent (Holick, 2007). This propensity to Vitamin D deficiency is related in part to the fact that dark skin pigmentation reduces the synthesis of Vitamin D generated from sun exposure. As a result, individuals with dark skin are more dependent on dietary Vitamin D intake to maintain normal Vitamin D levels. Moreover, there is evidence that many African Americans have a lower dietary intake of dairy products, a major dietary source of Vitamin D. It is speculated that the high propensity to Vitamin D deficiency among African Americans combined with a diet characterized by high sodium:low potassium:low calcium may contribute to the high prevalence of hypertension in this population.

Overall, there is a striking positive relationship between socioeconomic status and dietary consumption of healthy foods associated with cardiovascular risk reduction and prevention of hypertension, such as fruits, vegetables, calcium, potassium, and foods with low energy density (Kant, Graubard, & Kumanyika, 2007). Social determinants of dietary habits and access to healthy foods are important contributors to racial/ethnic disparities in hypertension.

Socioeconomic Status and Social Capital

Several studies have documented an inverse relationship between socioeconomic status (SES) and blood pressure (Diez-Roux, Northridge, Morabia, Bassett, & Shea, 1999). The higher prevalence of hypertension among African Americans is related in part to the disproportionate representation in lower socioeconomic classes (Diez-Roux et al., 1999). Gillum, Mussolino, and Madans (1998) similarly found that low family income and low educational levels were significantly associated with elevated systolic blood pressure among African American men (Gillum et al., 1998).

A series of multilevel analyses have identified compelling links between environmental influences and neighborhood characteristics as important determinants of health. The context in which individuals live can modulate individual risk factors for cardiovascular disease. Recent studies indicate that residents of neighborhoods with better walkability, availability of healthy foods, greater safety, and more social cohesion were less likely to be hypertensive (Mujahid et al., 2008). The disproportionate concentration of African Americans in segregated neighborhoods with low social capital creates a context that may aggravate an individual's predisposition to hypertension.

Sleep

Several recent studies have implicated poor sleep quality and/or short sleep duration in the development of cardiovascular complications. It has been reported that poor sleep quality is also related to hypertension in middle-aged adults (Cappuccio et al., 2007). Similar studies indicate a relationship between sleep and incident pre-hypertension among adolescents. Recent studies by our group and others indicate that African Americans have a relatively high prevalence of poor sleep quality in comparison with members of other racial/ethnic groups (Durrence & Lichstein, 2006). Although the etiology of this disparity remains to be clarified, it is postulated that poor sleep quality may be related to psychosocial factors such as high stress, social conditions such as shift work, and neighborhood characteristics such as high-density housing, noise, and crime. It remains to be determined whether interventions that ameliorate poor sleep quality might reduce the incidence of hypertension.

Blood pressure exhibits circadian variation in which levels peak in the morning upon awakening and fall to their lowest levels at night during sleep. Recent studies suggest that many individuals with poor sleep quality fail to exhibit the nocturnal fall or "dipping" of blood pressure (Yilmaz et al., 2007). A number of investigations have documented ethnic differences in blood pressure dipping, with African Americans exhibiting a smaller nocturnal decline in blood pressure (Gretler, Fumo, Nelson, & Murphy, 1994; Harshfield, Pulliam, Somes, & Alpert, 1993; Harshfield, Wilson, Treiber, & Albert, 2002; James, 1981; Murphy, Fumo, Gretler, Nelson, & Lang, 1991; Sherwood, Steffen, Blumenthal, Kuhn, & Hinderliter, 2002). A meta-analysis of ethnic differences in blood pressure dipping among adults and adolescents concluded that African Americans display blunted nocturnal decreases in blood pressure in comparison with individuals of European descent (Profant & Dimsdale, 1999; Harshfield & Treiber, 1999). Given that blunted blood pressure dipping has been associated with increased left ventricular mass and other complications, this difference may have implications for understanding the greater virulence of hypertension among African Americans (Rizzoni et al., 1992; Belsha et al., 1998).

HYPERTENSION AND CARDIOVASCULAR COMPLICATIONS: RACIAL DISPARITIES

Stroke

Several population-based studies have documented that African Americans and some Hispanic Americans have a higher stroke incidence than whites. For example, the Atherosclerosis Risk in Communities (ARIC) Study documented that African Americans had an incidence of stroke 38 percent higher than that of whites (Rosamond et al., 1999). Similarly, the Greater Cincinnati/Northern Kentucky community-based study documented that stroke and transient ischemic attack incidence rates are higher for blacks at every age, with the greatest risk (two- to five-fold) seen in young and middle-aged African Americans (<65 years of age) (Kleindorfer et al., 2005; Pandey & Gorelick, 2005). These investigators did not observe racial differences in case fatality rates, so they concluded that the higher incidence of strokes is the primary determinant of higher stroke mortality among blacks. In addition, racial differences have been noted in the incidence of various sub-types of ischemic stroke. African Americans are nearly twice as likely as whites to have small-vessel strokes and strokes of undetermined origin. In contrast to some older studies, more recent evidence with state-of-the-art clinical characterization indicates that African Americans have a significant proportion of ischemic strokes due to large vessel disease and cardioembolism (Pandey & Gorelick, 2005).

Racial differences in rates of ischemic strokes are paralleled by similar patterns in hemorrhagic strokes. Surveillance studies in northern Manhattan documented significantly higher incident rates of subarachnoid hemorrhage among African Americans and Hispanics than among whites (Labovitz et al., 2006). Similarly, the risk of intracerebral hemorrhage is substantially higher in African Americans than whites. One community-based study in the United States noted an excess risk of hemorrhagic strokes of four- to nine-fold among relatively young individuals aged 35 to 54. Similarly, a community-based study in South London in the United Kingdom observed much higher rates of intracerebral hemorrhage among African American immigrants from either the Caribbean or sub-Saharan Africa as compared with whites (Smeeton et al., 2007).

Taken together, most analyses suggest that the striking racial disparities in rates of both ischemic and hemorrhagic strokes in relatively young and middle-aged adults can be attributed primarily to pre-stroke hypertension that is inadequately diagnosed, treated, and controlled. In addition, there is a growing body of evidence that genetic factors contribute to the predisposition to stroke. We have reported stroke susceptibility genetic variants associated with stroke in the phosphodiesterase 4D gene in African Americans (Song et al., 2006). The high stroke risk among blacks is further compounded by the higher prevalence of additional stroke risk factors such as obesity and diabetes.

Left Ventricular Hypertrophy and Heart Failure

The incidence of heart failure increases exponentially in the seventh decade of life and beyond, with an overall lifetime risk of approximately 20 percent. Although heart failure is generally considered a disease of the elderly, it is notable that African Americans often experience an earlier onset of the disease. Prospective, population-based studies have documented that age-adjusted incident heart failure is related to the development of myocardial infarction as well as the influence of cardiovascular risk factors such as hypertension, obesity, and diabetes. Community-based studies and clinical trials have documented a striking pattern in which the etiology of heart failure in whites is typically related to ischemic heart disease, whereas African Americans tend to have a greater proportion of hypertension-induced heart failure (Yancy, 2005).

The age-dependent, progressive development of heart failure reflects a process of pathological cardiac remodeling that is influenced by the hemodynamic load imposed by systolic blood pressure as well as the pro-inflammatory, neurohumoral milieu characteristic of obesity and diabetes. The initial "adaptive" development of left ventricular hypertrophy in response to the hypertensive state gradually transitions toward contractile dysfunction and the eventual clinical manifestations of heart failure. Most studies indicate that African Americans have a higher prevalence of left ventricular hypertrophy than whites even after adjustment for other risk factors such as systolic blood pressure and body mass index. African Americans manifest a higher prevalence of the major risk factors for developing heart failure: hypertension, obesity, diabetes, and left ventricular hypertrophy. Indeed, the multivariate model analysis of the ARIC cohort indicates that the higher risk of heart failure among African Americans is primarily related to the higher prevalence of hypertension, diabetes, and lower socioeconomic status (Loehr et al., 2008). The inclusion of socioeconomic factors in the model suggests the potential influence of access to quality health care and the effective diagnosis and management of risk factors (for example, hypertension) as an important determinant of health disparities related to heart failure.

Renal Failure

Studies involving population-based cohorts as well as clinical trials have documented a striking disparity in the incidence of end-stage renal failure in African Americans and whites. This health disparity is related in large part to the higher prevalence of risk factors for kidney disease, such as hypertension and diabetes, among African Americans (McClellan, 2005). However, it is also noteworthy that recent studies have identified genetic variants in African Americans that appear to predispose them to glomerular injury, scarring, and the progression of renal disease (Kopp et al., 2008). It is speculated that the more rapid decline in renal function in response to the injury imposed by factors such as hypertension may explain the very high incidence of end-stage renal failure in African Americans.

Analysis of the NHANES dataset has documented significant racial/ethnic disparities in the prevalence of micro-albuminuria as an early marker of renal injury and the development of kidney disease. In multivariate models that adjusted for confounding factors, nondiabetic African Americans had a two-fold higher risk and Mexican-Americans were at 1.8-fold higher risk of albuminuria compared with whites. It is also notable that the major factors associated with albuminuria were related to socioeconomic factors involving access to quality care and/or indices of effective management risk factors such as the level of glycemic control among diabetics, systolic blood pressure, income, diuretic use, and hypertensive treatment status (Bryson, Ross, Boyko, & Young, 2006).

African American men with chronic kidney disease progress to end-stage renal disease more rapidly than whites. Of note, cross-sectional analysis of approximately ten thousand participants in the Kidney Early Evaluation Program documented a higher prevalence of poorly controlled hypertension among African American men, providing evidence in support of the postulate that uncontrolled hypertension accelerates the progression of renal disease and contributes to racial disparities in the progression of kidney disease (Duru et al., 2008).

One of the challenges in the prevention of chronic kidney disease is the relative lack of awareness of the scope of the problem in black communities. In a recent population-based survey of approximately two thousand randomly selected African Americans within urban centers in the Midwestern and Southeastern regions of the United States, only 23.5 percent reported that they had been screened for kidney disease within the last year. Although almost half (43.7%) of African Americans had a chronic kidney disease risk factor, only 2.8 percent reported that kidney disease was a top health concern. Almost half knew the correct definition of kidney disease (48.6%), but relatively few knew there was a test to diagnose kidney disease (23.7%) or were aware that African Americans were at greater risk than whites of developing chronic kidney disease (18.1%). African Americans with either a higher level of education, recent contact with a physician, or a major risk factor for kidney disease were the most likely to have a correct perception of their disease risk (Waterman et al., 2008). These findings indicate that there is a critical need for health education on cardiovascular risk factors and complications of hypertension such as renal failure.

TREATMENT OF HYPERTENSION: MULTILEVEL INTERVENTIONS IN AFRICAN AMERICAN COMMUNITIES

Advances in the detection, treatment, and control of hypertension have contributed substantially to the decline in cardiovascular mortality in many developed countries over the past thirty years. However, the decline in cardiovascular deaths in the United States has not been uniformly distributed across racial groups (Whitworth, 2003; Burt, Whelton, et al., 1995). Half of the mortality disparity between African Americans and whites is directly attributable to hypertension (Wolz et al., 2000). These mortality disparities reflect differences in social and cultural influences such as health behaviors, access to quality health care, and environmental exposures that may affect blood pressure (Fields et al., 2004; Burt, Cutler, et al., 1995; Chobanian et al., 2003; Hajjar & Kotchen, 2003; Ostechega, Yoon, Hughes, & Louis, 2008; Ostechega, Dillon, Hughes, Carroll, & Yoon, 2007).

Few researchers have performed in-depth analyses of the levels of awareness, treatment, and control of hypertension within an African American community-based sample, but a good example is the Jackson Heart Study (Wyatt et al., 2008). Among the 5,249 participants, 62.9 percent were classified as having hypertension. Women and persons at least 65 years old were more likely to have hypertension. Similarly, lower socioeconomic status, low physical activity, obesity, hypercholesterolemia, diabetes, and chronic kidney disease were associated with an increased likelihood of having hypertension. A high proportion of the hypertensive participants (87.3%) were aware of their hypertension diagnosis. Awareness significantly increased with age, female sex, presence of any major co-morbid condition, and obtaining preventive care. A high proportion of the hypertensive patients in the sample were receiving treatment (83.2%). Treatment rates were highest among women, older individuals, those with health insurance, patients who access preventive care, and patients with any major comorbid condition. Blood pressure control was achieved in just over half (53%) of all the hypertensive participants, regardless of treatment status. Within this African American sample, women and individuals with higher socioeconomic status were more likely to reach blood pressure control levels than were men and less affluent participants. The overall blood pressure distribution among the Jackson Heart Study cohort compared favorably with that of the national probability sample of African Americans in the NHANES survey. Hypertension prevalence and awareness estimates were similar; yet treatment and control rates appeared to be higher in the Jackson Heart Study cohort.

Collectively, this information indicates that higher rates of control can be achieved among African Americans. These results also suggest that public health efforts to increase awareness and treatment among African Americans can contribute to more effective control rates of hypertension within high-risk African American communities such as Jackson, Mississippi.

Community-based Interventions

Beginning in the early 1970s, conventional wisdom guided by theoretical concepts and new scientific information ushered in a new wave of community-based randomized control trials (Davis, 2004). These trials were designed to comprehensively lower multiple behavioral risk factors associated with the onset of cardiovascular diseases, including hypertension. The trials included the Stanford Five-City Project (Farquhar et al., 1985), the Minnesota Heart Health Program (Blackburn et al., 1984), and the Pawtucket Heart Health Program (Carleton, Lasater, Assaf, Lefebre, & McKinlay, 1987). These were investigator-initiated research and demonstration studies that included different aspects of health-promotion education as the primary intervention tool delivered through multiple channels. Various iterations have emerged over the past thirty-five years; however, the basic premise remains the same: risk reduction intervention at the community level will create a diffusion effect that improves individual and subsequent community health by lowering the overall incidence of heart attacks and strokes.

The first generation of community-based intervention trials were large in scope and long-term in duration (ranging from ten to fourteen years) (Stone, 1991). Each adopted a clinical trial approach with community randomization assignments to treatment and control groups. The incongruent nature of this quasi-experimental design prevented investigators from creating a truly "controlled" environment. In retrospect, this design inevitably contributed to the modest or negative results obtained (Carleton, Lasater, Assaf, Feldman, & McKinlay, 1995; Farquhar et al., 1990; Luepker et al., 1994). Despite less than anticipated outcomes, lessons learned from these initial intervention studies helped shape the development of subsequent, more successful second-generation projects with implications gleaned for a new wave of targeted community intervention trials.

Unlike their predecessors, smaller second-generation community trials on heart attack and stroke prevention report positive outcomes (Fulwood, Guyton-Krishnan, Wallace, & Sommer, 2006). Moreover, net effects were achieved with a reduced budget and shorter duration of intervention exposure. The Bootheel Heart Health Project provides an example. This project was implemented in six counties in Missouri and used exercise groups, heart-healthy cooking demonstrations, and several risk-reduction education components as interventions (Brownson et al., 1996). Study subjects were exposed to interventions over a three-year period. The investigators intentionally selected this particular area of Missouri as the location for the interventions because of the demographic characteristics of the region. The area is rural and has a high concentration of African Americans who are medically underserved and have high rates of poverty and low levels of educational attainment. The investigators reported significant population-wide improvement in fruit and vegetable consumption and prevalence of cholesterol screening. Improvements in physical activity, blood pressure, smoking cessation, fruit and vegetable consumption, weight reduction, and cholesterol screening were also reported in African Americans.

Unlike the previous studies, Bootheel incorporated coalition building that guided the development of tailored community interventions within counties. Individual behavioral change was evaluated as the primary unit of analysis rather than the community. The presence of a health coalition in a community was also used as an indicator to determine the degree of intervention exposure as opposed to random assignments of individuals or communities to treatment and control groups. Counties with a low coalition presence were compared with those having a higher degree of coalition building to evaluate the effect of interventions on risk-factor behavior change. Positive changes resulted from the project at a relatively low annual cost of approximately $105,000. Evaluation expenses were minimized by collecting self-reported behavioral estimates and limiting physiologic indicators.

The Centers for Disease Control and Prevention (CDC) have responded to health disparities related to racial and ethnic minority status by launching Racial and Ethnic Approaches to Community Health (REACH). The REACH program is a cornerstone of CDC's efforts to identify, reduce, and ultimately eliminate health disparities. The REACH grant based in Atlanta was administered through the Fulton County Department of Health and Wellness and designed to address cardiovascular disease among African Americans. REACH for Wellness has served more than twenty-four thousand predominantly African American people in the Atlanta Renewal Community, and improvements have been reported since the program began. The program offers free, community-based services such as nutrition education classes, physical activity programs, empowerment groups for men and women, cardiovascular wellness centers in churches, and cardiovascular resource centers in barbershops and beauty salons. After the program was implemented, medication adherence among adults with high blood pressure increased from 79.1 percent in 2002 to 80.5 percent in 2004 (Centers for Disease Control and Prevention, 2007). Although they are not randomized control trials, projects such as REACH include a community-based participatory dimension in their design.

It is anticipated that effective control of hypertension in African American communities will require a multipronged approach that includes community-level interventions as well as patient empowerment efforts to enhance self-management of this disorder.

Hypertension Treatment: Patient-Level Interventions

Medication Adherence Differences in the effectiveness of blood pressure control achieved in African American communities are a major determinant of racial disparities in hypertension-related mortality. Poor adherence to prescribed antihypertensive medications has been noted as a major barrier to blood pressure control (Chobanian et al., 2003). Prior studies have demonstrated lower medication adherence rates among African American hypertensive patients than among whites (Bosworth et al., 2008). The African American Study of Kidney Disease and Hypertension (AASK) trial found that 48 percent of the hypertensive patients enrolled had a poor rate of medication adherence (Lee et al., 1996). Similarly, Bosworth and colleagues (2008) confirmed higher rates of inadequate blood pressure control among African Americans as well as a greater prevalence of non-adherence to the medical regimen.

Many barriers impede successful antihypertensive medication adherence in African American communities (Ogedegbe et al., 2004). Non-adherence to medical regimens often reflects a failure in communication that may involve issues of health literacy or health beliefs. For example, on often-cited reason for non-adherence is that the patient "felt better" or "felt cured" and failed to recognize hypertension as a chronic disorder requiring lifelong treatment. Evidence to date suggests that successful interventions aimed at increasing antihypertensive medication adherence include addressing psychological barriers (for example, the patient's beliefs and concerns about medication), providing emotional support during visits to physicians, and teaching patients strategies that increase self-efficacy to overcome barriers to adherence ((Fahey et al., 2006;

Ogedegbe et al., 2004; Krousel-Wood et al., 2005). It remains questionable whether provider-level interventions such as physician-targeted educational efforts or "pay-for-performance" are the most effective approaches to eliminating racial disparities in hypertension control (Fahey et al., 2005). The most promising approaches focus on empowering and/or enabling patients to enhance their self-management skills. Specifically, interventions involving support from peers or family members are thought to be potential avenues of success (Friday, 1999; Krousel-Wood et al., 2005).

Social Support   Overall, most research has shown that increased morbidity and mortality are both related to a lack of social support (Litwin & Shiovitz-Ezra, 2006; Everson-Rose & Lewis, 2005; Seeman, 2000). By contrast, some literature states that social support can be negatively related to healthy aging if it is filled with critical or demanding interactions (Seeman, 2000). Strong socially supportive networks have been associated with healthy aging and the reduction of cardiovascular mortality (Seeman, 2000; Vogt, 1992; Michael, 1999; Litwin & Shiovitz-Ezra, 2006). However, there are mixed results on the protective nature of social support in women compared with men (Sato et al., 2008). Lyyra and Heikkinen (2006) found that perceived social support is not associated with mortality among men. Interestingly, there are a number of studies that support the old adage "it's better to give than receive." Recently, several studies have found that those who frequently volunteer or provide support to others had lower mortality (Krause, 2006; Harris & Thorensen, 2005; Brown et al., 2003; Sato et al., 2008). Moreover, marital status was more important than other socially supportive relationships with regard to mortality (Rutledge et al., 2003; Brown et al., 2003).

The family unit constitutes a naturally occurring network for social support. Other social networks include friends, neighbors, religious organizations, and community groups (Litwin & Shiovitz-Ezra, 2006). Interventions such as those that seek to utilize already occurring supports and resources have the potential to successfully support long-term behavior change. Programs with an emphasis on social support can help families maintain and strengthen support systems as they work through an intervention strategy together. One model for the use of family support combines both naturally occurring (family) and "constructed" (friends) support. While lack of social support may be an equally important risk factor for many racial/ethnic groups, mechanisms for social support may be different between blacks, whites, and Hispanics (Boden-Albala & Sacco, 2002). Socioeconomic status and traditional versus modern kin groupings may have varying impacts on racial/ethnic groups.

Culture and Family Interventions

In this chapter, we use the term *culture* to refer to an individual's lifestyle behaviors, values, and beliefs. These cultural factors are distinctly different from the self-identified categorization by race/ethnicity or the sociologically determined group to which an individual may be assigned. Cultural factors play a major role in whether new behaviors are adopted and maintained. The collective historical and social experience of African Americans has had an influence on the cultural values and core beliefs within this racial/ethnic population. Barriers to successful interventions in black populations include a mistrust of the health care system, socioeconomic disadvantage, inadequate awareness, and communication barriers. The core cultural values common in African American communities include commitment to immediate family and extended family relationships, communalism, religion/spirituality, education, and expressiveness (Resnicow et al., 1999; Kumpfer et al., 2002). The resilience and salutary aspects of African American communities provide excellent opportunities for programs aimed toward enhancing health. Furthermore, it has been suggested that culturally sensitive interventions for minority populations should pay attention to several important factors during the planning and execution phases: (1) degree of family influence; (2) level of acculturation and identity; (3) differential family member acculturation leading to family conflict; (4) family migration and relocation history; (5) trauma, loss, and possible post-traumatic stress due to relocation; (6) work and financial stressors; and (7) language preferences and impediments due to English as a second language, and level of literacy in the native language. These complex issues related to cultural sensitivity reinforce the importance of family-based interventions to address cardiovascular risk factor reduction.

Lifestyle Modifications and Family Interventions

Cardiovascular risk behaviors are learned early in life from family members. Moreover, risk factor status among family members is often very similar due to family practices shared in the home environment. Similarly, behavioral risk factors correlate highly with objective cardiovascular disease (CVD) risk factors such as elevated blood pressure, obesity, low levels of high-density lipoprotein cholesterol, and high levels of low-density lipoprotein cholesterol and triglycerides among family members (Bush et al., 1991; Knuiman et al., 1996; Perusse et al., 1997; Iannotti et al., 1999). Since this interaction between genetics and environment begins early in life and therefore has a long time to become ingrained, attempting to change behavior in adulthood is difficult. Research has shown that adults with a parent or sibling suffering from a cardiovascular event (e.g., heart attack or stroke) are not necessarily motivated to change behavioral risk factors learned early in life (Kip et al., 2002; Becker et al., 2005; Mosca et al., 2008). Kip and colleagues (2002) found that the occurrence of a heart attack or a stroke in an immediate family member did not lead to self-initiated changes in behavioral risk factors (smoking, exercise, lipids, body weight, and blood pressure). Similarly, Becker and colleagues found it difficult to change behavior and objective risk factors following the hospitalization of a family member with a CVD-related event (Becker et al., 2005; Mosca et al., 2008). Nevertheless, some success has been achieved in achieving blood pressure reduction through behavioral interventions. For example, the PREMIER trial demonstrated that relatively intensive behavioral interventions incorporating a goal-driven approach to weight loss, sodium reduction, increased physical activity, and limited alcohol intake are effective in promoting significant reductions of blood pressure (Lien et al., 2007).

In contrast with efforts to promote behavioral change in high-risk adults, an alternative and potentially more effective approach is to begin teaching healthy lifestyle habits to young children before they form unhealthy habits that are resistant to change.

A number of programs are attempting to teach young children healthy lifestyle habits through their high-risk parents. The Families Implementing Good Health Traditions for Life (FIGHT for Life) program, implemented by one of the authors of this chapter in Atlanta from 2004 to 2007, was a pilot study whose aims included reducing blood pressure and lipid levels through improved physical activity and nutritional habits in black families. The study used a three-group, cluster-randomized design, with families rather than individuals assigned to treatment conditions. Participants in the study were recruited from a variety of locations, including primary care clinics. In addition, motivational interviewing was used to aid families in achieving behavioral change. Seventy-one percent of the families assigned to the class intervention attended 75 percent or more of the sessions. Preliminary results reveal some promising changes made on the part of the participants. Specifically, parents significantly increased their fruit intake per week (+7.9 servings/wk; $p < .01$) and minutes of vigorous activity per week (+55 min/wk; $p < .04$). Results also included trends toward significance for minutes of walking per week (+205 min/wk; $p < .06$); diastolic blood pressure (–4 mm Hg; $p < .09$); and total cholesterol (–8 mg/dL; $p < .06$). Based on these results and post-intervention feedback, it appears that family interventions are a very promising method for improving lifestyle behaviors not only in parents but in their children.

Dietary Intervention

The development of hypertension in susceptible individuals is related to aging and prolonged exposure to adverse lifestyles including excessive dietary intake of sodium and high-fat foods as well as relatively deficient intake of fiber, potassium, calcium, and Vitamin D. Many studies have evaluated the efficacy of implementing dietary changes as a means of reducing blood pressure. Controlled trials have documented that a variety of dietary modifications are achievable and effective in reducing blood pressure (BP) (DASH-Sodium Collaborative Research Group, 2001; Appel et al., 1997; Appel et al., 2003; Appel et al., 2005; Writing Group of the PREMIER Collaborative Research Group, 2003). In most cases, dietary interventions that focus on a single nutrient have yielded either equivocal (dietary calcium) or relatively modest sustained blood pressure decreases (dietary sodium) (Dickinson et al., 2006). An alternative strategy manipulates the intake of multiple micronutrients and recognizes that many foods have salutary effects based on uncharacterized elements such as endogenous antioxidants. The Seventh Report of the Joint National Committee on the Prevention, Detection, Evaluation, and Treatment of High Blood Pressure (JNC VII) has recommended that blood pressure be lowered by adoption of the Dietary Approach to Stop Hypertension (DASH) eating plan (Chobanian et al., 2003). The DASH eating plan emphasizes the importance of a diet rich in fruits, vegetables, low-fat dairy products, potassium, and calcium with a reduced content of dietary cholesterol and sodium for lowering blood pressure. The DASH diet has been shown to enhance sodium excretion in association with reducing blood pressure in both blacks and whites. Indeed, African Americans tend to exhibit the most robust blood-pressure-lowering response to this dietary intervention. Unfortunately, the benefits of DASH have not been successfully translated into everyday practice.

Underutilization of current knowledge is evident in data indicating that only 35 percent of individuals with hypertension in the United States report being counseled by a health professional to modify their diet (Mellen et al., 2004). Additionally, the average sodium content of a typical American diet is reported at 4,000 mg, a level far exceeding the current recommended daily allowance of 2,400 mg (Chobanian et al., 2003). Furthermore, only 23 percent of Americans report eating five or more servings of fruits and vegetables daily (CDC, 2006). Thus, it is clear that effective interventions such as the DASH eating plan, shown to reduce blood pressure and the risk of heart disease and stroke, need to implemented beyond the experimental research setting to reach individuals and families in communities. Previous studies that have attempted to translate DASH into everyday practice have met with limited success, perhaps because they have not incorporated the skill building that is necessary to increase self-efficacy for preparing DASH-like meals (Appel et al., 2003; Writing Group of the PREMIER Collaborative Research Group, 2003). However, adhering to a DASH diet is a standard treatment recommendation, either as a first-line intervention or adjunct to drug therapy, in patients with hypertension. While the efficacy of the DASH eating plan in achieving control of blood pressure in research settings is well documented, there is little or no data on its impact on blood pressure reduction in community-based settings. Future research and new demonstration models are needed to develop ways to integrate either community-level or family-level interventions with the DASH diet to prevent and/or eliminate hypertension in African American communities.

Hypertension Treatment: Medical Interventions

In accordance with standard clinical practice and guidelines, the medical treatment of hypertension must include lifestyle modifications as the foundation of treatment. It is well established that weight loss or changes in diet can yield blood pressure reductions that rival most pharmaceutical agents. As noted above, dietary changes such as the DASH eating plan can potentiate the response to pharmacologic treatments of hypertension (Conlin et al., 2003). Thus, clinicians must address nonpharmacologic factors that will affect the efficacy of antihypertensive treatment.

The high-risk profile that typifies many African Americans with hypertension mandates a holistic approach that is appropriately aggressive in reducing the risk of cardiovascular complications. African Americans tend to develop elevations in blood pressure at an earlier age and suffer a more virulent clinical course with vascular complications such as stroke and renal failure. Compared with other racial/ethnic groups, African Americans are more likely to have severe forms of hypertension that typically require three or more antihypertensive medications to achieve control. It has been postulated that there are significant genetic and pathobiological differences in the etiologic basis of hypertension among African Americans as compared with other groups. For example, there is suggestive evidence that African Americans tend to exhibit greater salt sensitivity, higher aldosterone levels, relative suppression of the circulating renin-angiotensin system, and more volume-dependent hypertension. This has led to a tendency among clinicians to prescribe diuretics and calcium channel blockers as the major classes of antihypertensive agents in African Americans. This approach to single-drug therapy is supported to some extent by a comparative clinical trial performed within the Veterans Administration (VA) medical care system (Cushman et al., 2000).

Although these findings tend to guide race-based therapeutics, it is important to emphasize that they are generalizations based on relatively modest intergroup differences in mean blood pressure response. Moreover, many are relatively small studies in which there were inadequate controls for confounding factors such as socioeconomic status. In general, there is much greater variance in drug response *within* racial groups than *between* them. Skin color remains a very crude proxy for predicting antihypertensive therapeutic response in the individual patient. Indeed, it is noteworthy that in the VA's comparative drug trial, one of the largest differentials in drug response was between blacks living in the Southeastern United States (lower responsiveness to angiotensin-converting enzyme inhibition) and African Americans in the rest of the nation (higher responsiveness). This finding indicates that behavioral and environmental factors are as important as biological factors in determining drug response. For example, it has been documented that the response to blockade of the renin-angiotensin system is blunted in patients who are obese and/or consume a high-sodium, low-potassium diet (Mokwe et al., 2004). It is speculated that the high prevalence of obesity and high-sodium, low-potassium diets among African Americans (particularly those living in the Southeastern United States) may explain the apparent "racial" differences seen in various studies. The failure to account for the confounding influences of social, cultural, and behavioral factors has tended to perpetuate the clinical stereotypes that underlie many race-based therapeutic strategies. It is anticipated that the advent of biomarkers and pharmacogenetics will enable clinicians to move beyond skin color and incorporate more refined tools to predict biological responses. Emerging genomic tools hold the potential to reflect and correlate with biogeographic ancestry while yielding insights into biological differences that move beyond the superficial social construct of "race."

In most circumstances the debate about differences in response to single-agent therapy becomes moot once it is recognized that most patients will require two or more medications to achieve optimal blood pressure control. In most situations, patients will need a combination that includes blockade of the renin-angiotensin system (with an angiotensin-converting enzyme [ACE] inhibitor or angiotensin receptor blocker) in combination with either a diuretic or calcium channel blocker. Recent evidence suggests a particular efficacy of the ACE inhibitor/calcium channel blocker in conferring mortality benefit (Jamerson et al., 2008). This can be an effective combination in African American patients and may be less likely to induce metabolic disturbances that predispose to the development of diabetes that can occur in diuretic-based treatment regimens.

SUMMARY

Hypertension is the most common and most significant modifiable disorder that causes racial disparities in mortality in the United States. The weight of evidence supports the thesis that hypertension is caused by a complex interplay of genetic, psychosocial, behavioral, cultural, and environmental factors. It is also evident that individual lifestyle options and choices play a critical role in the development of hypertension. It should be recognized that circumstances of social context can contribute to the development of hypertension through pathways involving psychosocial stresses and constraints on salutary behaviors. Nevertheless, interventions that promote physical fitness, limit excess adiposity, minimize sodium and alcohol intake, and promote a DASH-like diet can prevent hypertension or facilitate the control of blood pressure. It is conceivable that a multipronged approach that engages communities, social networks, families, health care providers, and individuals to adopt these salutary habits could effectively reduce racial disparities in morbidity and mortality by enhancing awareness, treatment, and control of hypertension.

REFERENCES

Anderson, N. B., & Armstead, C. A. (1995). Toward understanding the association of socioeconomic status and health: A new challenge for the biopsychosocial approach. *Psychosomatic Medicine, 57*, 213–225.

Appel, L. J., Champagne, C. M., et al. (2003). Effects of comprehensive lifestyle modification on blood pressure control: Main results of the PREMIER clinical trial. *Journal of the American Medical Association, 289*, 2083–2093.

Appel, L. J., Moore, T.J., et al. (1997). A clinical trial of the effects of dietary patterns on blood pressure. *New England Journal of Medicine, 336*, 1117–1124.

Appel, L. J., Sacks, F.M., et al. (2005). Effects of protein, monounsaturated fats and carbohydrate intake on blood and serum lipids. Results of the Omni Heart Randomized Trial. *Journal of the American Medical Association. 294*, 2455–2464.

Becker, D. M., Yanek, L., Johnson, W. R., Garrett, D., Moy, T. F., Reynolds, S. S., et al. (2005). Impact of a community-based multiple risk factor intervention on cardiovascular risk in black families with a history of premature coronary disease. *Circulation, 111*, 1298–1304.

Belsha, C. W., Wells, T. G., McNiece, K. G., Seib, P. M., Pummer, J. K., & Berry, P. L. (1998). Influence of diurnal blood pressure variations on target organ abnormalities in adolescents with mild essential hypertension. *American Journal of Hypertension, 11*, 410–417.

Blackburn, H., Luepker, R. V., Kline, F. G., Bracht, N., Carlaw, R., Jacobs, D., et al. (1984). The Minnesota Heart Health Program: A research and demonstration project in cardiovascular disease prevention. In J. D. Matarazzo et al. (Eds), *Behavioral health: A handbook of health enhancements and disease prevention*. New York: Wiley.

Boden-Albala, B., & Sacco, R. L. (2002, January). Socioeconomic status and stroke mortality: Refining the relationship. *Stroke, 33*(1), 274–275.

Bosworth, H. B., Powers, B., Grubber, J. M., Thorpe, C.T., Olsen, M.K., Orr, M., & Oddone, E. Z. (2008). Racial differences in blood pressure control: Potential explanatory factors. *Journal of General Internal Medicine, 23*(5), 692–698.

Brown, S. L., Nesse, R. M., Vinokur, A. D., & Smith D. M. (2003). Providing social support may be more beneficial than receiving it: Results from a prospective study of mortality. *Psychological Science, 14*(4), 320–327.

Brownson, R. C., Smith, C. A., Pratt, M., Mack, N. E., Jackson-Thompson, J., Dean, C. G., et al. (1996). Preventing cardiovascular disease through community-based risk reduction: The Bootheel Heart Health Project. *American Journal of Public Health, 86*, 206–213.

Bryson, C. L., Ross, H. J., Boyko, E. J., & Young, B. A. (2006). Racial and ethnic variations in albuminuria in the US: Third National Health and Nutrition Examination Survey (NHANES III) population: Associations with diabetes and level of CKD. *American Journal of Kidney Disease, 48*(5), 720–726.

Burt, V. L., Cutler, J. A., Higgins, M., Horan, M. J., Labrathe, D., Whelton, P., et al. (1995). Trends in the prevalence, awareness, treatment, and control of hypertension in the adult US population. Data from the health examination surveys, 1960 to 1991. *Hypertension, 26*, 60–69.

Burt, V. L., Whelton, P., Roccella, E. J., Brown, C., Cutler, J. A., Higgins, M., et al. (1995). Prevalence of hypertension in the US adult population. Results from the Third National Health and Nutrition Examination Survey, 1988–1991. *Hypertension, 25*, 305–313.

Bush, P. J., Iannotti, R. J., et al. (1991). Relationships among black families' cardiovascular disease risk factors. *Preventive Medicine, 20*(4), 447–461.

Campbell, M. C., & Tishkoff, S. A. (2008). African genetic diversity: Implications for human demographic history, modern human origins, and complex disease mapping. *Annual Review of Genomics and Human Genetics, 9*, 403–433.

Cappuccio, F. P., Stranges, S., Kandala, N. B., Miller, M. A., Taggart, F. M., Kumari, M., et al. (2007). Gender-specific associations of short sleep duration with prevalent and incident hypertension: The Whitehall II Study. *Hypertension, 50*(4), 693–700.

Carleton, R. A., Lasater, T. M., Assaf, A. R., Lefebre, R. C., & McKinlay, S. M. (1987). The Pawtucket Heart Health Program: An experiment in population-based disease prevention. *Rhode Island Medical Journal, 70*, 533–538.

Carleton, R. A., Lasater, T. M., Assaf, A. R., Feldman, H. A., & McKinlay, S. (1995). The Pawtucket Heart Health Program: Community changes in cardiovascular risk factors and projected disease risk. *American Journal of Public Health, 85*, 777–785.

Centers for Disease Control and Prevention (CDC). (2006). *Behavioral risk factor surveillance system survey data*. Atlanta: U.S. Department of Health and Human Services, Centers for Disease Control and Prevention.

Centers for Disease Control and Prevention (CDC). (2007). *The power to reduce health disparities: Voices from REACH communities*. Atlanta: U.S. Department of Health and Human Services, Centers for Disease Control and Prevention.

Chichlowska, K. L., Rose, K. M., Diez-Roux, A. V., Golden, S. H., McNeill, A. M., & Heiss, G. (2008). Individual and neighborhood socioeconomic status characteristics and prevalence of metabolic syndrome: The Atherosclerosis Risk in Communities (ARIC) Study. *Psychosomatic Medicine, 70*(9), 986–992.

Chiolero, A., Bovet, P., Paradis, G., & Paccaud, F. (2007). Has blood pressure increased in children in response to the obesity epidemic? *Pediatrics, 119*, 544–553.

Chobanian, A. V., Bakris, G. L., Black, H. R., Cushman, W. E., Green, L. A., Izzo, J. L., et al. (2003). Seventh report of the Joint National Committee on Prevention, Detection, Evaluation, and Treatment of High Blood Pressure. *Hypertension, 290*, 1206–1252.

Collins, R., & Winkleby, M. (2002). African American subgroups at high and low risk for hypertension: A signal detection analysis of NHANES III, 1988–1991. *Preventive Medicine, 35*, 303–312.

Conlin, P. R., Erlinger, T. P., Bohannon, A., Miller, E. R., III, Appel, L. J., Svetkey, L. P., et al. (2003). The DASH diet enhances the blood pressure response to losartan in hypertensive patients. *American Journal of Hypertension, 16*(5, Pt 1), 337–342.

Cook, N. R., Obarzanek, E., Cutler, J. A., Buring, J. E., Rexrode, K. M., Kumanyika, S. K, et al. (2009). Trials of Hypertension Prevention Collaborative Research Group. Joint effects of sodium and potassium intake on subsequent cardiovascular disease: The Trials of Hypertension Prevention follow-up study. *Archives of Internal Medicine, 169*(1), 32–40.

Cowley, A.W., Jr. (2008). Renal medullary oxidative stress, pressure-natriuresis, and hypertension. *Hypertension, 52*(5), 777–786.

Cruickshank, J. K., & Beevers, D. G. (1982). Epidemiology of hypertension: Blood pressure in blacks and whites. *Clinical Science* (London), *62*, 1–6.

Cushman, W. C., Reda, D. J., Perry, H. M., Williams, D., Abdellatif, M., & Materson, B. J. (2000). Regional and racial differences in response to antihypertensive medication use in a randomized controlled trial of men with hypertension in the United States. Department of Veterans Affairs Cooperative Study Group on Antihypertensive Agents. *Archives of Internal Medicine, 160*(6), 825–831.

Cutler, J. A., Sorlie, P. D., Wolz, M., Thom, T., Fields, L. E., & Roccella, E. J. (2008). Trends in hypertension prevalence, awareness, treatment, and control rates in United States adults between 1988–1994 and 1999–2004. *Hypertension, 52*, 818–827.

DASH-Sodium Collaborative Research Group. (2001). Effects on blood pressure of reduced dietary sodium and the Dietary Approaches to Stop Hypertension (DASH) Diet. *New England Journal of Medicine. 344*, 3–10.

Davis, S. K. (2004). Cardiovascular risk-reduction community intervention trials. In D. S. Blumenthal & R. J. DiClemente (Eds.), *Community-based health research: Issues and methods.* New York: Springer, 199–213.

Denton, N. A., & Massey, D. S. (1991). Patterns of neighborhood in a multiethnic world: US metropolitan areas, 1970–1980. *Demography, 28*, 41–63.

Dickinson, H. O., Mason, J. M., Nicolson, D. J., Campbell, F., Beyer, F. R., Cook, J. V., et al. (2006). Lifestyle interventions to reduce raised blood pressure: A systematic review of randomized controlled trials. *Journal of Hypertension, 24*(2), 215–233.

Diez-Roux, A. V., Merkin, S. S., Arnett, D., Chambless, L., Massing, M., Nieto, F. J., et al. (2001). Neighborhood of residence and incidence of coronary heart disease. *New England Journal of Medicine, 345*, 99–106.

Diez-Roux, A. V., Northridge, M. E., Morabia, A., Bassett, M. T., & Shea, S. (1999). Prevalence of social correlates of cardiovascular disease risk factors in Harlem. *American Journal of Public Health, 89*, 302–307.

Din-Dzietham, R., Liu, Y., Bielo, M., & Shamsa, F. (2007). High blood pressure trends in children and adolescents in national surveys, 1963 to 2002. *Circulation, 116*, 1488–1496.

Dubowitz, T., Heron, M., Bird, C. E., Lurie, N., Finch, B. K., Basurto-Dávila, R., et al. (2008). Neighborhood socioeconomic status and fruit and vegetable intake among whites, blacks, and Mexican Americans in the United States. *American Journal of Clinical Nutrition, 87*(6), 1883–1891.

Durrence, H. H., & Lichstein, K. L. (2006). The sleep of African Americans: A comparative review. *Behavioral Sleep Medicine, 4*(1), 29–44.

Duru, O. K., Li, S., Jurkovitz, C., Bakris, G., Brown, W., Chen, S. C., et al. (2008). Race and sex differences in hypertension control in CKD: Results from the Kidney Early Evaluation Program (KEEP). *American Journal of Kidney Disease, 51*(2),192–198.

Everson-Rose, S. A., & Lewis, T. T. (2005). Psychosocial factors and cardiovascular diseases. *Annual Review of Public Health, 26*, 469–500.

Fahey, T., Schroeder, K., & Ebrahim, S. (2005). Educational and organisational interventions used to improve the management of hypertension in primary care: A systematic review. *British Journal of General Practice, 55 (520)*, 875–882.

Fahey, T., Schroeder, K., Ebrahim, S. (2006, October). Interventions used to improve control of blood pressure in patients with hypertension. *Cochrane Database of Systematic Reviews, 18*(4), CD005182.

Farquhar, J. W., Fortmann, S. P., Flora, J. A., Taylor, C. B., Haskill, W. L., Williams, P. T., et al. (1990). Effects of community-wide education on cardiovascular disease risk factors: The Stanford Five-City Project. *Journal of the American Medical Association, 18*, 359–365.

Farquhar, J. W., Fortmann, S. P., Maccoby, N., Haskell, W. L., Williams, P. T., Flora, J. A., et al. (1985). The Stanford Five-City Project. Design and methods. *American Journal of Epidemiology, 122*, 323–334.

Fields, L. E., Burt, V. L., Cutler, J. A., Hughes, J., Roccella, E. J., & Sorlie, P. (2004). The burden of adult hypertension in the United States, 1999 to 2000: A rising tide. *Hypertension, 44*, 398–404.

Friday, G. H. (1999). Antihypertensive medication compliance in African-American stroke patients: Behavioral epidemiology and interventions. *Neuroepidemiology, 18*(5), 223–30.

Friday, G., Alter, M., et al. (2002). Control of hypertension and risk of stroke recurrence. *Stroke, 33*, 2652–2657.

Frisancho, A. R., Leonard, W. R., & Bollettino, L. A. (1984). Blood pressure in blacks and whites and its relationship to dietary sodium and potassium intake. *Journal of Chronic Disease, 37*, 515–519.

Fulwood, R., Guyton-Krishnan, J., Wallace, M., & Sommer, E. (2006). Role of community programs in controlling blood pressure. *Current Hypertension Report, 8*(6), 512–520.

Geronimus, A. T., Bound, J., Waidmann, T. A., Hillemeier, N. M., & Burns, P. B. (1996). Excess mortality among blacks and whites in the United States. *New England Journal of Medicine, 335*, 1552–1558.

Gillum, R. F., Mussolino, M. E., & Madans, J. H. (1998). Coronary heart disease risk factors and attributable risks in African American women and men: NHANES I epidemiologic follow-up study. *American Journal of Public Health, 88*, 913–917.

Gretler, D. D., Fumo, M. T., Nelson, K. S., & Murphy, M. B. (1994). Ethnic differences in circadian hemodynamic profile. *American Journal of Hypertension, 7*, 7–14.

Grim, C. E., Luft, F. C., Miller, J. Z., McNeely, G. R., Batterbee, H. D., Hames, C. G., et al. (1980). Racial differences in blood pressure in Evans County, Georgia: Relationship to sodium and potassium intake and plasma renin activity. *Journal of Chronic Disease, 33*, 87–94.

Guyton, J. R. (2002). Clinical assessment of atherosclerotic lesions: Emerging from angiographic shadows. *Circulation, 106*, 1308–1309.

Haan, M., Kaplan, G. A., & Camacho, T. (1987). Poverty and health. *American Journal of Epidemiology, 125*, 989–998.

Hajjar, I., & Kotchen, T. A. (2003). Trends in prevalence, awareness, treatment, and control of hypertension in the United States, 1988–2000. *Journal of the American Medical Association, 290*, 199–206.

Harrel, J. P., Hall, S., & Taliaferro, J. (2003). Physiological responses to racism and discrimination: An assessment of the evidence. *American Journal of Public Health, 93*, 243–247.

Harris, A. H., & Thorensen, C. E. (2005). Volunteering is associated with delayed mortality in older people: Analysis of the longitudinal study of aging. *Journal of Health Psychology, 10(6)*, 739–52.

Harshfield, G. A., Pulliam, D. A., Somes, G. W., & Alpert, B. S. (1993). Ambulatory blood pressure patterns in youth. *American Journal of Hypertension, 6*, 968–973.

Harshfield, G. A., & Treiber, F. A. (1999). Racial differences in ambulatory blood pressure monitoring: Derived 24 h patterns of blood pressure in adolescents. *Blood Pressure Monitoring, 4*, 107–110.

Harshfield, G. A., Wilson, M. E., Treiber, F. A., & Albert, B. S. (2002). A comparison of ambulatory blood pressure patterns across populations. *Blood Pressure Monitoring, 7*, 265–269.

Holick, M. F. (2007). Vitamin D deficiency. *New England Journal of Medicine, 357(3)*, 266–281.

Howard, G., Prineas, R., Moy, C., Cushman, M., Kellum, M., Temple, E., et al. (2006). Racial and geographic differences in awareness, treatment, and control of hypertension: The reasons for geographic and racial differences in stroke study. *Stroke, 37*, 1171–1178.

Hypertension Detection and Follow-up Program Cooperative Group. (1997). *Journal of the American Medical Association, 277*, 157–166.

Iannotti, R. J., Zuckerman, A. E., et al. (1999). Intrafamilial relations of cardiovascular disease risk factors in African-Americans: Longitudinal results from DC SCAN. *Preventive Medicine, 28(4)*, 367–377.

Jamerson, K., Weber, M.A., Bakris, G.L., Dahlöf, B., Pitt, B., Shi, V., et al. (2008). ACCOMPLISH trial investigators: Benazepril plus amlodipine or hydrochlorothiazide for hypertension in high-risk patients. *New England Journal of Medicine, 359(23)*, 2417–2428.

James, G. D. (1981). Race and perceived stress independently affect the diurnal variation of blood pressure in women. *American Journal of Hypertension, 4*, 383–384.

Kant, A. K., Graubard, B. I., & Kumanyika, S. K. (2007). Trends in black-white differentials in dietary intakes of U.S. adults, 1971–2002. *American Journal of Preventive Medicine, 32(4)*, 264–272.

Kaplan, G. A. (1999). What is the role of the social environment in understanding inequalities in health? *Annals of the New York Academy of Science, 896*, 116–119.

Kip, K. E., McCreath, H. E., et al. (2002). Absence of risk factor change in young adults after family heart attack or stroke. *American Journal of Preventive Medicine, 22(4)*, 258–266.

Kleindorfer, D., Panagos, P., Pancioli, A., Khoury, J., Kissela, B., Woo, D., et al. (2005). Incidence and short-term prognosis of transient ischemic attack in a population-based study. *Stroke, 36(4)*, 720–723.

Knuiman, M. W., Divitini, M. L., et al. (1996). Familial correlations, cohabitation effects, and heritability for cardiovascular risk factors. *Annals of Epidemiology, 6(3)*, 188–194.

Kopp, J. B., Smith, M. W., Nelson, G. W., Johnson, R. C., Freedman, B. I., Bowden, D. W., et al. (2008). MYH9 is a major-effect risk gene for focal segmental glomerulosclerosis. *Nature Genetics, 40(10)*, 1175–1184.

Kramer, H., Han, C., Post, W., Goff, D., Diez-Roux, A., Cooper, R., et al. (2004). Racial/ethnic differences in hypertension and hypertension treatment and control in the multi-ethnic study of atherosclerosis (MESA). *American Journal of Hypertension, 17(10)*, 963–970.

Krause, N. (2006). Church-based social support and mortality. *Journals of Gerontology Series B–Psychological Sciences & Social Sciences, 61(3)*, S140–6.

Krieger, N., Williams, D. R., & Moss, N. M. (1997). Measuring social class in US public health research: Concepts, methodologies, and guidelines. *Annual Review of Public Health, 18*, 341–378.

Krousel-Wood, M., Hyre, A., Muntner, P., & Morisky, D. (2005). Methods to improve medication adherence in patients with hypertension: Current status and future directions. *Current Opinion in Cardiology, 20(4)*, 296–300.

Kumpfer, K., Alvarado, R., Smith, P., & Bellamy, N. (2002). Cultural sensitivity and adaptation in family-based prevention interventions. *Prevention Sciences, 3*(3), 241–246.

Labovitz, D. L., Halim, A. X., Brent, B., Boden-Albala, B., Hauser, W. A., & Sacco, R. L. (2006). Subarachnoid hemorrhage incidence among Whites, Blacks and Caribbean Hispanics: The Northern Manhattan Study. *Neuroepidemiology, 26*(3),147–150.

Lanford, H. G., Watson, R. L., & Douglas, B. H. (1980). Factors affecting blood pressure in population groups. *Transactions of the Association of American Physicians, 63*, 135–146.

Lee, J. Y., Kusek, J. W., et al. (1996). Assessing medication adherence by pill count and electronic monitoring in the African American study of kidney disease and hypertension (AASK) pilot study. *American Journal of Hypertension, 9*(3), 715–725.

Lien, L. F., Brown, A. J., Ard, J. D., Loria, C., Erlinger, T. P., Feldstein, A. C., et al. (2007). Effects of PRE-MIER lifestyle modifications on participants with and without the metabolic syndrome. *Hypertension 50*(4), 609–616.

Lillie-Blanton, M., & LaVeist T. (1996). Race/ethnicity, the social environment and health. *Social Science & Medicine, 43*, 83–91.

Litwin, H., and Shiovitz-Ezra, S. (2006). Network type and mortality risk in later life. *The Gerontologist, 46*(6), 735–743.

Loehr, L. R., Rosamond, W. D., Chang, P. P., Folsom, A. R., & Chambless, L. E. (2008). Heart failure incidence and survival (from the Atherosclerosis Risk in Communities study). *American Journal of Cardiology, 101*(7), 1016–1022.

Luepker, R. V., Murray, D. M., Jacobs, D. R. Jr, Mittelmark, M. B., Bracht, N., Carlaw, R., et al. (1994). Community education for cardiovascular disease prevention: Risk factor changes in the Minnesota Heart Health Program. *American Journal of Public Health, 84*, 1383–1393.

Lyyra, T. M., & Heikkinen, R. L. (2006). Perceived social support and mortality in older people. *Journals of Gerontology Series B–Psychological Sciences and Social Sciences, 61*(3), S147–S152.

Mathew, B., Patel, S. B., Reams, G. P., Freeman, R. H., Spear, R. M., & Villarreal, D. (2007). Obesity-hypertension: Emerging concepts in pathophysiology and treatment. *American Journal of Medical Science, 334*(1), 23–30.

McCarron, D. A., Morris, C. D., & Cole, C. (1982). Dietary calcium in human hypertension. *Science, 217*, 267–269.

McClellan, W. M. (2005). Epidemiology and risk factors for chronic kidney disease. *Medical Clinics of North America, 89*(3), 419–445.

Mellen, P. B., Palla, S. L., Goff, D. C., & Bonds, D. E. (2004). Prevalence of nutrition and exercise counseling for patients with hypertension, United States, 1999 to 2000. *Journal of General Internal Medicine, 19*(9): 917–924.

Michael, Y. L. (1999). Health behaviors, social networks, and healthy aging: Cross-sectional evidence from the Nurses' Health Study. *Quality of Life Research, 8*(8), 711–722.

Mokwe, E., Ohmit, S. E., Nasser, S. A., Shafi, T., Saunders, E., Crook, E., et al. (2004). Determinants of blood pressure response to quinapril in black and white hypertensive patients: The Quinapril Titration Interval Management Evaluation Trial. *Hypertension, 43*(6),1202–1207.

Mosca, L., Mochari, H., Liao, M., Christian, A. H., Edelman, D. J., Aggarwal, B., et al. (2008). A novel family-based intervention trial to improve heart health: FIT heart. *Circulation: Cardiovascular Quality and Outcomes, 1*, 98–106.

Mujahid, M. S., Diez-Roux, A. V., Morenoff, J. D., Raghunathan, T. E., Cooper, R. S., Ni, H., et al. (2008). Neighborhood characteristics and hypertension. *Epidemiology, 19*(4), 590–598.

Murphy, M. B., Fumo, M. T., Gretler, D. D., Nelson, K. S., & Lang, R. M. (1991). Diurnal blood pressure variation: Differences among disparate ethnic groups. *Journal of Hypertension* Supplement, *9*, S45–S47.

Obisesan, T. O., Vargas, C. M., & Gillum, R. F. (2000). Geographic variation in stroke risk in the United States: Region, urbanization, and hypertension in the Third National Health and Nutrition Examination Survey. *Stroke, 31*, 19–25.

Ogedegbe, G., Harrison, M., et al. (2004). Barriers and facilitators of medication adherence in hypertensive African Americans: A qualitative study. *Ethnicity and Disease, 14*, 3–12.

Ostechega, Y., Dillon, C. F., Hughes, J., Carroll, M., & Yoon, S. (2007). Trends in hypertension prevalence, awareness, treatment, and control in older US adults: Data from the National Health and Nutrition Examination Survey, 1988–2004. *Journal of the American Geriatrics Society, 55*, 1056–1065.

Ostechega, Y., Yoon, S. S., Hughes, J., & Louis, T. (2008). *Hypertension awareness, treatment and control: Continued disparities in adults, United States, 2005–2006.* NCHS data brief no 3. Hyattsville, MD: National Center for Health Statistics.

Pandey, D. K., & Gorelick, P. B. (2005). Epidemiology of stroke in African Americans and Hispanic Americans. *Medical Clinics of North America, 89*(4), 739–752.

Perusse, L., Rice, T., et al. (1997). Familial resemblance of plasma lipids, lipoproteins and postheparin lipoprotein and hepatic lipases in the HERITAGE Family Study. *Arteriosclerosis and Thrombosis Vascular Biology, 17*(11), 3263–3269.

Pickering, G. (1981). Position paper: Dietary sodium and human hypertension. In J. Laragh, F. Bahler, & D. Seldin (Eds.), *Frontiers in hypertension research* (pp. 37–42). New York: Springer-Verlag.

Profant, J., & Dimsdale, J. E. (1999). Race and diurnal blood pressure patterns: A review and meta-analysis. *Hypertension, 33*, 1099–1104.

Resnicow, K., Baranowski, T., Ahluwalia, J.S., & Braithwaite, R.L. (1999). Cultural sensitivity in public health: Defined and demystified. *Ethnicity and Disease, 9*, 10–21.

Rizzoni, D., Muiesan, M. L., Montani, G., Zulli, R., Calebich, S., & Agabiti-Rosei, E. (1992). Relationship between initial cardiovascular structural changes and daytime and nighttime blood pressure monitoring (erratum *American Journal of Hypertension 6*, 177). *American Journal of Hypertension, 5*, 180–186.

Rosamond, W. D., Folsom, A. R., Chambless, L. E., Wang, C. H., McGovern, P. G., Howard, G., et al. (1999). Stroke incidence and survival among middle-aged adults: 9-year follow-up of the Atherosclerosis Risk in Communities (ARIC) cohort. *Stroke, 30*(4), 736–743.

Rossier, B. C., Pradervand, S., Schild, L., & Hummler, E. (2002). Epithelial sodium channel and the control of sodium balance: Interaction between genetic and environmental factors. *Annual Review of Physiology, 64*, 877–897.

Rutledge, T., Matthews, K., Lui, L. Y., Stone, K. L., & Cauley, J. A. (2003). Social networks and marital status predict mortality in older women: Prospective evidence from the Study of Osteoporotic Fractures (SOF). *Psychosomatic Medicine, 65*(4), 688–694.

Sato, T., Kishi, R., Suzukawa, A., Horikawa, N., Saijo, Y., & Yoshioka E. (2008). Effects of social relationships on mortality of the elderly: How do the influences change with the passage of time? *Archives of Gerontology and Geriatrics, 47*(3), 327–339.

Seeman, T. E. (2000). Health-promoting effects of friends and family on health outcomes in older adults. *American Journal of Health Promotion, 14*(6), 362–370.

Seftel, H. C., Johnson, S., & Muller, E. A. (1980). Distribution and biosocial correlations of blood pressure levels in Johannesburg blacks. *South African Medical Journal, 57*(9), 313–320.

Sherwood, A., Steffen, P. R., Blumenthal, J. A., Kuhn, C., & Hinderliter, A. L. (2002). Nighttime blood pressure dipping: The role of the sympathetic nervous system. *American Journal of Hypertension, 15*, 111–118.

Smeeton, N. C., Heuschmann, P. U., Rudd, A. G., McEvoy, A. W., Kitchen, N. D., Sarker, S. J., et al. (2007). Incidence of hemorrhagic stroke in black Caribbean, black African, and white populations: The South London stroke register, 1995–2004. *Stroke, 38*(12), 3133–3138.

Song, Q., Cole, J. W., O'Connell, J. R., Stine, O.C., Gallagher, M., Giles, W. H., et al. (2006). Phosphodiesterase 4D polymorphisms and the risk of cerebral infarction in a biracial population: The Stroke Prevention in Young Women Study. *Human Molecular Genetics, 15*(16), 2468–2478.

Sorlie, P. D., Backland, E, & Keller, J. B. (1995). US mortality by economic, demographic, and social characteristics: The National Longitudinal Mortality Study. *American Journal of Public Health, 85*, 949–956.

Sorof, J. M., Lai, D., Turner, J., Poffenbarger, T., & Portman, R. (2004). Overweight, ethnicity, and the prevalence of hypertension in school-aged children. *Pediatrics, 113*, 475–482.

Stamler, R., Stamler, J., Riedlinger, W. F., Algera, G., & Roberts, R. H. (1978). Weight and blood pressure: Findings in hypertension screening of 1 million Americans. *Journal of the American Medical Association, 240*, 1607–1610

Stone, E. J. (1991). Comparison of NHLBI community-based cardiovascular research studies. *Journal of Health Education, 22*, 134–136.

Vogt, T. M. (1992). Social networks as predictors of ischemic heart disease, cancer, stroke and hypertension: Incidence, survival and mortality. *Journal of Clinical Epidemiology, 45*(6), 659–666.

Waterman, A. D., Browne, T., Waterman, B. M., Gladstone, E. H., & Hostetter, T. (2008). Attitudes and behaviors of African Americans regarding early detection of kidney disease. *American Journal of Kidney Disease, 51*(4), 554–562.

Whitworth, J. A. (2003). World Health Organization, International Society of Hypertension Writing Group, 2003 World Health (WHO)/International Society of Hypertension (ISH) statement on management of hypertension. *Journal of Hypertension, 21*, 1983–1992.

Williams, D. R., & Collins, C. (1995). US socioeconomic and racial differences in health: Patterns and explanations. *Annual Review of Sociology, 21*, 349–389.

Williams, R. B., Barefoot, J. C., Blumenthal, J. A., Helms, M. J., Luecken, L., Pieper, C. F., et al. (1997). Psychosocial correlates of job strain in a sample of working women. *Archives of General Psychiatry, 54*, 543–548.

Wolz, M., Cutler, J., Roccella, E. J., Rhode, F., Thom, T., & Burt, V. (2000). Statement from the National High Blood Pressure Education Program: Prevalence of hypertension. *American Journal of Hypertension, 13*, 103–104.

Writing Group of the PREMIER Collaborative Research Group. (2003). Effects of comprehensive lifestyle modification on blood pressure control: Main results of the PREMIER clinical trial. *Journal of the American Medical Association, 89*, 2083–2093.

Wyatt, S. B., Akylbekova, E. L., Wofford, M. R., Coady, S. A., Walker, E R., Andrew, M. E., et al. (2008). Prevalence, awareness, treatment, and control of hypertension in the Jackson Heart Study. *Hypertension 51*, 650–656.

Yancy, C. W. (2005). Heart failure in African Americans. *American Journal of Cardiology, 96*(7B), 3i-12i.

Yilmaz, M. B., Yalta, K., Turgut, O. O., Yilmaz, A., Yucel, O., Bektasoglu, G., et al. (2007). Sleep quality among relatively younger patients with initial diagnosis of hypertension: Dippers versus non-dippers. *Blood Pressure, 16*(2), 101–105.

Young, J. H., Chang, Y. P., Kim, J. D., Chretien, J. P., Klag, M. J., Levine, M. A., et al. (2005). Differential susceptibility to hypertension is due to selection during the out-of-Africa expansion. *Public Library of Science Genetics, 1*(6), e82.

Zemel, M. B., Gualdonia, S. M., Walsh, M. E., et al. (1986). Effects of sodium and calcium on calcium metabolism and blood pressure regulation in hypertensive black adults. *Journal of Hypertension, 4*, S364.

Zhu, H., Yan, W., Ge, D., Treiber, F. A., Harshfield, G. A., Kapuku, G., et al. (2008). Relationships of cardiovascular phenotypes with healthy weight, at risk of overweight, and overweight in US youths. *Pediatrics, 121*, 115–122.

Zhu, X., & Cooper, R. S. (2007). Admixture mapping provides evidence of association of the VNN1 gene with hypertension. *Public Library of Science ONE, 2*(11), e1244.

CHAPTER

13

A GENERAL OVERVIEW OF CANCER IN THE UNITED STATES

Incidence and Mortality Burden Among African Americans

SHEDRA AMY SNIPES
DONELLA J. WILSON
ANGELINA ESPARZA
LOVELL A. JONES

Each year about 565,650 Americans die of cancer, making it the second leading cause of death in the United States (American Cancer Society [ACS], 2008a; Sedjo et al., 2007). In 2008 alone, 1,437,180 new cancer cases were diagnosed in the United States (745,180 men and 692,000 women) (ACS, 2008a). Still, news regarding cancer is becoming more hopeful; current trends suggest a steady increase in expected cancer survival and decreasing incidence of some cancer types (Sedjo et al., 2007). In fact, millions of Americans are currently living with or are in a state of remission from cancer due to advances in prevention, screening, and treatments. Recent work by Sedjo et al. (2007) suggests that between 1992 and 2004, overall cancer incidence declined by 0.6 percent each year. Reductions in cancer rates are most significant in cancers of the prostate, cervix, breast, lung (males only), and colon (ACS, 2008a; Sedjo et al.,

2007). Similar trends are observed for cancer survival. The best five-year survival rates are observed in cancers of the prostate (98.4%), thyroid (96.7%), testis (95.4%), melanoma (91.1%), and breast (88.6%) (ACS, 2008a). Conversely, the poorest five-year survival rates are observed in cancers of the pancreas (5%), liver (10.8%), lung and bronchus (15%), and esophagus (15.6%) (ACS, 2008a). A more descriptive list of cancer survival rates is included in Table 13.1. Please note, however, that while survival rates inform us about those who live past their cancers, results represent only the percentage of cancer patients who are alive after five years. Survival rates fall short of distinguishing among patients who are in remission, those who have relapsed, and

TABLE 13.1   **Five-Year Relative Survival Rates* for all Malignancy Stages at Diagnosis, 1996–2003.**

Site	%	Site	%
Breast (female)	88.6	Ovary[§]	44.9
Colon and rectum	64.0	Pancreas	5.0
Esophagus	15.6	Prostate[¶]	98.4
Kidney[†]	65.5	Stomach	24.3
Larynx	62.9	Testis	95.4
Liver[‡]	10.8	Thyroid	96.7
Lung and bronchus	15.0	Urinary bladder	79.5
Melanoma of the skin	91.1	Uterine cervix	71.6
Oral cavity and pharynx	59.1	Uterine corpus	82.9

*Rates are adjusted for normal life expectancy and are based on cases diagnosed in the SEER 17 areas from 1996–2003, followed through 2004.
[†]Includes renal pelvis.
[‡]Includes intrahepatic bile duct.
[§]Recent changes in classification of ovarian cancer, specifically excluding borderline tumors, have affected survival rates.
[¶]The rate for local stage represents local and regional stages combined.
Source: Ries, L. A. G., Melbert, D., Krapcho, M., et al. (Eds). (2007). SEER Cancer Statistics Review, 1975–2004, National Cancer Institute, Bethesda, MD. http://www.seer.cancer.gov/csr/1975_2004/ Permission to use granted by the American Cancer Society, Surveillance Research, 2008.

those who are still in treatment. Thus, five-year relative survival rates do not fully represent the proportion of people whose cancers have been completely in remission during the measured five-year survival period.

SCREENING GUIDELINES

Proper screening is one of the most effective ways to prevent and treat cancer. Regular screening exams enable health care professionals to diagnose cancers at an early stage when they are most treatable, and to detect and remove precancerous growths. Screening methods that can detect precancerous lesions and prevent malignant tumors from forming are available for cancers of the cervix, colon, and rectum. Prevention is achieved by allowing removal of precancerous tissue before it becomes malignant. Regular screening can also detect cancers of the breast, colon, rectum, cervix, prostate, oral cavity, and skin at early stages when treatment is most successful.

In general, early detection of any cancer will reduce risk of mortality. However, not all cancers have early detection screening guidelines. The only cancers for which there are recommended guidelines for screening and early detection for asymptomatic individuals are breast, prostate, colon and rectum, and cervix-uterus. Table 13.2 summarizes American Cancer Society recommendations for screening and early detection of cancers in asymptomatic individuals, including a general cancer-related check-up.

Since some cancers, such as those of the lung and bronchus, have no screening tests available for the general population, periodic surveillance of high-risk groups may be the only form of detection. There are also some risk factors that an individual can control, including diet, physical activity, and not smoking. For example, smoking is a risk factor for cancers of the lungs, mouth, throat, larynx, bladder, and several other organs. Currently, the American Cancer Society recommends a healthy diet, at least 30 minutes of regular physical exercise to achieve and maintain a healthy weight, and avoidance of cigarette smoking or exposure to secondhand smoke to reduce overall cancer risk (see the ACS website at www.cancer.org).

Molecular Aspects of Cancer in the Twenty-First Century

Developing biomarkers that detect early stages of cancer or that determine the likelihood of cancer progression will be crucial to controlling this disease. Identification of disease genes via genetic profiling—i.e., the identification of a tumor's unique genetic fingerprint—may lead to options for personalized medicine based on an individual's own DNA.

On the outside most tumors can appear pretty much alike, yet genetic profiling reveals that tumors are hugely variable at the level of the genome and suggests that those variations can be exploited to develop powerful cancer therapies on a personalized level (National Cancer Institute [NCI], 2009). Cancers from every organ system—notably lung, breast, prostate, blood, kidney, and colon—have been shown to be genetically different and susceptible to genetically tailored therapy. For example, two types of lymphoma that look the same under the microscope but respond differently to

TABLE 13.2 **Screening Guidelines for the Early Detection of Cancer in Asymptomatic People.**

Site	Recommendation
Breast	Yearly mammograms starting at age 40. The age at which screening should be stopped should be individualized by considering the potential risks and benefits of screening in the context of overall health status and longevity.
	Clinical breast exam should be part of a periodic health exam about every 3 years for women in their 20s and 30s and every year for women 40 and older.
	Women should know how their breasts normally feel and report any breast change promptly to their health care providers. Breast self-exam is an option for women starting in their 20s.
	Screening MRI is recommended for women with an approximately 20%–25% or greater lifetime risk of breast cancer, including women with a strong family history of breast or ovarian cancer and women who were treated for Hodgkin disease.
Colon & rectum	Beginning at age 50, men and women should begin screening with one of the examination schedules below:
	■ A fecal occult blood test (FOBT) or fecal immunochemical test (FIT) every year
	■ A flexible sigmoidoscopy (FSIG) every 5 years
	■ Annual FOBT or FIT and flexible sigmoidoscopy every 5 years*
	■ A double-contrast barium enema every 5 years
	■ A colonoscopy every 10 years
Prostate	The PSA test and the digital rectal examination should be offered annually, beginning at age 50, to men who have a life expectancy of at least 10 years. Men at high risk (African American men and men with a strong family history of one or more first-degree relatives diagnosed with prostate cancer at an early age) should begin testing at age 45. For both men at average risk and high risk, information should be provided about what is known and what is uncertain about the benefits and limitations of early detection and treatment of prostate cancer so that they can make an informed decision about testing.
Uterus	Cervix: Screening should begin approximately 3 years after a woman begins having vaginal intercourse, but no later than 21 years of age. Screening should be done every year with regular Pap tests or every 2 years using liquid-based tests. At or after age 30, women who have had 3 normal test results in a row

TABLE 13.2 *(Continued)*.

Site	Recommendation
	may get screened every 2 to 3 years. Alternatively, cervical cancer screening with HPV DNA testing and conventional or liquid-based cytology could be performed every 3 years. However, doctors may suggest a woman get screened more often if she has certain risk factors, such as HIV infection or a weak immune system. Women aged 70 and older who have had 3 or more consecutive normal Pap tests in the last 10 years may choose to stop cervical cancer screening.
	Screening after total hysterectomy (with removal of the cervix) is not necessary unless the surgery was done as a treatment for cervical cancer.
	Endometrium: The American Cancer Society recommends that at the time of menopause all women should be informed about the risks and symptoms of endometrial cancer and strongly encouraged to report any unexpected bleeding or spotting to their physicians. Annual screening for endometrial cancer with endometrial biopsy beginning at age 35 should be offered to women with or at risk for hereditary nonpolyposis colon cancer (HNPCC).
Cancer-related checkup	For individuals undergoing periodic health examinations, a cancer-related checkup should include health counseling and, depending on a person's age and gender, might include examinations for cancers of the thyroid, oral cavity, skin, lymph nodes, testes, and ovaries, as well as for some nonmalignant diseases.

*Combined testing is preferred over either annual FOBT or FIT, or FSIG every 5 years, alone. People who are at moderate or high risk for colorectal cancer should talk with a doctor about a different testing schedule.

American Cancer Society guidelines for early cancer detection are assessed annually in order to identify whether there is new scientific evidence sufficient to warrant a reevaluation of current recommendations. If evidence is sufficiently compelling to consider a change or clarification in a current guideline or the development of a new guideline, a formal procedure is initiated. Guidelines are formally evaluated every 5 years regardless of whether new evidence suggests a change in the existing recommendations. There are 9 steps in this procedure, and these "guidelines for guideline development" were formally established to provide a specific methodology for science and expert judgment to form the underpinnings of specific statements and recommendations from the Society. These procedures constitute a deliberate process to ensure that all Society recommendations have the same methodological and evidence-based process at their core. This process also employs a system for rating strength and consistency of evidence that is similar to that employed by the Agency for Health Care Research and Quality (AHCRQ) and the US Preventive Services Task Force (USPSTF). Permission to use granted by the American Cancer Society, Inc.

standard therapy were discovered to be distinguishable from each other at a molecular level (Edwards et al., 2005; ASCO, 2006).

Progress in diagnosing cancer at the molecular level has been most significant for breast and prostate cancer. Research teams have been able to pin down recently discovered cancer markers by sharing their data. A collaborative effort through the Cancer Genetic Markers of Susceptibility (CGEMS) initiative discovered a variation found in a DNA region called 8q24 that predicts as much as 20 percent of the risk of prostate cancer in white men (Schumacher et al., 2007; Yeager et al., 2007; ASCO, 2006; Laxman et al., 2008). They also confirmed an earlier identification of a separate, nearby variation that accounts for about 7 percent of the prostate cancer risk in men of European heritage and about 16 percent of prostate cancer risk among men of African heritage (Schumacher et al., 2007; Yeager et al., 2007; ASCO, 2006; Laxman et al., 2008). In addition, researchers have identified a recurring pattern of abnormal rearrangements of chromosomes that induce specific prostate genes and cancer genes to fuse together. This gene fusion involves the prostate-specific gene TMPRSS2 and the cancer-causing oncogenes ERG and ETV (Schumacher et al., 2007; Yeager et al., 2007; ASCO, 2006; Laxman et al., 2008). With this type of information, scientists are developing a diagnostic test that checks specifically for the presence of these fused genes or their protein products in the blood or urine as a means of early detection (Schumacher et al., 2007; Yeager et al., 2007; ASCO, 2006; Laxman et al., 2008).

Targeted therapy drugs such as tamoxifen and herceptin are being used along with genetic evidence to fight breast cancer. It is now routine to categorize breast tumors by their genetic profiles: for example, estrogen receptor-positive, progesterone receptor-positive, or Her2/neu-positive (Finn et al., 2007). Overexpression of these receptors in breast cancer tumors opens the possibility of treatment either by discontinuation of the hormones that fuel their growth, such as estrogen or progesterone, or through the administration of agents such as tamoxifen and raloxifene that block the hormone receptors present in these tumors (Finn et al., 2007). During the 1970s, a failed contraceptive, tamoxifen, was used to block the tumor-inducing properties of estrogen in tumors that carried protein complexes known as estrogen receptors. In 1978, the U.S. Food and Drug Administration (FDA) approved tamoxifen for treating estrogen receptor positive breast cancer, estimated to account for about three-fourths of all breast tumors. Pioneering work on HER2/neu in the late 1980s led to FDA approval in 1998 for use of the drug trastuzumab (Herceptin) against specific, genetically driven types of metastatic breast cancer. Herceptin works by shutting down the protein receptors produced by the HER2/neu gene and has given hope to more than twenty-seven thousand women diagnosed each year with HER2/neu-positive tumors, which account for as many as 15 percent of breast cancers (Finn et al., 2007). Originally approved for treatment of metastatic tumors, Herceptin is now indicated for women with early-stage breast cancer.

In other areas of cancer research, development of a vaccine against cervical cancer, Gardasil, is an example of how cancer research provides drugs that are targeted against it. Gardasil contains factors that use the body's own immune system to immunize against four types of human papilloma virus (HPV) known to cause most forms of cervical cancer (Kornblau et al., 2009). Two of these HPV strains cause benign genital warts, diagnosed in up to one million Americans each year; the other two cause 70 percent of all cervical cancer cases worldwide (Kornblau et al., 2009). While this vaccine offers a promising new approach to the prevention of cervical cancer, it cannot replace other prevention strategies since it does not treat women who have already been exposed to the virus and does not cover all strains of HPV that cause cancer (Kornblau et al., 2009).

While more research needs to be done, advances in cancer therapy have been made using biomarkers. Genomic medicine is moving to advance cancer treatment by exploring ways to detect and even prevent disease based on an individual's own DNA. As an increasing number of cancer-related genes are being discovered with attempts to correlate them to a particular disease prognosis, these advances in cancer treatment will likely serve as paradigms to develop our understanding of all cancer types, ultimately providing a scientific basis for more personalized care.

CANCER BURDEN AMONG AFRICAN AMERICANS

Despite new and exciting developments in modern medicine, cancer health disparities continue to exist for nearly every racial and ethnic minority in the United States. These disparities are particularly striking for African Americans, who experience the highest cancer death rates and the lowest survival rates of any racial/ethnic group (ACS, 2008b) (see Tables 13.3 and 13.4). The most recent statistics indicate that cancer death rates for African American men are 35 percent higher and cancer death rates for African American women are 18 percent higher than the rates for every other racial group combined (ACS, 2008b).

Reasons for the disproportionate burden of cancer among African Americans include inadequate access to health care or preventive services and higher rates of overall health problems relative to white Americans (NCI 1999; Haynes & Smedley, 1999; Smedley, Stith, & Nelson, 2003; Gross et al., 2008; Virnig et al., 2009). In the "Unequal Treatment" report issued by the United States Institute of Medicine (IOM), Smedley et al. (2003) discussed barriers within the health system and in patient-physician clinical encounters. Examples of health care system barriers cited in the IOM report include linguistic and cultural barriers on the part of providers, lack of a stable relationship between patient and provider (mistrust), financial limitations of poor and minority patients, and fragmentation of the health care system. These factors, along with disproportionate employment in high-risk occupations and exposure to prejudice and discrimination, may contribute to higher rates of cancer incidence and mortality among African American populations (Bacquet & Ringen, 1986; Jones, 1989; Smedley et al., 2003).

Despite an increased burden of cancer incidence and death among African Americans, limited research has been conducted among African American populations in comparison with non-Hispanic whites. This dearth of knowledge, unfortunately, contributes to a lack of biological, cultural, and social understanding of the reasons for cancer disparities. In fact, many barriers still prevail that prevent African Americans

TABLE 13.3   **Cancer Incidence Rates* by Site, Race, and Ethnicity, United States, 2000–2004.**

Incidence	White	African American	Asian American and Pacific Islander	Native American and Alaska Native[†]	Hispanic/ Latino[‡§]
All sites					
Males	556.7	663.7	359.9	321.2	421.3
Females	423.9	396.9	285.8	282.4	314.2
Breast (female)	132.5	118.3	89.0	69.8	89.3
Colon and rectum					
Males	60.4	72.6	49.7	42.1	47.5
Females	44.0	55.0	35.3	39.6	32.9
Kidney and renal pelvis					
Males	18.3	20.4	8.9	18.5	16.5
Females	9.1	9.7	4.3	11.5	9.1
Liver and bile duct					
Males	7.9	12.7	21.3	14.8	14.4
Females	2.9	3.8	7.9	5.5	5.7
Lung and bronchus					
Males	81.0	110.6	55.1	53.7	44.7
Females	54.6	53.7	27.7	36.7	25.2
Prostate	161.4	255.5	96.5	68.2	140.8

(*Continued*)

TABLE 13.3 *(Continued)*.

Incidence	White	African American	Asian American and Pacific Islander	Native American and Alaska Native[†]	Hispanic/ Latino[‡§]
Stomach					
Males	10.2	17.5	18.9	16.3	16.0
Females	4.7	9.1	10.8	7.9	9.6
Uterine cervix	8.5	11.4	8.0	6.6	13.8

*Per 100,000, age adjusted to the 2000 US standard population.

[†]Data based on Contract Health Service Delivery Areas (CHSDA), 624 counties comprising 54 percent of the U.S. American Indian/Alaska Native population; for more information, please see: Espey, D. K., Wu, X. C., Swan, J., et al. *Annual report to the nation on the status of cancer, 1975–2004,* featuring cancer in American Indians and Alaska Natives.

[‡]Persons of Hispanic/Latino origin may be of any race.

[§]Data unavailable from the Alaska Native Registry and Kentucky.

[¶]Data unavailable from Minnesota, New Hampshire, and North Dakota.

Source: Ries, L. A. G., Melbert, D., Krapcho, M., et al. (Eds.). (2007). SEER Cancer Statistics Review, 1975–2004. Bethesda, MD: National Cancer Institute, http://www.seer.cancer.gov/csr/1975_2004/ 2007. Permission to use granted by the American Cancer Society, Surveillance Research, 2008.

TABLE 13.4 Cancer Mortality Rates* by Site, Race, and Ethnicity, United States, 2000–2004.

Mortality	White	African American	Asian American and Pacific Islander	Native American and Alaska Native[†]	Hispanic/ Latino[‡¶]
All sites					
Males	234.7	321.8	141.7	187.9	162.2
Females	161.4	189.3	96.7	141.2	106.7
Breast (female)	25.0	33.8	12.6	16.1	16.1
Colon and rectum					
Males	22.9	32.7	15.0	20.6	17.0
Females	15.9	22.9	10.3	14.3	11.1

(Continued)

TABLE 13.4 (*Continued*).

Mortality	White	African American	Asian American and Pacific Islander	American Indian and Alaska Native[†]	Hispanic/ Latino[‡¶]
Kidney and renal pelvis					
Males	6.2	6.1	2.4	9.3	5.4
Females	2.8	2.8	1.1	4.3	2.3
Liver and bile duct					
Males	6.5	10.0	15.5	10.7	10.8
Females	2.8	3.9	6.7	6.4	5.0
Lung and bronchus					
Males	72.6	95.8	38.3	49.6	36.0
Females	42.1	39.8	18.5	32.7	14.6
Prostate	25.6	62.3	11.3	21.5	21.2
Stomach					
Males	5.2	11.9	10.5	9.6	9.1
Females	2.6	5.8	6.2	5.5	5.1
Uterine cervix	2.3	4.9	2.4	4.0	3.3

*Per 100,000, age adjusted to the 2000 U.S. standard population.

[†]Data based on Contract Health Service Delivery Areas (CHSDA), 624 counties comprising 54 percent of the U.S. American Indian/Alaska Native population; for more information, please see Espey, D. K., Wu, X. C., Swan, J., et al., *Annual report to the nation on the status of cancer, 1975–2004,* featuring cancer in American Indians and Alaska Natives.

[‡]Persons of Hispanic/Latino origin may be of any race.

[§]Data unavailable from the Alaska Native Registry and Kentucky.

[¶]Data unavailable from Minnesota, New Hampshire, and North Dakota.

Source: Ries, L. A. G., Melbert, D., Krapcho, M., et al. (Eds.). (2007). *SEER Cancer Statistics Review, 1975–2004.* Bethesda, MD: National Cancer Institute, http://www.seer.cancer.gov/csr/1975_2004/ Permission to use granted by the American Cancer Society, Surveillance Research, 2008.

and other minority populations from participating in cancer research. For example, African Americans and other minorities tend to have more negative attitudes towards participating in cancer studies than whites due to mistrust of the scientific community. Many African Americans and members of other minority groups believe that scientists who conduct health research should not be trusted since their main interest lies in conducting research rather than in helping those they are studying (Mouton et al., 1997; Paskett et al., 1996; Paskett et al., 2008). This skepticism and doubt of researchers may stem from negative past experiences or from mistrust that the scientific community has instilled in these populations through the years. For example, many members of the African American community remember the unethical Tuskegee Institute Syphilis Study, which was one of the most horrible scandals in American scientific history. It authorized scientists and medical professionals to monitor untreated syphilis among 400 African American men over a period of forty years (Brant, 1978). The men who participated in the study were never told they were participating in an experiment, and they were denied treatment for their condition. During the study, some men died and others became permanently blind or bore children with congenital syphilis (Brant, 1978).

In 1972, details about the Tuskegee Syphilis study were released in the national press (Brant, 1978). The Department of Health, Education and Welfare immediately stopped the experiment. Negative beliefs within minority populations still exist surrounding the Tuskegee Study. Such beliefs need to be acknowledged and then addressed through sincere efforts on behalf of scientists to reestablish trust. Otherwise, mistrust will continue to impede the recruitment, participation, and retention of African Americans and other minorities in cancer research.

RISK FACTORS, SYMPTOMS, AND TREATMENT OPTIONS FOR THE FOUR LEADING CANCERS

The following four sections review current epidemiological information regarding the four leading cancers—lung and bronchus, breast, prostate, and colon and rectum—with emphasis on the status of African Americans. Much of the information presented here has been gleaned from the American Cancer Society's *Facts and Figures* published in 2008. Specific data on cancer incidence and mortality rates for African Americans are shown in Tables 13.3 through 13.6.

Cancer of the Lung and Bronchus

It was estimated that 215,020 new cases of cancer involving the lung and bronchus would be diagnosed in 2008, accounting for 15 percent of all cancer diagnoses (ACS, 2008a). Although the incidence of these cancers is continuing to decline in the general population, rates among women are starting to plateau. This leveling off comes after increases over many years. There are two general classifications of lung cancer: small cell and non-small cell. Of these two types, non-small cell is more prevalent, accounting for 87 percent of all cases (ACS, 2008a).

TABLE 13.5 **Top Ten New Cancer Diagnoses among African Americans, 2007 Estimates.**

	Male			Female		
Rank	Site	Cases	%	Site	Cases	%
1	Prostate	30,870	37	Breast	19,010	27
2	Lung and bronchus	12,490	15	Lung and bronchus	9,060	13
3	Colon and rectum	7,860	9	Colon and rectum	8,580	12
4	Kidney and renal pelvis	3,280	4	Uterine corpus	3,420	5
5	Non-Hodgkin lymphoma	2,640	3	Pancreas	2,310	3
6	Oral cavity and pharynx	2,590	3	Kidney and renal pelvis	2,310	3
7	Pancreas	2,080	3	Non-Hodgkin lymphoma	2,240	3
8	Urinary bladder	2,050	3	Myeloma	1,920	3
9	Myeloma	1,940	2	Uterine cervix	1,910	3
10	Liver and intrahepatic bile duct	1,880	2	Ovary	1,770	3
	All sites	83,240		All Sites	69,660	

* Excludes basal and squamous cell skin cancers and in situ carcinoma except urinary bladder.
Note: Estimates are rounded to the nearest 10. Permission to use granted by the American Cancer Society, Surveillance Research, 2007.

Lung cancer accounts for the greatest number of cancer-related deaths for both sexes. It was estimated that more than 160,000 people would die of lung cancer in 2008, for a total of 29 percent of all cancer deaths occurring during that year (ACS, 2008a). It is important to note that lung cancer kills more women than breast cancer. Lung cancer death rates have been declining over the last decade. This decline is attributed to the decreased smoking rates over the past thirty years.

Although the incidence rates for lung cancer in African American males have declined in recent years, they remain significantly higher (110.6) than the rates for members of other racial or ethnic groups (whites, 81; Asian/Pacific Islanders, 55.1; Hispanics, 53.7; and Native Americans, 44.7), as shown in Table 13.3 (ACS, 2008b). Researchers

TABLE 13.6 **Top Ten Causes of New Cancer Deaths among African Americans, 2007 Estimates.**

		Male			Female		
Rank	Site	Cases	%	Site	Cases	%
1	Lung and bronchus	9,970	31	Lung and bronchus	6,730	22
2	Prostate	4,240	13	Breast	5,830	19
3	Colon and rectum	3,420	11	Colon and rectum	3,650	12
4	Pancreas	1,700	5	Pancreas	2,000	6
5	Liver and intrahepatic bile duct	1,430	5	Ovary	1,290	4
6	Stomach	1,130	4	Uterine corpus	1,220	4
7	Leukemia	980	3	Myeloma	990	3
8	Esophagus	950	3	Leukemia	890	3
9	Myeloma	860	3	Stomach	820	3
10	Oral cavity and pharynx	840	3	Uterine cervix	720	2
	All sites	22,120		All Sites	24,140	

Note: Estimates are rounded to the nearest 10. Permission to use granted by the American Cancer Society, Surveillance Research, 2007.

have tried to discover reasons for the high incidence of lung and bronchus cancers in African American males by hypothesizing about physiological differences. For example, some conclude that African Americans may be at a higher risk of developing lung and bronchus cancer because they tend to metabolize serum cotinine (a major metabolite of nicotine) at a lower rate than members of other racial or ethnic groups, suggesting that it is more difficult for this minority population to quit smoking (Perez-Stable et al., 1998). Other studies that have examined the role of genetic factors as a predisposing factor for lung and bronchial cancer found that smoking patterns and not polymorphic gene variance was a greater determining factor for the increased risk among African Americans (Guillemette, 2003). Nevertheless, these biological and inherited differences warrant further investigation before they are used as the basis for definite conclusions.

Cancer of the Breast

For the year 2008, 182,460 new cases of breast cancer were expected to occur in the United States, and of these, approximately 1,990 were expected to occur among men (ACS, 2008a). Excluding cancers of the skin, breast cancer is the most frequently diagnosed cancer in women. White women have higher rates of breast cancer than women in any other group. However, the incidence of breast cancer in white women is highest among those who are 40 years and older, while African American women have a higher incidence of cancer at age 40 and under (ACS, 2008b). Incidence and mortality rates for both white and African American women remain higher than the rates for women in other ethnic and racial groups. Between these two groups, the incidence is higher in white women, but death rates are greater among African American women.

African American women suffer from the highest mortality rate for breast cancer of all ethnic groups, and they are less likely than white women to survive five years post-diagnosis (ACS, 2008b). The five-year survival rate for white women is 90 percent, while African American women have a survival rate of only 77 percent (ACS, 2008b). Differences in survival observed among these two racial groups may be attributed to stage at diagnosis, tumor characteristics, comorbidity, socioeconomic factors, and difficulty accessing the health care system (health literacy) (ACS, 2008b). Thus, increased availability of screening, improved health literacy, and access to a continuum of care among African American women may help to improve their survival rates.

Disparities in breast cancer rates may also have biological implications. A national breast cancer survey conducted by the American College of Surgeons compared data from 2,400 African American women and 24,000 white women with breast cancer (Natarjan et al., 1999). The results indicated that African American women were less likely to have positive estrogen receptors in their primary tumors. In addition, African American women have poorer survival rates when matched with white women who have the same tumor stage and estrogen receptor status (Houchens & Merajver, 2008). Significant differences were also observed between African American and white female patients for family history of breast cancer, age at first pregnancy, number of pregnancies, and age at menopause. This has led to the question of whether there are differences between these groups on other variables, such as oncogene patterns.

Preliminary data from current, ongoing work conducted by Dr. Lovell A. Jones et al. (unpublished) indicate that non-protein bound and albumin bound estradiol serum fractions may be higher in young African American women than in white women. It is possible that all of these hormonal differences may be related to cultural variables such as diet. Therefore, further study of the influence of cultural practices on biomarkers may provide new insights into the etiology of cancer among the general population.

Cancer of the Prostate

Prostate cancer is the most common type of cancer among American men. The American Cancer Society estimated that about 186,320 new cases of prostate cancer would be diagnosed in the United States in 2008 and about 28,660 men would die of the disease (ACS, 2008a). One man in six will get prostate cancer during his lifetime, and one man in thirty five will die of this disease (ACS, 2008a). However, African American men have a far higher death rate from prostate cancer than members of any other racial or ethnic group in the United States (ACS, 2008b).

Differences in incidence and survival rates among African American men with prostate cancer may be linked to differences in treatment. African American men with advanced prostate cancer are less likely than white men to receive surgical treatment (ACS, 2008b). Lack of access to the most effective treatment options may account for the higher mortality rate observed in African American men with advanced disease. Thus, the health care industry may also contribute to the poor outcomes observed in racial and ethnic minority populations with regard to cancer survival.

Prostate cancer can often be found early by testing the amount of PSA (prostate-specific antigen) in the blood. Prostate cancer also can be found at an early stage when the doctor does a digital rectal exam (DRE). Because the prostate gland lies just in front of the rectum, during the DRE the doctor can detect any bumps or hard places on the prostate. These tests are not perfect, however. Uncertain or false test results could cause confusion and anxiety. There is no question that the PSA test can help spot prostate cancer, but it cannot tell how dangerous the cancer is. Some prostate cancers are slow-growing and may never cause problems.

Due to these issues, screening for prostate cancer has become a topic of lively discussion. While the American Cancer Society does not recommend routine testing for prostate cancer at this time, many health professionals continue to do routine testing. In any case, it is important to discuss the pros and cons of testing with men so that each man can decide if testing is right for him. If a man chooses to be tested, the tests should include a PSA blood test and DRE (digital rectal exam) yearly, beginning at age 50, for men at average risk who can be expected to live at least 10 more years. For men deemed to be at higher risk, including African American men, discussion of testing should begin as early as age 40.

Cancer of the Colon and Rectum

The American Cancer Society estimated that about 108,070 new cases of colon cancer and 40,740 new cases of rectal cancer would be diagnosed in the United States in 2008 and that about 49,960 people would die from the disease. The incidence of colorectal cancer has decreased over the last two decades, with the improvement attributed mostly to increased screening for the disease and removal of precancerous polyps (ACS, 2008a). The death rate from colorectal cancer has been going down for the past twenty-four years among both men and women. Not only has early detection played a role, but improved therapies may have had an impact. However, there are racial differences in mortality rates for African Americans and whites.

Prior to 1980, colorectal cancer death rates were higher in whites than in African American men; numbers were similar in women of both races. Since then, researchers have seen a marked divergence: while colorectal cancer incidence and death rates have plummeted among whites, rates among African Americans and members of other minority groups have declined far more slowly. In 2005, the mortality rates were about 48 percent higher in African American men and women than in whites (ACS, 2008b).

In addition to lagging screening numbers, studies have shown that insurance status plays a big role in survival. A report published by the American Cancer Society found that uninsured Americans were less likely to receive screening for cancer, more likely to be diagnosed with an advanced stage of the disease, and less likely to survive that diagnosis than their privately insured counterparts (Ward, 2008). This report also showed that among African Americans, the five-year survival rate for colorectal cancer was 30 percent higher among patients who were privately insured than for those without health insurance (Ward, 2008).

Studies have also shown that African American patients are more likely than whites to be diagnosed when the disease is in its later stages; they are also less likely to receive the recommended surgery, chemotherapy, and radiation treatment after a cancer diagnosis. As indicated in Tables 13.3 and 13.4, more African Americans develop and die from colon and rectum cancer than members of all the other groups, with rates almost three times those of Native Americans and twice those of Hispanics. Among both male and female African Americans, colon and rectum cancer is the third leading cancer diagnosis. In the United States, colorectal cancer mortality decreased between 1975 and 1989 among whites but increased among African American males (26%) and females (20%). Today, mortality rates among African Americans are still higher than those of any other racial or ethnic group (ACS, 2008a).

NEEDED ACTIONS—IMPLICATIONS FOR AFRICAN AMERICANS AND OTHER MINORITY POPULATIONS

To reduce the incidence and mortality of cancer and improve survival rates among the African American population, many improvements are needed. First, research efforts must shift from simply identifying the existence of cancer disparities to finding ways to address the unique barriers, beliefs, and discrimination concerns of the African American population (Blocker et al., 2006; Wray et al., 2009). We strongly urge that culturally appropriate strategies be developed to attract African American participants into clinical and epidemiological cancer studies. For example, we recommend that researchers take into account religiosity and spirituality among African Americans (Katz et al., 2004; Husaini et al., 2008; Kinney et al., 2009), community resources (Caburnay et al., 2008), and the important roles played by family members and spouses (Blocker et al., 2006).

We also encourage researchers to consider geographic and regional characteristics that may differentiate African Americans from other populations in the United States. All too often, much emphasis is placed on the racial classification with little regard to ethnic or geographical differences among African Americans. Jones et al. (2006) indicate that data often fails to capture existing regional and ethnic differences in the African American population, as well as other ethnic groups. African Americans are as diverse as other ethnic and racial populations, as reflected by Americans of African heritage from Nigeria, Ethiopia, South Africa, or the West Indies, in addition to

Hispanics and others. It can also be argued that geographic differences within the United States may have significant impact on outcomes, the availability of resources, and standards of care. Being an African American in west Alabama can mean something culturally and regionally very different from being African American in the San Francisco Bay Area or in Atlanta. Thus, the current system of research does not satisfactorily elucidate the racial, ethnic, or geographical differences observed.

In addition, mistrust of the scientific community by African Americans must be taken into consideration. Such beliefs need to be acknowledged and addressed through ongoing positive interactions and relationships. The "face" of the scientific community should also change. Cancer institutions conducting research need to include investigators who reflect the racial or ethnic composition of their study participants to foster trust and manifest a caring attitude toward minority populations (Mouton et al., 1997; Paskett et al., 2008). If these changes are not made, mistrust will continue to obstruct the recruitment and participation of African Americans in cancer studies.

Lack of health insurance is another important factor that must be addressed to reduce cancer incidence and mortality and to improve survival rates. African Americans, other minority populations, and the economically disadvantaged may suffer disproportionately from lack of health insurance coverage. Finally, disadvantages in health insurance coverage exist among the unemployed, as most Americans are insured through an employer. Survival of cancer and other serious illnesses is related to insurance and employability, as people who develop such illnesses may not be able to keep their jobs and thus are likely to lose their insurance coverage.

Our specific recommendations include the following:

1. Development of improved health policy about health insurance coverage that includes screening and treatment components. Insurance coverage should be available and affordable for all, include a simple and fair policy for coverage, and be sustainable for those who lose employment because of a serious illness.

2. Examination of the relationship between cancer and the cancer risks associated with the African American population through quality behavioral and epidemiological research.

3. Initiation of improved descriptive and analytic cancer studies recognizing that African Americans are not all alike, either genetically or culturally, and collection of data emphasizing these differences.

4. Development of culturally sensitive methodologies that provide appropriate cancer information to the African American population.

5. Equal inclusion of African Americans in clinical and behavioral cancer research trials. Inclusion should be properly enforced by withdrawing funding from institutions that are guilty of non-compliance.

6. Increased efforts to build trust in African American communities, resulting in more successful recruitment and retention of African Americans in cancer clinical trials.

7. Increased hiring of qualified investigators who reflect the racial or ethnic composition of the study participants to improve trust levels and create a perception of a caring attitude toward members of minority groups.

8. Dissemination of research findings in a manner that can be made available to the African American community at large.

If cancer research among African Americans is redesigned to incorporate these recommendations, accurate cancer information may be obtained to ultimately decrease the higher incidence and mortality rates while improving the poor survival rates of the African American population.

REFERENCES

American Cancer Society. (2008a). *Cancer facts & figures 2008*. Atlanta: Author.

American Cancer Society. (2008b). *Cancer facts & figures for African Americans 2007–2008*. Atlanta: Author.

American Society of Clinical Oncology (ASCO). (2006). *Understanding tumor markers*. Retrieved February 6, 2009, from www.cancer.net/patient/Library/Cancer.Net+Features/Treatments%2C+Tests%2C+and+Procedures/Understanding+Tumor+Markers.

Bacquet, C., & Ringen, K. (1986). Cancer among blacks and other minorities. Washington, DC: National Institutes of Health.

Blocker, D. E., Romocki, L. S., Thomas, K. B., Jones, B. L., Jackson, E. J., Reid, L., et al. (2006). Knowledge, beliefs, and barriers associated with prostate cancer prevention and screening behaviors among African American men. *Journal of the American Medical Association, 98*, 8.

Brant A. (1978). Racism and research: The case of the Tuskegee Syphilis Study. *The Hastings Center Magazine* Hudson, NY: The Hastings Center Institute of Society, Ethics and the Life Sciences.

Caburnay, C. A., Kreuter, M. W., Cameron, G., Luke, D. A., Cohen, E. L., McDaniels, L., et al. (2008). Black newspaper as a tool for cancer education in African American communities. *Ethnicity & Disease 18*, 488–495.

Edwards, B. K., Brown, M. L., Wingo, P. A., et al. (2005). Annual report to the nation on the status of cancer, 1975–2002, featuring population-based trends in cancer treatment. *Journal of the National Cancer Institute, 97*, 1407–1427.

Espey, D.K., Wu, X. C., Swan, J., et al. (2007). Annual report to the nation on the status of cancer, 1975–2004, featuring cancer in Native Americans and Alaska Natives. *Cancer, 110*(10): 2119–2152.

Finn, R. S., Dering, J., Ginther, C., Wilson, C. A., Glaspy, P., Tchekmedyian, N., et al. (2007). Dasatinib, an orally active small molecule inhibitor of both the src and abl kinases, selectively inhibits growth of basal-type/ "triple-negative" breast cancer cell lines growing in vitro. *Breast Cancer Research and Treatment, 105*(3), 319–326.

Gross, C. P., Smith, B. D., Wolf, E., & Anderson, M. (2008). Racial disparities in cancer therapy: Did the gap narrow between 1992 and 2002? *Cancer, 112*(4):900–908.

Guillemette, C. (2003). Pharmacogenomics of human UDP-glucuronosyltransferase enzymes. *Pharmacogenomics Journal, 3*, 136–158.

Haynes, M. A.., & Smedley, B. D. (Eds.). (1999). *The unequal burden of cancer: An assessment of NIH research and programs for ethnic minorities and the medically underserved*. Washington, DC: National Academies Press.

Houchens, N. W., & Merajver, S. D. (2008). Molecular determinants of the inflammatory breast cancer phenotype. *Oncology (Williston Park), 22* (14): 1556–1561, discussion 1561, 1565–1568, 1576.

Husaini, B. A., Reece, M. C., Emerson, J. S., Scales, S., Hull, P. C., & Levine, R. S. (2008). A church-based program on prostate cancer screening for African American men: Reducing health disparities. *Ethnicity & Disease, 18*, S2-179–S2-184.

Jones, L. A. (Ed.). (1989). *Minorities and cancer*. New York: Springer-Verlag, 1989.

Jones, L. A., et al. (2006). Between and within: International perspectives on cancer and health disparities. *Journal of Clinical Oncology, 24*(14), 2204–2208.

Katz, M. L., James, A. S., Pignone, M. P., Hudson, M. A., Jackson, E., Oates, V., et al. (2004). Colorectal cancer screening among African American church members: A qualitative and quantitative study of patient-provider communication. *BMC Public Health, 4*, 62.

Kinney, A. Y., Coxworth, J. E., Simonson, S. E., & Fanning, J. B. (2009). Religiosity, spirituality, and psychological distress in African-Americans at risk for having a hereditary cancer predisposing gene mutation. *American Journal of Medical Genetics, Part C, 151C*, 13–21.

Kornblau, S. M., Tibes, R., Qiu, Y.H., Chen, W., Kantarjian, H. M., Andreeff, M., et al. (2009). Functional proteomic profiling of AML predicts response and survival. *Blood, 113*(1), 154–64.

Laxman, B., Morris, D. S., Yu, J., Siddiqui, J., Cao, J., Mehra, R., et al. (2008). A first-generation multiplex biomarker analysis of urine for the early detection of prostate cancer. *Cancer Research, 68*(3), 645–649.

Mouton, C. P., Harris, S.. Rovi, S., et al. (1997). Barriers to black women's participation in cancer clinical trials. *Journal of the National Medical Association, 89*(11), 721–727.

Natarjan, N., Nemoto, T., Mettlin, C., & Murphy, G. P. (1999). Race-related differences in breast cancer patients. *Cancer, 56*, 1704–1709.

National Cancer Institute. (1999). *Cancer care issues in the United States: Quality of care, quality of life*. President's Cancer Panel, January 1, 1997–December 31, 1998. Bethesda, MD: National Cancer Program.

National Cancer Institute. (2009). Tumor markers: Questions and answers. Retrieved February 6, 2009, from www.cancer.gov/cancertopics/factsheet/Detection/tumor-markers

Paskett, E. D., DeGraffinreid, C., Tatum, C. M., & Margitic, S. E. (1996). The recruitment of African-Americans to cancer prevention and control studies. *Preventive Medicine, 25*(5), 547–553.

Paskett, E. D., Reeves, K. W., McLaughlin, J. M., Katz, M. L., McAlearney, A., Ruffin, M. T., et al. (2008). Recruitment of minority and underserved populations in the United States: The centers for population health and health disparities experience. *Contemporary Clinical Trials, 28*(6), 847–861.

Perez-Stable, E. J., Herrera, B., Jacob, P., & Benowitz, N. L. (1998). Nicotine metabolism and intake in black and white smokers. *Journal of the American Medical Association, 280*, 152–156.

Ries, L. A. G., Melbert, D., Krapcho, M., Stinchcomb, D. G., Howlader, N., Horner, M. J., et al. (2007). *SEER Cancer Statistics Review, 1975–2005*. Bethesda, MD: National Cancer Institute.

Schumacher, F. R., Feigelson, H. S., Cox, D. G., Haiman, C. A., Albanes, D., Buring, J., et al. (2007). A common 8q24 variant in prostate and breast cancer from a large nested case-control study. *Cancer Research, 67*(7), 2951–2956.

Sedjo, R. L., Byers, T., Barrera, E., Cohen, A., Fontham, E. T. H., et al. (2007). A midpoint assessment of the American Cancer Society challenge goal to decrease cancer incidence by 25% between 1992 and 2015. *Cancer Journal for Clinicians, 57*, 326–340.

Smedley, B. D., Stith, A. Y., & Nelson, A. R. (2003). *Unequal treatment: Confronting racial and ethnic disparities in healthcare*. Washington, DC: Institute of Medicine, The National Academies Press.

Virnig, B. E., Baxter, N. N., Habermann, E. B., Feldman, R. D., & Bradley, C. J. (2009). A matter of race: Early-versus late-stage cancer diagnosis. *Health Affairs, 28*, 1.

Ward, E. (2008) Association of insurance with cancer care utilization and outcomes. *CA: A Cancer Journal for Clinicians, 58*(1).

Wray, R. J., McClure, S., Vijaykumar, S., Smith, C., Ivy, A., Jupka, K., et al. (2009). Changing the conversation about prostate cancer among African Americans: Results of formative research. *Ethnicity & Health, 14*(1), 27–43.

Yeager, M., Orr, N., Hayes, R. B., Jacobs, K. B., Kraft, P., Wacholder, S., et al. (2007). Genome-wide association study of prostate cancer identifies a second risk locus at 8q24. *Nature Genetics, 39*(5), 645–649.

14

HEALTH DISPARITIES: THE CASE FOR DIABETES

GREGORY STRAYHORN

Diabetes mellitus pis a spectrum of diseases in which a significant elevation of blood glucose (sugar) causes deleterious effects on multiple body systems. Diabetes can be divided into three major insulin deficits: production, action, or both. Failure to produce insulin in the pancreas, known as Type I diabetes or juvenile diabetes, occurs when the body's immune system destroys pancreatic beta cells where insulin is produced and secreted. Type I diabetes represents between 5 and 10 percent of all cases of diabetes mellitus. The most prevalent form of diabetes mellitus, Type II, represents between 90 and 95 percent of all cases. Type II diabetes is caused initially by the failure of cells to properly use insulin, known as insulin resistance. Over time, as the pancreas increases its production of insulin to compensate for insulin resistance, pancreatic beta cells become exhausted and lose their ability to produce insulin. Thus, both a deficit in insulin production and a dysfunction in insulin action ensue. If not managed, the resulting high levels of glucose lead to serious health complications and contribute to premature death. A third form of diabetes mellitus, gestational diabetes, involves insulin resistance during pregnancy. If not effectively managed, gestational diabetes increases chances of complications to pregnant women and their infants. In 2007, direct medical costs of diabetes amounted to approximately $116 billion, which is 2.3 times the total medical expenditures for non-diabetic patients. Indirect costs such as disability, work loss, and premature mortality added up to $58 billion (CDC, 2009c).

EPIDEMIOLOGY AND DISPARITIES OF DIABETES PREVALENCE

In 2007, the Centers for Disease Control and Prevention (CDC) estimated that 23.6 million people, or 7.8 percent of the U.S. population, had diabetes. Of these cases, 17.9 million were diagnosed and 5.7 million undiagnosed. Before diagnosis, people may have diabetes for eight to ten years. The prevalence of diabetes increases with age, comprising 10.7 percent of people over 20 years of age and 23.1 percent of people over the age of 60 years. The prevalence of diabetes in men and women over the age of 20 years is similar: 11.2 percent and 10.2 percent, respectively. The vast majority of patients diagnosed with diabetes are between 40 and 59 years old. Non-Hispanic blacks tend to be diagnosed at an average age of 49.7 years, as compared with 51.8 years for non-Hispanic whites. Although the prevalence of diagnosed diabetes in people younger than 20 years is 0.2 percent, the diagnosis of Type II diabetes in this group is increasing, especially in the 10–19-year-old age group. The rate of newly diagnosed Type II diabetes cases is higher among minority populations in this age group. Over the past 15 years the prevalence of diagnosed diabetes has more than doubled and is expected to double again by 2050 (CDC, 2008).

In comparison with non-Hispanic whites aged 20 years or older, the prevalence of diagnosed diabetes in non-Hispanic blacks is 1.5 times greater—9.8 percent versus 14.5 percent, respectively. The disparities in diagnosed diabetes cases between non-Hispanic whites and non-Hispanic blacks remain until age 65 years. Diabetes prevalence in non-Hispanic black women aged 65 to 74 years is 34.0 percent—more than double the rate of 15.2 percent for black women 40 to 64 years old. Thus, middle-aged and older non-Hispanic black women are at a significantly high risk of developing Type II diabetes (CDC, 2008).

Prediabetes, or impaired glucose tolerance or impaired fasting glucose, is a progenitor of Type II diabetes that also portends increased risk of heart disease and stroke. Prediabetes indicates that glucose levels are higher than normal but do not meet the criteria for diabetes. Among adults 20 years or older, 26 percent had impaired fasting glucose. The prevalence of prediabetes among non-Hispanic blacks does not significantly differ from that of non-Hispanic whites: 21.1 percent versus 25.1 percent (CDC, 2008).

ADVERSE EFFECTS OF DIABETES

Diabetes is the seventh leading cause of death in the United States, and for those with diabetes, age-adjusted risk of death is double the risk of those without diabetes. Diabetes also is associated with a significant disease burden. Adults with diabetes have a significantly higher risk of stroke, hypertension, blindness, kidney disease including kidney failure requiring dialysis, nervous system disease that leads to impaired sensation and pain in feet and hands, gastrointestinal dysfunction, erectile dysfunction and other nerve problems, lower extremity amputations, dental disease, complications of pregnancy, peripheral vascular disease that impairs walking and other activities of movement, increased death from pneumonia and influenza, and life-threatening acute problems such as diabetic ketoacidosis and hyperosmolar coma (CDC, 2009a).

Age-adjusted death rates related to diabetic ketoacidosis, an acute complication of diabetes that is life-threatening if not aggressively and immediately treated, declined significantly from 1980 to 2001. However, the 2001 death rate from this condition among non-Hispanic black men (56.5/100,000) remained significantly higher than that for other sex-race groups (3.5 times greater than non-Hispanic white women and 2.5 times greater than non-Hispanic white men and non-Hispanic black women). The death rate from this condition among non-Hispanic black women (22.6/100,000) is similar to that of non-Hispanic white men (21.7/100,000), with the lowest death rate among non-Hispanic white women (15.3/100,000). The disparity among non-Hispanic black men may be attributed to poorer self- and medical management of diabetes, insufficient access to medical care, and delay of adequate treatment (CDC, 2009a).

Non-Hispanic black men and women with diabetes have similar prevalence of self-reported cardiovascular disease conditions. Non-Hispanic black women have the lowest prevalence (28.9%) while non-Hispanic white men have the highest prevalence (38.7%). Non-Hispanic white women and black men have similar prevalence: 30.7 percent versus 31.3 percent, respectively (CDC, 2009a).

Age-adjusted hospital discharge diagnosis rates for diabetic non-Hispanic blacks and whites declined steadily from 1993 to 1999. However, there was a gradual upturn in the rate from 2001 to 2003. During these periods, non-Hispanic blacks had consistently higher rates than non-Hispanic whites. In 2003, the rate for non-Hispanic blacks was 17.3 percent, compared with 12.9 percent for non-Hispanic whites (CDC, 2009a; Jiang et al., 2009).

The 2002 age-adjusted incidence of end-stage renal disease (ESRD) per 100,000 diabetic patients was significantly higher among non-Hispanic black men and women than among non-Hispanic white men and women. Non-Hispanic black men had the highest incidence of ESRD. The 2005 age-adjusted prevalence of visual impairment among diabetes patients was similar for non-Hispanic black (18.0%) and white adults (17.7%) (CDC, 2009a). With some exceptions, the quality-of-life effects of diabetes on non-Hispanic black and white patients were similar. In 2005, between 37 and 58 percent of diabetic patients reported mobility limitations. More than 50 percent of non-Hispanic black and white women reported mobility limitations, while non-Hispanic black men reported the lowest prevalence, 37.7 percent, as compared with non-Hispanic white men at 44.6 percent. Of non-Hispanic blacks and whites with diabetes, 35 percent reported an inability to do usual activities at least one day during the past 30 days. In 2004, non-Hispanic black and white diabetic patients reported similar prevalence of poor mental health in the past 30 days: 41.9 percent and 43.6 percent, respectively (CDC, 2009a).

PREVENTION OF DIABETES

Evidence from randomized controlled trials demonstrates that the onset of Type II diabetes mellitus can be delayed or prevented in prediabetic individuals. The Diabetes

Prevention Research Group conducted a multicenter randomized controlled trial in the United States that sought to determine whether an intensive lifestyle intervention (prescribed exercise regimen, diet, and weight loss expectations) or treatment with metformin (a medication used to treat Type II diabetes), compared to placebo, would decrease the incidence of Type II diabetes. Over a four-year period non-Hispanic black participants, who represented approximately 20 percent of the 3,234 participants, showed similar reductions of Type II diabetes incidence in comparison with non-Hispanic whites. This study showed the efficacy of a structured intensive lifestyle intervention with participants of multiple ethnicities, but the long-term effectiveness of such an approach has not been determined in community and clinical setting (Diabetes Prevention Program Research Group, 2002; Bank, 2009). The cost of such a program could be prohibitive in usual clinical settings (Bank, 2009; Russell, 2009; Goetzel, 2009). Based on the current evidence from randomized controlled clinical trials, the American Diabetes Association offers the following recommendations for prediabetic individuals (American Diabetes Association, 2008a):

- Screen high-risk patients for impaired glucose intolerance (IGT) or impaired fasting glucose (IFG) every three years;

- Refer patients with IGT or IFG to support programs for weight management with a goal for overweight or obese patients to lose 5 to 10 percent of body weight and increase their participation in moderate physical activities to at least 150 minutes per week;

- Provide follow-up counseling;

- Consider the use of metformin in high-risk patients who are younger than 60, obese, have elevated lipids, hypertension, and family history of diabetes;

- Conduct annual monitoring for diabetes.

Modifiable Risk Factors to Prevent or Limit Diabetes-Related Medical Complications

Numerous medical and behavioral risk factors can be modified to limit medical complications associated with diabetes. Preventive strategies include effective management of hypertension, reduction of high cholesterol, weight control, increased physical activity; and smoking cessation. Between 2003 and 2004, the reported prevalence of these risk factors among non-Hispanic black and white diabetic patients was high, and for some, similar (CDC, 2009a).

The reported prevalence of high cholesterol was 50.9 percent and 50.8 percent and smoking was 23.4 percent and 23.9 percent, respectively, for non-Hispanic black and white diabetic patients. The prevalence of combined overweight and obesity (87.3% versus 82.4%), obesity (59.7% versus 53.1%), hypertension (63.1% versus 51.9%), and physical inactivity (38.3% versus 32.0%) tended to be higher for non-Hispanic black patients than for non-Hispanic white diabetic patients, respectively (CDC, 2009a).

Prevention of the Adverse Health Outcomes of Diabetes Mellitus

Once there is an established diagnosis of diabetes, success in decreasing the prevalence and incidence of adverse health outcomes, morbidity, and mortality depends on maintaining glucose levels in an acceptable range and reducing modifiable risk factors. Procedures for meeting these goals have been established through evidence-based clinical guidelines recommended by organizations such as the American Diabetes Association (ADA), the National Committee for Quality Assurance (NCQA), and the Agency for Healthcare Research and Quality (AHRQ). The recommended guidelines can be categorized as clinical, preventive, and self-management (Table 14.1).

Affordable and accessible health care and support services are important factors in assisting diabetic patients to follow the recommended guidelines and decrease their risk for diabetes-associated adverse health outcomes. Looking at three recommended services (hgb A1c, retinal eye examination, and foot examination) from 2002 to 2004, there was no interval change in the proportion of non-Hispanic blacks and whites who complied with the three recommendations. According to AHRQ, in 2004 there were no significant black-white differences in rates of compliance with these recommendations: 46.7 percent compared with 47.4 percent, respectively. However, studies in

TABLE 14.1   **Recommendations for Preventing Adverse Health Outcomes of Diabetes Mellitus.**

Clinical
- Annual dilated eye examinations
- Annual comprehensive foot examination
- Annual assessment of lipid control and management
- Three- to six-month assessment of glucose control using hemoglobin A1c and management
- Annual assessment of kidney function
- Assessment of blood pressure control and management

Preventive
- Annual influenza vaccination
- Pneumococcal vaccination
- Daily use of aspirin

Self-Management/Lifestyle Modification
- Diabetes education
- Regular self-management of blood glucose
- Moderate regular physical activity
- Weight control
- Daily self-exam of feet
- Smoking cessation

managed care settings have shown that the measurement of Hemoglobin A1c levels is significantly lower among non-Hispanic blacks. Non-Hispanic blacks who are enrolled in managed care settings, including Medicare managed care, receive dilated eye examinations, nephropathy assessment, and foot examinations at similar or higher rates than non-Hispanic whites (U.S. Department of Health and Human Services, 2008).

Receipt of recommended services is important for the control and improvement of intermediate clinical parameters (control of glucose level, lipids, and hypertension) that can help patients avoid diabetes-associated adverse clinical outcomes. The proportion of non-Hispanic blacks with control of diabetes as measured by hgb A1c and recommended by clinical guidelines did not significantly change between 1988–1994 and 1999–2004. Non-Hispanic blacks had a slight decline in achievement of hgb A1c levels at or below the recommended level, with only 36.6 percent achieving this level between 1999 and 2004. Non-Hispanic whites saw a significant improvement during the same period, from 40 percent to 55.7 percent. Both non-Hispanic black and white diabetic patients had significant increases in the proportion with cholesterol levels at or below the recommended level. However, the gap between non-Hispanic blacks and whites remained the same, although it was not statistically significant. Yet, in studies where the recommended services are considered good and controlled for in multivariate analyses, non-Hispanic blacks are significantly less likely to have control of their glucose and lipid levels at the recommended levels (U.S. DHHS, 2008).

With regard to preventive services, non-Hispanic blacks are significantly less likely than whites to receive the influenza vaccination. This difference appears to be related to their refusal to receive the vaccination rather than to limitations in its availability. Non-Hispanic blacks are more likely to express concerns about the adverse effects of the vaccination, especially if they know someone who developed a serious influenza infection after receiving the vaccine. Studies in managed care settings find no disparity in aspirin use between non-Hispanic black and white diabetic patients in managed care settings (Kenrick et al., 2006; Hebert et al., 2005; Schneider et al., 2001). Comparing behavioral recommendations, non-Hispanic blacks have higher rates of daily glucose self-monitoring and lower rates of smoking (CDC, 2009a; Self-monitoring, 2007). However, they tend to be more obese and less physically active (CDC, 2009a). In controlled trials that include nutrition and physical activity interventions, non-Hispanic black participants show similar improvements in diabetes and lipid control and weight decline (Diabetes Prevention Program Research Group, 2002).

ACCESS TO HEALTH CARE RESOURCES

Although access to affordable and quality health care is key to the receipt of recommended serves for diabetes care and the prevention of diabetes-associated adverse health outcomes, disparities continue to exist in health care settings where cost and access to care should not pose barriers. In health care settings that implemented recommended strategies to improve the quality of diabetes care (physician reminders, physician feedback, and diabetes registries), researchers found that disparities of care depended on the intensity of the strategy but that there were no consistent disparity patterns. Examples of disparities include non-Hispanic blacks being less likely to receive influenza vaccination, regardless of the intensity of care, across all strategies. While non-Hispanic blacks were less likely to receive LDL-cholesterol testing in programs with low-intensity use of physician feedback and diabetes registries, they were also less likely to receive this testing in settings with high-intensity use of physician reminders. Similarly, non-Hispanic blacks were less likely to receive hgb A1c testing in settings with high-intensity use of physician reminders and low-intensity use of physician feedback. Comparing black-white differences in medication management of hgb A1c, non-Hispanic blacks were less likely to receive the expected management in programs with high-intensity use of registries and physician reminders and low-intensity use of physician feedback. Non-Hispanic blacks tended to receive recommended medical management of systolic blood pressure across all strategy approaches and levels of intensity, but not for medication management of LDL cholesterol. Thus, disparities in care of intermediate clinical outcomes showed no consistent pattern related to differences in the intensity of care using various recommended strategies (Kenrick et al., 2006).

Most studies that have been conducted to date demonstrate that improved access to diabetes care for non-Hispanic blacks narrows or eliminates disparities related to the processes of diabetes care. However, limited or no effects are found with regard to the improvement of disparities in the intermediate outcomes (glucose, lipids, and hypertension) that are important for the prevention of adverse health outcomes associated with cardiovascular diseases (Trivedi et al., 2005; Chou et al., 2005; Safford et al., 2003; Adams et al., 2005; Selby et al., 2007). Continued disparities in these intermediate outcomes are generally attributed to factors related to individual patients and their environmental conditions outside of medical care resources. Management of intermediate outcomes depends on patients' ability to afford recommended actions and activities. Income and out-of-pocket expenses have been shown to have similar effects on medication underuse by non-Hispanic black and white patients (Tseng et al., 2008; American Diabetes Association, 2008b; Karter et al., 2003). Neighborhood characteristics (crime, trash, litter, poor lighting at night, and lack of access to exercise facilities, transportation, and supermarkets) are associated with health behaviors and diabetes outcomes of adult diabetic patients in managed care. A cross-sectional study found that the most problematic neighborhoods were associated with higher rates of smoking, less physical activity, poor blood pressure control, and lower scores on perception of physical and mental health among non-Hispanic black patients (Gary et al., 2008).

INTERVENTIONS TAILORED TO THE PATIENT'S CULTURAL BACKGROUND AND LITERACY LEVEL

Tailoring clinical interventions to patients' cultural backgrounds and levels of literacy show variable results. Most interventions focus on diabetes self-management education. ADA provides ten national standards for diabetes self-management education and lifestyle modification. Standard 7 recommends that educational plans should be individualized and incorporate cultural influences, beliefs and attitudes, and health literacy levels (American Diabetes Association, 2008a). Interventions that are individualized to take into account each participant's readiness for change, that use support groups composed of participants with similar demographic backgrounds (including race, sex, socioeconomic status, and education levels), and that employ lay community health advisors and/or educators from similar backgrounds to provide the education and follow-up programs, have shown significant improvements in diabetes knowledge and self-management skills, behavioral change (such as diet and weight loss), and improvements in lipid levels, but have shown modest improvements in glucose control (Norris et al., 2006; Glasgow et al., 2002).

The National Diabetes Education Program (NDEP)

The NDEP, a multifaceted program launched in 1997, is the result of a collaboration between the CDC and NIH to reduce diabetes-associated morbidity and mortality. The program is based on three major scientific studies that demonstrated the efficacy of tight management of diabetes to reduce associated complications and programs that prevented or delayed the onset of diabetes. The NDEP seeks to raise awareness of diabetes as a serious disease and to facilitate management at the provider and patient level through awareness campaigns, community interventions, partnership networks, and a focus on special populations and the health system. The NDEP partnered with over 200 professional organizations, communities, consumer groups, and private-sector organizations who provided input into the program's design, implementation, and dissemination of messages and educational tools. The NDEP provides educational and promotional resources to local and state public health agencies. The NDEP reports that over a ten-year period the percentage of Americans who believe that diabetes is a serious disease increased from 8 percent to 89 percent. The program's effectiveness in improving diabetes intermediate outcomes and reducing complications has not been established (CDC, 2009b).

ECONOMIC IMPLICATIONS OF DIABETES PREVENTION AND MANAGEMENT

Studies to date have focused on the efficacy of interventions that sought to prevent diabetes or to improve intermediate outcomes and thereby prevent complications that lead to morbidity and mortality. These interventions have focused on individuals and health professionals in traditional health care settings rather than on changing social norms related to health behaviors. In comparison with medical management, improved health behaviors are more efficacious in preventing diabetes and its complications. The most effective interventions that modify health behaviors of groups involve policies and regulations that influence social norms (Bank, 2009; Russell, 2009; Goetzel, 2009).

The recommendations of many efficacy studies would be cost-prohibitive to implement as part of routine medical care or in community settings. The Diabetes Prevention Program Study demonstrated the efficacy of lifestyle intervention on the delay or prevention of diabetes among prediabetic people; however, the estimated cost of such an approach is $192,999 per healthy year. Less intense and costly interventions that incorporate similar principles are recommended, but their effectiveness is not guaranteed. Goetzel (2009) suggests that approaches to prevention of diseases that are heavily influenced by behavior and their associated morbidity and mortality should focus on environmental, policy, and regulatory interventions that promote changes in social and behavioral norms. Examples include policies and regulations that have led to the reduced rates of smoking by 50 percent over the last 40 years. By contrast, obesity rates have progressively increased in recent years in response to the high prevalence of sedentary lifestyles and eating habits that promote weight gain. Options presented for reducing obesity include the following:

> *labeling nutritional value of food at restaurants, supermarkets, school cafeterias, and vending machines; developing walkable communities and parklands; building bicycle lanes; removing soda machines from schools and requiring daily physical activity by students; and supporting effective media campaigns that counterbalance the marketing of high-fat, low-nutrition food products. Meaningful social norms can be achieved through coordinated efforts involving multiple stakeholders (for example, urban planners, food growers and distributors, educators, government officials, civic leaders, and health care officials) without exclusively relying on expensive medical personnel for improving health (Goetzel, 2009).*

Workplace interventions that support the development of social norms to promote healthy lifestyles have been shown to reduce medical cost and absenteeism while producing combined cost savings of approximately nine dollars for every dollar invested in these programs (Goetzel, 2009).

How might such approaches affect diabetes-related health disparities? Interventions such as the Diabetes Prevention Program Study that focused on health behavior changes have demonstrated similar results for both non-Hispanic blacks and whites. Thus, cost savings associated with changes in social norms across diverse populations should be expected.

CONSIDERATIONS FOR FUTURE RESEARCH AND POLICY IMPLICATIONS

Access to affordable health care resources in culturally sensitive settings can be expected to decrease health disparities among non-Hispanic black patients. However, studies in managed care settings where access to quality health care is controlled have shown variable outcomes in reducing health disparities. Studies that extend beyond the medical setting and include culturally focused programs that incorporate support from peer or lay health advisors have shown promise in improving self-management knowledge and efficacy but have not demonstrated consistent effectiveness in achieving intermediate health outcomes that are associated with reducing diabetes health complications. Sources of variability are attributed to individual characteristics, environmental characteristics that are external to the health care setting, and patients' inability to afford the recommended treatment regimens. Future research should focus on identifying intrapersonal, environmental, and cost barriers and developing interventions that ameliorate these barriers.

Most intervention studies are short-term in duration, usually lasting no longer than twelve months. As a result, longer-term effects are not known. Longer-term effectiveness studies are needed to determine whether the results of short-term efficacy studies are generalizable and sustainable.

Since there is strong evidence that the prevention of diabetes and its complications depends on behavioral and lifestyle changes that are affected by social and environmental norms, studies that focus on policy and regulatory changes that promote healthy lifestyles should be pursued. Examples include health-promoting policies and regulations in the workplace; media campaigns that focus on the benefits of healthy lifestyles; improvement of community resources that promote healthy lifestyles; and reduction of environmental barriers such as crime, poor street lighting, and limited access to facilities for physical activities. Health disparities may also be attenuated through financial support to move health promotion activities from traditional and expensive health care settings into homes and schools, as well as programs that use less costly health personnel or trained community peer or lay advisors and incorporate cultural considerations (Health Promotion Advocates, 2009).

REFERENCES

Adams, A. S., Fang, Z., Mah, C., et al. (2005). Race differences in long-term diabetes management in an HMO. *Diabetes Care, 28*(12), 2844–2849.

American Diabetes Association. (2008a). Standards of medical care in diabetes—2008. *Diabetes Care, 31*, Supplement 1, S12–S54.

American Diabetes Association. (2008b). Third-party reimbursement for diabetes care, self-management education, and supplies. *Diabetes Care, 31*, Supplement, S95–S96.

Bank, S. (2009). The Diabetes Prevention Program: How the participants did it. *Health Affairs, 28*(1), 57–62.

Centers for Disease Control and Prevention. (2008). *National diabetes fact sheet: General information and national estimates on diabetes in the United States, 2007.* Atlanta, GA: U.S. Department of Health and Human Services, Centers for Disease Control and Prevention.

Centers for Disease Control and Prevention. (2009a). Diabetes data and trends. Retrieved May 21, 2009, from http://apps.nccd.cdc.gov/ddtstrs/

Centers for Disease Control and Prevention. (2009b). Diabetes public health resource. Retrieved May 21, 2009, from http://www.cdc.gov/DIABETES/ndep/index.htm

Centers for Disease Control and Prevention. (2009c). Diabetes: Successes and opportunities for population-based prevention and control. National Center for Chronic Disease Prevention and Health Promotion. Retrieved May 21, 2009, from http://www.cdc.gov/nccdphp/publications/aag/ddt.htm

Chou, A. F., Brown, A. F., Jensen, R. E., et al. (2005). Gender and racial disparities in the management of diabetes mellitus among Medicare patients. *Women's Health Issues, 17*, 150–161.

Diabetes Prevention Program Research Group. (2002). Reduction in the incidence of Type 2 diabetes with lifestyle intervention or Metformin. *New England Journal of Medicine, 346*(6), 393–403.

Gary, T. L., Safford, M. M., Gerozoff, R. B., et al. (2008). Perception of neighborhood problems, health behaviors, and diabetes outcomes among adults with diabetes in managed care. *Diabetes Care, 31*, 273–278.

Goetzel, R. Z. (2009). Do prevention or treatment services save money? The wrong debate. *Health Affairs, 28*(1), 37–41.

Glasgow, R. E., Toobert, D. J., Hampson, S. E., & Strycker, L. A. (2002). Implementation, generalization and long-term results of the "choosing well" diabetes self-management intervention. *Patient Education and Counseling, 48*, 115–122.

Health Promotion Advocates. (2009). Briefing Document: Background for the Health Promotion FIRST (Funding Integrated Research, Synthesis and Training) Act and the Healthy Workforce Act. Retrieved May 21, 2009, from http://www.healthpromotionadvocates.org/resources/presentation.htm.

Hebert, P. L., Frick, K. D., Kane, R. L., et al. (2005). The causes of racial and ethnic differences in influenza vaccination rates among elderly medicare beneficiaries. *Health Services Research, 40*, 517–537.

Jiang, H. J., Andrews, R., Stryer, D., & Friedman, B. (2005). Racial/ethnic disparities in potentially preventable readmissions: The case of diabetes. *American Journal of Public Health, 95*(9), 1561–1568.

Karter, A. J., Stevens, M. R., Herman, W. H., et al. (2003). Out-of-pocket costs and diabetes preventive services. *Diabetes Care, 26*, 2294–2299.

Kenrick, D., et al. (2006). The association between clinical care strategies and the attenuation of racial/ethnic disparities in diabetes care: The Translating Research Into Action for Diabetes (TRIAD) study. *Medical Care, 44*(12), 1121–1128.

Norris, S. L., Chowdhury, F. M., Le, K. V., et al. (2006). Effectiveness of community health workers in the care of persons with diabetes. *Diabetes Medicine, 23*, 544–556.

Russell, L. B. (2009). Preventing chronic disease: An important investment, but don't count on cost savings. *Health Affairs, 28*(1), 42–45.

Safford, M., Eaton, L., Hawley, G., et al. (2003). Disparities in use of lipid-lowering medications among people with type 2 diabetes mellitus. *Archives of Internal Medicine, 163*: 922–928.

Schneider, E. C., Cleary, P. D., Zaslavsky, A. M., et al. (2001). Racial disparities in influenza vaccination: Does managed care narrow the gap between African Americans and Whites? *Journal of the American Medical Association, 286*, 1455–1460.

Selby, V., Swain, B. E., & Geroff, R. B. (2007). Understanding the gap between good processes of diabetes care and poor intermediate outcomes. *Medical Care, 45*, 1144–1153.

Self-monitoring of blood glucose among adults with diabetes—United States, 1997–2006. (2007). *Morbidity and Mortality Weekly Report, 56*(43), 1133–1137.

Trivedi, N. A., Zaslavsky, A. M., Schneider, E. C., et al. (2005). Trends in the quality of care and racial disparities in Medicare managed care. *New England Journal of Medicine, 353*(7), 692–700.

Tseng, C. W., Tierney, E. F., Gerzoff, R. B., et al. (2008). Race/ethnicity and economic differences in cost-related medication underuse among insured adults with diabetes. *Diabetes Care, 31*, 261–266.

U.S. Department of Health and Human Services (USDHHS), Agency for Healthcare Research and Quality. (2008, February). *2007 national healthcare disparities report*. Rockville, MD: U.S. Department of Health and Human Services, Agency for Healthcare Research and Quality. AHRQ Pub. No. 08-0041.

CHAPTER

15

SYSTEMIC LUPUS ERYTHEMATOSUS

S. SAM LIM
CHARMAYNE DUNLOP-THOMAS
CRISTINA DRENKARD

Systemic lupus erythematosus (known as lupus or SLE) is a chronic, autoimmune disorder without known cause or cure. Unlike other autoimmune conditions such as thyroiditis or type 1 diabetes, lupus is not organ-specific. Every organ system in the body can be affected, from mild inflammatory skin rashes to internal organ involvement. Patients with lupus are affected by a diverse array of clinical manifestations that can accumulate over time.

Despite the diversity of clinical presentation, what unites those with lupus is the attribution of symptoms and signs to the production of autoantibodies and subsequent activation of the immune system. Laboratory tests are routinely available for the detection of certain autoantibodies. The most commonly used screening test for lupus is the antinuclear antibody (ANA), which is positive in nearly all cases of lupus. However, it is not very specific, meaning that it is also found in patients with other chronic conditions as well as a small percentage of otherwise asymptomatic people. Different autoantibody tests suffer from other limitations. Therefore, a lupus diagnosis cannot be made from laboratory tests alone. The gold standard for diagnosis comes from the assessment of an experienced clinician (e.g., a rheumatologist). Classification criteria have been developed by the American College of Rheumatology (ACR) to serve as a case definition for clinical trials and epidemiologic studies (Table 15.1). The ACR

TABLE 15.1 **The 1997 Updated American College of Rheumatology Criteria for the Classification of Systemic Lupus Erythematosus.**

Criterion	Definition
1. Malar "butterfly" rash	Fixed erythema, flat or raised, over the malar eminences, tending to spare the nasolabial folds
2. Discoid rash	Erythematosus raised patches with adherent keratotic scaling and follicular plugging; atrophic scarring may occur in older lesions
3. Photosensitivity	Skin rash as a result of unusual reaction to sunlight, by patient history or physician observation
4. Oral ulcers	Oral or nasopharyngeal ulceration, usually painless, observed by a physician
5. Arthritis	Nonerosive arthritis involving two or more peripheral joints, characterized by tenderness, swelling, or effusion
6. Serositis	Pleuritis (convincing history of pleuritic pain or rub heard by physician or evidence of pleural effusion) *OR* Pericarditis (documented by ECG, rub or evidence of pericardial effusion)
7. Renal disorder	Persistent proteinuria (>0.5 grams/day or >3+ if quantitation not performed) *OR* Cellular casts (may be red cell, hemoglobin, granular, tubular or mixed)
8. Neurologic disorder	Seizures (in the absence of offending drugs or known metabolic derangements; e.g. uremia, ketoacidosis or electrolyte imbalance) *OR* Psychosis (in the absence of offending drugs or known metabolic derangements; e.g. uremia, ketoacidosis or electrolyte imbalance)
9. Hematologic disorder	Hemolytic anemia (with reticulocytosis) *OR* Leukopenia (<4000/ml total on two or more occasions) *OR* Lymphopenia (<1500/ml on two or more occasions) *OR* Thrombocytopenia (<100,000/ml in the absence of offending drugs)
10. Immunologic disorder	Anti-DNA (antibody to native DNA in abnormal titer) *OR* Anti-Sm (presence of antibody to Sm nuclear antigen) *OR*

(Continued)

TABLE 15.1 *(Continued)*.

Criterion	Definition
	Positive finding of antiphospholipid antibodies based on 1) an abnormal serum level of IgG or IgM anticardiolipin antibodies; 2) a positive test result for lupus anticoagulant using a standard method; or 3) a false-positive serologic test for syphilis known to be positive for at least 6 months and confirmed by *Treponema pallidum* immobilization (TPI) or fluorescent treponemal antibody (FTA) absorption test
11. Antinuclear antibody (ANA)	Abnormal titer of ANA by immunofluorescence or an equivalent assay at any point in time and in the absence of drugs known to be associated with "drug-induced lupus" syndrome

Sources: Hochberg (1997); Tan et al. (1982).

criteria reflect major clinical features of the disease, incorporate associated laboratory findings, and can often be used for diagnostic purposes as well. A person is classified as having lupus if he or she is documented as having four or more of the eleven criteria, either serially or simultaneously, during any interval of observation. It is important to emphasize that each feature must be attributed to lupus and not another cause.

The diagnosis of lupus can initially be challenging for both the physician and the patient. In a study of patients who developed lupus while in the military, it took an average of over one and a half years from the onset of lupus symptoms for a diagnosis to be made (Heinlen et al., 2007). In this population with universal access to health care that underwent regular medical examinations, initial symptoms were nonspecific enough to significantly delay physician diagnoses. This delay is magnified even more in the general population, particularly members of certain vulnerable groups, such as those who are from a lower socioeconomic level with barriers to health care access.

There is no cure for lupus. However, as with other chronic diseases, its symptoms can be managed. More than forty years ago, lupus was felt to be a severe disease that almost always led to hospitalization and premature death. However, with better recognition of the disease and improved treatments, survival and quality of life have improved. The cornerstone of any chronic illness is patient education. Lupus can be difficult to understand and manage without proper guidance. With often unpredictable waxing and waning of disease, it is even more important for patients to be aware of their condition and be equipped with methods to manage their disease under the guidance of a physician. Though the cause of many disease flares is unknown, there are a few known potential precipitants of disease activity that can be avoided, including medication non-adherence, exposure to sunlight, drugs, and exogenous hormones.

Since each patient with lupus is unique, the treatment is tailored to the type and degree of disease activity. The main goal of treatment is to reverse the inflammatory process without causing permanent damage or side effects. Various immunosuppressive medications are often used. Unfortunately, current medications are often not entirely effective in controlling disease activity in many patients and come with their own side effects, some of which can be quite significant. In addition, as time passes, accumulation of irreversible damage and other related comorbidities can add to disease burden, complicating treatment and disease outcomes. No new drugs have been approved for lupus in more than fifty years, and a renewed search for more effective treatments with less toxicity is underway.

RELEVANT AND RECENT EPIDEMIOLOGY

Gender/Age

Lupus is much more frequent among women than among men, with ratios reported as high as 14:1. The preponderance of women with lupus probably reflects, in part, the role of sex hormones in the pathogenesis of the disease. The peak incidence in women is during their reproductive years, which also coincides with their period of peak career development. The disease also tends to flare during periods of hormonal changes, particularly during pregnancy and hormone use (oral contraceptives and hormone replacement therapy).

Although lupus is regarded as primarily a disease of women of childbearing age, it can afflict all ages. Pediatric-onset lupus is described as the development of the disease before age 18. This accounts for approximately 8 to 15 percent of all lupus diagnoses. It is, however, rarely seen before the age of five, being more common after age ten. Blacks, as well as Hispanics, have been found to have more active disease at an earlier age, predisposing them to less favorable long-term outcomes (Alarcon et al., 1999).

Ethnicity

Special attention should be given to different ethnic groups with appropriate stratified rates. Recently, summarized data showed that some of the lowest rates can be seen among white Americans, Canadians, and Spaniards, with incident rates of 1.4, 1.6, and 2.2 cases per 100,000 people, respectively (Danchenko, Satia, & Anthony, 2006). In predominantly white populations, which tend to have less severe disease for longer durations, prevalence rates may be underestimated if milder cases or patients in remission are not ascertained. The data from Northern European countries are excellent resources in understanding the burden of lupus among this group.

Incidence and prevalence rates are consistently higher among ethnic minorities across studies from different countries. It is a striking and consistent observation that lupus has a predilection for those of African origin. In England, for example, the annual incidence rate in people of Afro-Caribbean ethnicity was 31.9 cases per 100,000 for both genders in Nottingham, and 25.8 cases per 100,000 for females in Birmingham, whereas whites showed rates of 3.4 and 4.3 per 100,000, respectively (Hopkinson, Doherty, & Powell, 1994; Johnson, Gordon, Palmer, & Bacon, 1995). The reasons for this disparity are unclear. The "Prevalence Gradient Hypothesis" suggests that there is an increase in disease in those of African origin as they migrated from Africa to North America or Europe (Bae, Fraser, & Liang, 1998). The implication is that genetic and environmental factors may be important in the cause and prognosis of lupus in a way that may not be too dissimilar to how diet influenced coronary artery disease in people from Japan as they migrated to North America by way of Hawaii (Robertson et al., 1977).

Although those of African origin have higher rates of lupus, epidemiologic studies of lupus often have reported proportionally lower numbers of blacks than whites. Many studies do not report ethnicity at all (Tables 15.2 and 15.3). An early study in Alabama and New York City reported an incidence of 6.3 per one million during a ten-year period for white girls less than 15 years old (Siegel, Holley, & Lee, 1970). This was based on only two hospitalized cases, with no cases in black girls being reported. A study of Allegheny County, Pennsylvania, determined an incidence rate of 3 and 3.4 per 100,000 per year among white and black girls between the ages of 12 and 19 years, respectively (McCarty et al., 1995). This was based on twelve white and three black children. The lowest annual incidence rate of 0.5 per 100,000 per year was reported in Baltimore, Maryland, where ten black patients younger than 15 years old were found from hospital discharge records (Hochberg, 1985).

Epidemiologic Methods

Estimates of the incidence and prevalence of lupus in the United States have varied widely (Table 15.2). This is likely to be due to the use of different case definitions, limited sources for case ascertainment, small source populations, and different demographic groups targeted, as well as the protean characteristics of the disease, poor reliability of self-report, lack of reliability in diagnosis and coding in health system databases, and issues related to access to health care by high-risk populations. Estimates for other types of lupus (e.g., primary discoid lupus) are even less well-defined.

The most commonly accepted definition of lupus in epidemiologic studies is the updated 1997 ACR Criteria for the Classification of SLE (Table 15.1). Although the use of ACR criteria enhances study comparability, there are some drawbacks. Notably, the sensitivity of the criteria was shown to be only 83 percent in an external population versus 96 percent in the test population (Tan et al., 1982). Additionally, the criteria tend to be skewed toward limited detection of mild cases of lupus or incident cases at early stages of their prodrome. Not only would the population size be underestimated, but the cases would be biased toward those of longer disease duration and greater severity. With four of the eleven criteria referring to skin, the ACR criteria are also overly biased toward cutaneous manifestations of lupus. Because of these limitations, the Systemic Lupus International Collaborating Clinics (SLICC) group is currently revising the ACR criteria.

Lupus patients interact with the health care system at many different points. In order to assess the full spectrum of disease, cases should be ascertained from a wide

TABLE 15.2 Lupus Epidemiologic Studies from the United States and Canada.

Reference	Study Location/ Country	Study Years	Population at Risk	Number of Lupus Cases by Ethnicity	Annual Incidence*	Prevalence**
Siegel et al., 1970	New York City and Jefferson County, AL/U.S.	1956–1965	1,165,700	Total 193 White 124 Black 69	2.0ˆ (overall)	19.3ˆ (overall)
Fessel, 1974	San Francisco, CA/ U.S.	1965–1973	121,444 members of Kaiser	Total 74 White 41 Black 22	7.6 (overall)	50.8 (overall)
Michet, McKenna, Elveback, Kaslow, & Kurland, 1985	Rochester, MN/U.S.	1950–1979	56,447	Total 46 ethnic rates not reported; from population 99% White	1.8ˆ (definite) 2.1ˆ(suspected)	40.0 (overall)
Hochberg, 1985	Baltimore, MD/U.S.	1970–1977	Not given	Total 302 White 79 Black 223	4.6ˆ (overall)	ND
McCarty et al., 1995	Allegheny County, PA/U.S.	1985–1990	1,336,449	Total 191 White 141 Black 48 Other 2	2.4 (overall)	ND
Uramoto et al., 1999	Rochester, MN/U.S.	1950–1992	Rochester population	Total 48 ethnic rates not reported; from population 94% White, 1% Black	3.06+ (overall) 5.56+(1980–92) 1.51+(1950–79)	122ˆ (Jan 1992)

Study	Location	Year	Population	Cases / Ethnicity	Incidence	Prevalence
Walsh et al., 2001	Nogales, AZ/U.S.	1997	19,489	Total 26 from population 92% Mexican-American	ND	94 (overall)
Ward, 2004	NHANES III (sample of the U.S. population)	2000	20,050	40 self-report, ethnic rates not reported; from population 42.3% White and 27.4% Black	ND	241 self-report 53.6 SLE drugs
Naleway, Davis, Greenlee, Wilson, & McCarty, 2005	Rural area Wisconsin/ U.S.	1991–2001	77,280	Total 117 ethnic rates not reported; from population 97% White	5.1ˆ (overall)	78.5ˆ (overall)
Bernatsky et al., 2007	Quebec/Canada	1994–2003	~7.5 million	3,825 in 2003 ethnic rates not reported	3.0 (PB) 2.8 (HDD)	32.8 (PB) 31.9 (HDD) 51.0 (Composite) 44.7 (Bayesian model)

*per 100,000 per year
**per 100,000
ˆage adjusted to national or regional population
+age and sex-adjusted
Abbreviations: ARA, American Rheumatism Association; ND, not determined; DB, database; PB, physician billing; HDD, hospital discharge data.

TABLE 15.3 Lupus Epidemiologic Studies from Europe.

Author/Year (Reference)	Study Location/ Country	Study Years	Population at Risk	Number of Lupus Cases by Ethnicity	Annual Incidence*	Prevalence**
Hopkinson et al., 1994	Nottingham/UK	1989–1990	601,693	Total 147 White 117 Afro-Car 21 Asian 7 Chinese 2	4.0+ (overall) 3.4+ 31.9+ 4.1+ ND	24.7+(overall) 20.3+ 207.0+ 48.8+ 92.9+
Johnson et al., 1995	Birmingham and Solihull Districts/UK	1991–1992	872,877	Total 242 White 155 Afro-Car 50 Asian 36 Chinese 1	3.8ᶜ (overall)	27.7ᶜ(overall) 20.7ᶜ 111.8ᶜ 46.7ᶜ ND
Nightingale, Farmer, & de Vries, 2006, 2007	Nationwide/UK	1992–1998	12,911,216 person-years	Incident 390 Prevalent 1,538 (ethnic rates not reported)	3.0 (overall)	25.0 (1992) 40.7 (1998)
Somers, Thomas, Smeeth, Schoonen, & Hall, 2007	Nationwide/UK	1990–1999	33,666,320 person-years	Total 1,638 (ethnic rates not reported)	4.7+(overall)	ND
Govoni, Castellino, Bosi, Napoli, & Trotta, 2006	Ferrara District/Italy	1996–2002	~346,000	Total 201 (from mostly white population)	2.01 (2000) 1.15 (2001) 2.60 (2002)	57.9 (overall)

Lopez, Mozo, Gutierrez, & Suarez, 2003	Asturias/North Spain	1998–2002	1,073,971	Total 367 (from mostly white population)	2.15 (overall)	34.1 (2002)
Nossent, 2001	Finnmark and Troms Counties/Norway	1978–1996	224,403	Total 105 (from mostly white population)	2.9* (overall) 2.4 (1978–86) 2.7 (1987–95)	49.7* (1996)
Stahl-Hallengren, Jonsen, Nived, & Sturfelt, 2000	Lund and Orup Districts/South Sweden	1986–1991	174,952	Incident 1987–91: 41 Prevalent 1986: 121 (from mostly white population)	4.8 (1987–91) 4.5 if patients with ≥ 4 ACR are assessed	42.0 (1986) 68.0 (1991)
Voss, Green, & Junker, 1998	Funen County/Denmark	1980–1994	387,841	Definite: 107 Incomplete:20 (from mostly white population)	1.0 (1980) 3.6 (1994)	22.2+ (overall definite) 5.2 (overall incomplete)

*per 100,000 per year
**per 100,000
+age standardized to national or regional population
^age standardized to European population
Abbreviations: CTD, connective tissue disease; ND, not determined; GP, general practitioners; DB, database; HDD, hospital discharge data; MR, medical record.

range of sources. Obtaining potential cases at several points improves maximal case ascertainment. Furthermore, as disease manifestations change for a particular patient or as certain types of damage predominate, patients with lupus may be more likely to be found at different types of facilities. Rheumatologists and hospitals have been the common, logical sources for many studies. However, nephrologists and dermatologists also see many potential cases. Patients with end-stage renal disease for several years often have less active systemic disease activity and, therefore, are less likely to be found at a rheumatologist's office. Cutaneous manifestations of lupus are frequent. Other specialists, such as hematologists, cardiologists, and obstetricians, may also encounter patients with lupus. University databases, though an important source of cases, are biased subsets of patients. Access to clinical and pathology (particularly skin and renal) laboratories would be a high-yield source for locating additional patients. Identifying the presumably milder cases of SLE that can be found only in the primary care arena has never been adequately addressed at a population level.

Although children have been identified in population-based epidemiologic studies of lupus, child-related efforts have not been focused or consistent. Historically, lupus was erroneously thought to be primarily an adult disease. Pediatric lupus is an important subgroup of lupus that deserves special attention. In general, these patients are found in pediatric hospitals and in the practices of specialists (e.g., pediatric rheumatologists and nephrologists). These sources should be included in case ascertainment if pediatric rates are to be valid. Some studies from the United States and Europe included pediatric patients of all ages, whereas others included only those 15 years of age and older. Although some U.S. studies reported pediatric lupus rates, case ascertainment efforts have not been broad enough or the numbers have been too small to be considered valid.

Researchers should define and target the population from whom incidence and prevalence rates are being determined and the geographic area in which they live. Significant numbers of people at risk for the disease should be captured. It would not be appropriate for countries with a heterogeneous mix of ethnicities, such as the United States, to extrapolate national rates based on a single study. Multiple studies are needed in areas that contain significant high-risk ethnic populations. This "sampling" of rates in different ethnic groups would contribute to a more accurate national estimate.

BLACK DISPARITIES IN LUPUS

The predominance of lupus in the black community is an overarching theme, underneath which exist various levels of health disparities.

Disease Activity and Damage

The clinical course of lupus can range from various minor manifestations occurring over time to catastrophic onset of organ damage and failure. It is not possible to accurately predict in an individual to what degree his or her disease will be active. However, in general, blacks, compared to whites, accumulate disease activity faster (Arbuckle et al., 2003), have more disease activity (Alarcon et al., 1999), and have more frequent renal (Alarcon et al., 2002), neurological, and serosal involvement (Ward & Studenski, 1990). Blacks exhibit more irreversible scarring as a result of active disease, including kidney damage (Rivest et al., 2000).

Mortality

Population-based and inception cohort studies have shown significant improvement in the survival of lupus patients over the last five decades. In the early 1950s and before the advent of steroid treatments, when lupus was considered a rapidly fatal disease, the first survival study with lupus patients showed that less than 50 percent were alive five years after diagnosis (Merrell & Shulman, 1955). Recent studies from developed countries have shown that over 95 percent, 90 percent, and 75 percent of lupus patients are alive after five, ten and fifteen years, respectively (Cervera et al., 2003; Hochberg, 1990; Pistiner, Wallace, Nessim, Metzger, & Klinenberg, 1991; Uramoto et al., 1999). The decrease in mortality rates of lupus patients has been attributed to earlier diagnosis, recognition of mild forms, advances in management of flares, and better treatment of complications and comorbid conditions, such as hypertension, infection, and renal failure. Although mortality has greatly improved, death rates for patients with lupus remain three to five times higher than in the general population (Bernatsky et al., 2006; Uramoto et al., 1999). Mortality in lupus patients is burdened by marked age, gender, and ethnic disparities (Bernatsky et al., 2006).

In the United States, the disparity in mortality suffered by ethnic minorities with lupus is prominent. Blacks and other minority ethnic groups with lupus show overall mortality rates two to three times higher than whites, and they die at younger ages (Krishnan & Hubert, 2006). Based on national statistics, trends in lupus mortality for black and white women differed and racial disparities in overall mortality from lupus enlarged during the latter half of 1968–1991 (Walsh, Algert, Gregorio, Reisine, & Rothfield, 1995) and during 1979–1998 (CDC, 2002). In white females, total lupus mortality has been constant since the late 1970s at an average annual rate of 4.6 deaths per million. Stable incidence and prolonged survival among younger women shifted lupus mortality to older women in the American white population (Figure 15.1). This shift suggests that lupus among whites has become a chronic disease with significant comorbid conditions contributing to long-term mortality. Among black women, mortality has increased more than 30 percent since the late 1970s and more than 70 percent among women aged 45 to 64 years. Racial disparities in early diagnosis, access to care, disease severity, and response to and compliance with therapeutic regimens are some of the factors that may explain the lack of improvement in the survival of young blacks with lupus.

The inequities in mortality rates among minority populations arise from the interplay of known and unrecognized environmental and genetic factors. Biological factors have been associated with more active disease, higher prevalence of severe lupus manifestations, and higher mortality rates from lupus in blacks and Hispanics compared with whites (Alarcon et al., 2006). Although lupus mortality is most frequently caused by active lupus or by associated organ failure, infection, or cardiovascular disease

FIGURE 15.1 *Systemic Lupus Erythematosus Death Rates (Per 10 Million Population) among Females, by Age Group and Ethnicity—United States, 1979–1998.*

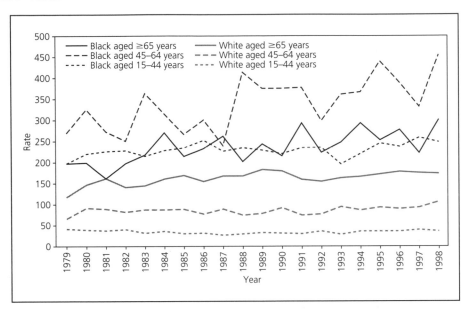

Source: Centers for Disease Control (CDC). (2002). Trends in deaths from systemic lupus erythematosus—United States, 1979–1998. *Morbidity and Mortality Weekly Report, 51,* 371–374.

from accelerated atherosclerosis, some studies suggest that renal disease might account for excess lupus-related deaths among blacks (Korbet, Schwartz, Evans, & Lewis, 2007). Additionally, several studies have shown that poverty, educational level, psychosocial factors, and access to health care are environmental risk factors associated with higher mortality in lupus, regardless of ethnicity (Alarcon et al., 2001; Duran, Apte, & Alarcon, 2007; Liang et al., 1991). Geographic distribution of clusters with higher mortality rates are concentrated in areas with high rates of poverty and numbers of ethnic minorities, indicating that environmental factors are likely implicated, in part, in the outcomes of lupus (Walsh & Gilchrist, 2006). Because racial inequities in survival of patients with lupus appear to be multidimensional, reducing the gap requires a better understanding of the interdependence between biological and environmental risk factors, and the implementation of multilevel interventions on modifiable factors.

Health-Related Quality of Life

Lupus patients experience a wide range of problems with physical, psychological, and social functioning. These experiences are not always captured by descriptions of physiological measures. In order to characterize the wide spectrum of the effects of lupus on patients, a comprehensive assessment should be used to measure both health and quality of life outcomes. Health-related quality of life outcomes refer to the impact of a disease and its treatment on an individual's ability to function and self-perceived well-being in physical, mental, and social domains of life (Panopalis & Clarke, 2006). Previous studies have identified psychosocial (e.g., social support) and behavioral variables (e.g., helplessness, coping with illness) as being associated with quality of life in patients with lupus. Assessments of quality of life in patients with lupus have been shown to be lower than in patients with other chronic diseases (Kuriya, Gladman, Ibanez, & Urowitz, 2008).

Quality of life assessments have become increasingly important as new treatments are developed and introduced to lupus patients. It has been an ongoing challenge to identify instruments that will accurately and reliably assess this outcome. The goal of quality of life research is to determine health outcomes from the perspective of the patient. Most authors agree on the existence of four major domains (Tsokos et al., 2007):

- Physical status and functional abilities
- Psychological status and well-being
- Social interactions
- Economic and/or vocational status and factors

The socioeconomic status (SES) of individuals with chronic diseases such as lupus can influence several disease-related outcomes including health-related quality of life. Alternatively, the characteristics and course of the disease can have a strong impact on the socioeconomic status of individuals with lupus. SES is difficult to measure directly. Surrogate markers such as occupation, educational level, or income are often used. As it relates to a chronic disease, education remains constant, but income may decline, adding to the complexity of this measurement. There are important links between economic resources and health status. Some important influential aspects include access to health insurance, transportation to clinic visits, and payment for medications.

Racial/ethnic and gender effects may be intricately related to lupus (Sule & Petri, 2006). As the epidemiology and clinical/laboratory features of lupus differ with ethnicity, there is an ongoing debate regarding the relationship of ethnicity and SES to poor outcomes in patients with lupus (Karlson et al., 1997). This relationship can be seen with particular clarity in children with lupus. In one study, SES and self-concept correlated significantly with both quality of life and physical function, indicating the importance of these factors in assessing children with chronic diseases (Moorthy, Peterson, Onel, Harrison, & Lehman, 2005). The researchers concluded that disease activity, physical function, and quality of life are different constructs, with partial overlap, and cannot be used as proxies for one another (Moorthy, Harrison, Peterson, Onel, & Lehman, 2005).

Self-assessed health status is an important indicator of the general health of the population. It is generally recognized as a valid measure for predicting future health outcomes. According to the 2003 National Center of Health Statistics, blacks had the largest percentage of persons indicating that they have fair to poor health (LaVeist, 2005).

THE GEORGIA LUPUS REGISTRY

Given the predilection of the disease for those of African origin and the paucity of large studies focusing on the black population, it is imperative that better and more accurate epidemiologic data be gathered. In keeping with the goals of the *National Arthritis Action Plan: A Public Health Strategy* (NAAP) (Meenan, Callahan, & Helmick, 1999), the Centers for Disease Control and Prevention (CDC) Arthritis Program is funding a population-based registry in Atlanta, the Georgia Lupus Registry (GLR), to better define the incidence and prevalence of diagnosed lupus and to better characterize individuals with this disease. Atlanta was chosen in part because of its relatively large black population. The catchment area has over 1.6 million people, almost half of whom are black. A sister project is also underway in Michigan.

A fundamental strategy for the success of the GLR is the partnership of the state health department with its academic counterpart, Emory University. The academic partner provides on-site expertise in lupus to conduct the registry. The state health department provides surveillance expertise and can use its "surveillance exemption" from the HIPAA Privacy Rule (CFR Parts 160 and 164) to designate the university as a public health authority for this specific project, permitting it to collect protected health information (PHI) without written patient authorization. Otherwise, obtaining individual consent for case finding and medical record reviews would be prohibitively costly, time-consuming, and result in severe underreporting. Collecting PHI is needed to determine if diagnosed cases meet case definition criteria and to provide enough information to prevent duplicate entry of patients, since the same patient may be encountered in multiple facilities. The registry meets all requirements as laid out in the Office for Civil Rights HIPAA guidelines. In addition, all pertinent local, university, state, and CDC IRB reviews and approvals have been obtained.

To maximize ascertainment of potential cases, a broad range of case finding sources are being utilized (Figure 15.2). Once a potential case is identified, more than 200 data elements are potentially abstracted for each patient at each facility, with core data including all elements required for various lupus classification criteria, including the ACR criteria (Table 15.1). A snapshot of the status of abstracting at target facilities and practices is provided in Table 15.4, and the numbers of diagnosed lupus cases meeting classification criteria are reported in Table 15.5, stratified by gender and ethnicity (black and white). The GLR will estimate the incidence and prevalence rates for the entire spectrum of diagnosed lupus cases meeting standard classification criteria utilizing one of the largest groups of lupus patients ever assembled.

The GLR also represents a unique opportunity to understand the burden and disparities of lupus across ethnic and socioeconomic groups. Because of the large number

FIGURE 15.2 *Sources of Potential Cases in the Georgia Lupus Registry.*

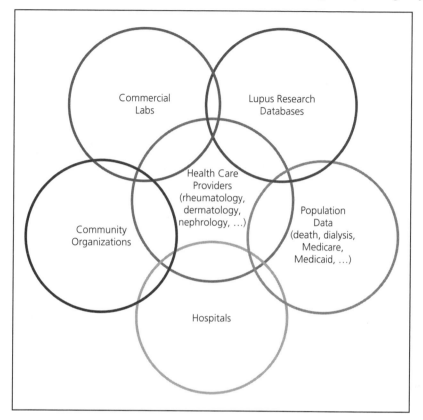

TABLE 15.4   **Major Facilities that Serve as Sources of Potential Cases in the Georgia Lupus Registry (as of December 2008).**

| | Georgia Lupus Registry | | |
Facilities	Total Number	Number Completed or Ongoing	Percent Complete
Hospitals	19	17	89
Rheumatologists	34	25	74
Nephrologists	79	38	48
Dermatologists	103	21	20

TABLE 15.5 Preliminary, Minimum Estimates for the Georgia Lupus Registry (as of July 2008).

		Catchment Area Population[1]	Number of Validated Lupus Patients[2,3]
Georgia[4]			
Overall		1,489,683	1,345
Whites	Total	684,544	261
	Male	351,176	28
	Female	333,368	233
Blacks	Total	740,031	1,033
	Male	346,139	103
	Female	393,892	930

[1] Population estimates, year 2003, Dekalb and Fulton Counties, United States Department of Health and Human Services (US DHHS), Centers for Disease Control and Prevention (CDC), National Center for Health Statistics (NCHS), Bridged-Race Population Estimates, United States. Vintage 2004: Years 2000–2004, April 2006 online database, based on the September 8, 2005, data release.
[2] Meeting either (1) ≥ 4 of 11 revised 1982 ACR criteria or (2) 3 ACR criteria with a final diagnosis of lupus by a rheumatologist
[3] 2002–2004
[4] Fulton and DeKalb counties

of black lupus patients already abstracted by the registry, preliminary descriptions of health issues in the black community and disparities affecting them are available and published in abstract format with peer-reviewed publications soon to follow. For instance, recent GLR data showed that there were no significant differences in the prevalence of disease manifestations between recently diagnosed black patients in indigent versus private facilities, suggesting that any observed differences with longer follow-up may be attributed to environmental factors (Lim, Easley, Shenvi, Chhitwal, & Drenkard, 2006). More severe disease and poorer outcomes among adult black males compared with females have been found, and future studies are needed to determine whether these differences are associated with biological or psychosocial factors. Ethnic disparities have been found in health care system utilization and costs. In recently diagnosed patients with lupus, blacks had higher rates of hospital admissions and emergency room visits with longer length of stay for emergency room and hospital services compared with whites (Lim et al., 2008). In addition, the GLR represents a unique source from which to acquire population-based descriptions of childhood-onset lupus in the United States (Lim, Easley, Shenvi, Vogler, & Drenkard, 2006). Disparities in early disease expression patterns among black pediatric and adult lupus patients have been described from the registry data, showing more cutaneous manifestations and vasculitis and less serosal involvement in the pediatric group (Drenkard, Rossello, Vogler, & Lim, 2006).

With over 1,300 lupus cases already registered in Atlanta, estimates will be more statistically precise than those that were previously available, and meaningful analyses of the disparate impact of lupus on blacks will be feasible from a population-based setting. This registry does not address other important racial/ethnic populations thought to potentially be of high risk for lupus in the United States, particularly Hispanics, Asians, and Native American/Alaska Natives. Currently, early planning is underway to establish additional registry sites in areas that would better capture these persons and ultimately allow for the formulation of more comprehensive and generalizable national estimates.

POLICY IMPLICATIONS AND RECOMMENDATIONS FOR CLOSING THE DISPARITY GAP

Among rheumatic diseases, lupus appears on the surface to have been relatively extensively studied with regard to health disparities according to race, ethnicity, and SES. However, these studies are often drawn from university-affiliated rheumatology or lupus clinics and tend to have biased representation of people with lupus (sicker, with more complications). The numbers of patients in these studies often lack the size to allow for adequate evaluation of many aspects of health disparities. As mentioned in this chapter, studies often are underpowered to evaluate disparities in blacks compared with other ethnic groups and sometimes do not report ethnicity at all. Greater research funding should be directed toward understanding the factors, both biological and social, that lead to the higher prevalence among blacks and disparity of outcomes between blacks and whites. The funding of the Georgia Lupus Registry by the Centers for Disease Control and Prevention is an excellent step toward more accurately describing health disparities in the black community through accurate epidemiologic information.

Education and awareness programs need to be targeted to reach high-risk populations, especially those in the black community. At the time of this publication, the Office of Women's Health, in partnership with the Ad Council, has developed the Campaign to Raise Lupus Awareness, which is an integrated public service campaign with the objective of getting lupus on the radar of young women of color, particularly blacks, Latinas, and Asian Americans in their childbearing years (18 to 44 years old). Radio, TV, and print materials are being disseminated in these communities. Patient advocacy organizations, such as the Lupus Foundation of America, will play a key role during this campaign and in sustaining these efforts into the future.

Current health care access options to serve the most vulnerable lupus patients must be maximized. Because of the potentially complex nature of the disease and the special clinical experience needed to best manage the disease, support for dedicated lupus clinics can assist in this endeavor. In May 2003, a dedicated lupus clinic was started within Grady Hospital. Located in Atlanta, Georgia, it is one of the largest public hospital systems in the Southeast serving the medically indigent in a predominantly black population. In recent years, the clinic has grown to over 650 patients, one of the largest cohorts of lupus patients in the country. Years of fostering a trusting relationship between clinicians/staff and patients has created an ideal environment from which to treat and learn about lupus.

A dedicated lupus clinic in a lower-SES, black community also affords a unique opportunity to create, adapt, and evaluate culturally sensitive health education as a way to improve outcomes and close the disparity gap. Cultural sensitivity is the incorporation of the ethnic and cultural experiences, values, beliefs, and behavioral patterns of a targeted population and the acknowledgment of the historical, environmental, and social forces in the design, delivery, and evaluation of research tools and health promotion materials and programs (Braithwaite & Taylor, 2001). Acknowledgment of the differences of the correlates and predictors of health behaviors amongst racial and ethnic populations and understanding of the most appropriate channels and settings to deliver the materials and programs are the foundations to the cultural adaptation of research measures and interventions to subpopulations. Although health education is an important part of the optimal care of chronic diseases, tailored materials and programs targeting ethnic minorities of low socioeconomic level with lupus are rare in our country. Not only are minorities with lupus underrepresented in research studies, there are also no studies addressing the benefits of culturally appropriate educational programs in working with black lupus patients. Moreover, available educational resources regarding lupus, such as small group counseling, websites, printed materials, and public lectures are mostly designed to target middle-class whites with a medium-high literacy level. Culturally sensitive materials, research tools, and behavioral programs targeting minorities with lupus are greatly needed to understand and reduce health disparities in lupus.

REFERENCES

Alarcon, G. S., Bastian, H. M., Beasley, T. M., Roseman, J. M., Tan, F. K., Fessler, B. J., et al. (2006). Systemic lupus erythematosus in a multi-ethnic cohort (LUMINA) XXXII: [Corrected] contributions of admixture and socioeconomic status to renal involvement. *Lupus, 15*(1), 26–31.

Alarcon, G. S., Friedman, A. W., Straaton, K. V., Moulds, J. M., Lisse, J., Bastian, H. M., et al. (1999). Systemic lupus erythematosus in three ethnic groups: III. A comparison of characteristics early in the natural history of the LUMINA cohort. LUpus in MInority populations: Nature vs. Nurture. *Lupus, 8*(3), 197–209.

Alarcon, G. S., McGwin, G., Jr., Bastian, H. M., Roseman, J., Lisse, J., Fessler, B. J., et al. (2001). Systemic lupus erythematosus in three ethnic groups. VII [correction of VIII]. Predictors of early mortality in the LUMINA cohort. LUMINA Study Group. *Arthritis and Rheumatism, 45*(2), 191–202.

Alarcon, G. S., McGwin, G., Jr., Petri, M., Reveille, J. D., Ramsey-Goldman, R., & Kimberly, R. P. (2002). Baseline characteristics of a multiethnic lupus cohort: PROFILE. *Lupus, 11*(2), 95–101.

Arbuckle, M. R., James, J. A., Dennis, G. J., Rubertone, M. V., McClain, M. T., Kim, X. R., et al. (2003). Rapid clinical progression to diagnosis among African-American men with systemic lupus erythematosus. *Lupus, 12*(2), 99–106.

Bae, S. C., Fraser, P., & Liang, M. H. (1998). The epidemiology of systemic lupus erythematosus in populations of African ancestry: A critical review of the "prevalence gradient hypothesis." *Arthritis and Rheumatism, 41*(12), 2091–2099.

Bernatsky, S., Boivin, J. F., Joseph, L., Manzi, S., Ginzler, E., Gladman, D. D., et al. (2006). Mortality in systemic lupus erythematosus. *Arthritis and Rheumatism, 54*(8), 2550–2557.

Bernatsky, S., Joseph, L., Pineau, C. A., Tamblyn, R., Feldman, D. E., & Clarke, A. E. (2007). A population-based assessment of systemic lupus erythematosus incidence and prevalence: Results and implications of using administrative data for epidemiological studies. *Rheumatology (Oxford), 46*(12), 1814–1818.

Braithwaite, R. L., & Taylor, S. E. (2001). *Health issues in the Black community* (2nd ed.). San Francisco: Jossey-Bass.

Centers for Disease Control (CDC). (2002). Trends in deaths from systemic lupus erythematosus—United States, 1979–1998. *Morbidity and Mortality Weekly Report, 51*, 371–374.

Cervera, R., Khamashta, M. A., Font, J., Sebastiani, G. D., Gil, A., Lavilla, P., et al. (2003). Morbidity and mortality in systemic lupus erythematosus during a 10-year period: A comparison of early and late manifestations in a cohort of 1,000 patients. *Medicine (Baltimore), 82*(5), 299–308.

Danchenko, N., Satia, J. A., & Anthony, M. S. (2006). Epidemiology of systemic lupus erythematosus: A comparison of worldwide disease burden. *Lupus, 15*(5), 308–318.

Drenkard, C., Rossello, L., Vogler, L., & Lim, S. S. (2006). The Georgia Lupus Registry: Differences between pediatric and adult SLE among recently diagnosed black patients. *Arthritis and Rheumatism, 54*(Suppl.), S437.

Duran, S., Apte, M., & Alarcon, G. S. (2007). Poverty, not ethnicity, accounts for the differential mortality rates among lupus patients of various ethnic groups. *Journal of the National Medical Association, 99*(10), 1196–1198.

Fessel, W. J. (1974). Systemic lupus erythematosus in the community. Incidence, prevalence, outcome, and first symptoms; the high prevalence in black women. *Archives of Internal Medicine, 134*(6), 1027–1035.

Govoni, M., Castellino, G., Bosi, S., Napoli, N., & Trotta, F. (2006). Incidence and prevalence of systemic lupus erythematosus in a district of north Italy. *Lupus, 15*(2), 110–113.

Heinlen, L. D., McClain, M. T., Merrill, J., Akbarali, Y. W., Edgerton, C. C., Harley, J. B., et al. (2007). Clinical criteria for systemic lupus erythematosus precede diagnosis, and associated autoantibodies are present before clinical symptoms. *Arthritis and Rheumatism, 56*(7), 2344–2351.

Hochberg, M. C. (1985). The incidence of systemic lupus erythematosus in Baltimore, Maryland, 1970–1977. *Arthritis and Rheumatism, 28*(1), 80–86.

Hochberg, M. C. (1990). Systemic lupus erythematosus. *Rheumatic Disease Clinics of North America, 16*(3), 617–639.

Hochberg, M. C. (1997). Updating the American College of Rheumatology revised criteria for the classification of systemic lupus erythematosus. *Arthritis and Rheumatism, 40*(9), 1725.

Hopkinson, N. D., Doherty, M., & Powell, R. J. (1994). Clinical features and race-specific incidence/prevalence rates of systemic lupus erythematosus in a geographically complete cohort of patients. *Annals of the Rheumatic Diseases, 53*(10), 675–680.

Johnson, A. E., Gordon, C., Palmer, R. G., & Bacon, P. A. (1995). The prevalence and incidence of systemic lupus erythematosus in Birmingham, England. Relationship to ethnicity and country of birth. *Arthritis and Rheumatism, 38*(4), 551–558.

Karlson, E. W., Daltroy, L. H., Lew, R. A., Wright, E. A., Partridge, A. J., Fossel, A. H., et al. (1997). The relationship of socioeconomic status, race, and modifiable risk factors to outcomes in patients with systemic lupus erythematosus. *Arthritis and Rheumatism, 40*(1), 47–56.

Korbet, S. M., Schwartz, M. M., Evans, J., & Lewis, E. J. (2007). Severe lupus nephritis: Racial differences in presentation and outcome. *Journal of the American Society of Nephrology, 18*(1), 244–254.

Krishnan, E., & Hubert, H. B. (2006). Ethnicity and mortality from systemic lupus erythematosus in the US. *Annals of the Rheumatic Diseases, 65*(11), 1500–1505.

Kuriya, B., Gladman, D. D., Ibanez, D., & Urowitz, M. B. (2008). Quality of life over time in patients with systemic lupus erythematosus. *Arthritis and Rheumatism, 59*(2), 181–185.

LaVeist, T. A. (Ed.). (2005). *Minority populations and health: An introduction to health disparities in the United States*. San Francisco: Jossey-Bass.

Liang, M. H., Partridge, A. J., Daltroy, L. H., Straaton, K. V., Galper, S. R., & Holman, H. R. (1991). Strategies for reducing excess morbidity and mortality in blacks with systemic lupus erythematosus. *Arthritis and Rheumatism, 34*(9), 1187–1196.

Lim, S. S., Easley, K., Shenvi, N., Chhitwal, N., & Drenkard, C. (2006). The Georgia Lupus Registry: Recently diagnosed blacks with SLE receiving indigent care do not have worse disease compared to blacks receiving private care. *Arthritis and Rheumatism, 54*(Suppl.), S438.

Lim, S. S., Easley, K., Shenvi, N., Vogler, L., & Drenkard, C. (2006). The Georgia Lupus Registry (GLR): Population-based description of childhood SLE from Atlanta. *Arthritis and Rheumatism, 54*(Suppl.), S101.

Lim, S.S., Jamal, A., Bayakly, R., Easley, K., Shenvi, N., & Drenkard, C. (2008). The Georgia Lupus Registry: The high utilization and direct cost of emergency care and hospital admissions in early SLE by ethnicity and gender. *Arthritis and Rheumatism, 58*(Suppl.), S882.

Lopez, P., Mozo, L., Gutierrez, C., & Suarez, A. (2003). Epidemiology of systemic lupus erythematosus in a northern Spanish population: Gender and age influence on immunological features. *Lupus, 12*(11), 860–865.

McCarty, D. J., Manzi, S., Medsger, T. A., Jr., Ramsey-Goldman, R., LaPorte, R. E., & Kwoh, C. K. (1995). Incidence of systemic lupus erythematosus: Race and gender differences. *Arthritis and Rheumatism, 38*(9), 1260–1270.

Meenan, R. F., Callahan, L. F., & Helmick, C. G. (1999). The National Arthritis Action Plan: A public health strategy for a looming epidemic. *Arthritis Care Research, 12*(2), 79–81.

Merrell, M., & Shulman, L. E. (1955). Determination of prognosis in chronic disease, illustrated by systemic lupus erythematosus. *Journal of Chronic Disease, 1*(1), 12–32.

Michet, C. J., Jr., McKenna, C. H., Elveback, L. R., Kaslow, R. A., & Kurland, L. T. (1985). Epidemiology of systemic lupus erythematosus and other connective tissue diseases in Rochester, Minnesota, 1950 through 1979. *Mayo Clinic Proceedings, 60*(2), 105–113.

Moorthy, L. N., Harrison, M. J., Peterson, M., Onel, K. B., & Lehman, T. J. (2005). Relationship of quality of life and physical function measures with disease activity in children with systemic lupus erythematosus. *Lupus, 14*(4), 280–287.

Moorthy, L. N., Peterson, M., Onel, K. B., Harrison, M. J., & Lehman, T. J. (2005). Quality of life in children with systemic lupus erythematosus. *Current Rheumatology Report, 7*(6), 447–452.

Naleway, A. L., Davis, M. E., Greenlee, R. T., Wilson, D. A., & McCarty, D. J. (2005). Epidemiology of systemic lupus erythematosus in rural Wisconsin. *Lupus, 14*(10), 862–866.

Nightingale, A. L., Farmer, R. D., & de Vries, C. S. (2006). Incidence of clinically diagnosed systemic lupus erythematosus 1992–1998 using the UK General Practice Research Database. *Pharmacoepidemiology and Drug Safety, 15*(9), 656–661.

Nightingale, A. L., Farmer, R. D., & de Vries, C. S. (2007). Systemic lupus erythematosus prevalence in the UK: Methodological issues when using the General Practice Research Database to estimate frequency of chronic relapsing-remitting disease. *Pharmacoepidemiology and Drug Safety, 16*(2), 144–151.

Nossent, H. C. (2001). Systemic lupus erythematosus in the Arctic region of Norway. *Journal of Rheumatology, 28*(3), 539–546.

Panopalis, P., & Clarke, A. E. (2006). Quality of life in systemic lupus erythematosus. *Clinical Developments in Immunology, 13*(2–4), 321–324.

Pistiner, M., Wallace, D. J., Nessim, S., Metzger, A. L., & Klinenberg, J. R. (1991). Lupus erythematosus in the 1980s: A survey of 570 patients. *Seminars in Arthritis and Rheumatism, 21*(1), 55–64.

Rivest, C., Lew, R. A., Welsing, P. M., Sangha, O., Wright, E. A., Roberts, W. N., et al. (2000). Association between clinical factors, socioeconomic status, and organ damage in recent onset systemic lupus erythematosus. *Journal of Rheumatology, 27*(3), 680–684.

Robertson, T. L., Kato, H., Gordon, T., Kagan, A., Rhoads, G. G., Land, C. E., et al. (1977). Epidemiologic studies of coronary heart disease and stroke in Japanese men living in Japan, Hawaii and California. Coronary heart disease risk factors in Japan and Hawaii. *American Journal of Cardiology, 39*(2), 244–249.

Siegel, M., Holley, H. L., & Lee, S. L. (1970). Epidemiologic studies on systemic lupus erythematosus: Comparative data for New York City and Jefferson County, Alabama, 1956–1965. *Arthritis and Rheumatism, 13*(6), 802–811.

Somers, E. C., Thomas, S. L., Smeeth, L., Schoonen, W. M., & Hall, A. J. (2007). Incidence of systemic lupus erythematosus in the United Kingdom, 1990–1999. *Arthritis and Rheumatism, 57*(4), 612–618.

Stahl-Hallengren, C., Jonsen, A., Nived, O., & Sturfelt, G. (2000). Incidence studies of systemic lupus erythematosus in Southern Sweden: Increasing age, decreasing frequency of renal manifestations and good prognosis. *Journal of Rheumatology, 27*(3), 685–691.

Sule, S., & Petri, M. (2006). Socioeconomic status in systemic lupus erythematosus. *Lupus, 15*(11), 720–723.

Tan, E. M., Cohen, A. S., Fries, J. F., Masi, A. T., McShane, D. J., Rothfield, N. F., et al. (1982). The 1982 revised criteria for the classification of systemic lupus erythematosus. *Arthritis and Rheumatism, 25*(11), 1271–1277.

Tsokos, G. C., Gordon, C., & Smolen, J. S. (Eds.). (2007). *Systemic lupus erythematosus: A companion to rheumatology*. Philadelphia: Mosby Elsevier.

Uramoto, K. M., Michet, C. J., Jr., Thumboo, J., Sunku, J., O'Fallon, W. M., & Gabriel, S. E. (1999). Trends in the incidence and mortality of systemic lupus erythematosus, 1950–1992. *Arthritis and Rheumatism, 42*(1), 46–50.

Voss, A., Green, A., & Junker, P. (1998). Systemic lupus erythematosus in Denmark: Clinical and epidemiological characterization of a county-based cohort. *Scandinavian Journal of Rheumatology, 27*(2), 98–105.

Walsh, B. T., Pope, C., Reid, M., Gall, E. P., Yocum, D. E., & Clark, L. C. (2001). SLE in a United States–Mexico border community. *Journal of Clinical Rheumatology, 7*(1), 3–9.

Walsh, S. J., Algert, C., Gregorio, D. I., Reisine, S. T., & Rothfield, N. F. (1995). Divergent racial trends in mortality from systemic lupus erythematosus. *Journal of Rheumatology, 22*(9), 1663–1668.

Walsh, S. J., & Gilchrist, A. (2006). Geographical clustering of mortality from systemic lupus erythematosus in the United States: Contributions of poverty, Hispanic ethnicity and solar radiation. *Lupus, 15*(10), 662–670.

Ward, M. M. (2004). Prevalence of physician-diagnosed systemic lupus erythematosus in the United States: Results from the third national health and nutrition examination survey. *Journal of Women's Health (Larchmont), 13*(6), 713–718.

Ward, M. M., & Studenski, S. (1990). Clinical manifestations of systemic lupus erythematosus: Identification of racial and socioeconomic influences. *Archives of Internal Medicine, 150*(4), 849–853.

CHAPTER

16

ORAL HEALTH

RUEBEN C. WARREN
ALLAN J. FORMICOLA
CASWELL A. EVANS

Clifford O. Dummett Sr., in his book entitled *Afro-Americans in Dentistry: Sequence and Consequence*, writes about the beginnings of dentistry for African Americans:

> *[In1740] The first reference to an Afro-American in health and medical practice is to be found in an early account of dental practice. The reference is to a Negro male named Simon who was regarded as being able to "bleed and draw teeth" and as "one who pretended to be a great doctor among his people" (Dummett & Dummett, 1977).*

Later in the book, Dummett writes about Robert Tanner Freeman, who was one of six men recommended for the D.M.D. degree from Harvard University's School of Dental Medicine. In 1869, Dr. Freeman was the first African American to receive the dental doctorate in the United States. From those early beginnings until today, assuring the oral health of African Americans has been a challenge not only for African American dentists, but for the dental profession and the nation as a whole (Dummett, 1974). Chronicling what has occurred to assure oral health for African Americans, in principle, is no different than for other populations. However, discerning emphasis and priority requires targeting the history and current activities in salient areas related to oral health, dental education, and oral health care delivery. This chapter reviews oral health and craniofacial research, dental education, and dental service (oral health care delivery) in general, and specifically for the African American population. The chapter will also recommend strategies for improving oral health, dental education, and oral health care delivery.

RESEARCH: ACQUISITION AND APPLICATION OF KNOWLEDGE

Much is published in the scientific literature and the popular press about "dental" diseases (Borrell, Burt, Neighbors, & Warren, 2006; Gross & Genco, 1998; Perkins & Perkins, 2000; Enwonwu & Saunders, 2000). Over the years, dental concerns have broadened beyond teeth and dental-related structures and functions to include oral health and many other craniofacial diseases, as well as the relationship between oral health and systemic health (Warren, 1990; Taylor, 2000; Hodge, 2000). Interest in these relationships, while not new, has tremendous potential for eliminating racial and ethnic health disparities that have led to growing numbers of excess deaths experienced by African Americans (U.S. Department of Health & Human Services [U.S. DHHS], 1985). These excess deaths are largely preventable and have yet to be fully explained by biomedical and public health research (Otten et al., 1990). The 1985 Report of the Secretary's Task Force on Black and Minority Health calculated 60,000 excess deaths among African Americans. These excess deaths were additional, presumably preventable and unnecessary deaths among African Americans. The sex- and age-adjusted death rate of their white, non-Hispanic counterparts was used as a baseline of what would have occurred if the death rates of the two populations had been the same. In 1985, 80 percent of these excess deaths among African Americans were attributed to six categories of causes: cardiovascular disease and stroke; cancer; cirrhosis; diabetes; homicide and unintentional injury; and infant mortality (U.S. DHHS, 1985). In 1992, HIV/AIDS was recorded as a seventh cause of excess deaths among African Americans (U.S. DHHS, 1990).

In a 2005 article on health disparities published in *Health Affairs* by a team of scientists, it was reported that the 60,000 excess deaths recorded in 1985 had, by 2002, risen to 83,000 (Satcher et al., 2005). Satcher, the senior author of the article, was the surgeon general in 2000 when the surgeon general's report on Oral Health was published. Interestingly, one major and overriding theme in the surgeon general's report on Oral Health was that "oral health means much more than healthy teeth" and that "oral health is integral to general health" (U.S. DHHS, 2000). It is becoming increasing clear that major oral diseases have an adverse biological impact on selected systemic conditions. What remains to be determined is whether those influences are bidirectional; whether the impact is more than biological (i.e. social, psychological, etc.); whether the relationships are merely associational or traceable to predictable cause-effect interactions; and whether this oral and systemic relationship has an equal impact on oral and systemic health.

There is growing evidence of biological associations between oral and systemic diseases (Joshipura, 2002; Danesh, 1999; Janket, Baird, Chuang, & Jones, 2003). In a 2000 symposium entitled "Exploring the Relationship Between Oral and Systemic Health Within the African American Population," cosponsored by the National Dental Association Foundation, the National Dental Association, Colgate-Palmolive Companies, and the National Institute of Dental and Craniofacial Research, National Institutes of Health, scientists, academicians, and health policy makers were challenged to relate oral diseases to the seven leading causes of excess deaths among African Americans. The purpose of the symposium was to discuss how to ensure that African Americans and other underserved populations benefit equitably from research addressing the associations between oral and systemic diseases (Moise, 2000). In earlier years, similar forums were held to address the same topic areas. However, there was limited focus on the experiences of people of color who disproportionately suffer from both oral and systemic diseases. The 2000 symposium intentionally focused on the research that undergirded what was known about the relationships between oral and systemic diseases in relation to conditions that disproportionately affect African Americans. Moreover, one of the presuppositions of the symposium was that there was an association between oral and systemic health, as well as oral and systemic diseases, that needed investigation. Thus, the emphasis at this symposium was on population-based health promotion and public health prevention, in addition to disease, dysfunction, and premature death. The symposium was hosted by Howard University's College of Dentistry because of the university's long history of educating African American dental professionals.

The organizers of the symposium used the 1985 federal publication entitled The Report of the Secretary's Task Force on Black and Minority Health and the 2000 U.S. Surgeon General's Report on Oral Health as foundational documents to organize the symposium. The 1985 report was published in response to ongoing disparities in health status between people of color in the United States and their non-Hispanic white counterparts. In introducing the report, then-Secretary of the Department of Health and Human Services Margaret Heckler wrote,

> [T]here was a continuing disparity in the burden of death and illness experienced by Black and other minority Americans as compared with our nation as a whole. That disparity has existed ever since accurate Federal recordkeeping began more than a generation ago, and although our health charts do itemize steady gains in the health of minority Americans, the stubborn disparity remained . . . an affront to both our ideals and to the ongoing genius of American medicine (U.S. DHHS, 1985).

The Task Force report was the first time that the federal government acknowledged that health disparities could be chronicled by race and ethnicity, which was an important precursor to addressing this longstanding problem. The 2000 U.S. surgeon general's report on Oral Health was also timely because it highlighted five key questions and answers related to oral and systemic diseases and their interconnectedness: (1) What is oral health? (2) What is the status of oral health in the United States? (3) What is the relationship between oral health and general health and well-being? (4) How is oral health promoted and maintained, and how are oral diseases prevented? and (5) What are the needs and opportunities to enhance oral health?

What Is Oral Health?

The surgeon general's report emphasized a broad definition of oral health that included all aspects of the dental, oral, and craniofacial complex. The report also emphasized the interaction, interconnectedness, and inseparable aspects of oral and systemic health, which also represents "the very essence of our humanity. To speak and smile; sigh and kiss; smell, taste, touch, chew, and swallow; cry out in pain; and convey a world of feelings and emotions through facial expressions transcends the false separation which is often omitted in understanding what it is to be truly human" (Evans & Kleinman, 2000). The report also described the biomedical intricacies of oral health from birth to death and the uniqueness of oral-facial tissues and how they interact with other systems in the body.

What Is the Status of Oral Health in the United States?

The report broadened the scope of what is usually considered when addressing common dental diseases (i.e., dental caries, periodontal diseases, etc.) by discussing selected major oral and craniofacial diseases such as oral cancer and disorders such as cleft lip and cleft palate. For example, Figure 16.1 highlights the decline in edentulism over the past twenty years (National Center for Health Statistics, 1975, 2000), yet dental caries remains one of the most common diseases of childhood (Figure 16.2) (National Center for Health Statistics, 2000). Disparities in the five-year relative survival rates for oral and pharyngeal cancer are documented in Figure 16.3 (Reis et al., 1999), and the prevalence of cleft lip and cleft palate is recorded in Figure 16.4 (Schulman, Edmonds, McClearn, Jensrold, & Shaw, 1993). Rates of all of these adverse conditions differ markedly between non-Hispanic whites and African Americans.

FIGURE 16.1 *Rates of Edentulism in U.S. Adults, 1971–1974 Versus 1988–1994.*

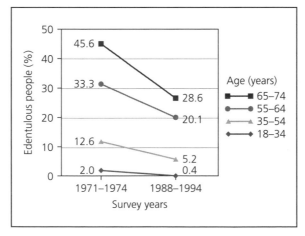

The percentage of people without any teeth has declined among adults during the past 20 years.
Source: National Center for Health Statistics (1975).

FIGURE 16.2 *Most Common Diseases Among 5-to-17-year-olds, 1996.*

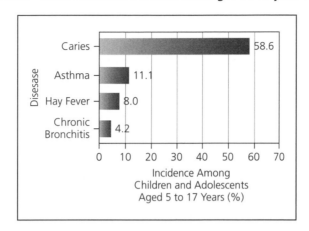

Data for dental caries include decayed or filled primary and/or decayed, filled, or missing permanent teeth. Data for asthma, chronic bronchitis, and hay fever are based on reports of household respondents about the sampled 5-to-17-year-olds.
Source: National Center for Health Statistics (1975, 2000).

FIGURE 16.3 *Five-Year Relative Survival Rates for Blacks and Whites with Oral and Pharyngeal Cancers.*

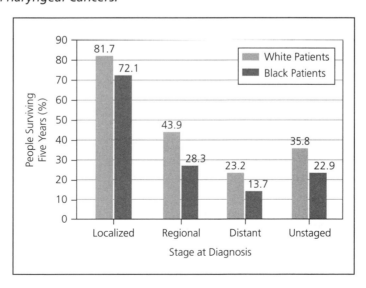

Source: Ries et al. (1999).

FIGURE 16.4 *Most Common Congenital Malformations Among Whites and Blacks.*

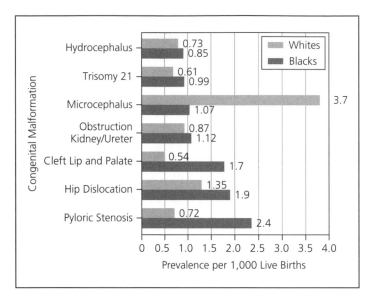

Source: Schulman et al. (1993).

The numbers of untreated decayed teeth in poor people and non-poor people also show disparities (Figure 16.5) (National Center for Health Statistics, 2000). Racial identity (i.e., African American) and low-income status are risk markers for selected dental diseases (Otten et al., 1990). Combining these risk markers places low-income African Americans at additional risk, resulting in a layering effect. Finally, the surgeon general's report revealed that the common symptom of pain accompanies many conditions affecting oral health, reducing quality of life and restricting daily functions.

There is an assumed linear relationship between oral health, dental care, and oral health care. While some portion of health can be attributed to care, much more involves factors beyond the perimeters of the health care delivery system. What is clear, nonetheless, is that the more disease is present, the more professional care is needed; few dental diseases heal independent of care. In this regard, because race/ethnicity and income are related to oral health status, and African Americans experience disproportionately high prevalence of dental and oral diseases, more dental professionals are needed to provide badly needed care. Moreover, because the race/ethnicity of the dentist is positively associated with the race/ethnicity of patient profiles, increasing the number of minority dentists will undoubtedly increase the oral health services that are available and accessible to underserved populations (Linn, 1972; Montoya, Hayes-Bautista, Gonzales, & Smeloff, 1978; Warren, 1979, 1980).

FIGURE 16.5 *Percentages of Poor People Versus Non-poor People with at Least One Untreated Decayed Tooth, by Age.*

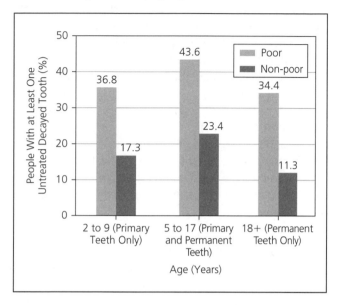

Source: National Center for Health Statistics, 1996.

What Is the Relationship Between Oral Health and General Health and Well-Being?

The surgeon general's report made it clear that numerous systemic diseases and conditions, as well as many pharmaceutical therapies, have oral manifestations. In addition, the report applied criteria for assessing the quality of the published scientific evidence regarding associations between oral health and conditions and events such as diabetes, heart disease, stroke, and adverse pregnancy outcomes. Further research is needed to determine whether these associations are causal or coincidental. This portion of the report also described the relationship between oral health and quality of life. Oral health affects speech, eating, self-esteem, social interaction, education, career development, and emotional state. The report noted that oral health clearly is related to well-being and quality of life when measured in functional, psychological, and economic dimensions. Diet, nutrition, sleep, and work are all affected by oral health status, and the overall societal burden that results from poor oral health is significant. Most of the available preventive approaches are focused on dental caries and periodontal diseases, and further research is needed to develop measures to prevent other oral diseases and conditions.

How Is Oral Health Promoted and Maintained, and How Are Oral Diseases Prevented?

The report described the unique and sometimes overlapping contributions of the dental, medical, and public health components of professional provision of oral health care. Some dentists, such as those who participate in lifestyle behavior modification programs, are involved in all three components. Estimates of national expenditures for dental health care and financing and reimbursement mechanisms demonstrate that Americans do invest substantially in oral health care services, the costs of which totaled an estimated $60 billion in 2000 (Health Care Financing Administration, 2000). However, this estimate does not include the many services rendered by other health care providers. The report also explored factors that affect the nation's capacity to improve oral health, such as the need to add oral health topics to curricula for all health professions, the need for additional faculty members in dental schools, and the need for the dental workforce to reflect the racial/ethnic and gender demographics of the U.S. population.

What Are the Needs and Opportunities to Enhance Oral Health?

Determinants of health affect members of society across all life stages. The surgeon general's report discussed how a complex interplay of factors—individual biology, physical and socioeconomic environment, personal behaviors and lifestyles, organization of health care services—bears on the level of oral health a person achieves throughout life. Dental professionals can become more effective in their contribution to improvements in the oral health of Americans, particularly children, elderly, and persons with disabilities. The report noted that access to care makes a difference in oral health status and that barriers to access must be reduced and eliminated. Eliminating barriers to access will require informed public and knowledgeable policymakers, integrated and culturally competent programs of care, and sufficient resources to pay and reimburse for care.

The report noted that many factors need to be addressed to increase access to care. Although the availability of insurance increases that access, there are 108 million Americans who do not have any form of dental insurance coverage. For every person without medical insurance, there are 2.7 people without dental insurance in the United States. Federal and state assistance programs for selected oral health services exist, but they are limited in scope. Moreover, the reimbursement levels are low in comparison with the usual fees for care. Reducing some of these barriers to care would have a profound effect on the numbers of people seeking needed dental care. In addition, the promise of science in creating new technologies for prevention, treatment, restoration, and rehabilitation of oral and craniofacial disorders and conditions also may increase access to care.

As previously indicated, this chapter addresses challenges and successes in improving and sustaining oral health in the black community. The chapter is divided into three interconnected areas: research, education, and service.

Research in oral health is conducted in at least four overlapping venues: academia, industry, the dental profession, and government. Most research in oral health, however, is either conducted or supported by the National Institute of Dental and Craniofacial Research (NIDCR). The dental institute is one of thirteen institutes and centers at the U.S. National Institutes of Health (NIH). The mission of NIDCR is to "promote the general health of the American people by improving their oral, dental, and craniofacial health." Biomedical research has done well in clarifying the basic science mechanisms that are associated with the major morbidities and mortalities facing the U.S. population. However, the research challenges that are associated with racial and ethnic, oral, and systemic health disparities reach far beyond biomedical science into investigations that seek to understand why biomedical discoveries are not equitably available, accessible, and acceptable to all segments of the U.S. population.

Research is defined by federal government as "a systematic investigation including research development, testing, and evaluation, designed to develop or contribute to generalizable knowledge" (http://www.hhs.gov/ohrp/humansubjects/guidance/45cfr46 .htm#46.102).

For the purpose of this chapter, research will be described consistent with the reported research mission at NIH, which systematically uses science to pursue fundamental knowledge about the nature and behavior of living systems and to apply that knowledge to extend healthy life and reduce the burdens of illness and disability by (1) fostering fundamental creative discoveries, innovative research strategies, and their applications as a basis to advance significantly the nation's capacity to protect and improve health; (2) developing, maintaining, and renewing scientific human and physical resources that will assure the nation's capability to prevent disease; (3) expanding the knowledge base in medical and associated sciences in order to enhance the nation's economic well-being and ensure a continued high return on the public investment in research; and (4) exemplifying and promoting the highest level of scientific integrity, public accountability, and social responsibility in the conduct of science (National Institutes of Health, 2009).

Two basic categories of human subject research are biomedical or basic research and applied research. While the equipment, training, and methods are sometimes similar in both research areas, the fundamental difference involves research questions. Biomedical investigators often derive their research questions from previous work drawn from the confines of the laboratory. This research is often funded as a result of an investigator, on his or her own, submitting a research application. This research is known as unsolicited research; its opposite is targeted research. Questions from this type of research are usually investigator-initiated. Applied research, on the other hand, is designed to solve practical problems rather than to acquire knowledge for knowledge's sake (http://www.lbl.gov/Education/ELSI/research-main.html).

The applied researcher's "laboratory" is often outside of a controlled setting (laboratory), and investigators frequently must deal with a series of uncontrollable factors that require adjusting research protocols in order to sustain the rigor needed for valid and reliable results. The latter investigations generally are included in population-based public health research starting with epidemiology. One relatively new area of applied research, which has tremendous potential to improve the oral health of African Americans, is community-based participatory research.

Community-based participatory research (CBPR) focuses on social, structural, and physical environmental inequities through active involvement of community members, organizational representation, and researchers in all aspects of the research process (Israel et al., 1998). The CBPR process is scientific inquiry conducted in partnership between a traditionally trained practitioner and lay participants. In CBPR projects, the community participates fully in all aspects of the research process. The "expert" practitioner and the lay participant are co-equal partners in a CBPR process. This method requires that the views, concerns, and interests of all participants receive equal weight in determining the focus of the research question, the approach employed in attempting to identify answers and solutions, and the use and significance of the products of the research endeavor (http://en.wikipedia.org/wiki/Community-based_participatory_ research).

The work of CBPR combines three activities: investigation, learning, and action. It is a method of social investigation of problems involving participation in problem formulation and resolution. It is a learning process for the researcher and participants, who analyze the structural causes of named problems through collective discussion and interaction. Finally, it is a way for researchers and lay communities to engage in concerted action, both short- and long-term (Merzel & D'Afflitti, 2003). The direct link between research and action is a unique aspect of participatory research. By combining the creation of knowledge with concrete action, the traditional research dichotomy between knowing and doing is dissolved. Because the community is a full partner in the process, translating knowledge acquisition into effective action is more fluid and cost effective.

Using the basic knowledge created by biomedical and behavioral science research and translating that knowledge through population-based applied research methodologies to improve the human condition should generate new strategies to eliminate oral health disparities among African Americans. Equally important, an enhanced, targeted research agenda focused specifically on promoting oral health among African Americans should improve their systemic health as well. Moreover, improving the oral health of African Americans will likely also provide *lessons learned* for other underserved groups. Better-informed oral health research outcomes for African Americans can also translate into an enhanced teaching and learning environment for educating dental professionals of all racial and ethnic groups.

Historically, African American dentists have disproportionately served African Americans (Linn, 1972; Warren, 1979). In the foreseeable future, more African American dentists will be needed if access to oral health care and improved oral health among African Americans and other underserved populations are expected (Sullivan Commission, 2004). However, increasing the number of African American dentists has been persistently problematic. African American dentists have come almost singularly from U.S. dental schools, in contrast with dentists from other minority groups who, in addition to graduating from U.S. undergraduate dental schools, have migrated from other countries where many of them received their dental education.

EDUCATION: THE RELATIONSHIP BETWEEN ORAL HEALTH AND LACK OF PRACTITIONERS OF COLOR

As indicated previously, the comprehensive surgeon general's report on oral health in America, published in 2000 (U.S. DHHS, 2000), revealed that there has been an improvement in the oral health of the nation, but significant public health problems remain. Pointing to a disparity in oral disease based on income, race, and ethnicity, the surgeon general's report linked poor oral health in persons of color to a lack of practitioners of color. The report issued the discouraging data that there is only one black practitioner for every 6,140 black patients, as compared with one non-Hispanic white practitioner for every 1,452 non-Hispanic white patients—a huge discrepancy in access to care. Creating greater numbers of African American practitioners becomes a critical way to resolve this problem.

Subsequent to the surgeon general's report, two other national reports (Smedley, Stith, & Bristow, 2004; Sullivan Commission, 2004) carefully documented the lack of diversity in all of the health professions and urged renewed efforts to rectify the problem. It is also clear that all practitioners must be prepared to treat all patients regardless of their race or ethnicity. However, in a landmark study (Smedley, Stith, & Nelson, 2002), it was shown that there were worse health outcomes in African Americans and Hispanics when there was discordance between the racial or ethnic makeup of practitioners and their patients. Further, it was suggested that practitioner biases could affect the outcome of treatment. This Institute of Medicine (IOM) report studied several disease categories including cardiovascular disease, and although the study did not specifically look at oral disease, the Study Panel concluded that the findings were strong enough to recommend that all practitioners receive cultural competence training to increase their awareness of the role that biases play in the outcome of treatment.

To improve the oral health of African Americans, Hispanics, and other people of color, it is important to examine the role that education plays in preparing a sufficient workforce to treat all segments of society. To better understand the educational system for dentistry, this section on education will broadly review three periods of dental education: (1) the formative years from the 1920s to 1959, (2) an awakening period of social consciousness from the 1960s to 1980s, and (3) an activist period from the 1990s to the present geared toward addressing inadequate access and lack of diversity in the dental workforce. Our aim in describing these three periods is to explore why the current configuration exists and to show how racial and ethnic diversity in the enrollment of students became the current focus of the profession. The challenges of increasing the representation of African Americans as well as Hispanics and Native Americans in the dental profession remain significant, as indicated in the final section.

The Formative Years: 1920s to 1959

The formative years of U.S. dental education set the stage for a long period of educating African American dentists, mainly at Howard University's College of Dentistry and at the School of Dentistry at Meharry Medical College. The medical and dental professions in the United States in the twentieth century were guided by two landmark reports based on studies conducted in the early part of the century and supported by the Carnegie Foundation for the Advancement of Education. Prior to the issuing of these reports by Flexner in 1910 (Flexner, 1910), and Gies in 1926 (Gies, 1926), training of physicians and dentists was substandard and conducted by for-profit schools unaffiliated with universities. Both reports were credited with raising standards including admissions standards for entering students and developing dental schools as part of the university system in the United States. College-level education became a prerequisite for entry to the professional schools, and national accrediting agencies developed and standardized entrance examinations. As a result of the Flexner report, only two of the eight black medical schools remained open: Howard University in Washington, DC, and Meharry Medical College in Nashville, Tennessee. Fortunately, these two medical schools also had dental schools. The Gies report's vision was for the dentists to be the highest-level licensed practitioners to manage the oral health of the public and that general practitioners would be assisted by a range of specialists. Both of these reports recognized the importance of Howard University and the Meharry Medical College in the field of medicine and dentistry for the education of African American practitioners. Howard's dental school (organized in 1884) and Meharry's dental school (organized in 1886) were recognized as critical institutions for educating African American practitioners, and Gies recommended that both dental schools be supported.

The Gies report indicated that an inadequate number of African American dentists were being educated and that the ratio of African American dentists to the African American population was 1 to 8,500 in comparison with 1 to about 1,700 white dentists to the white population. In 1924, Howard was enrolling a class of approximately 45 students and Meharry about 90 students. Enrollment of African American dental students was not keeping up with yearly increases of the African American population. The total enrollment of African American dental students in the period from 1919 to 1925 was 608. Given the segregated system of education in the nation, it was surprising that in 1925, twenty-five dental schools had an enrollment of both white and black students. But, instead of recommending that all dental schools enroll students of both races, the report noted the prevailing attitude of the time in the following statement: "General growth of sentiment for segregation has increased the tendency, in many dental schools, to restrict the attendance to white students" (Gies, 1926, pp. 292 and 549).

From this beginning the die was cast, and in subsequent decades the inadequacy of the number of African American students enrolled in dental schools in the United States continued. Howard and Meharry have produced and continue to educate the greatest number of African American dentists. Table 16.1 shows that little progress was made during the twentieth century in addressing the inadequacy of the production of African American dentists (Gies, p. 91; U.S. DHHS, 2000, Table 98, p. 237).

The largely segregated system of education in the United States prevailed, and it was not until the Great Society programs of the 1960s and 1970s that higher education was challenged by the federal government to open its doors to women and minorities.

TABLE 16.1   **Population Ratios of White and African American Dentists in 1926 vs. 1996.**

	White	African American
1926	1:1,700	1:8,500
1996	1:1,452	1:6,140

Source: 1926 data: the Gies report; 1996 data: the surgeon general's report.

Affirmative action rules were enacted, leading to a new chapter with ups and downs in including minorities in the nation's universities, colleges, and professional schools.

The Period of Awakening: 1960s–1980s

During the period of awakening, the United States became socially aware of the limitations it had placed in denying women and minorities access to higher education. Affirmative action became the way to remedy this problem. It is important to briefly review the history of affirmative action in order to understand the action or inaction that higher education and professional schools pursued during the period of awakening. The era of affirmative action was ushered in when President John F. Kennedy in 1961 issued Executive Order 10925 requiring federal contractors to take affirmative action to ensure representation of minorities in employment. Later, extended by the 1964 Civil Rights Act and backed up by federal governmental enforcement agencies (OFCCP and the EEOC), institutions of higher education established affirmative action programs to increase the number of women and minorities in their student bodies and within their faculties.

Affirmative action programs have met several challenges, but the most important cases that have reached the Supreme Court are the 1978 *Bakke v. Regents of the University of California* and more recently, in 2000 and 2001 respectively, *Gratz* and *Grutter v. Bollinger*, two cases at the University of Michigan. The results of the Supreme Court action on these cases indicate that it is lawful to take race into account in admissions decisions, but that it must be done in a narrowly tailored way to achieve diversity. Quota systems are not permitted. The Supreme Court decisions also endorse the goal of achieving diversity rather than remedying past racial discrimination. Two other state actions have also influenced what universities and professional schools have (or have not) done with regard to affirmative action. *Hopwood v. State of Texas* and Proposition 209 in California dampened and eliminated, respectively, the use of affirmative action in admissions decisions. However, the recent Supreme Court rulings in 2003 indicate that affirmative action plans must show that there is an important and persuasive reason to use race as a factor and that taking race into account is the only way to achieve the goal (*Affirmative Action Compliance in Higher Education*, 2008).

Dental statistics make it clear that the oral health of African Americans is much worse than that of non-Hispanic Whites. Practice patterns also demonstrate that

African American practitioners treat a higher proportion of African Americans than do other practitioners (U.S. DHHS, 2000, p. 236; Solomon, Williams, & Sinkford, 2001). Taken together, these two facts provide a firm basis for dental schools to take affirmative action in making admissions decisions to enroll African Americans. Public institutions and state-supported dental schools must take into account the African American population in relation to the number of practicing dentists when developing their affirmative action plans. As mentioned previously, Table 16.1 indicates that the national ratio of African American dentists to the African American population in 1996 was 1:6,140, as compared with a ratio of 1:1,452 for white dentists and the white population. The ratio will vary by state, and in states where the population of African Americans is high and there is a paucity of African American practitioners it should be expected that state-supported schools have strong affirmative action programs. However, from a national perspective it is essential that all dental schools have affirmative action programs to admit greater numbers of African American students as well as Hispanic and Native Americans, two groups that suffer from the same lack of practitioners—ratios of 1:5,425 Hispanic dentists to population and 1:10,072 Native American dentists to population.

The lack of progress made in graduating African American practitioners (as well as Hispanics and Native Americans) was noted in the Sullivan Commission report (Sullivan Commission, 2004). Approximately 55 to 59 accredited dental schools were operating between 1976 and 2003. These schools, on average, graduated a total of only 202 African American students per year. That number includes Meharry and Howard, which account for about 120 of those students. Further, only 5 percent of students in the nation's specialty dental programs are African American. Similarly, persons of color have been inadequately represented among the teachers of future health care professionals. In 2002–2003, of the 4,805 full-time faculty, 5.5 percent or 267 were African American, 4.84 percent or 233 were Hispanic/Latino, and 16 or 0.33 percent were Native American. The Sullivan report concluded, "The data for medicine, nursing, and dentistry . . . demonstrate the failure of these professions to keep pace with the changing demographics of the nation. If unchanged, these data draw a roadmap to a health care system that remains inherently unequal, bearing little resemblance to the nation at large, and directly contributory to the health disparities faced by minority populations." After examining the lack of progress of enrolling and graduating minority practitioners in nursing, medical, and dental schools, the Sullivan Commission made several recommendations. Many of the recommendations of the IOM and Sullivan Commission reports have been taken into account in programs that have been stimulated by national foundations that recognize the need to take action. The following three key recommendations from the Sullivan Commission report formulate important guidelines for schools of nursing, medicine, and dentistry:

> *Colleges, universities, and health professions schools should support socioeconomically disadvantaged college students who express an interest in the health professions and provide these students with an array of support services, including*

mentoring, test-taking skills, counseling on application procedures, and interviewing skills. (Sullivan Commission report, recommendation 4.5)

The Association of American Medical Colleges, the American Association of Colleges of Nursing, the American Dental Education Association, and the Association of Academic Health Centers should promote the review and enhancement of health professions schools admissions policies and procedures to: a) enable more holistic, individualized screening processes; b) ensure a diverse student body with enhanced language competency and cultural competence for all students; and c) develop strategies to enhance and increase the pool of minority applicants. (Sullivan Commission report, recommendation 4.8)

Diversity should be a core value in the health professions. Health professions schools should ensure that their mission statements reflect a social contract with the community and a commitment to diversity among their students, faculty, staff, and administration. (Sullivan Commission report, recommendation 4.10)

Taken collectively, the reports of the surgeon general, the IOM, and the Sullivan Commission document the need for new action to recruit and enroll greater numbers of underrepresented minority (URM) students into dentistry, medicine, and nursing programs. These reports have led to educational reforms targeted to improving diversity.

The Activist Period: 1990s to the Present

The need to increase the enrollment of underrepresented minority (URM)[1] students has become a national priority for dentistry during the activist period. As the twentieth century came to a close and the twenty-first century dawned, the U.S. began to recognize that the minority population would by mid-century be the majority. Businesses began to recognize the need to diversify their workforce. In the health professions, the majority schools took stock of the failed efforts of the past to enroll more URM students and started new efforts. Fueling those new efforts were the three national reports referred to above: the IOM report entitled In the Nation's Compelling Interest, the Sullivan Commission report, Missing Persons, and the IOM report, Unequal Treatment. Taken together, these three reports urged the nation's schools of medicine, dentistry, and nursing to undertake new efforts to increase their enrollment of URM students and improve the cultural competence of all students. As indicated above, the surgeon general's report on the oral health of the nation linked the lack of practitioners of color to the poorer oral health of racial and ethnic minorities.

---

[1] URM students are those students whose representation in U.S. dental schools is far below their respective groups' percentage in the U.S. population. African American, Hispanic, and Native American students are the groups defined as underrepresented. For example, in 1996 African Americans made up 12.0 percent of the population but only 2.2 percent of active dentists (surgeon general's report, p. 236), and Hispanics were similarly underrepresented with only 2.8 percent of dentists but 10.7 percent of the population.

The activist period is also characterized by several new initiatives. They include university mission statements aspiring to diversity; support from major foundations for demonstration projects; and efforts by individual schools to increase enrollment of URM students. These initiatives adhere to the recommendations cited above from the Sullivan Commission report. Most universities today include in their mission statements that they wish to become a diverse institution in student enrollment and faculty. These mission statements are important because they create an expectation that individual schools and colleges will adopt similar statements that will guide policy on hiring of faculty and admitting students. The idea that diversity within an educational institution is a benefit to the learning environment has been proven by classroom studies (Gurin, Lehman, & Lewis, 2007). There is more active learning—e.g., a broader range of discussion—in classes that include a diverse group of students. Leadership at the school level is able to draw upon university resources to design and implement programs to promote diversity. A number of universities have appointed Diversity Officers that often report directly to the President of the University. Similarly, the more enlightened dental schools have followed up by appointing assistant or associate deans for diversity and/or multicultural affairs.

Three major U.S. foundations have focused attention on developing programs designed to increase applications and enrollment by URM students. The largest such initiative ever undertaken in the nation has been the Robert Wood Johnson Foundation's (RWJF) Pipeline, Profession & Practice: Community-Based Dental Education (Dental Pipeline) program (Bailit, Formicola, D'Abreu, Stavisky, & Zamora, 2005). Collaborating with the RWJF initiative are The California Endowment and the W. K. Kellogg Foundation. The Dental Pipeline program has had two major overlapping goals: to improve the cultural awareness and sensitivity of all dental students through community-based education, and to increase the enrollment of underrepresented minority students. In the first phase of this program (2002–2007) 15 dental schools[2] received funds to change their curricula to add cultural awareness through didactic course work and by sending students into facilities in underserved communities to learn about the problems confronting community residents. It has been shown (Smith et al., 2006) that students will carry out as practitioners what they learn in dental school, so if students are educated to appreciate the problems of the underserved they are more likely to open their practices to patients from all economic and racial/ethnic groups.

The URM initiative under the Dental Pipeline program includes initiatives to attract college students into careers in dentistry through summer enrichment programs; post-baccalaureate programs to enhance applicants' opportunities to enroll in dental

---

[2]The 15 dental schools funded were at the following institutions: Boston University, University of Connecticut, Howard University, University of Illinois at Chicago, Loma Linda University, Meharry Medical College, University of North Carolina, Ohio State University, University of the Pacific, Temple University, University of California at Los Angeles and at San Francisco, University of Southern California, University of Washington, and West Virginia University. The National Program Office for the program is located at Columbia University. Additional information can be obtained at www.dentalpipeline.org.

school and to implement changes in admissions policies; and procedures that go beyond examining standardized test scores and college grade point averages to programs designed to mentor students interested in dentistry as a career. Guiding the development of the RWJF Dental Pipeline program was a study of problems and challenges faced by college students and enrolled dental students when considering a dental career (Veal, Perry, Stavisky, & D'Abreu-Herbert, 2004). The study found that college students were receiving little guidance regarding the entry requirements and the application process for dental school and that enrolled students of color found that the lack of faculty mentors of color caused great challenges.

To address these issues, the Dental Pipeline schools established summer enrichment programs to better prepare URM students for entry to dental school. Seven summer enrichment programs are offered by Dental Pipeline schools. Another finding was that there was a need to develop post-baccalaureate programs for students who need an extra year to prepare for dental school after completing college. Dental Pipeline schools now offer six such programs. These schools reached out to URM students on college campuses and to the pre-health advisors to increase the number of URM students applying to dental schools. Two recruitment collaboratives were formed—one in California and the other in the northeast—to improve the coordination of recruitment on college campuses and to provide consistent outreach effort to college students.

One of the important findings of the Dental Pipeline program was the need to employ new methods of reviewing applicants' credentials. For too long, colleges and professional schools have relied on standardized test scores as a major component of assessing whether students will be successful members of society. Bowen and Bok (1998) have shown that SAT scores do not predict who will be successful in society. Many universities have shifted from an overemphasis on SAT scores, and some have even eliminated them in admissions consideration. Professional schools, however, have continued to rely on standardized admissions tests and in many schools excellent candidates have been eliminated based on their scores. Most of the Dental Pipeline schools have learned that a more balanced approach to considering the qualifications of candidates includes taking account of other factors such as disadvantaged educational status, work and family obligations, leadership skills, and commitment to service. When these characteristics are factored into the admissions review appropriately with college grade point averages and the standardized Dental Admission Test scores, a wider range of students from a variety of backgrounds are considered and admitted.

As a result of these changes, enrollment of URM students in the Dental Pipeline schools (not including Meharry and Howard) rose 57 percent from 2002–2003 to 2007–2008 (Formicola et al., 2009). The actual increase in numbers was from 90 to 142 URM students enrolled in the 13 majority schools. At the beginning of the program several of these schools enrolled no URM students at all, and by the end of the project all of the schools enrolled URM students and some of the schools in one year or another had enrollment of URM students as 20 percent of their first-year class. This Dental Pipeline program clearly demonstrates that outreach and recruitment efforts on campuses that have large numbers of URM students and newer methods of evaluating applicants for admission improve the enrollment of students of color. These programs are producing best practices that other schools can employ to improve diversity in their student bodies.

The Dental Pipeline program is currently in its second phase, funding eight additional dental schools to replicate the results from Phase I. Four of the Phase II schools[3] are concentrating on improving their recruitment and enrollment of URM students. In addition, the American Dental Education Association (ADEA) is creating a network of admissions officers who are better prepared to assist their schools to achieve diversity in student enrollment and to strengthen the accreditation requirements for diversity. The National Dental Association (NDA) is developing a national mentoring program to assist dental schools to work with local chapters of the NDA to provide mentors for applicants. In addition, and unrelated to the Dental Pipeline program, the American Dental Association has adopted programs designed to improve outreach to minority students and to improve diversity in leadership. These national associations enhance the work done by the individual schools.

Another important national program to assist students is a summer enrichment program for college students who are interested in medical school, for which the Robert Wood Johnson Foundation has provided funding since 1987. Three years ago, the program was expanded to include students interested in dentistry. The six-week program is operated on twelve college campuses and consists of enrichment courses in the basic sciences and preparation for applying to medical and dental school. Instruction includes improving study skills, interviewing, and test preparation for entrance examinations. Currently, the twelve campuses enroll a total of approximately 600 pre-medical students and 200 pre-dental students who have completed their first or second year of college.

Another major effort is underway in the United States to improve the enrollment of URM students in dental education. The Bridging the Gap (BTG) Program was conceived under the W. K. Kellogg Foundation's national Community Voices: Health Care for the Underserved program (Kellogg Foundation, 2006). This effort is creating partnerships of colleges that enroll large numbers of URM students with dental schools in three states: Georgia, New Mexico, and New York. An 18-month (2007–2009) planning grant from the Josiah Macy Jr. Foundation is being used to design a new pathway for URM students into dental school through early identification of students in high school followed by admission into a combined college–dental school coordinated program. Dentistry often loses well-prepared URM students to the field of medicine, and this pathway has been created to recruit such students into the field. Whether these three regional programs will progress beyond the planning stage into actual implementation is unknown. However, the fact that the planning grant is underway underscores the importance of national foundation support for efforts to advance the work of bringing diversity into the health care fields.

---

[3]The four RWJF Phase II schools focusing on improving the enrollment of URM students are Baylor College of Dental Medicine, A.T. Still School of Dentistry in Arizona, Virginia Commonwealth University School of Dentistry, and Creighton University School of Dentistry.

Individual school efforts often lead to widespread adoption. The Dental Pipeline program was shaped in part from leadership institutions that had already built strong recruitment and enrollment programs to increase the diversity of students coming from college into dental school. Similarly, it is important to deal with the other issues, such as encouraging diversity in the faculty. One route into faculty positions is through postgraduate training in the dental specialties. Hospital dental services in urban areas also require more URM staff.

One way to develop diversity in faculty and hospital staffs was demonstrated through a special program in New York City. The Harlem Hospital Dental Service lacked dental specialists to treat the complex needs of the population surrounding the hospital while its affiliated dental school at Columbia University wished to increase the diversity of its faculty. Through a combined effort between the general practice residency program at Harlem Hospital and the postgraduate specialty program at Columbia, twenty one mainly African American dentists were trained in six different dental specialty fields over a period of approximately ten years (Formicola et al., 2003). Of the graduates, fifteen hold academic appointments: four full-time at Columbia, one full-time at Case Western Reserve University, and ten part-time at Columbia. Nine of the graduates hold joint appointments at the Harlem Hospital and two have full-time positions at the hospital. One of the graduates is employed full-time at the Veterans Administration Hospital and three are full-time practitioners. In many cases, these individuals were the first fully trained African American practitioners in their specialty fields in New York City. There is an ongoing need for greater representation of URM dentists in postgraduate fields in dentistry and on the faculty of most dental schools. This program demonstrates that institutions can address diversity needs when there is harmony between the defined need and planning of programs to improve diversity. Finally, the American Dental Education Association is providing grants to increase the number of URM faculty. Funded by the W. K. Kellogg Foundation, seven grants have been awarded to facilitate the training and career development of URM faculty. These initiatives will eventually lead to improving the representation of African Americans as well as other URM practitioners in the field of dentistry. However, it is important to keep in mind the challenges that confront these efforts.

THE CHALLENGES IN DENTAL EDUCATION

The challenges faced by dental education in achieving greater diversity are evident in statistics regarding applications and enrollment. Figure 16.6 shows that the number of applicants to dental schools has had two major peaks—one in the mid- to late 1970s when there were 15,734 applicants, and another in the 2000–2005 period when there were 13,742 applicants. The growth in total applications since 1990 has been 59 percent. At the same time the number of first-year students enrolled in dental schools decreased significantly between these two peak periods, declining from 6,301 to 4,733. So there are at least three applicants for each position and deciding which applicants to

FIGURE 16.6 *U.S. Dental School Applicant and First-Year Enrollment Trends, 1955–2007.*

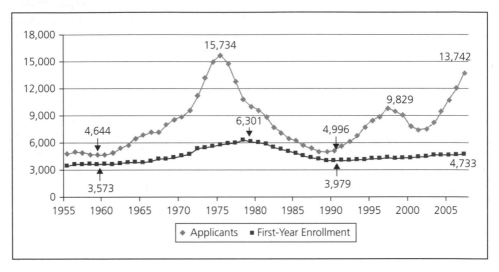

Source: Courtesy of American Dental Education Association, *Official Guide to Dental Schools, 2005–2006.*

accept has become a complex and complicated matter for all schools. All applicants are finding it difficult to gain admission to dental school.

Figure 16.7 shows the number of minority applicants to dental schools. After a relatively flat period during the 1990s, there has been a steady increase in URM student applications. Applications by African Americans have more than doubled, going from 316 in 1990 to 807 in 2006. As can be seen, the most recent upsurge in applications began around 2003. Recent applicant growth can be attributed to implementation of programs to increase the applicant pool and a national effort by organized dentistry to place diversity in the profession as the number one issue alongside improvement in access to care for underserved population groups. The National Dental Association has long championed the need to increase representation of African American students in the nation's majority schools. So too has the American Dental Education Association; however, the American Dental Association has more recently made this a priority issue.

Figure 16.8 demonstrates how far we have yet to travel to increase the enrollment of URM students. It shows that there has been a small increase between 1990 and 2006 from 215 to 279 African American students entering dental schools and similarly for Hispanics from 245 to 323. The data indicate a slow but steady increase in enrollment following a low point in 1999, but it is clear that more progress is needed to bring representation of African American students in dental school closer to this group's proportion of the population.

FIGURE 16.7 *Minority Applicants to U.S. Dental Schools, 1990–2007.*

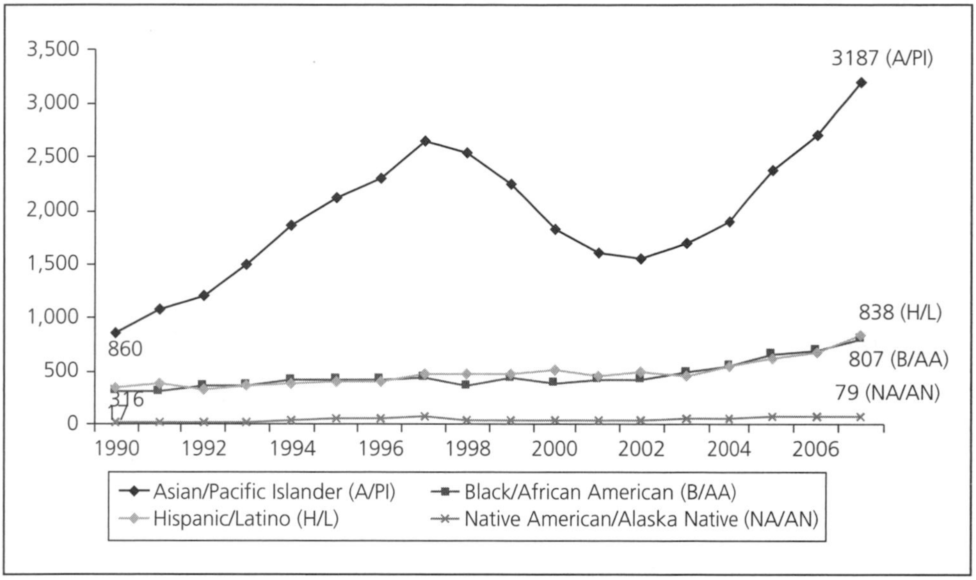

Source: Courtesy of American Dental Education Association, *Official Guide to Dental Schools, 2005–2006.*

Another major challenge that all students confront when applying and enrolling in dental school is the high cost of the education and the debt students accumulate by the time they complete four years of college and four years of dental school. Resident and nonresident fees in 2003–2004 for first-year dental students averaged between $18,607 and $20,034 and $29,803 and $31,483, respectively. There is a wide range in tuition, depending on whether students enroll in a state-financed school or a private school and whether students are residents or nonresidents of the state. For example, first-year tuition in 2007–2008 was $25,000 at the University of California–Los Angeles, a state school, and $61,900 at the University of Southern California, a private school in the same city (American Dental Association, 2008). The average debt load for graduates in 2006 was $162,155. The percent of students with debt of $100,000 or more did not differ between URM students and white students (Chmar et al., 2007). Many students from families of modest means cannot conceive of incurring such high levels of debt. However, an ADEA survey showed that only 17 percent of graduates needed to extend the usual 10-year loan repayment period, while 27 percent were able to pay off their loans early. Between 1999 and 2001, new dentists' annual net income averaged $142,461, and dentists are in the top 5 percent of earners in the United States (American Dental Education Association, 2006). All dental schools have financial aid officers who assist students with arranging loans or grants/scholarships. It is important that college

FIGURE 16.8 *First-Time, First-Year Minority Enrollees in U.S. Dental Schools, 1990–2007.*

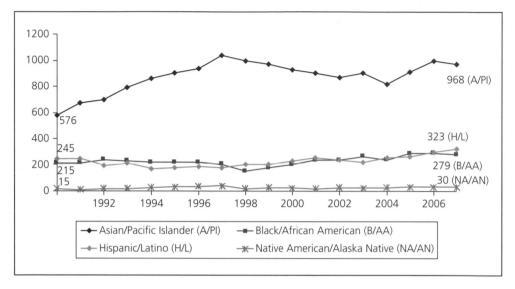

Source: Courtesy of American Dental Education Association, *Official Guide to Dental Schools, 2005–2006.*

students become familiar with this information, as they may otherwise reject the idea of becoming a dentist because they have heard that the costs are too high. The financial challenges are not insurmountable. There are programs underway to address them, and new ones will be developed in the future that lead eventually to a greater representation of African Americans and other underrepresented minorities in dentistry. As URM students continue to enter the field of dentistry, they will serve as role models for the next generation of students, further encouraging them to consider dentistry as a career.

SERVICE: PUBLIC AND PRIVATE; COMMUNITY, GROUP, AND INDIVIDUAL

From an ideal perspective, promoting and protecting health and preventing diseases at the community and/or group levels, as well as promoting and protecting health and preventing diseases for the individual should be the initial set of considerations for members of the dental profession. Concerns regarding access to dental care and receipt of systemic and other oral health services can then be approached in the context of community, group, and individual health promotion, protection, and disease prevention efforts and outcomes. However, the literature clearly documents that ideal circumstances may not prevail, particularly for African Americans and other underserved populations (Walker, Mays, & Warren, 2004). In some instances, due to a plethora of disease, access to care may be the compelling concern. Moreover, even when access to care is available, it may not be accessible or acceptable. Therefore, availability, accessibility, and acceptability are reasonable constructs that can provide a meaningful way to discuss the provision of oral health services.

With reference to health care, oral and general, these three major constructs frame an evaluation of the quality of care delivered. Availability means the service is suitable and ready to use; accessibility means the service is able to be used, entered, or reached; and acceptability means the service achieves minimal requirements (Warren, 1999). The literature is also clear that all of these levels are seldom realized simultaneously, particular with regard to the underserved or populations that are disproportionately ill.

Guidelines for the types of health care that are available and needed have been highlighted as three levels of prevention: primary, secondary, and tertiary. Primary prevention occurs when disease is absent and health promotion and education are enough. Secondary prevention occurs when disease is at a minimum and early treatment will usually resolve the problem. Tertiary prevention requires major surgery and rehabilitation. These measurements provide an operational framework for individuals and groups to manage their health care (Leavell & Clark, 1965). However, by starting with community efforts, the best clinical, cost-effective, and efficacious strategies for maximum oral health benefits can be realized.

Community-Level Health Promotion, Protection, and Disease Prevention Initiatives

When thinking about oral health, one must address an array of dental and craniofacial issues. However, preventing dental caries has been the major focus of concern related to oral health, and reducing dental caries is the major example of success in the dental profession. Community water fluoridation is the scientific innovation principally responsible for the success, and it is the initiative most reported and recorded. The proper use of fluoride reduces dental decay and even reverses the progression of existing dental caries. In general, the use of fluoride has been a major contributor to the overall decline of dental decay and reductions in the severity of this disease in the United States and other developed countries. Based on community-level research conducted during the 1940s, fluoride has subsequently and routinely been added to community drinking water supplies as a public health measure to reduce dental decay. Studies conducted by numerous researchers in many communities over a fifty-year period have verified the safety and the effectiveness of this measure. These studies have consistently demonstrated reduction in dental decay in the range of 15 to 60 percent depending on the particular circumstances of the study population and community. These reductions are achieved at fluoride levels of 0.07 to 1.2 parts per million of fluoride to water (CDC, 1999). The contrast between the cost of water fluoridation and the cost of professionally restoring decayed teeth is so staggering that it can be visualized by comparing one penny with a $10,000 stack of pennies. In 2006, 69.2 percent of the U.S. population served by community water systems received optimally fluoridated water, an increase from 62.1 percent in 1992 and from 65.0 percent in 2000. State-specific percentages in 2006 ranged from 8.4 percent in Hawaii to 100 percent in DC (median: 77.0%). In 2006, the *Healthy People 2010* target of 75 percent had been met by twenty-five states and Washington, DC. Overall, approximately 184 million persons served by community water systems received fluoridated water; of that number, approximately eight million persons received water with sufficient naturally occurring fluoride concentrations (American Medical Association, 2008). Because the fifty largest cities are heavily populated with African American residents, the African American population receives substantial benefit from community water fluoridation. Other community, or population-based, uses of fluorides have also demonstrated effectiveness. For example, schools have proven to be effective sites for fluoride use for the purpose of reducing dental cavities among school children. Tablets containing proper amounts of fluoride can be chewed and swallowed, or fluoride-containing solutions can be used as a mouth rinse. In some limited instances, particularly in rural or remote sites, fluoride can be added directly to the water supply of a school. Each of these measures has been proven effective when the intervention is applied correctly and in appropriate settings. While the opposition to community fluoridation remains strong, the opposition to fluoride tablets and fluoride mouth rinses has been much less vocal and resistant. However, the cost effectiveness and efficiency of tablets and mouth rinses have been less impressive. Nonetheless, an impressive array of preventive measures have enhanced the oral health of the public (Truman, Gooch, & Evans, 2002). The challenge is to assure that all benefit equitably from what research has discovered and education has taught.

Personal Actions to Prevent Dental Diseases

Across the life span of individuals and throughout families, the most effective measures to reduce oral diseases are simple preventive interventions that can be applied daily. These measures exert a substantial influence over the eventual need for curative care and the extent and effectiveness of that care (CDC, 1998). Brushing teeth daily with a fluoridated toothpaste is a basic measure that serves to decrease development of dental cavities; flossing along with brushing helps prevent the development of periodontal diseases (gum disease) and deterioration. Periodontal diseases affect the soft tissues surrounding the teeth and also result in erosion of the bone (Dye & Thornton-Evans, 2007). The use of dental floss is an important component of personal oral hygiene. Dental floss is used primarily to clean the areas between teeth and remove bacteria from between the teeth and surrounding gum tissue. Dietary uses of fluoride supplements in fluoride-deficient communities or fluoride mouth rinses are also among the actions under the control of individuals and families.

Diet plays a critical role in determining levels of dental disease, particularly the processes leading to dental cavities, and consequently is another focal point for personal action. Candy, sweets in general, soda pop, and other foods that contain high level of refined sugars contribute to the development of cavities in teeth. To prevent or reduce the need for curative dental care and restoration, such foods should be avoided or minimally consumed. When these items are eaten, care should be taken to brush the teeth as soon as possible.

The use of sports mouth guards is another simple step that can reduce the need for dental care that might result from trauma and collisions. These devices typically require fabrication by a dentist and trained dental personnel; however, their consistent use is a matter of personal action and commitment. Research has proven that craniofacial injuries in football, basketball, soccer, and other contact sports can be greatly reduced if mouth guards are used consistently, particularly with children (Warren, 1999).

Smoking has a deleterious effect on oral and systemic health and can lead to the need for care. The components of cigarette smoke damage the gums and other soft tissue and can contribute to the development and progression of soft tissue diseases. Cigarette smoking is also associated with the development of certain forms of cancer. Pipe smoking, in particular, can lead to cancer of the lips and tongue. The practices of chewing tobacco and placement of "snuff" in the mouth are closely associated with development of dental diseases, particularly oral cancers. Cessation of smoking and other tobacco use can prevent oral diseases and reduce the need for curative care, as well as potentially saving one's life. Other actions that can be taken to prevent oral diseases and adverse conditions require service provided by trained professionals. Several types of service will be highlighted to provide examples of additional steps that can be taken to prevent or reduce the need for curative care.

Professional-Level Services to Prevent Disease

Professional services that prevent oral disease are rendered by a dentist, dental hygienist, or other dental auxiliary under the direction of a dentist. Examples of these services include professional-level tooth cleaning (prophylaxis) and care for the gums, instructions in optimal home care and tooth brushing techniques, fluoride applications including fluoride gels, dietary guidance, smoking cessation assistance, mouth guard fabrication, and oral health and disease risk assessment, among others.

A particularly important preventive measure that necessarily entails the services of a trained oral health professional is the application of dental sealants. Dental sealants are applied to the chewing surfaces of teeth to seal off naturally occurring pits and fissures where the vast majority of cavities start. Sealing these areas has been shown in numerous studies to have a profound effect on reducing cavities on the chewing surfaces of molar teeth, particularly in children. Application of dental sealants is a service that can be provided individually or at the community level. School districts and dental care provider organizations sponsor school-based dental sealant programs in many communities.

Despite the best preventive efforts by individuals, most people will eventually require oral health services and dental care provided by a trained professional. In fact, regular dental examinations and oral health assessments have been shown to be beneficial for all people across the life span.

Professional Dental Services

Private Practice   There are approximately 155,000 professionally active dentists in the United States today. Of this group, there are about 5,300 African American dentists and roughly the same number of Hispanic dentists. The vast majority (92%) of active dentists are in private practice. Women constitute about 14 percent and "minorities" account for about 11 percent of practicing dentists. Whereas in medicine 40 percent of physicians are in primary care practices, approximately 80 percent of dentists are in general practice. The remaining dentists are trained specialists in one or more of nine dental specialty areas: orthodontics, oral and maxillofacial surgery, oral and maxillofacial radiology, periodontics, pediatric dentistry, endodontics, prosthodontics, dental public health, and oral and maxillofacial pathology. About 69 percent of dental practices consist of one dentist, and another 20 percent entail two dentists. The remaining 11 percent are group practices comprising three or more dentists. Dental practices may be established in community settings, and many can be found in large complexes of medical offices.

Fee policies in dental practices vary. Some accept direct payment for service from the patient only. Others may accept payment from insurance companies but are selective and restrictive among those companies. Some practices accept Medicaid payment, but unfortunately most do not. Depending on the state, only 10 to 20 percent of dentists accept patients enrolled in the Medicaid program. However, a large number of African American dentists treat low-income people, and the reimbursement arrangements also vary (Montoya et al., 1978, Warren, 1979).

Finding a dental practice suitable for one's needs can be a matter of asking for a referral from a friend, coworker, relative, or neighbor. The local Yellow Page guide also lists dental practices. Communities are served by component dental societies of the American Dental Association (ADA). Local and state components of the National Dental Association (NDA) may also be present. The NDA is notable in representing the interests of African American dentists and the oral health interests of the African American community over many decades. The Hispanic Dental Association (HDA) may also have a local presence in some communities. Each of these organizations can be found via the Internet and through local telephone directories. These dental societies can provide contact information for the offices of area dentists.

Dental societies may sponsor or otherwise support services at the community level that provide a means for accessing care that might not otherwise be available. For example, the Give Kids A Smile Program, sponsored by the ADA, enables many low-income children to receive needed dental care in communities across the country. The National Dental Association has been supportive of Head Start, a federal preschool program for low-income children that provides dental care for all of its enrollees. However, the need for care far outstrips the available resources to provide care. Dental societies can also be contacted to determine what services they provide or sponsor and to obtain specific details regarding their programs.

Area Hospitals   Some hospitals provide dental services. For example, emergency rooms are typically utilized for true dental emergencies such as those resulting from trauma to the mouth and face. However, services from hospital emergency rooms often are also sought for toothache from a long-neglected condition. Emergency rooms may not be equipped or staffed to deal with such "emergencies" and often provide medication or a prescription for pain relief with possibly a referral for care at a later point. Some hospitals do provide outpatient dental care in addition to the inpatient care provided. Hospitals in a particular locale can supply information regarding the services they provide. However, a hospital is not an ideal place to obtain regular dental care, even though it may be the only place available or accessible.

Local and State Health Departments Many local (that is, city or county) health departments provide dental care services directly or have provisions for making dental care available to qualified patients through arrangements with local dental care providers. Some state health departments also provide or sponsor dental care services. Specific health departments can be contacted to determine what types of services are available.

Local, State, and National Civic Groups and Philanthropies A search of local, state, and national organizations would reveal many that provide oral health and dental services as part of their mission. The qualifications for patients, age groups or limits, as well as other unique features of these programs would vary by organization. However, many communities offer these resources. Examples of such services may include dentist volunteer clinics, services for the homeless, mobile dental clinic service, night ministry clinics, service for street youths, and the like.

Community and "Free" Clinics Many communities have what are generically described as "community clinics" or possibly known as "free clinics." These clinics vary in their range of service, hours of operation, protocols, and operational procedures. Locating these clinics may require some additional effort, as many are not high-profile. An area organization such as a primary care association or community health center should be able to provide details regarding clinics in the community.

Dental Schools In communities where dental schools are located, the schools can serve, and many times elect to serve, as a resource for dental care. An important consideration in these facilities is that not all patients present conditions suitable for care provided by a student-dentist. Consequently, not all persons seeking care will become patients. However, most dental schools have some provision for walk-in emergencies. Dental school fees for services would typically be less than those established in private practice. In addition, as a part of the teaching and training program, specialty care provided by residents is available and is an excellent source for care.

Federally Supported Clinical Services More than a thousand Federally Qualified Health Centers (FQHCs) provide health services across the country. These FQHCs represent more than 5,000 service delivery sites nationally. The FQHC model of health service delivery was created more than forty years ago. Currently, FQHCs are located in all states and the District of Columbia, serving urban and rural populations.

Their mission is to provide quality health services to anyone who requires it, regardless of their ability to pay for care. Based on their federal subsidy, FQHCs are obligated to serve medically underserved areas and populations. About 70 percent of the FQHCs provide dental services.

SUMMARY

Various dental services are available, and professional care should meet individual and community needs. While the dental profession has the responsibility to assure that standards are met, individuals must take responsibility for their own health. Oral health cannot be fully realized by assuring systemic or general health. These two components must be complemented with considerations of the social, psychological, and spiritual well-being of the individual and the group in their physical and social environments (Warren, 2007). This chapter describes a continuum of research, education, and service to frame a paradigm for oral health. Separation of these essential elements has resulted in a fragmented, dysfunctional, and expensive health care system and major health and oral health disparities. Combining them seamlessly should create valid and reality-based information that can be taught in a culturally competent and proficient manner to a racially and ethnically diverse group of students preparing for careers in the health professions. Upon graduation, these professionals will deliver evidence-based care to promote health, prevent disease, and provide care to all people regardless of their demographic and economic backgrounds. African Americans will be a part of a system that connects individual well-being to that of groups, communities, and nations, resulting in health systems that span the globe as disease, dysfunction, and premature death currently do.

REFERENCES

Affirmative Action Compliance in Higher Education. (2008). Education Encyclopedia. Retrieved November 10, 2008, from http://www.answers.com/topic/affirmative-action-compliance-in-higher-education

American Dental Association. (2008, March). *2007–2008 survey of dental education: Tuition, admission, and attrition, Volume 2.* Chicago: American Dental Association Survey Center.

American Dental Education Association (ADEA). (2006). *Official guide to dental schools* (p. 37). Washington, DC: American Dental Education Association.

American Medical Association (AMA). (2008). Populations receiving optimally fluoridated public drinking water—United States, 1992–2006. *Journal of the American Medical Association, 300*(8), 892–894.

Bailit, H. L., Formicola, A. J., D'Abreu, K., Stavisky, J., & Zamora, G. (2005). The origin and design of the Dental Pipeline Program. *Journal of Dental Education, 69*(2), 232–238.

Borrell, L., Burt, B. A., Neighbors, W., & Warren, R. C. (2006). The role of individual and neighborhood social factors on periodontitis: The Third National Health and Nutrition Examination Survey. *Journal of Periodontology, 77*(3), 444–453.

Bowen, W., & Bok, D. (1998). *The shape of the river.* Princeton, NJ: Princeton University Press.

Centers for Disease Control (CDC). (1998). Preventing and controlling oral and pharyngeal cancer: Recommendations from a national strategic planning conference. *Morbidity and Mortality Weekly Report, 47*(RR-14),1–12.

Centers for Disease Control (CDC). (1999). Achievements in public health, 1900–1999: Fluoridation of drinking water to prevent dental caries. *Morbidity and Mortality Weekly Report, 48*(41), 933–940.

Chmar, J., et al. (2007). Annual survey of dental school seniors. *Journal of Dental Education, 71*(9), 1228–1253.

Danesh J. (1999). Coronary heart disease, helicobacter pylori, dental disease, chlamydia pneumoniae, and cytomegalovirus: Meta-analyses of prospective studies. *American Heart Journal, 138*(5, Pt. 2), S434-S437.

Dummett, C. O. (1974). Dentistry's beginnings among blacks in the United States. *Journal of the National Medical Association, 66*(4), 321–327.

Dummett, C.O., & Dummett, L. D. (1977). *Afro-Americans in dentistry: Sequence and consequence of events.* Los Angeles: Author.

Dye, B. A., & Thornton-Evans, G. (2007). A brief history of national surveillance efforts for periodontal disease in the United States. *Journal of Periodontology, 78*(7, Suppl.), 1380–1386.

Enwonwu, C. O., & Saunders, C. (2000). Nutrition: Impact on oral and systemic health. *Compendium*, Special Issue, 22(3), 12–18.

Evans, C. A., & Kleinman, D. (2000). The Surgeon General's report on America's oral health: Opportunities for the dental profession. *Journal of the American Dental Association, 131*(12), 1721–1728.

Flexner, A. (1910). Medical education in the United States: A report to the Carnegie Foundation on Higher Education. Washington, DC: Science and Health Publications, Inc.

Formicola, A., Klyvert, M., McIntosh, J., Thompson, A., Davis, M., & Cangialosi, T. (2003). Creating an environment for diversity in dental schools: One school's approach. *Journal of Dental Education, 67*(5), 491–499.

Formicola, A., et al. (2009). The Dental Pipeline Program's impact on access and student diversity. *Journal of the American Dental Association. 140*, 346–353.

Gies, W. J. (1926). *Dental education in the United States and Canada: A report of the Carnegie Foundation for the Advancement of Teaching* (p. 137). Boston: Merrymount Press.

Gross, S. G., & Genco, R. J. (1998). Periodontal disease and diabetes mellitus: A two-way relationship. *Journal of Periodontology, 3*(1), 51–61.

Gurin, P., Lehman, J., & Lewis, E. (2007). *Defending diversity: Affirmative action at the University of Michigan* (pp. 118–128). Ann Arbor: University of Michigan Press.

Health Care Financing Administration. (2000). *National health and expenditures projects: 1998–2008.* Retrieved April 2000 from http://www.cms.hhs.gov/HealthCareFinancingReview/Downloads/99winterpg165.pdf

Hodge, C. E. (2000). HIV/AIDS: Impact on the African American community. *Compendium*, Special Issue, 22(3), 52–56.

Israel, B., Schulz, A., et al. (1998). Review of community-based research: Assessing partnership approaches to improve public health. *Annual Review of Public Health, 19*, 173–302.

Janket, S. J., Baird, A. E., Chuang, S. K., & Jones, J. A. (2003). Meta-analysis of periodontal disease and risk of coronary heart disease and stroke. *Oral Surgery, Oral Medicine, Oral Pathology, Oral Radiology, and Endodontics, 95*(3), 559–569.

Joshipura, K. (2002). The relationship between oral conditions and ischemic stroke and peripheral vascular disease. *Journal of the American Dental Association, 133* (Suppl.), 23S–30S.

Kellogg Foundation Community Voices Study Committee. (2006, May). Bridging the gap: Partnerships between dental schools and colleges to produce a workforce to fully serve America's diverse communities. *Community Voices, 610.*

Leavell, H., & Clark, E. (1965). *Preventive medicine for the doctor in his community.* New York: McGraw-Hill.

Linn, E. (1972). Professional activities of black dentists. *Journal of the American Dental Association, 82*, 118.

Merzel, C., & D'Afflitti, J. (2003). Reconsidering community-based health promotion: Promise, performance and potential. *American Journal of Public Health*, 93(4), 557–574.

Moise, D. (2000). Periodontal disease, race, and vascular disease. *Compendium*, Special Issue, 22(3), 34–41.

Montoya, R., Hayes-Bautista, D., Gonzales, L., & Smeloff, E. (1978). Minority dental school graduates: Do they serve minority communities? *American Journal of Public Health, 68*(10), 1017–1019.

National Center for Health Statistics. (1975). *First National Health and Nutrition Examination Survey (NHANES I).* Hyattsville, MD: Author.

National Center for Health Statistics. (1996). *Third National Health and Nutrition Examination Survey (NHANES III).* Reference manuals and report (book on CD-ROM). Hyattsville, MD: Author.

National Institutes of Health. (2009). Mission Statement. Retrieved May 23, 2009, from http://www.nih.gov/about/index.html

Otten, M. W., Jr., Teutsch, S. M., Williamson, D. F., et al. (1990). The effect of known risk factors on the excess mortality of black adults in the United States. *Journal of the American Medical Association, 263*(6), 845–850.

Perkins, T. M., & Perkins, I. (2000). Chronic alcoholism: A common risk factor in oral cancer alcoholic cirrhosis. *Compendium*, Special Issue, 22(3), 49–51.

Reis, L. A., Kosary, C. L., Hankey, B. F., et al. (Eds.). (1999). *SEER Cancer Statistics Review, 1973–1996*. Bethesda, MD: National Cancer Institute.

Satcher, D., Fryer, G. E., Jr., McCann, J., et. al. (2005, March/April). What if we were equal? A comparison of the black-white mortality gap in 1990 and 2000. *Health Affairs, 24*(2), 459–464.

Schulman, J., Edmonds, L. D., McClearn, A. B., Jensrold, N., & Shaw, G. M. (1993). Surveillance for and comparison of birth defects prevalence in two geographic areas: United States, 1983–88. *Morbidity and Mortality Weekly Report*, CDC Surveillance Summary, *42*(1), 1–7.

Smedley, B., Stith, A., & Bristow, L. (Eds.). (2004). *In the nation's compelling interest: Ensuring diversity in the health care workforce*. Washington, DC: National Academies Press.

Smedley, B., Stith, A., & Nelson, A. (Eds.). (2002). *Unequal treatment: Confronting racial and ethnic disparities in health care*. Washington, DC: National Academies Press.

Smith, C., et al. (2006). Dental education and care for underserved patients: An analysis of students' intentions and alumni behavior. *Journal of Dental Education, 70*, 398.

Solomon, E. S., Williams, C. R., & Sinkford, J. C. (2001). Practice location characteristics of black dentists in Texas. *Journal of Dental Education, 65*(6), 571–574.

Sullivan Commission on Diversity in the Health Care Workforce. (2004). *Missing persons: Minorities in the health professions*. Retrieved May 24, 2009, from http://www.aacn.nche.edu/Media/pdf/SullivanReport.pdf

Taylor, G. (2000). Exploring interrelationships between diabetes and periodontal disease in African Americans. *Compendium*, Special Issue, *22*(3), 42–48.

Truman, B. I., Gooch, B. F., & Evans, C. A. Jr. (Eds.). (2002). The guide to community preventive services: Interventions to prevent dental caries, oral and pharyngeal cancers, and sports-related craniofacial injuries. *American Journal of Preventive Medicine, 23*(1, Supp).

U.S. Department of Health and Human Services. (1985). Report of the Secretary's Task Force on Black and Minority Health [Executive Summary]. Washington, DC: U.S. Government Printing Office.

U.S. Department of Health and Human Services. (1990). *Health, United States*. Washington, DC: U.S. Government Printing Office.

U.S. Department of Health and Human Services. (2000). *Oral health in America: Report of the Surgeon General*. Rockville, MD: National Institutes of Health.

Veal, K., Perry, M., Stavisky, J., & D'Abreu-Herbert, K. (2004). The pathway to dentistry for minority students: From their perspective. *Journal of Dental Education, 68*(9), 938–946.

Walker, B., Mays, V. M., & Warren, R. C. (2004, October). The changing landscape for the elimination of racial/ethnic health status disparities. *Journal of Health Care for the Poor and Underserved, 15*(1).

Warren, R. C. (1979, October). A descriptive study of black Meharry dental graduates, 1960–1974. *Quarterly of the National Dental Association, 38*, 1.

Warren, R. C. (1980). The barriers in setting up a dental practice in areas of high need. In A. Tryon and S. Silberman (Eds.), *Post-graduate dental handbook series*. Minneapolis: Publishing Sciences Group.

Warren, R. C. (1990). Oral health for the poor and underserved. *Journal of Health Care for the Poor and Underserved, 1*(1), 169–180.

Warren, R. C. (1999). *Oral health for all: Policy for available, accessible, and acceptable care*. Washington, DC: Center for Policy Alternatives.

Warren, R. C. (2007). The impact of horizontal and vertical dimensions of faith on health and health care, *Journal of the Interdenominational Theological Center*, 71–85.

PART

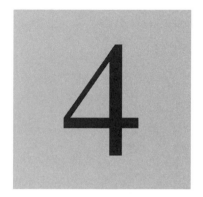

4

LIFESTYLE
BEHAVIORS

CHAPTER

17

SUBSTANCE USE DISORDERS IN THE AFRICAN AMERICAN COMMUNITY

JEAN J. E. BONHOMME
RONALD L. BRAITHWAITE
MELITA MOORE

Drug use in the United States has been stereotyped in the media and framed in the public mind as a disproportionate problem of African American youth (SAMHSA, 2004). The National Survey on Drug Use and Health conducted in 2004 by the Substance Abuse and Mental Health Services Administration (SAMHSA) to estimate the prevalence of illicit drug use in the United States found that among youth aged 12 to 17 years, rates of current illicit drug use varied significantly by major racial/ ethnic group (see Table 17.1). However, the rate was actually highest for Native American or Alaska Native youth (26.0 %). Rates were 12.2 percent for youth reporting two or more races, 11.1 percent for white youth, 10.2 percent for Hispanic youth, but only 9.3 percent for African American youth and 6.0 percent for Asian youths. Native American, multiracial, white, and Latino youth all reported higher drug use rates than African American youth.

TABLE 17.1 **Prevalence of Illicit Drug Use Among Youth Ages 12 to 17, 2004.**

Native American or Alaska Native	26.0%
Youth reporting two or more races	12.2%
Whites	11.1%
Latinos/Hispanics	10.2%
African Americans	9.3%
Asians	6.0%

SCOPE OF SUBSTANCE USE IN THE UNITED STATES

Substance abuse, dependence, and addiction are major public health issues. In 2004, 22.5 million Americans aged 12 years or older were classified with substance dependence or abuse within the past year (9.4% of the population). Of the 22.5 million, 3.4 million were classified with dependence on or abuse of both alcohol and illicit drugs, 3.9 million were dependent on or abused illicit drugs but not alcohol, and 15.2 million were dependent on or abused alcohol but not illicit drugs.

An estimated 19.1 million Americans age 12 years or older were current users of illicit drugs in 2004, meaning they had used an illicit drug at least once during the 30 days prior to being interviewed. This represents 7.9 percent of the population aged 12 or older. When specific substances are considered (see Table 17.2), there were 2 million current cocaine users, 467,000 of whom used crack, and 929,000 users of hallucinogens. An estimated 166,000 individuals were current heroin users. The number of current users of Ecstasy (Methylenedioxymethamphetamine, or MDMA) was 450,000. Marijuana is the most commonly used illicit drug, with a rate of 6.1 percent (14.6 million users). Between 2002 and 2004, past-month marijuana use declined for male youths aged 12 to 17 years (9.1% in 2002, 8.6 percent in 2003, and 8.1 percent in 2004), but it remained level for female youths (7.2%, 7.2%, and 7.1%, respectively) during the same span. In 2004, 6 million persons were current users of psychotherapeutic drugs taken nonmedically (2.5%). These include 4.4 million who used opiate pain relievers, 1.6 million who used tranquilizers, 1.2 million who used stimulants, and 300,000 who used sedatives.

As reported at the thirty-ninth annual conference of the American Society of Addiction Medicine (ASAM) in 2008, substance abuse is an especially important issue because of its huge financial costs to society (Mental Health America, 2009). In the

TABLE 17.2   **U.S. Population Estimates, Current Users of Specific Drugs, 2004.**

Total cocaine users	2,000,000
Crack cocaine users	467,000
Heroin users	166,000
Ecstasy (MDMA) users	450,000
Marijuana users	14,600,000
Total non-medically taken drug users	6,000,000
Opiate pain reliever users	4,400,000*
Tranquilizer users	1,600,000*
Stimulant users	1,200,000*
Sedative users	300,000*

*Some used more than one type of drug; thus, non-medically taken total exceeds 6,000,000.

United States, substance abuse is estimated to cost $535 billion a year, more than the estimated yearly societal costs for cancer ($210 billion/year) and diabetes ($132 billion/year) combined. Also, employment status was found to have a bearing on drug use, which is noteworthy because African Americans have traditionally suffered higher rates of unemployment than the general population. In 2004, 19.2 percent of unemployed adults aged 18 or older were current illicit drug users compared with 8.0 percent of those employed full time and 10.3 percent of those employed part time. However, of the 16.4 million illicit drug users aged 18 or older in 2004, 12.3 million (75.2%) were employed either full or part time.

DEPENDENCE VERSUS ADDICTION

In understanding substance use among African Americans, it is important to consider that more recent literature in addiction medicine is making a new and vitally important distinction between addiction and dependence (Graham et al., 2007). Both addiction and dependence are distinct from abuse, in which a substance is used in a manner other than its intended purpose but without compulsion or actual need to maintain normal function. Addiction is defined as continued substance use in the face of adverse consequences. Addiction is characterized by overriding compulsion, using drugs and/ or alcohol to the point of intoxication and grossly impaired function. For example, a person gets arrested for drunken driving and the person's license is confiscated. Two days later the same person is on the road again and drunk again. Punishment appears to have little or no effect as a deterrent. The key to recognizing addiction is that the use of the substance leads to *deteriorating* function. By contrast, dependence is defined as a state in which the mind and/or body relies on a substance for normal functioning. For example, a person may have a ruptured lumbar disk, with pain so severe that the person cannot work or take care of his or her children. When that person is given an opiate pain medication, the pain subsides to a degree at which the person can function normally. The key to recognizing dependence (as opposed to addiction) is that in the presence of the substance, function *improves*. Distinguishing between addiction and dependence is crucially important. The *Diagnostic and Statistical Manual of Mental Disorders*, Volume IV (DSM-IV) does not make any distinction here, and unfortunately, usually neither do the criminal courts. African Americans tend to suffer harsher treatment in the legal system for drug offenses.

SOCIOECONOMIC STATUS: THE IMPACT ON SUBSTANCE ABUSE

Substantial evidence supports the general consensus that socioeconomic (SES) is a major contributor to disparities in morbidity and mortality attributed to a multitude of physical and psychiatric illnesses (Strickland & Clark, 2001). Williams and Collins (1995) reviewed evidence of the known SES gradient in health. Consistent racial differences in health exist in most epidemiologic reports. There is unequivocal evidence of disproportionate morbidity and mortality among the lower SES groups, and low-SES African Americans suffer a greater burden of morbidity and mortality than Americans of all other racial/ethnic groups. Factors driving this inverse SES-health relationship include greater exposure to pathogenic social and environmental conditions (Commission for Racial Justice, 1987), greater life stress burdens (Kessler, 1979), more negative health behavior profiles (Kessler, 1995), and lack of access to or utilization of quality health care (Blendon et al., 1989; Williams, 1990).

There is further evidence that lower SES is associated with earlier substance use initiation, shorter transition from recreational drug use to regular use and abuse, and greater prevalence of use of the more neurotoxic drugs such as crack cocaine (Lillie-Blanton, Anthony, & Schuster, 1994). In addition, with lower SES there is evidence of more negative outcomes from the use of legal substances such as tobacco (Sterling & Weinkam, 1989) and alcohol (Djata, 1987).

MECHANISMS OF ADDICTION AND DEPENDENCE

Different classes of drugs have different mechanisms of action, but all potentially addictive drugs increase the activity of the reward pathway in the brain by increasing dopamine transmission. Different parts of the brain are responsible for addiction as opposed to dependence. For example, the areas in the brain underlying addiction to morphine are the reward pathway (including the ventral tegmental area [VTA], nucleus accumbens, and cortex). Areas underlying dependence on morphine are the thalamus and brainstem. Thus, it is possible to be dependent on morphine without being addicted. This is especially true for people being treated for chronic diseases with opiates—for example, alleviation of pain associated with terminal cancer. They may be dependent, because if the drug is stopped, they suffer reemergence of pain and/or a withdrawal syndrome. However, there is no compulsive use, and the prescribed use is short-lived. Most people treated with opiates in medical settings for pain control (e.g., after surgery) are unlikely to become addicted. Although they may feel some euphoria, the analgesic and sedating effects predominate.

The emergence of new forms of drugs that can be smoked has led to more widespread use and greater potential for the development of addiction. This has been particularly true in the African American community with the advent of crack cocaine. In addition, there has been a growing problem with ice (smokeable methamphetamine) in many regions. Smoking is much more socially acceptable behavior than using needles or snorting drugs, given our long history of accepting tobacco smoking. For this reason, when a drug is presented in smokeable form, a major social barrier to the initiation of its use (e.g., needle aversion) is removed.

Smoking is actually potentially the most addictive route of drug administration. Behavioral science has demonstrated that the faster a reward (or punishment) follows an action, the greater its effectiveness in reinforcing (or extinguishing) similar future behavior. In addition, smoking gets high levels of a drug into the blood faster than any other method of drug ingestion. When a drug is snorted, it takes 30 to 120 seconds to get into the blood, and high blood levels are rarely attained. When a drug is injected in the arm, it takes a long circulatory pathway, going up the arm, into the right side of the heart, into the lungs, back into the left side of the heart, and up the carotid arteries into the brain. This process takes about eighteen seconds, and high blood levels of the drug are commonly achieved. However, when a drug is smoked, it takes a short circulatory path into the lungs, into the left side of the heart, and into the carotid arteries to the brain. Because of the enormous surface area of the lungs, high blood levels of the drug are commonly attained. This process takes only about *seven* seconds. If you were training a dog with food rewards, which would be most effective—giving the food in 7 seconds, in 18 seconds, or in 30 to 120 seconds? Hence, rapidity of onset of the action of a drug is strongly associated with addictive potential. That is in part why it is so hard to give up smoking tobacco, and why cocaine addiction grew exponentially when the smokeable crack form was introduced. This may appear counterintuitive because solids seem more substantial than liquids, and liquids seem more substantial than vapors. However, of the three, vapors can access the brain the most rapidly following drug use.

The withdrawal/abstinence syndrome is defined as the physical and mental effects resulting from discontinuation of addictive substances by persons who have become habituated to their use. Withdrawal symptoms may include severe cravings as well as physiological and psychological reactions that occur when the drug is no longer taken. Tolerance is defined as the phenomenon of decreased effect of a drug with repeated exposure. Thus, with prolonged use the drug must be taken in increasing quantities to achieve the same level of response achieved initially, whether that effect is euphoria or simply preventing withdrawal symptoms. Tolerance is one of the primary determinants of substance abuse. Tolerance is among the diagnostic criteria for alcoholism noted in DSM-IV. However, tolerance does not necessarily lead to addiction.

During the 2008 annual ASAM conference, Jag H. Khalsa, PhD, chief of the medical consequences branch in the division of pharmacotherapies and medical consequences of drug abuse at the National Institute on Drug Abuse (NIDA), indicated that "Drug addicts have major medical problems in addition to drug addiction." Many drug addicts inject drugs intravenously or intramuscularly and acquire multiple co-occurring infections such as HIV, hepatitis C, tuberculosis, and sexually transmitted diseases. An addict can also have cardiovascular, hepatic, or immunologic complications that need to be treated, Khalsa noted.

According to Robert Drake, MD (2003), 37% of alcohol abusers and 53 percent of drug abusers also have at least one serious mental illness. Also, of all people diagnosed as mentally ill, 29 percent abuse either alcohol or drugs. Problems commonly observed in dual diagnosis include depressive disorders, such as depression and bipolar disorder; anxiety disorders, including generalized anxiety disorder, panic disorder, obsessive-compulsive disorder, and phobias; and other psychiatric disorders, such as schizophrenia and personality disorders.

THE IMPACT OF NICOTINE AND ALCOHOL

Nicotine is legal and not commonly thought of as a drug, but it is responsible for a greater number of deaths in the United States than any other drug, with more than 400,000 Americans dying yearly from tobacco-related diseases. Smokers die an average of 13 to 14 years earlier than nonsmokers. Many smoking-related diseases affect African Americans disproportionately. Diseases known to be linked to smoking include cancer of the bladder, esophagus, larynx, lung, mouth, and throat, as well as chronic lung disease (chronic bronchitis and emphysema), chronic heart and cardiovascular disease, and reproductive problems.

According to the Centers for Disease Control and Prevention (1999), "Tobacco use is the single most preventable cause of death and disease in our society. Most people begin using tobacco in early adolescence, typically by age 16; almost all first use occurs before high school graduation. Children buy the most heavily advertised brands, and are three times more affected by advertising than adults." A marketing barrage, including sexually oriented advertising, fruit flavors, menthol, glamour, hip-hop culture, and celebrity role models, particularly targets minority youth.

On August 19, 2004, Morehouse School of Medicine (MSM) reported that minority youth in Atlanta were specifically being targeted by companies flooding new products using lures from the black culture that were decidedly "hip-hop" and youth oriented. Former presidents of MSM James Gavin III, MD, Louis Sullivan, MD (also former secretary of the U.S. Department of Health and Human Services), and David Satcher, MD (also former CDC director and U.S. Surgeon General) called upon tobacco companies to remove their products from store shelves. Tobacco companies refused, claiming to be in compliance with the tobacco settlement agreements. RJ Reynolds, a major tobacco manufacturer, markets "New Kool Mixx, Kool Smooth Fusion, and Camel Exotic Blends." Phillip Morris, another tobacco manufacturer, markets "Marlboro Menthol 72 millimeter," to black, Latino, and other minority youth. The National Youth Tobacco Survey (NYTS) (2004) found that 12.8% of middle school students and 34.8 percent of high school students use tobacco. Bidis and kreteks—cheap, highly toxic, small rolled and flavored cigarettes made from tobacco residue—are becoming increasingly popular among youth. Among middle school students, black students were significantly more likely than white students to smoke cigars (8.8% and 4.9 percent, respectively).

Alcohol is also legal and not usually thought of as a drug, but it is responsible for 150,000 deaths per year in the United States. Alcohol acts as a central nervous system depressant but may falsely appear to be a stimulant due to its depression of inhibitory control mechanisms in the brain. In addition to the risks of alcohol addiction, alcohol increases the risks of chronic liver disease; falls, drownings, and other accidents; fetal alcohol syndrome; head, neck, stomach, and breast cancers; homicide, victim or perpetrator; motor vehicle accidents; risky sexual behaviors, including unplanned or unwanted pregnancy and contraction of sexually transmitted diseases (STDs); and suicide.

PERFORMANCE-ENHANCING SUBSTANCES: SUBSTANCE ABUSE AMONG ATHLETES

A category of substances less commonly recognized as substances of potential abuse are performance-enhancing drugs. There has been little research examining the magnitude of the problem in the African American community, but use of performance-enhancing substances among certain African-American athletes has received considerable media attention.

The mounting use of performance-enhancing substances (PESs) among athletes is an escalating concern among the general public. "Doping" has become a hot topic of recent debate, although its history can be traced to the inception of competitive sport itself: the Greek Olympics of 776 BC. Ancient Greek athletes were known to ingest special stimulating potions containing mushrooms, roots, and animal extracts designed to enhance their athletic prowess. The word "doping" is thought to be derived from the Afrikaans word *dop*, the name of an alcoholic beverage made of grape skins used as a stimulant by the Zulu warriors of South Africa to enhance their performance during battle. However, during the twentieth century performance-enhancing substances became more sophisticated, ranging from all-natural concoctions to scientifically formulated pharmacologic products.

Doping in sport is defined as the presence in the human body of substances or methods of administration that are included on the "Prohibited List" published by the World Anti-Doping Agency (WADA). These include anabolic agents, hormones and related substances, Beta-2 agonists, hormone antagonists and modulators, diuretics and masking agents, stimulants, substances designed to enhance oxygen transfer, chemical and physical manipulation, and gene doping.

It has been well documented that the use of performance-enhancing substances by athletes is increasing exponentially. There has been some debate, however, as to whether there has been an actual increase in usage of these banned substances or whether the seeming increase can be attributed to the fact that detection and subsequent reporting have been vastly improved. In any event, PESs have dominated conversation in the sports world, captured the attention of the medical community, and preoccupied athletes. The United States Congress has weighed in on this topic, and it has become a focal point for politicians, as evidenced by the Mitchell Report, which provided a newfound impetus for investigation into PESs in Major League Baseball.

The prevalence of these banned substances has prompted many studies among and between classes of athletes, including, but not limited to, utilization by members of various ethnic/racial groups. While limited data currently exist to support or refute such allegations, it does appear that African American athletes, on all levels, have escaped the stereotypical labeling usually accorded to their communities. According to a report issued by the Centers for Disease Control and Prevention in 2007, African American students in grades 9 through 12 were less likely than Hispanic or white students to have engaged in lifetime illegal steroid or methamphetamine use.

With the escalating pressure to "win by any means necessary," athletes of all ages and levels of competition have turned to anabolic-androgenic steroids (AASs). Popularized by the East German Olympic athletes in the 1950s and common in weight-lifting and wrestling, AASs have permeated professional sports, most notably baseball, football, and track and field. In the United States, an estimated 1 to 3 million people have used anabolic steroids (Sjoqvist, Garle, & Rane, 2008). Nationwide, 5.1 percent of high school boys and 2.7 percent of high school girls have used steroids (CDC, 2007; Gregory & Fitch, 2007). In 2009, a self-reported survey found that 1 in 10 retired NFL players had used AASs while still playing (Horn, Gregory, & Guskiewicz, 2009). AASs are synthetic derivatives of testosterone. Studies have shown that these drugs can influence lean body mass, muscle size and strength, protein metabolism, bone metabolism, and collagen synthesis (Kerr & Congeni, 2007). However, the risk of potential side effects outweighs the benefits. AASs affect the function of cardiovascular, hepatic, endocrine/reproductive, psychiatric, and dermatologic systems. Hypertension, myocardial infarction, cardiomyopathy, and sudden cardiac death are possible cardiac complications.

The psychiatric component of AAS use is commonly known and includes aggression ("roid rage"), psychosis, anxiety, and depression. Decreased testosterone, gynecomastia, and testicular atrophy in men, as well as masculinization, clitoral hypertrophy, and decreased menstruation in women, are documented endocrine effects. Elevation in liver function tests, cholestasis, and hepatocellular adenomas have been noted; and premature baldness and acne can occur. Adolescents have been found to be more susceptible than adults to the adverse effects of anabolic steroid use, with effects that include accelerated maturation and earlier development of secondary sexual characteristics and premature closure of growth plates in long bones (Casavant et al., 2007).

Although nutritional supplements are considered safe because they are natural substances used to augment the diet, the misuse and overuse of supplements can cause significant detrimental health issues and even death. The Dietary Supplement Health and Education Act (DSHEA, Public Law 103-417) defines a dietary supplement as a product intended to supplement the diet that contains one of the following ingredients: vitamin, mineral, herb or other botanical, amino acid of a concentrate, metabolite, constituent, extract, or combination of any ingredient. Stimulants are commonly used in supplements but go underrecognized. Common stimulants include caffeine, epehedrine, pseudoepehedrine, New-Synephrine, amphetamines, and methamphetamines. These can be found in coffee, colas, energy drinks, cold medication, muscle-building or weight-loss supplements, ADHD medications, and diet pills, according to the Dietary Supplement Health and Education Act of 1994 (see http://www.fda.gov/Food/DietarySupplements/default.htm).

Ephedra was banned in 2004 because of adverse cardiovascular effects—the first nutritional supplement to be banned in the United States. It had been popularized as a performance-enhancing supplement due to its stimulant effects. Ephedra has a chemical structure similar to amphetamine and reportedly improved athletic performance, enhanced weight loss, and boosted energy levels (Keisler & Hosey 2005). Haller and Benowitz (2000) examined cases related to ephedra use and concluded that adverse effects included hypertension, arrhythmia, myocardial infarction, hemorrhagic stroke, seizure, and death.

Other supplements are consumed by athletes to help repair muscle damage or increase muscle mass. Creatine is a protein supplement commonly used to increase strength among athletes (Kraemer & Volek, 1999). Creatine is an amino acid compound that is produced by the liver, kidneys, and pancreas and can be found in beef, pork, and fish. It provides a fast but short-lived energy surge, and athletes use it in the hope of improving performance and increasing strength. Energy stored in adenosine triphosphate (ATP) is used in the first second of activity, while energy stored in creatine phosphate is used in the next ten seconds (Matich, 2007). A double-blind study provided 20 grams per day of creatine monohydrate for five days to qualified sprinters and jumpers who performed 45 seconds of continuous jumping and 60 seconds of continuous treadmill running. Supplementation enhanced performance in the jumping test by 7 percent for the first 15 seconds and 12 percent for the next 15 seconds, but there was no difference for the final 15 seconds. There was a 13 percent improvement in the time of intensive running to exhaustion (Bosco, 1997). Normal dietary intake of creatine is 1 to 2 grams per day, but manufacturers generally recommend ingesting 10 to 20 grams per day. Taking doses greater than the daily recommended dose can lead to side effects such as muscle cramping, unwanted weight gain, seizure, vomiting, cardiac arrhythmia, myopathy, deep vein thrombosis, and death, according to the Center for Food Safety and Applied Nutrition Special Nutritionals Adverse Event Monitoring System (1997).

DRUG USE COMORBIDITIES

Many comorbid conditions associated with substance use such as hepatitis C affect African Americans disproportionately. In the United States, approximately 4 million persons have been exposed to hepatitis C (El-Serag, 2008), and about 2.8 million carry the virus chronically. Possible consequences of chronic viral hepatitis include cirrhosis and liver cancer. Hepatitis C is spread by contact with the blood of infected individuals, primarily through injected drugs.

Chronic hepatitis C virus (HCV) is known to be the most common blood-borne infection in the United States (Feckenstein, 2004). The highest prevalence of infection exists among African Americans at 3.2 percent, with African Americans accounting for 22 percent of HCV cases in the United States. Data were collected from five blood centers in different regions of the United States on a total of 862,398 volunteer blood donors with one or more donations from March 1992 through December 1993 (Murphy et al., 1996). Of this group, 3,126 donors were confirmed HCV-positive, for a crude prevalence of 3.6 per 1,000. The rate was higher for African Americans (odds ratio, 1.7) and Latinos (odds ratio, 1.3). Seropositivity for human T-lymphotropic virus types I and II, HIV, or hepatitis B core antigen is associated with HCV seropositivity (odds ratio, 10.4) (Feckenstein, 2004).

DRUGS AND SEXUAL BEHAVIOR

Human immunodeficiency virus (HIV) is another infection that is commonly drug-related (or associated with high-risk sexual activity related to drugs) that affects African Americans disproportionately. The CDC estimates that one in fifty African American men and one in 160 African American women in the United States is HIV positive. The most common route of HIV transmission worldwide is sex between men and women. In most countries outside Africa, injection drug use is a major second transmission route. Needle use can cause HIV to spread explosively through drug-using populations. Part of the reason is that injection drug users often form very tight-knit groups with close social contacts for distribution. HIV transmission has been reported with many non-opiate injected drugs including cocaine, methamphetamine, body-building steroids, and even drugs injected for medicinal purposes. Injecting drug users also remain susceptible to other HIV transmission vectors, including unprotected sex with an infected partner.

A substantial amount of heterosexual HIV transmission, especially among women and minorities, is related to sex with injecting drug users. Drug-associated sexual risk behavior can occur with or without injection drugs, including sex for drug exchanges, sex for money to buy drugs, and sex with other people who have HIV risk factors as a result of social networks among drug users. Non-injected mind-altering substances (including alcohol and marijuana) can impair judgment and lead to risky sexual behavior. The presence of other sexually transmitted diseases, especially those that create ulcers in the genital tract (herpes, syphilis, gonorrhea, etc.), increases the risk of HIV transmission by sexual exposure. One STD increases approximately fourfold the risk of transmission from a single sexual exposure, and two STDs increase the risk as much as sixteenfold.

Sexually transmitted infections (STIs) are common among drug users. A cross-sectional survey on STIs and risky behaviors was conducted among 407 drug abusers in treatment facilities in 1998 (Hwang et al., 2000). Infections with human immuno-deficiency virus (HIV), hepatitis B virus (HBV), hepatitis C virus (HCV), herpes simplex virus type 2 (HSV-2), syphilis, chlamydia, and gonorrhea were detected by testing. High prevalences of STIs among drug abusers were discovered. Out of 407 subjects, approximately 62 percent demonstrated markers for STIs. The percentages of patients testing positive were as follows: HSV-2 antibodies 44.4 percent; HCV antibodies 35.1 percent; HBV antibodies 29.5 percent; HIV antibodies 2.7 percent; syphilis antibodies 3.4 percent; chlamydia nucleic acid 3.7 percent; gonorrhea nucleic acid 1.7 percent. Logistic regression identified several demographic and behavioral associations. HIV infection was associated with African American race, use of smoke-able freebase (crack) cocaine, and STI history. HBV infection was associated with age over 30 years, IDU, needle sharing, history of drug abuse treatment, and African American race. HCV infection was associated with age over 30 years, injecting drugs, and needle sharing. HSV-2 infection was associated with age over 30 years, female sex, and African American race. Syphilis was associated only with a history of STIs.

Given the increased prevalence of both HIV and HCV among African Americans, co-infection (defined as the presence of both HIV and HCV in the same individual at the same time) becomes an especially common problem. In the United States, approximately 4 million people test positive for HCV antibodies (Feckenstein, 2004) and about 1.3 million are HIV positive. More than 400,000 HIV-positive individuals (approximately 40%) also have HCV. As many as 50 to 90 percent of people who got HIV through IDU also picked up HCV because HIV and HCV share a common route of infection, contact with human blood and blood products. The health complications of HCV may be serious, especially in the case of HIV co-infection. Hepatitis C treatment is often more difficult when HIV is present. HIV/HCV co-infected mothers' risk of HCV transmission to children increases from 5 percent to 17 percent. HIV and HCV influence one another. HIV reduces the body's ability to fight HCV and can speed up the progression to cirrhosis, liver cancer, and liver failure from HCV to less than ten years unless treated. HCV-associated liver complications are one of the leading causes of death among HIV-positive persons. The liver is critically important for processing many HIV medicines, so liver function must be preserved as much as possible for optimal HIV treatment.

Hepatitis B (HBV) is associated with drug use and has an infection pattern much like HIV. HBV is transmitted by blood contact with infected blood, semen, or vaginal fluids. Up to 10 percent of infected persons become carriers, and about 1.25 million are currently infected in the United States, some with chronic hepatitis. HBV/HIV co-infection is more common than HIV/HCV co-infection, but HBV is less likely to cause chronic disease. Chronic HBV/HIV co-infection is very likely to contribute to end-stage liver disease.

SUBSTANCE USE AND TUBERCULOSIS

Tuberculosis (TB) is yet another disease commonly associated with drug use that takes a greater toll on the black community than the general population. Substance users are at especially high risk, most notably alcoholics. The HIV/AIDS pandemic, which has been fueled in large measure in the United States by substance abuse–driven risk behaviors, has dramatically increased incidence. HIV-positive persons are highly susceptible to infection, and it is more difficult to treat TB in the presence of HIV. Recent increases in TB morbidity in the United States have been concentrated in racial and ethnic minorities, foreign-born persons, and persons with HIV.

Substance users are at higher risk for TB infection due to drug-related immune system derangements, poor nutrition, and general lack of a health-conscious lifestyle. In addition, relapsing drug users diagnosed with TB often fail to comply with TB treatment regimens. Treatment regimens for TB normally have cure rates in excess of 95 percent. However, failure of compliance with antituberculosis medications has resulted in an increasing rate of multiple-drug-resistant tuberculosis (MDR-TB), which responds poorly to therapy (Bloch et al., 1994). MDR-TB is defined as a form of tuberculosis that is resistant to two or more of the primary drugs (isoniazid [INH] and rifampin) used for TB treatment. Treatment involves drug therapy over many months or years and may require surgery. Despite the longer course of treatment, the cure rate decreases from over 90 percent for nonresistant strains of TB to 50 percent or less for MDR-TB. In 2005, the CDC reported that 7.8 percent of tuberculosis cases in the United States were resistant to INH and that 1.2 percent of tuberculosis cases in the United States were resistant to both INH and rifampin. Over 70 percent of primary MDR-TB cases occurred in foreign-born persons.

Bloch et al. (1994) assessed antituberculosis drug resistance patterns, geographic distribution, demographic characteristics, and risk factors of reported TB patients in the United States. Resistance was found to INH and/or rifampin in 9.5 percent of cases whose isolates were tested, and such cases were found in 107 counties in 33 states. Resistance to both INH and rifampin (MDR-TB) was found in 3.5 percent of cases whose isolates were tested against both drugs; such cases were found in 35 counties in 13 states. New York City accounted for 61.4 percent of the nation's MDR-TB cases. The three-month population-based incidence rate of MDR-TB in New York City was 52.4 times (95% confidence interval [CI], 35.5 to 78.3) that of the rest of the nation (9.559 versus 0.182 cases per million population). Compared with the rates in the rest of the nation, the relative risk of MDR-TB in New York City was 39.0 in non-Hispanic whites, 299.3 in Hispanics, 420.9 in Asian/Pacific Islanders, and 701.0 in non-Hispanic blacks.

ETHNICITY AND SENTENCING FOR DRUG OFFENSES

Considerable controversy exists as to how much of the observed overrepresentation of African American males in the criminal justice system represents actual differences in criminal behavior as opposed to differential treatment under the criminal justice system. Existing racial disparities may have been exacerbated by sentencing policy changes adopted throughout the 1980s and early 1990s requiring mandatory minimum sentences for a variety of drug-related offenses. A 1990 RAND study found that while defendants in California received generally comparable sentences for comparable offenses regardless of race, this was not the case with respect to drug offenses. These policy changes resulted in a significant increase in drug offenders sentenced to prison and in longer prison terms (Klein, Petersilia, & Turners, 1990). Overall, the number of black drug offenders sentenced to prison increased by 707 percent between 1985 and 1995, while the number of white drug offenders increased by 306 percent (Mumola & Beck, 1997). Drug offenders accounted for 42 percent of the rise in the African American state prison population compared with 26 percent of the rise in the white state prison population during that same ten-year period (Mumola & Beck, 1997).

Differential sentencing for drug possession based on the form of drug commonly used by a specific ethnic group is dramatically increasing the percentage of ethnic minorities in correctional facilities (Braithwaite & Arriola, 2009). African Americans and Latinos are more likely to use cocaine in its "crack" form than in its powder form. Crack is simply cocaine powder processed by heating with common baking soda, but possession of crack typically incurs a much harsher sentence. Federal guidelines call for a mandatory minimum five-year sentence to a possible maximum of twenty years for possession of five grams of crack (the weight of two pennies). In striking contrast, a similar weight of powder cocaine is only a misdemeanor with no mandatory minimum sentence and maximum penalty of one year in jail. Half a kilogram of powder cocaine is required to carry the same punishment as possession of only five grams of crack. Since 500 grams of powder cocaine has a much greater street value than five grams of crack, is addictive, and could be readily converted into crack with common household items, a sentencing differential of this magnitude does not seem rational or justifiable.

According to U.S. District Judge Clyde S. Cahill of Missouri, the federal guidelines for possession of crack have "been directly responsible for incarcerating nearly an entire generation of young black American men." The U.S. Sentencing Commission reported that the racial breakdown of cocaine powder convictions in 2000 was 17.8 percent white defendants, 30.5 percent black, and 50.8 percent Latino. During the same time period, the distribution of crack cocaine convictions was 5.6 percent white defendants, 84.7 percent black, and 9.0 percent Latino, a conviction rate 15 times greater for blacks than for whites caught with the same basic chemical substance. Federal sentencing guideline penalties for crack cocaine offenses generally are three to six times as long as the penalties for powder cocaine offenses involving equivalent quantities of the drug. Advocates for social justice and equity consider such sentencing guidelines to be a form of racial profiling and racial discrimination.

INCARCERATION AND DRUG-RELATED INFECTIOUS DISEASES

The high incarceration rates of African Americans may fuel the spread of drug-related infectious diseases in the African American community. There is more injection drug use (IDU) in correctional facilities than in drug treatment centers (Decker et al., 1985). Although the first major risk factor identified for AIDS was male homosexual activity, IDU was always the most prevalent risk factor among the incarcerated. Inmate populations are drawn heavily from the IDU population outside of prison. Up to 25 percent of inmates report IDU even while in prison. The use of contaminated needles in a prison environment may pose an especially great risk for a number of blood-borne infections. Restrictions on the availability of needles, which were intended to reduce the prevalence of drug use, may instead increase sharing of the few available needles. In addition, tattooing is a high-risk activity in prisons, since this is often done with guitar strings, light bulb filaments, and other nonsterile but expedient materials (Braithwaite, Hammett, & Mayberry, 1996). Sharing of improperly cleaned injection solutions, containers, cotton, and other paraphernalia also contribute to transmission of blood-borne infections. When needles are not available, articles such as pieces of ballpoint pens and light bulb filaments may be used by inmates to inject drugs and to tattoo (Mahon, 1994). Access to illegal drugs continues to be prevalent in many U.S. correctional facilities. Since the majority of inmates eventually return to communities, and given that they represent a captive population while incarcerated, a unique opportunity exists to provide them with information during their incarceration and the pre-release phase that may facilitate successful reintegration into their respective communities (Braithwaite et al., 1996). Such information could include job skills, health care referrals, and STD, HIV, and drug prevention and treatment. Such intervention has potentially far-reaching value for protecting public health and safety for the community at large.

The CDC issued a 2006 HIV/AIDS Surveillance Report that revealed some encouraging positive findings, according to H. Westley Clark, MD, director of the Center for Substance Abuse Treatment at the Substance Abuse and Mental Health Services Administration (SAMHSA) in Rockville, Maryland (CDC, 2006). This report showed that in 2006, transmission of HIV in adults and adolescents by injection drug use had declined to 13 percent, and among people newly diagnosed with HIV, the rate of transmission by injection drug use had decreased from 34 percent to less than 20 percent. In addition, the AIDS case rate for children under the age of 13 years had dropped substantially. "We have made important progress in the HIV arena for children under 13," said Dr. Clark. Successful results of efforts to combat HIV/AIDS can be attributed to a concerted effort among members of the community, people in recovery, and organizations such as the CDC and SAMHSA, noted Dr. Clark, adding, "We need to continue to work together if we are going to make sustained progress."

SUMMARY

Addiction is a public health issue of enormous consequence, carrying a huge financial, social, interpersonal and emotional burden to society. Crime, violence, accidents, family instability, HIV, hepatitis, tuberculosis, sexually transmitted diseases, lost time from work, diminished work productivity, unemployment, and many other social ills are all strongly associated with substance use. For this reason, it is an issue that concerns the well-being of the general population. We must recognize that the current predominantly criminal justice–oriented approach to the problem of substance use is ineffective and ultimately counterproductive. By definition, addiction is continued use in the face of negative consequences, and thus the threat of incarceration has not been a reasonable approach to deterrence. Inmates incarcerated for years on drug offenses may relapse immediately upon release, and some continue to use drugs even while incarcerated.

It is vitally important not to attach the label "addict" to every person with a chronic need for a drug. Some individuals are merely dependent, using medications even in large quantities safely and responsibly with measurable improvement in their quality of life, in contrast to the addicted person who cannot control or regulate drug use and cannot function effectively in day-to-day activities. Addiction is a real medical and psychiatric illness, with demonstrable and measurable physiological and psychological characteristics, and therefore must be addressed within the context of the disease model approach, with appropriate interventions and treatments.

Furthermore, addiction must be addressed within the specific culture of the addicted individual. African Americans have unique life circumstances that must be understood and addressed in order to successfully approach the problem in this population. Access to drug treatment must be provided. The costs of treatment are quite modest compared to the substantial expense of police work, drug trials, and incarceration. Moreover, the comorbidities of addiction must be addressed, given the enormous physical health burden that can affect not only the addict, but family members and the community in which they live.

Incarcerated individuals must be provided with drug treatment, and ongoing opportunities for treatment must be provided upon their release. Institutional forms of racial profiling such as massively unequal sentencing for crack cocaine as opposed to powder cocaine must be unmasked and actively opposed. Drug prevention education must be provided to children from elementary grades through high school. Many individuals have become involved with drugs in the tragically mistaken belief that drug use would solve their problems, and they might not have done so if they had been forewarned of the many potential negative consequences of drug experimentation.

REFERENCES

American Society of Addiction Medicine. (2008). ASAM's 39th Annual Medical-Scientific Conference April 10–13, 2008, in Toronto, Ontario, Canada.

Blendon, R. J., Aiken, L. H., Freeman, H. E., & Corey, C. R. (1989). Access to medical care for black and white Americans: A matter of continuing concern. *Journal of the American Medical Association, 261*(2), 278–281.

Bloch, A. B., Cauthen, G. M., Onorato, I. M., Dansbury, K. G., Kelly, G. D., Driver, C. R., et al. (1994). Nationwide survey of drug-resistant tuberculosis in the United States. *Journal of the American Medical Association, 271*(9), 665–671.

Bosco, C. (1997). Effect of oral creatine supplementation on jumping and running performance. *International Journal of Sports Medicine, 18*, 369–372.

Braithwaite, R. L., & Arriola, K. R. (2009). Health issues: Males of color in prison. Commentary submitted for publication in the *American Journal of Public Health,* Special Issue on Men's Health.

Braithwaite, R., Hammett, T., & Mayberry, R. (1996). *Prison and AIDS: A public health challenge.* San Francisco: Jossey-Bass.

Casavant, M. J., Blake, K., Griffith, J., Yates, A., & Copley, L. M. (2007). Consequences of use of anabolic androgenic steroids. *Pediatric Clinics of North America, 54*(4), 677–690.

Center for Food Safety and Applied Nutrition Special Nutritionals Adverse Event Monitoring System. (1997). Retrieved from http://www.ext.colostate.edu/safefood/newsltr/v2n3s03.html

Centers for Disease Control and Prevention (CDC). (1999). *Best practices for comprehensive tobacco control programs.* Washington, DC: Author.

Centers for Disease Control and Prevention (CDC). (2006). *HIV/AIDS surveillance report.* Washington, DC: Author.

Centers for Disease Control and Prevention (CDC). (2007). *Youth risk behavior surveillance—United States.* Washington, DC: Author.

Commission for Racial Justice. (1987). *Toxic wastes and race in the United States.* Report of the United Church of Christ (UCC).

Decker, M. D., Vaughn, W., Brodie, J. S., et al. (1985). Seroepidemiology of hepatitis B in Tennessee prisoners. *Journal of Infectious Diseases, 150*, 205–216.

Djata, B. (1987). The marketing of vices for black consumers. *Business and Society Review, 62*, 47–49.

Drake, R. (2003). Dual diagnosis and integrated treatment of mental illness and substance abuse disorder fact sheet. Retrieved May 25, 2009, from http://www.naminh.org/NAMI-Fact-Sheet-Dual.pdf.

El-Serag, H. B. (2008). Burden of Hepatitis C infection: Realities and challenges. *Medscape Gastroenterology,* Hepatitis C expert column. Posted 12/04/2008. Available at http://cme.medscape.com/viewarticle/584515

Fleckenstein, J. (2004, February). Chronic hepatitis C in African Americans and other minority groups. *Current Gastroenterology Reports, 6*(1), 66–70.

Graham, A. W., Schultz, T. K., Mayo-Smith, M. F., Ries, R. K. (Eds.), & American Society of Addiction Medicine (Producer). (2007). *Principles of addiction medicine* (3rd ed.). New York: Lippincott.

Gregory, A. J., & Fitch R. (2007). Sports medicine: Performance-enhancing drugs. *Pediatric Clinics of North America, 54*(4), 797–806.

Haller, C. A., & Benowitz, N. L. (2000). Adverse cardiovascular and central nervous system events associated with dietary supplements containing ephedra alkaloids. *New England Journal of Medicine 343*, 1833–1838.

Horn, S., Gregory, P., & Guskiewicz, K. (2009, March). Self-reported anabolic-androgenic steroids use and musculoskeletal injuries: Findings from the Center for the Study of Retired Athletes Health Survey of Retired NFL Players. *American Journal of Physical Medicine and Rehabilitation, 88*(3): 192–200.

Hwang, L., Ross, M. W., Zack, C., Bull, L., Rickman, K., & Holleman, M. (2000, October). Prevalence of sexually transmitted infections and associated risk factors among populations of drug abusers. *Clinical Infectious Diseases, 31*(4), 920–926.

Keisler, B. D., & Hosey, R. G. (2005). Ergogenic aids: An update on ephedra. *Current Sports Medicine Reports, 4*, 231–235.

Kerr, J. M., & Congeni, J. A. (2007). Anabolic-androgenic steroids: Use and abuse in pediatric patients. *Pediatric Clinics of North America, 54*(4), 771–785.

Kessler, R. C. (1979). Stress, social status and psychological distress. *Journal of Health and Social Behavior, 20*, 259–272.

Kessler, R. C. (1995). Epidemiology of psychiatric comorbidity. *Textbook of psychiatric epidemiology* (pp. 356–365). Baltimore: Williams & Wilkins.

Klein, S., Petersilia, J., & Turners, S. (1990). Race and imprisonment decisions in California. *Science, 247*, 812–816.

Kraemer, W. J., & Volek, J. S. (1999). Creatine supplementation: Its role in human performance. *Medicine and Science in Sports and Exercise 31*(8), 1147–1156.

Lillie-Blanton, M., Anthony, J. C., & Schuster, C. R. (1994). Probing the meaning of racial/ethnic group comparisons in crack cocaine smoking. *Journal of the American Medical Association, 269*(8), 993–997.

Mahon, N. (1994). Let's talk about sex and drugs: HIV transmission and prevention behind bars. *International Conference on AIDS, 10*(2), 335 (abstract no. PD0521, August 7–12).

Matich, A. J. (2007). Performance-enhancing drugs and supplements in women and girls. *Current Sports Medicine Report, 6*, 387–391.

Mental Health America. (2009). Fact sheet: Dual diagnosis. Retrieved May 25, 2009, from http://www.nmha.org/go/information/get-info/co-occurring-disorders/dual-diagnosis.

Mumola, C., & Beck, A. (1997). *Prisoners in 1996*. Washington, DC: U.S. Department of Justice, Bureau of Justice Statistics.

Murphy, E. L., Bryzman, S., Williams, A. E., Co-Chien, H., Schreiber, G. B., Ownby, H. E., et al. (1996). Demographic determinants of Hepatitis C virus seroprevalence among blood donors. *Journal of the American Medical Association, 275*(13), 995–1000.

National Youth Tobacco Survey, 2004. (2005, April 1). *Morbidity and Mortality Weekly Report, 54*(12), 297–301.

Sjoqvist, F., Garle, M., & Rane, A. (2008). Use of doping agents, particularly anabolic steroids, in sports and society. *Lancet, 371*(9627), 1872–1882.

Sterling, T. D., & Weinkam, J. J. (1989). Comparison of smoking-related risk factors among black and white males. *American Journal of Industrial Medicine, 15*(3), 319–333.

Strickland, T. L., & Clark, W. (2001). Substance abuse disorders among African American populations. In R. L. Braithwaite & S. E. Taylor (Eds.), *Health issues in the black community* (2nd ed.). San Francisco: Jossey-Bass.

Substance Abuse and Mental Health Services Administration (SAMHSA). (2004). National Survey on Drug Use and Health.

Williams, D. R. (1990). Socioeconomic differentials in health: A review and redirection. *Social Psychology Quarterly, 53*, 81–99.

Williams, D. R., & Collins, C. (1995). U.S. socioeconomic and racial differences in health: Patterns and explanations. *Annual Review of Sociology, 21*, 349–386.

CHAPTER

18

HIV/AIDS IN THE BLACK COMMUNITY

IVORY A. TOLDSON
ABA D. ESSUON
KAMILAH M. WOODSON

NATURE OF THE PROBLEM

The prevalence, burden, and mortality of HIV/AIDS are greater for African American people than for any other racial group in the United States. Since HIV/AIDS was first discovered in the early 1980s, the proportion of known cases has decreased among whites and increased among African Americans. By the mid-1990s, the rate of HIV/AIDS among African Americans exceeded the rate among whites. Currently, African Americans account for almost half (49%) of the people infected with HIV and AIDS (Hall et al., 2008). According to the Centers for Disease Control and Prevention (CDC), in 2005 the rate of AIDS diagnoses for African American adults and adolescents was ten times the rate for whites (CDC, 2007b). African American women are twenty-three times more likely to be diagnosed with AIDS than white women, and African American men are eight times more likely to be diagnosed than white men. By 2004, more than 200,000 African Americans had died from HIV/AIDS. HIV/AIDS is the leading cause of death in African American women aged 25 to 35 and the second leading cause of death in African American men aged 35 to 44.

There are no known genetic factors that place African American people at a greater risk for HIV/AIDS than other racial/ethnic groups. Across races, HIV/AIDS is spread through the exchange of blood, semen, and vaginal fluids through unprotected anal and vaginal intercourse, or puncturing the body with infected instruments, such as needles. Unlike most other deadly diseases, such as heart disease and cancer, HIV/AIDS has highly effective and uncomplicated methods of prevention, which can be described succinctly as practicing abstinence or using barrier methods, like condoms, during sexual intercourse and avoiding contact with dirty equipment during drug activity, such as needles, syringes, cookers, cotton, or rinse water.

Notwithstanding these straightforward methods of prevention, the rate of HIV/AIDS continues to rise in the African American community. The reasons for the rapid spread of HIV/AIDS in the African American community are not well understood (Hallfors, Iritani, Miller, & Bauer, 2007). Among all races, HIV/AIDS is most often spread by people who are unaware of their status with the virus, because HIV/AIDS is difficult to detect. HIV antibodies do not appear in the blood until about two weeks to six months after infection. In addition, HIV symptoms are inconsistent across infected individuals, with up to 60 percent of infected individuals exhibiting no symptoms of infection and others exhibiting symptoms that resemble those of other diseases. Some research evidence suggests that African American people are less likely to know their HIV status than members of other races, for reasons ranging from substandard health care to social stigma (Goosby, 2004).

Like men of other races, men in the African American community have more reported HIV/AIDS cases than women (Laurencin, Christensen, & Taylor, 2008). However, the racial disparity in HIV/AIDS is magnified by the relatively large number of cases among African American women, teenagers, and infants (Tuan, 2006). Most studies suggest that no single factor is responsible for the disproportionate number of HIV/AIDS infections in the African American community. Many circumstances unique to African American people increase the likelihood of exposure to the HIV/AIDS virus by disrupting normal life adjustment and relationship patterns (Adimora & Schoenbach, 2005). HIV antecedent factors include overrepresentation in impoverished areas, the disproportionate number of African American men in prison, inadequate access to health care, and social stigmas related to HIV. The conditions that contribute to HIV infections in the African American community are interrelated, creating a dynamic set of circumstances that place a greater percentage of African Americans at risk of infection.

Poverty

HIV/AIDS infection and survival are linked to socioeconomic levels (McDavid, Hall, Ling, & Song, 2007). Currently, the poverty rate for African Americans is 24.7 percent, compared to only 8.6 percent for non-Hispanic whites (Spriggs, 2006), a fact that accounts for much of the racial disparity in HIV/AIDS cases. Adimora and Schoenbach (2005) suggest that people who are segregated into high-poverty areas are likely to experience more life disruptions, including marital instability. Rapid HIV testing and other convenient means of detection are also less likely to be available in hospitals with fewer financial resources that serve high percentages of African Americans (Bogart et al., 2008).

Incarceration

Laurencin et al. (2008) suggest that high rates of incarceration among African American men may contribute to the spread of HIV/AIDS infections in the African American community. Although African Americans represent 13 percent of the U.S. population, they comprise nearly half of the inmates in state and federal prisons. A recent national study found that concurrent sexual relations were experienced more frequently among men who had been incarcerated for twenty-four hours or more in the preceding year (Adimora, Schoenbach, & Doherty, 2007). Men who reported concurrent sexual relationships were also more likely to engage in other behaviors associated with HIV/AIDS risk, including illicit drug use during sexual intercourse and sex with another man (Adimora, Schoenbach, & Doherty, 2007).

Drug Use

Injection drug use is the second leading cause of HIV infection for African American men and women. Needle-sharing behaviors associated with injection drug use, in which substances are delivered directly to the bloodstream, are an extremely efficient method of HIV transmission in that HIV-infected blood products can be directly delivered into the body through the use of dirty or improperly cleaned syringes (Mathers et al., 2008). In addition to the risks associated with injecting drugs, the use of non-injected drugs also increases the risk of HIV infection. Persons under the influence of drugs are more likely to have unprotected sex and to engage in unprotected sexual activity in exchange for drugs or money to buy drugs. One study, however, indicated a promising trend among African Americans. A recent multicity study indicated that between 1992 and 2004 the number of injection drug users declined 44 percent for African Americans as compared with a decline of 17 percent for whites (Broz & Ouellet, 2008). The study also revealed that younger African American heroin users were more likely to resist injection than younger white heroin users.

Access to Health Care

The relationship between high HIV rates and low socioeconomic status has been demonstrated by populations of color. With a poverty rate of one in four, African Americans are often faced with economic challenges that limit their access to high-quality health care. A recent survey found that 22 percent of African Americans with HIV had no medical coverage, compared with 17 percent of whites (Kaiser Family Foundation, 2006). In addition, African Americans were much less likely to have private insurance coverage: 14 percent compared with 44 percent of whites (Kaiser Family Foundation, 2006). African American people were more likely to delay medical treatment because of transportation difficulties or other competing needs. The lack of high-quality health care has been noted as one of the reasons why African Americans are more likely to be diagnosed in the later stages of HIV infection when treatment is less effective. For example, one study noted that white Medicaid enrollees who were HIV positive were more likely to receive highly active antiretroviral therapy (HAART) than African

American patients (King et al., 2008). Late diagnoses among African Americans have greatly contributed to the AIDS-related death rate of 55 percent.

EPIDEMIOLOGY

HIV has transitioned from being a disease of gay white males to an equal opportunity disease that is determined by one's behavior and has had a disproportionate impact on the African American community. From the beginning of the epidemic to 2005, 211,559 African Americans have died from AIDS-related illnesses. In the United States, approximately 1.1 million adults and adolescents are estimated to be living with diagnosed or undiagnosed HIV (CDC, 2008b). Of the estimated 1.1 million persons thought to be infected, one fourth (252,000 to 312,000) are believed to be unaware of their HIV-positive status (CDC, 2008b). In 2004, in terms of disease-related deaths, HIV (surpassed only by cancer and heart disease) was the fifth leading cause of death among women aged 35–44 and the sixth leading cause of death among women aged 25–34. In the same year, HIV was the leading cause of death for African American women aged 25–34, the third leading cause of death for African American women aged 35–44, and the fourth leading cause of death for African American women aged 45–54 and Hispanic women aged 35–44 (CDC, 2007b).

Although more than twenty-five years have passed since the beginning of the AIDS epidemic, persistently high rates of HIV transmission continue to make HIV prevention and treatment public health priorities. In the United States, the three primary modes of HIV transmission are male-to-male sexual contact (50%); high-risk heterosexual contact (33%), defined as heterosexual contact with a person known to have HIV infection or at least expected to be at high risk for the infection (e.g., injection drug users, persons who engage in unprotected sex with multiple partners, or men who have sex with men); and injection drug use (13%). HIV prevalence is greatest among males and persons aged 25–44, accounting for 74 percent and 57 percent of all HIV infections respectively (CDC, 2008b). Of the racial and ethnic groups in the United States, African Americans are disproportionably infected in that they account for the majority of all HIV/AIDS cases irrespective of sex, age, or mode of transmission, accounting for 43.9 percent of cases diagnosed among men and 67.2 percent of cases diagnosed among women (CDC, 2007b, 2008b).

The United States has an estimated nationwide HIV prevalence rate of 447.8 per 100,000 persons (CDC, 2008c). Among those living with HIV, African Americans represent 46.1 percent of the current provenance at 1,715.1 per 100,000, whites represent 34.6 percent at 224.3 per 100,000, Hispanics represent 17.5 percent at 585.3 per 100,000, Asian/Pacific Islanders represent 1.4 percent at 129.6 per 100,000, and American Indian/Alaska Natives represent 0.4 percent at 231.4 per 100,000 (CDC, 2008c). African Americans are contracting HIV/AIDS at a rate 10 times that of whites (CDC, 2007c). Despite accounting for nearly 50 percent of all reported HIV/AIDS cases, African Americans represent only 13 percent of the U.S. population; in contrast, whites represent 73 percent of the population and 29.3 percent of the reported HIV/

AIDS cases, and Hispanics represent 13 percent of the population and 18.1 percent of the HIV/AIDS cases (CDC, 2007b).

This disproportionate trend is most pronounced among African American teens and women. Among the U.S. teen population, wherein African Americans represent 16 percent of the total population, African American teens account for 69 percent of all reported HIV/AIDS cases. The majority of the HIV infections for both African American male and female adolescents have resulted from risky sexual activity with males (Harper, 2007). The primary mode of HIV infection for African American adolescent and young adult males aged 13–24, as well as for U.S. males in general, is male-to-male sexual contact at 49 percent, followed by injection drug use at 23 percent and high-risk heterosexual contact at 22 percent (Harper, 2007; CDC, 2008b).

With heterosexual contact at 74 percent followed by injection drug use at 24 percent as the primary modes of HIV infection for African American women, African American women have the fastest-growing rate of new HIV infections (CDC, 2008a). Although earlier in the epidemic the rate of HIV infection among women was underestimated because many of the women who became infected through injection drug use were never diagnosed, more accurate current estimates of HIV among women suggest that women account for more than one quarter of all new HIV/AIDS diagnoses (CDC, 2008a). While African American and Hispanic women represent only 24 percent of the total U.S. female population, they account for 82 percent of the total number of diagnosed AIDS cases among U.S. women in 2005 (CDC, 2008a). Even though the overall rate of new HIV infections is greatest among African American males, African American women are contracting HIV/AIDS at a rate 23 times greater than white women, representing 66 percent of reported cases among women (CDC, 2008a; Whitmore, Satcher, & Hu, 2005).

According to the CDC, the presence of certain sexually transmitted diseases (STDs) such as gonorrhea and syphilis greatly increases the chances of contracting and transmitting HIV, on the order of three- to fivefold increases. The highest rates of STDs are found among the African American population; for example, in 2005, African Americans were 18 times as likely as whites to have gonorrhea (representing 68% of the total number of cases in 2005) and approximately five times as likely to have syphilis (comprising 41% of all primary and secondary cases in 2005) (CDC, 2007b; Laurencin et al., 2008).

AIDS in black America has long represented a state of emergency, which has been made evident by the fact that 72 percent of all African Americans living with HIV/AIDS reside in nine U.S. states. Once concentrated in the Northeast and West Coast in large metropolitan urban areas with populations of 500,000 or more, the HIV/AIDS epidemic has settled in the smaller rural areas of the South, particularly in the Deep South (Foster, 2007; Wells Pence, Reif, & Whetten, 2007). The Deep South consists of six states—Louisiana, Mississippi, Alabama, Georgia, South and North Carolina—that share a history of cotton and tobacco production, together with slavery dependence and promotion. Despite representing only 19 percent of the region's population, African Americans in the Deep South account for 51 percent of persons living with HIV/AIDS and 56 percent of all newly diagnosed HIV cases in the region (CDC, 2002; Hammett & Drachman-Jones, 2006). From 2000 to 2005, although the rate of AIDS cases decreased by 6 percent in the rest of the nation, it increased 36 percent in the Deep South and 2 percent in the South (Wells Pence et al., 2007). In 2005, among the thirty-eight states with mandatory reporting, Southern states, consisting of sixteen states and the District of Columbia, ranked in the top eighteen for HIV/AIDS incidence, while the Deep South states ranked within the top sixteen (Reif & Whetten, 2006; Wells Pence et al., 2007). The six Deep South states also ranked among the fifteen states with the highest AIDS mortality rates (CDC, 2007a; Wells Pence et al., 2007).

The South accounts for 46 percent of all new AIDS diagnoses, with one third of all new cases occurring in the Deep South (Wells Pence et al., 2007). The high prevalence of HIV/AIDS in the Deep South has been attributed to high HIV occurrences among women, racial and ethnic minorities, the poor, and residents of rural areas. Although male-to-male sexual contact is the primary mode of transmission nationwide, in the Deep South male-to-male sexual contact and injection drug use are lesser modes of HIV transmission. The primary mode of HIV transmission in the Deep South is heterosexual sexual contact (Wells Pence et al., 2007).

CURRENT RESEARCH

Risk Factors and Barriers to Prevention

Although early research on HIV prevention focused almost exclusively on the impact of individual factors such as perceived risk and knowledge of HIV prevention, for many African Americans having awareness did not seem to translate into behavioral risk prevention. Consequently, recent research has focused on HIV risk in the context of broader social issues and constructs such as gender relationships, power dynamics, socioeconomic factors, sex roles, substance abuse, and experiences related to race and ethnicity (Jenkins, 2000). African American women at high risk for HIV are more often caught at the intersection of poverty and gender discrimination, and many report feeling powerless in protecting themselves against HIV (National Alliance of State and Territorial AIDS Directors [NASTAD], 2005). For African American males the intersection of HIV/AIDS with issues of sexuality creates a powerful dynamic. The 2005 NASTAD report further suggests that African American men who have sex with men must navigate many cultural, social, spiritual, sexual, racial, and economic issues that together pose a unique set of challenges.

Sexual Risk Factors

Researchers have suggested that the high rates of HIV in the African American population are directly linked to high rates of incarceration among African American men and their homosexual behaviors while incarcerated (Fullilove, 2001). According to Laurencin et al. (2008), the data show that African American women are most likely to be infected with HIV as a result of sex with men who are infected with HIV (CDC,

2007b). Studies have postulated lack of knowledge about their male partners' possible risk factors for HIV infection, including unprotected sex with multiple partners, intravenous drug use, or bisexuality, as driving influences for this predominant mode of transmission; thus, African American women are more likely than white women to have acquired HIV heterosexually (Laurencin et al., 2008). The predominant mode of transmission of HIV for African American men is through male to male sexual contact (CDC, 2007b; Laurencin et al., 2008).

The power dynamics between men and women represent an important aspect of HIV prevention for women (Amaro, 1995; Bradlock & Koniak-Griffin, 2007). Many studies focus on women, and a woman's ability to protect herself against HIV, within the context of an intimate relationship. This ability is directly related to empowerment and perceptions of efficacy in a woman's personal life (Guitierrez, Oh, & Gillmore, 2000). The impact of self-efficacy and empowerment on HIV is particularly significant because African American women often face multiple burdens of racism, sexism, and poverty that may increase feelings of powerlessness and hopelessness (Osmond et al., 1993; Quinn, 1993), making the practice of consistent condom use a challenge. Most often, many women do not experience the level of power in their relationship necessary to negotiate safer sex with their partner (Bradlock & Koniak-Griffin, 2007; Gutierrez et al., 2000).

A woman's sense of self and her beliefs about the fidelity of her partner represent another set of sexual risk factors. Cummings, Battle, Barker, and Krasnovsky (1999) suggest three major reasons for African American women's sexual risk taking: (1) Being in a relationship is a major source of self-validation and self-esteem, (2) Having unsafe sex (sex without a condom) helps women maintain their beliefs that their partners are faithful, and (3) African American women are often in denial about their vulnerability in relationships (Foreman, 2003). According to Thompson-Robinson et al. (2005), females felt uncomfortable discussing issues related to HIV/AIDS with their partners because they feared they would lose the intimate relationship with their partners as a result of HIV/AIDS discussions and self-advocacy (Thompson-Robinson et al., 2005).

Cultural values may further exacerbate risk. African American women tend to have cultural values that endorse relationships in which personal needs are sacrificed (Wyatt, 1992; Wyatt et al., 2000). The investigators suggest that for African American women, there are structural factors in relationships resulting in a lack of available mates. This shortage thereby increases their chances of remaining single and being unable to fulfill cultural expectations of marriage and children within a family context (Tucker & Mitchell-Kernan, 1995; Wilson, 1987; Wyatt et al., 2000). Wyatt et al. (2000) further suggest that as a consequence, African American women may be less likely to challenge cultural and relationship norms endorsing unprotected sex in order to avoid jeopardizing relationships through which they can satisfy these goals. Once these relationship goals are satisfied, married women tend to take greater sexual risks in their relationships (Wyatt et al., 2000). Requesting condom use within established relationships creates conflict and undermines trust by raising suspicions about sexually transmitted diseases and infidelity (Margillo & Imahori, 1998; Perrino, Fernandez, Bowen, & Arheart, 2006; Williams & Semanchuk, 1999; Wyatt et al., 2000).

Substance Use

Illicit drug use is the second leading cause of HIV infection for African American men and women (CDC, 2007b; Laurencin et al., 2008). Substance use has the potential to interfere with risk assessment, decision making, and negotiations around condom use (Perrino et al., 2006). Many studies have found that African American women who use alcohol or drugs are less likely to request the use of condoms (Bradlock & Koniak-Griffin, 2007; Hetherington, Harris, Bausell, & Kavanaugh, 1996; Perrino et al., 2006) and more likely to participate in sexual behavior that places them at greater risk for HIV infections (Perrino et al., 2006; Rees, Saitz, Horton, & Samet, 2001; Sikkema et al., 1995). Women who are under the influence of drugs may be less effective in their condom use attempts, and their intoxicated male partners may be less responsive to the women's condom use attempts (Perrino et al., 2006).

Lack of Awareness of HIV Serostatus

The high level of unrecognized HIV infections among African Americans is a public concern. As the CDC (2007a) points out, individuals who are unknowingly infected with HIV cannot benefit from earlier lifesaving therapies, nor can they protect their partners from becoming infected with HIV. The lack of screening is an even greater concern among African American men who have sex with men (Laurencin et al., 2008). Bing, Bingham, and Millett (2008) estimate that nearly half of all African American men who have sex with men and live in major U.S. cities are already infected with HIV (Bing, Bingham, & Millett, 2008), and they are much less likely to know (Mackellar, Valleroy, & Secura, 2005). Laurencin, Christensen, and Taylor (2008) further suggest that timely diagnosis is extremely critical, in that of all HIV infections diagnosed in African Americans in 2004, 40 percent progressed to an AIDS diagnosis within 12 months of their HIV diagnosis (CDC, 2007b; Laurencin et al., 2008).

Sexually Transmitted Diseases

Anatomical differences between men and women almost double the likelihood that a woman will contract HIV during unprotected vaginal intercourse with an infected partner as compared with a man's risk of contracting HIV from an infected female partner (NASTAD, 2008; Tuan, 2006). The presence of certain other STDs greatly increases the likelihood of acquiring or transmitting HIV infection (NASTAD, 2008), and an individual infected with both HIV and certain STDs has a greater chance of spreading HIV to others (Fleming & Wasserheit, 1999). Wyatt et al. (2000) found that African American women with an STD history were likely to take more risks in relationships, including engaging in unprotected vaginal intercourse (Wyatt et al., 2000).

Homophobia and Concealment of Homosexual Behavior

Homophobia and stigmatization can cause some African American men who have sex with men to identify themselves as heterosexual or not to disclose their sexual orientation (Laurencin et al., 2008). One reason cited for this nondisclosure is the notion that many in the African American community are less accepting of homosexuality than are members of other racial/ethnic groups. Other reasons include fears of social isolation, discrimination, and verbal/physical abuse (Thompson-Robinson et al., 2005). Consequently, this "masking" of behaviors contributes to the impact of HIV/AIDS in the African American community. According to Thompson-Robinson et al. (2005), in a study of 637 men who did not disclose their sexual orientation, 8 percent were HIV-infected; however, 61 percent of nondisclosing African American men reported engaging in unprotected sex with their female sex partners. During the initial phase of a relationship, women are more likely than men to disclose intimate details about themselves (Mays & Cochran, 1993). Research findings have indicated that men are significantly more likely than women to report having been dishonest with dating partners in order to have sexual relations (Cochran & Mays, 1990). Disclosing past sexual behaviors, same-sex sexual behaviors, or number of past sexual partners could be viewed as creating a high risk for embarrassment or potential loss of a relationship (Derelega & Chaikin, 1975; Mays & Cochran, 1993). Dishonest disclosures seem more acceptable than the possibility of rejection, and ironically these men perceive themselves to be at low risk for becoming infected with HIV (Thompson-Robinson et al., 2005).

Socioeconomic Issues

It is well documented that certain groups of women, specifically those who are young, poor, and African American, are at higher risk for unintended pregnancies, STDs, and HIV infection (Wyatt et al., 2000). A woman's vulnerability to the virus is attributable to deeply entrenched socioeconomic inequalities that further compound risk. Because 70 percent of the world's poor are women, they have fewer economic options than men and are far more vulnerable to engaging in transactional sex to pay for food, school fees, and other necessities (Bradlock & Koniak-Griffin, 2007). They are also vulnerable to coercive and forced sex; thus, they are often unable to negotiate condom use (Bradlock & Koniak-Griffin, 2007; Global Health Council, 2005). A woman who depends on money provided by her main partner to make ends meet may be in a position of reduced power when it comes to insisting on safer sex (Perrino et al., 2006).

Broader, contextual influences may also affect whether low-income African American women are able to effectively communicate with their main partners about condom use and protection against HIV infection (Perrino et al., 2006). Previous qualitative studies have indicated that economic, racial, and social factors have resulted in power differentials between African American men and women, in turn raising women's vulnerability to HIV infection (Fullilove, Fullilove, Haynes, & Gross, 1990; Margillo & Imahori, 1998; Perrino et al., 2006).

Prevention

Partner and relationship factors function as determinants of condom use among African American women who are at high risk of acquiring HIV through sexual contact (Perrino et al., 2006). Consequently, HIV infection prevention programs that target women individually have a distinct disadvantage when it comes to modifying partner behavior or relationship dynamics and patterns. El-Bassel et al. (2001) have described a "relationship-based" HIV infection intervention aimed at minority couples, rather than individual women, which targets relationship issues and communication patterns that influence condom use and safer sex (El-Bassel et al., 2001; Perrino et al., 2006).

The benefit of intervening at the relationship level is that both partners can become actively involved in establishing and meeting behavior change goals (Perrino et al., 2006), given that HIV/STI prevention research must take into consideration gender-specific variables such as a woman's fear of physical abuse (Perrino et al., 2006). According to Wyatt (1992), this type of intervention may be especially effective as well as highly sensitive and culturally appropriate (Perrino et al., 2006). Relative to men who have sex with men (MSM), interventions that promote earlier and more frequent HIV testing for African American MSM (CDC, 2002) or prevention outreach programs that target places that cater to MSM are extremely desirable. Another prevention strategy that would be favorable for MSM is creating access to more convenient testing methods such as rapid HIV tests or telephone results, which may help increase testing frequency and thereby reduce inadvertent transmission of HIV by African American MSM (NASTAD, 2005).

POLICY IMPLICATIONS

In many ways, U.S. policies on HIV/AIDS have been stalled in a political quagmire for more than a quarter of a century. Abject indifference characterized the U.S. government's earliest response to the AIDS crisis. AIDS was first reported as a national emergency in mainstream media in 1981, yet President Ronald Reagan did not speak publicly about the crisis until 1987, a year before his final year in office. From 1981 until the end of 1987 almost 28,000 people died of the disease.

Since 1987, every U.S. executive administration has devised formal strategies to combat HIV/AIDS. In 1988, President Reagan's 13-member Presidential Commission on the HIV Epidemic listened to testimony and proposed recommendations for a government policy on AIDS (Gebbie, 1989). However, most independent observers agree that the recommendations were largely disregarded (Collin, 2006). In 1991, President George H. W. Bush assembled the National Commission on AIDS (Perkins, 1993), which issued a scathing indictment of the U.S. response to the AIDS crisis in the report, "America living with AIDS: Transforming anger, fear, and indifference into action." The report lamented, "Workers on the front lines are struggling heroically to cope with illness and death, but their tools have been too few, their resources too constrained, and their logistics too crippled by the sabotage of disbelief, prejudice, ignorance, and fear" (National Commission on AIDS, 1991).

In 1995, President Bill Clinton established the Presidential Advisory Council on HIV/AIDS (PACHA) to provide more recommendations on the U.S. government's response to AIDS (Clinton, 1996). At a committee hearing, President Clinton acknowledged, "HIV infection is one of the most deadly health disparities between African Americans, Hispanics, and white Americans" and pledged a "$156-million initiative to stem the AIDS crisis in minority communities" (Clinton, 1998). However, the council was also criticized for offering too few recommendations, for simply reiterating the findings of predecessor commissions, and for allowing politics to overshadow priorities. Most notably, when President Clinton expressed opposition to a proposed needle exchange program after receiving evidence that the programs reduced the spread of HIV without promoting drug use, Dr. Mohammad N. Akhter, then the Executive Director of the American Public Health Association, stated, "Not releasing federal funds gives the impression that politics takes precedence over saving lives" (American Public Health Association, 1998).

President George W. Bush renewed PACHA's charter in 2001. Under President Bush, PACHA continued to field criticism for inactivity and political posturing. The most noted example was the controversial appointment to the Council of Dr. Joseph McIlhaney (Lawrence, 2004)—a physician with a dearth of published, peer-reviewed scientific research, who was a staunch opponent of condom education. Domestically, critics contended that President Bush's HIV policy was limited to strategies that primarily appealed to people who were politically conservative, such as abstinence-only education and faith-based initiatives. In a scathing critique, U.S. Representative Henry A. Waxman alleged that the Bush Administration routinely censored accurate scientific information, "gagged" scientists, and manipulated scientific advisory committees that did not fit within conservative ideologies (Waxman, 2006).

Internationally, President Bush has been lauded for the "President's Emergency Plan for AIDS Relief" (PEPFAR), which committed $15 billion over five years (2003–2008) to fight the global HIV/AIDS pandemic (Denny & Emanuel, 2008). Currently, PEPFAR has fifteen focus countries: Botswana, Côte d'Ivoire, Ethiopia, Guyana, Haiti, Kenya, Mozambique, Namibia, Nigeria, Rwanda, South Africa, Tanzania, Uganda, Vietnam, and Zambia. Ironically, the HIV/AIDS rate among African Americans is higher than that of half of the focus countries, yet PEPFAR does not allocate funding for domestic HIV/AIDS prevention programs.

President Barack Obama's *Factsheet on HIV/AIDS* outlines the strategies his administration will take to combat the pandemic, citing specific strategies for curbing the spread of HIV in the African American community. President Obama's plan calls for "measurable goals, timelines and accountability mechanisms" to monitor policy efficacy (Obama, 2008). President Obama's plan to help African American and other minority communities includes the following strategies: promoting innovative HIV/AIDS testing initiatives in minority communities; partnering with community leaders from churches and community organizations; targeting poverty and homelessness; addressing differences in access to health insurance coverage; promoting prevention and public health; and diversifying the health workforce (Obama, 2008). While President Obama's policy agenda is consistent with much of the current research and needs in the African American community, public health professionals and advocates have the responsibility of holding the new administration accountable and ensuring that campaign promises are converted into solutions.

U.S. HIV/AIDS policy is often weighed against the edicts from a 2001 United Nations General Assembly Special Session dedicated to HIV/AIDS (Collin, 2006).

Under the direction of the Soros Foundation, Collin (2006) offers policy recommendations designed to bring the United States into compliance with their UNGASS Declaration of Commitment on HIV/AIDS. Many of the findings are consistent with research presented in this chapter. Specifically, the report affirms the need for the United States to set benchmarks for reducing AIDS infection and associated racial disparities, expand interventions aimed at reducing stigma, and to deliver quality care more widely and equitably across racial and socioeconomic groups.

LESSONS LEARNED, BEST PRACTICES, AND RECOMMENDATIONS

Today, the United States struggles to redefine HIV/AIDS as a public health problem, after decades of futile moral invectives, bigotry, and arrogance. Detractors have propagated the myth that HIV/AIDS is restricted to a narrow and depraved segment of the population whose contemptible behaviors make them unworthy of a concerted public health agenda. As myths about HIV/AIDS dissipate, many leaders in the United States have focused on the pandemic abroad with a level of rigidity and chivalry that offers the illusion that domestic HIV problems are waning. National, state, and community leaders share some liability for creating a cultural climate of shame and apathy when responding to the HIV/AIDS epidemic at a time when the rate and scope of HIV/AIDS among African American people demand a reasoned and comprehensive public health agenda.

Like men of other races, men in the African American community have higher HIV/AIDS rates than women. However, African American women, teenagers, and infants are much more likely to contract HIV/AIDS than their counterparts in other racial/ethnic groups. Being African American does not increase the likelihood that a person will contract HIV/AIDS, but circumstances unique to the African American community increase chances of exposure to the HIV virus by disrupting normal life adjustment and relationship patterns. Some circumstances can increase an African American person's exposure to the virus, even in the absence of higher-risk behaviors. For example, although most studies suggest that African American people use drugs at lower rates than members of other groups, high rates of poverty can bring African American drug users into more frequent contact with infected instruments. A recent study supported by the National Institute of Drug Abuse found that young African Americans had elevated HIV risk even in the absence of high-risk sexual and drug use behavior (Hallfors et al., 2007).

Overall, current research on HIV/AIDS in the African American community supports a comprehensive public health agenda to reach all African Americans through education, clinical practice, and public policy. Increasing culturally congruent awareness, screening, testing and treatment services in traditional and nontraditional venues is essential to an inclusive national HIV/AIDS reduction policy. In the following paragraphs are specific recommendations that are consistent with the research presented in this chapter.

HIV policy should recognize the significant impact that social stigma has had in lowering the number of people who receive HIV tests and subsequent treatment.

Persons who are unaware of their HIV status are at great risk for spreading the virus. Since many African Americans must deal with strong social and environmental pressures within close-knit communities, greater emphasis should be placed on reducing stigma and the associated isolation among HIV-infected individuals.

Treatment providers and policymakers should also consider the nature and role of sexual relationships among African American people with regard to its influence on HIV prevention. Health policy that emphasizes the role of healthy sexual negotiation among heterosexual couples and men who have sex with men is essential to a comprehensive HIV/AIDS reduction strategy. Negotiating condom use, exploring sexual history, and getting tested are important aspects of this policy.

Research supports the role of drug prevention programs and harm reduction strategies in an HIV reduction program. Although African American people's use of drugs is not inconsistent with their representation in the population, the dangers of specific drug behaviors should be emphasized. Needle exchange programs should be implemented to reduce HIV risk among lower-income drug users.

Health policies should consider the social disadvantages faced by African American people who are overrepresented in low-income communities. Improving medical facilities in impoverished areas by providing resources to quickly and conveniently test and treat HIV is essential to achieving health parity. In addition, economic conditions affecting the African American community are central to higher rates of HIV infections. The declining availability of jobs with a livable wage that provide benefits such as health insurance disproportionately burdens the African American community. A safety net to provide health care during periods of unemployment, health crises, and family problems will be necessary to reduce the spread of HIV in the African American community.

High rates of incarceration and mortality among African American men have conceivably left a void in the African American community that has contributed to more loosely structured social networks and weakened sexual negotiation abilities among African American women. Current revisions of 25-year-old criminal justice policies and other remedial efforts should consider the intimate relationships of inmates reentering society.

Progressive and comprehensive HIV treatment and prevention programs should consider the use of nontraditional venues to render services, such as homes, schools, and churches. Community-based approaches could address African American people's reluctance to seek health care in traditional settings, reduce the ethnocentric biases among health care providers, and give care providers a more effective context for HIV prevention in African American communities.

REFERENCES

Adimora, A. A., & Schoenbach, V. J. (2005). Social context, sexual networks, and racial disparities in rates of sexually transmitted infections. *Journal of Infectious Diseases, 191*, S115–S122.

Adimora, A. A., Schoenbach, V. J., & Doherty, I. A. (2007). Concurrent sexual partnerships among men in the United States. *American Journal of Public Health, 97*(12), 2230–2237.

Amaro, H. (1995). Love, sex, and power. *American Psychologist, 50*, 437–447.

American Public Health Association. (1998). Administration, House say no federal funding for needle exchange programs. *Nation's Health, 28*(5), 1.

Bing, E. G., Bingham, T., & Millett, G. A. (2008). Research needed to more effectively combat HIV among African-American men who have sex with men. *Journal of the National Medical Association, 100*(1), 52–57.

Bogart, L. M., Howerton, D., Lange, J., Becker, K., Setodji, C. M., & Asch, S. M. (2008). Scope of rapid HIV testing in urban US hospitals. *Public Health Reports, 123*(4), 494–503.

Bradlock, A. R., & Koniak-Griffin, D. (2007). Relationship power and other influences on self-protective sexual behaviors in African American female adolescents. *Health Care for Women International, 28*, 247–267.

Broz, D., & Ouellet, L. J. (2008). Racial and ethnic changes in heroin injection in the United States: Implications for the HIV/AIDS epidemic. *Drug & Alcohol Dependence, 94*(1–3), 221–233.

Centers for Disease Control and Prevention. (2002). *HIV/AIDS surveillance report 2001*. Atlanta: U.S. Department of Health and Human Services.

Centers for Disease Control and Prevention. (2007a). *Sexually transmitted diseases surveillance, 2006*. Atlanta: U.S. Department of Health and Human Services.

Centers for Disease Control and Prevention. (2007b). Update to racial/ethnic disparities in diagnoses of HIV/AIDS—33 States, 2001–2005. *Morbidity and Mortality Weekly Report, 56*(9), 189–193.

Centers for Disease Control and Prevention. (2008a). *HIV/AIDS among women fact sheet revised August 2008*. Atlanta, GA: U.S. Department of Health and Human Services.

Centers for Disease Control and Prevention. (2008b). *HIV and AIDS in the United States: A picture of today's epidemic. Fact sheet revised August 2008*. Atlanta, GA: U.S. Department of Health and Human Services.

Centers for Disease Control and Prevention. (2008c). HIV prevalence estimates–United States, 2006. *Morbidity and Mortality Weekly Report, 57*(39), 1073–1076.

Clinton, W. J. (1996). Executive Order 13009—Amendment to Executive Order No. 12963 entitled Presidential Advisory. *Weekly Compilation of Presidential Documents, 32*(24), 1060.

Clinton, W. J. (1998). Remarks announcing the HIV/AIDS initiative in minority communities. *Weekly Compilation of Presidential Documents, 34*, 2166.

Cochran, S. D., & Mays, V. M. (1990). Sex, lies, and HIV [Letter to the editor]. *New England Journal of Medicine, 322*, 774–775.

Collin, C. (2006). *HIV/AIDS policy in the United States: Monitoring the UNGASS Declaration of Commitment on HIV/AIDS*. New York: Open Society Institute.

Cummings, G. L., Battle, R. S., Barker, J. C., & Krasnovsky, F. M. (1999). Are African American women worried about getting AIDS? A qualitative analysis. *AIDS Education and Prevention, 11*(4), 331–342.

Denny, C. C., & Emanuel, E. J. (2008). US Health Aid Beyond PEPFAR. *Journal of the American Medical Association* 300(17):2048–2051.

Derelega, V. J., & Chaikin, A. (1975). *Sharing intimacy: What we reveal to others and why*. Englewood Cliffs, NJ: Prentice-Hall.

El-Bassel, N., Witte, S. S., Gilbert, L., Sormanti, M., Moreno, C., & Pereira, L. (2001). HIV prevention for intimate couples: A relationship-based model. *Families, Systems & Health, 19*, 379–395.

Fleming, D. T., & Wasserheit, J. N. (1999). From epidemiological synergy to public health policy and practice: The contribution of other sexually transmitted diseases to sexual transmission of HIV infection. *Sexually Transmitted Infections, 75*, 3–17.

Foreman, F. E. (2003). Intimate risk: Sexual risk behavior among African American college women. *Journal of Black Studies, 33*(5), 637–653.

Foster, P. H. (2007). Use of stigma, fear, and denial in development of a framework for prevention of HIV/AIDS in rural African-American communities. *Family Community Health, 30*(4), 318–327.

Fullilove, M. T., Fullilove, R. E., Haynes, K., & Gross, S. (1990). Black women and AIDS prevention: A view towards understanding gender rules. *Journal of Sex Research, 27*, 47–64.

Fullilove, R. E. (2001). HIV prevention in the African American Community: Why isn't anybody talking about the elephant in the room? *Journal, 7*(1). Retrieved from http://www.aidscience.com/Articles/aidscience007.asp

Gebbie, K. M. (1989). The President's Commission on AIDS: What did it do? *American Journal of Public Health, 79*(7), 868–870.

Global Health Council. (2005). *Women's health*. Retrieved December 27, 2005, from http://www.globalhealth.org/womens_health/

Goosby, E. (2004). *Living with HIV/AIDS: The Black person's guide to survival.* Roscoe, IL: Hilton.

Gutierrez, L., Oh, H. J., & Gillmore, M. R. (2000). Toward an understanding of (em)power(ment) for HIV/AIDS prevention with adolescent women. *Sex Roles, 42*(7/8), 581–611.

Hall, H. I., Ruiguang, S., Rhodes, P., Prejean, J., Qian, A., Lee, L. M., et al. (2008). Estimation of HIV incidence in the United States. *Journal of the American Medical Association, 300*(5), 520–529.

Hallfors, D. D., Iritani, B. J., Miller, W. C., & Bauer, D. J. (2007). Sexual and drug behavior patterns and HIV and STD racial disparities: The need for new directions. *American Journal of Public Health, 97*(1), 125–132.

Hammett, T., & Drachman-Jones, A. (2006). HIV/AIDS, sexually transmitted diseases, and incarceration among women: National and southern perspectives. *Sexual Transmitted Diseases, 33*(7), S17–S22.

Harper, G. (2007, November). Sex isn't that simple: Cultural and context in HIV prevention intervention for gay and bisexual male adolescents. *American Psychologist*, 806–819.

Hetherington, S. E., Harris, R. M., Bausell, R. B., & Kavanaugh, K. H. (1996). AIDS prevention in high risk African American women: Behavioral, psychological and gender issues. *Journal of Sex and Marital Therapy, 22*, 9–21.

Jenkins, S. R. (2000). Toward theory development and measure evolution for studying women's relationships and HIV infection. *Sex Roles, 42* (7/8), 751–780.

Kaiser Family Foundation. (2006). *The HIV/AIDS epidemic in the United States.* HIV/AIDS Policy Fact Sheet. Retrieved in 2007 from http://www.kff.org/hivaids/3029.cfm

King, W. D., Minor, P., Kitchen, C. R., Ore, L. E., Shoptaw, S., Victorianne, G. D., et al. (2008). Racial, gender and geographic disparities of antiretroviral treatment among US Medicaid enrollees in 1998. *Journal of Epidemiology & Community Health, 62*(9), 798–803.

Laurencin, C. T., Christensen, D. M., & Taylor, E. D. (2008). HIV/AIDS and the African-American community: A state of emergency. *Journal of the National Medical Association, 100*(1), 35–43.

Lawrence, D. J. (2004). Policy trumps science in the Bush administration. *Journal of the Canadian Chiropractic Association, 48*(3), 195–197.

Mackellar, D. A., Valleroy, L. A., & Secura, G. M. (2005). Unrecognized HIV infection risk behaviors and perceptions of risk among young men who have sex with men. *Journal of Acquired Immune Deficiency Syndrome, 38*, 603–614.

Margillo, G. A., & Imahori, T. T. (1998). Understanding safer sex negotiation in a group of low-income African American women. In N. L. Roth & L. K. Fuller (Eds.), *Women & AIDS: Negotiating safer sex practices, care and representation* (pp. 43–69). New York: Haworth Press.

Mathers, B. M., Degenhardt, L., Phillips, B., Wiessing, L., Hickman, M., Strathdee, S. A., et al. (2008). Global epidemiology of injecting drug use and HIV among people who inject drugs: A systematic review. *Lancet, 372*(9651), 1733–1745.

Mays, V. M., & Cochran, S. D. (1993). Ethnic and gender differences in beliefs about sex partner questioning to reduce HIV risk. *Journal of Adolescent Research, 8*(1), 77–88.

McDavid, K., Hall, H. I., Ling, Q., & Song, R. (2007). Area socioeconomic factors and relative survival after a diagnosis of HIV, United States, 1996–2003. *Annals of Epidemiology, 17*(9), 739–740.

National Alliance of State and Territorial AIDS Directors (NASTAD). (2005). *A turning point: Confronting HIV/AIDS in African American communities.* Retrieved November 20, 2008, from http://www.nastad.org

National Alliance of State and Territorial AIDS Directors (NASTAD). (2008). The landscape of HIV/AIDS among African American women in the United States. *Issue Brief, 1*, 1–11. Retrieved from http://www.nastad.org

National Commission on AIDS. (1991). *America living with AIDS: Transforming anger, fear, and indifference into action.* Washington, DC: U.S. Government Printing Office.

Obama, B. (2008). *Barack Obama: Fighting HIV/AIDS worldwide.* Retrieved November 2008, from http://www.barackobama.com/pdf/AIDSFactSheet.pdf.

Osmond, M. W., Wambach, K. G., Harrison, D. E., Byers, J., Levine, P., Imershein, A., et al. (1993). The multiple jeopardy of race, class, and gender for AIDS risk among women. *Gender and Society, 7*(1), 99–120.

Perkins, J. E. (1993). Facing the health-policy challenge of HIV infection. *National Forum, 73*(3), 45.

Perrino, T., Fernandez, M. I., Bowen, G. S., & Arheart, K. (2006). Low-income African American women's attempts to convince their main partner to use condoms. *Cultural Diversity and Ethnic Minority Psychology, 12*(1), 70–83.

Quinn, S. C. (1993). AIDS and the African American woman: The triple burden of race, class, and gender. *Health Education Quarterly, 20*(3), 305–320.

Rees, V., Saitz, R., Horton, N. J., & Samet, J. (2001). Association of alcohol consumption and HIV sex and drug-risk behaviors among drug users. *Journal of Substance Abuse Treatment, 21*, 129–134.

Reif, S., & Whetten K. (2006). HIV infection and AIDS in the Deep South. *American Journal of Public Health, 96*(6), 970–973.

Sikkema, K. J., Koob, J. J., Cargill, V. C., Kelly, J. A., Desiderato, L. L., & Roffman, R. A. (1995). Levels and predictors of HIV risk behavior among women in low-income public housing developments. *Public Health Reports, 110*, 707–713.

Spriggs, W. E. (2006). Poverty in America: The poor are getting poorer. *Crisis, 113*(1), 14–19.

Thompson-Robinson, M. V., Richter, D. L., Shegog, M. L., Weaver, M., Trahan, L., Sellers, D., et al. (2005). Perception of partner risk and influences on sexual decision making or HIV prevention among students at historically black colleges and universities. *Journal of African American Studies, 9*(2), 16–28.

Tuan, N. (2006). *Young African American women and HIV*. Washington, DC: Advocates for Youth.

Tucker, M. B., & Mitchell-Kernan, C. (Eds.). (1995). *The decline of marriage among African Americans: Causes, consequences, and policy implications*. New York: Russell Sage Foundation.

Waxman, H. A. (2006). Politics and science: Reproductive health. *Health Matrix: Journal of Law Medicine, 16*(1), 5–25.

Wells Pence, B., Reif, S., & Whetten, K. (2007). Minorities, the poor, and survivors of abuse: HIV-infection patients in the US Deep South. *Southern Medical Association, 100*(11), 1114–1122.

Whitmore, S. K., Satcher, A. J., & Hu, S. (2005). Epidemiology of HIV/AIDS among non-Hispanic black women in the United States. *Journal of the National Medical Association, 97*, 19S–24S.

Williams, S. S., & Semanchuk, L. T. (1999). Perceptions of safer sex negotiation among HIV2 and HIV1 women at heterosexual risk: A focus group analysis. *International Quarterly of Community Health Education, 19*, 119–131.

Wilson, W. J. (1987). *The truly disadvantaged*. Chicago: University of Chicago Press.

Wyatt, G. E. (1992). The sociocultural context of African American and White American women's rape. *Journal of Social Issues, 48*, 77–91.

Wyatt, G. E., Vargas Carmona, J., Loeb, T., Guthrie, D., Chin, D., & Gordon, G. (2000). Factors affecting HIV contraceptive decision-making among women. *Sex Roles, 42* (7/8), 495–521.

CHAPTER

19

TOBACCO USE AND THE BLACK COMMUNITY IN THE UNITED STATES

A Community-Focused Public Health Model for Eliminating Population Disparities

ROBERT G. ROBINSON
RHONDA CONERLY HOLLIDAY

INTRODUCTION

The history of tobacco use within the black community in the United States has been the parallel story of two separate but interactive "movements"—one led by the tobacco industry and the other by the public health apparatus of tobacco prevention and control. This history has been fully documented (Robinson, Pertschuk, & Sutton, 1992; Robinson, 1998; USDHHS, 1998; Robinson & Headen, 1999; Headen & Robinson, 2001). The tobacco industry has engaged the black community with concentrated marketing efforts that include extensive targeted advertising and substantial promotions

(Thomas & Quinn, 2008). Targeted marketing is not a trivial matter, given the potential for fragmented opinions within the black community. King, Gebreselassie, Mallett, Kozlowski, and Bendel (2007) found that despite a clear understanding of tobacco industry intentions (i.e., improving its public image and increasing its profits by creating more smokers), one third of a randomly selected sample of African Americans believed tobacco companies donated money in order to help the community. It is also not trivial that tobacco industry promotions have led to ongoing cooptation of black community organizations and leaders (Barg, 2007). These dollars promote a façade of respectability. The most recent example is Lorillard's contribution of one million dollars in February 2009 to support an international civil rights center and museum in Greensboro, NC. Historically, targeted marketing and cooptation has meant the absence of advocacy emanating from the black community.

> The twenty-first century should be the "century of the community," and the emphasis of efforts to improve theory and practice ought to reflect this paradigm.
> —Robinson (2004)

Targeted advertising campaigns by the tobacco industry propelled the black community from a low prevalence of cigarette smoking to a position second only to that of Native Americans in the use of cigarettes—a phenomenon that persisted from the 1960s to 2001. As a result, tobacco-related morbidity and mortality rates among blacks became higher than those in any other ethnic group (USDHHS, 1998). A core focus of this chapter is the elimination of this disparity in 2001, providing the nation with perhaps the most significant public health example of the potential impact of comprehensive efforts on the elimination of population disparities. With regard to disparities between the black community and other groups, it is clear that tobacco industry advertising and promotions have been a contributing factor (Yerger, Przewonznik, & Malone, 2007).

As we will see in this chapter, the relationship between the black community and the tobacco prevention and control movement has had to overcome its own problems and challenges. In addition, the tobacco prevention and control movement, because of an absence of diversity and inclusiveness and a reliance on scientific models that facilitated the low prioritization of community and targeted initiatives, had consistently failed to fully engage black community interests.

In the years after the first Surgeon General's report on tobacco in 1964, the tobacco control movement was dominated by three major voluntary organizations: the American Cancer Society (ACS), the American Heart Association (AHA), and the American Lung Association (ALA). These organizations, in collaboration with the medical community, initially focused on cessation initiatives in the mainstream community and, with the success of these efforts, shifted to lower income strata where the effectiveness of cessation initiatives was less visible. The interests of the black community, despite the preponderance of low-income residents, were largely ignored.

The first critical focus resulting in a targeted intervention for blacks was the development in 1992 of Pathway to Freedom (PTF), a self-help cessation guide (Robinson,

Orleans, James, & Sutton, 1992). Prior to this effort, the tobacco prevention and control movement had little direct involvement with the black community. There was no representation by African Americans among the senior scientists involved in either the tobacco control section of the National Cancer Institute (NCI) or the Office on Smoking and Health (OSH) at the Centers for Disease Control and Prevention (CDC). This began to change in 1993 at OSH with the hiring of a black Associate Director and later at NCI with the infusion of senior black scientists. However, by this time a paradigm shift had occurred, with a movement away from cessation to policy interventions and a model of population-based science.

A focus on population-based approaches and subsequent prioritization of policy-related interventions certainly were of benefit to the black community, but these applications fell short in certain critical dimensions. Population-based interventions highlighted the critical importance of excise taxes, regulatory efforts designed to reduce secondhand smoke, and counter marketing with goals of prevention and protection of youth (CDC, 1999). These policy initiatives gained additional credibility by being designated as best practices (CDC, 1999). A negative consequence was failure to rigorously assess their impact on distinct race/ethnic communities. Indeed, a reliance on population-based approaches reinforced a disengagement with community and a disinclination to support targeted initiatives because of the prevailing assumption that a population-based approach encompassed everybody. This assumption is false, especially when the problem is one of disparities. The assumption does not adequately account for varied levels of effectiveness relative to heterogeneity, different types of needs, and the importance of competency; particularly for different race/ethnic communities.

The most comprehensive intervention effort, begun in the early 1990s, was NCI's and ACS's American Stop Smoking Initiative Study (ASSIST) that funded programs in seventeen states. A critique of ASSIST's non-responsiveness to the black community focuses on its emphasis on policy initiatives, partnership with State Health Departments ill-prepared to work with black organizations, lack of provision for direct services or material development, and inattention to fostering of community development as an important goal (Robinson, Pertschuk, & Sutton, 1992). These deficiencies were exacerbated by an evaluation design that depended on population-based analyses of ASSIST and non-ASSIST states. Because blacks constituted only 11.5 percent of the total ASSIST population of 90 million, impacts on black cessation rates were not needed in order to achieve a positive result. Substantive targeted outreach efforts to the black community were not carried out; subsequently, significant impacts, particularly with regard to alleviating population disparities, did not occur.

Similar weaknesses were present in the mid-1990s effort by the Robert Wood Johnson Foundation (RWJ), in partnership with the American Medical Association (AMA), to launch the SmokeLess States initiative (Robinson & Headen, 1999). Similar to ASSIST, the focus was statewide and directed toward policy goals related to excise taxes, regulation of secondhand smoke, and counter marketing. States with existing capacity and an environment ripe for policy development were prioritized. Once again, outreach to the black community was not prioritized and efforts toward community development were not integrated into the overall design. RWJ did not address this weakness until 2000, when funds were provided to support tobacco control national organizations in communities of color. However, this change followed trends that resulted in elimination of the black-white disparity in tobacco-use prevalence in 2001.

What happened to alter the impenetrability of the tobacco prevention and control movement? The change was brought about by concerted efforts on the part of the black community and its advocates and scientists. Ironically, the most significant impact resulted from a mistake made by the tobacco industry. R. J. Reynolds launched Uptown cigarette in 1990, the first tobacco product specifically targeted to the black community (Robinson & Sutton, 1994; Robinson & Headen, 1999). Philadelphia was chosen as one of two sites for a test market, and its black community rose up in fierce protest. This protest was based on the premise that a cigarette second only to R. J. Reynolds' unfiltered Camel in levels of tar and nicotine could not ethically be marketed without regard to the will of the community.

The protest, led by the Uptown Coalition, was the first time that the black community collectively rose to fight the tobacco industry, thereby transforming the tobacco prevention and control movement.[1] Whereas tobacco control traditionally chose health consequences as a major theme, the Uptown Coalition chose community empowerment. A community paradigm of empowerment meant that it was no longer an issue of smokers and nonsmokers but of everyone engaged in the protection of youth and the promotion of total community well-being. Because the Uptown Coalition was black-led, the tobacco industry was unsuccessful with its traditional ploy of trying to convince community members that any effort to protect individuals from "free choice" was paternalistic. Indeed, the Uptown Coalition's validation of the tobacco industry as the "enemy" gave credibility to California's emerging and ultimately nationally recognized media strategy in the 1990s, which also relied on the demonization of the tobacco industry. R. J. Reynolds removed Uptown cigarettes from merchant store shelves within thirteen days of the start of the protest.

It was no accident that concurrent with the Uptown revolt was the successful development of Pathway to Freedom (PTF) at Philadelphia's Fox Chase Cancer Center. The development of PTF led to critical research efforts that documented the guide's efficacy and underscored the importance of targeted materials and related-intervention initiatives. Two studies using and testing the PTF guide in conjunction with telephone "quit line" counseling to help black smokers quit were published jointly in 1998 (Boyd, Sutton, Orleans, et al., 1998; Orleans, Boyd, Bingler, et al., 1998). The two studies

---

[1] Core leadership of the Uptown Coalition were the following: Reverend Jesse Brown, Pastor of Christ Evangelical Lutheran Church and Chairperson of the Committee for Blacks Against Cancer; Carl Mansfield, MD, Chair of Radiation Oncology at Thomas Jefferson Hospital and Chair of the American Cancer Society (Philadelphia Chapter) Committee on the Socioeconomically Disadvantaged; Robert Robinson, PhD, Social Scientist at the Fox Chase Cancer Center and Chairperson of the National Black Leadership Initiative on Cancer (Philadelphia Chapter); and Charyn Sutton, Senior Communications Consultant.

tested a communications campaign designed to increase the number of calls from black smokers to a free telephone quit line for help to quit smoking. Boyd et al. (1998) demonstrated a dramatic increase in black call volumes. The PTF guide was rated more favorably than mainstream materials on several dimensions. Orleans et al. (1998) demonstrated statistically higher 12-month quit rates (25% versus 15.4%).

The Uptown victory and the development of PTF provided a foundation for black community advocacy that transformed the tobacco prevention and control movement. A movement that in 1990 had been predominantly white was diversified by the mid-1990s to include representation across the spectrum of U.S. communities. And though there continues to be a significant failure of inclusiveness in planning and decision making, the presence of multi-community representatives and organizations establishes tobacco prevention and control alongside other public health movements as grounded in the importance and ethical standard of diverse participation.

While these developments were critical in implementing diversification of the tobacco prevention and control movement, additional help was needed to make progress with respect to eliminating population disparities. In 1993, OSH launched a national initiative to support community development by establishing national organizations charged with pursuing tobacco prevention and control objectives in their respective communities (i.e., communities of color, youth, women, agricultural workers, low SES, and LGBT) (Robinson & Headen, 1999). The results were more than credible. National organizations such as the National Association of African Americans for Positive Imagery (NAAAPI) and the National Medical Association (NMA) were funded and laid the groundwork for national advocacy and communication efforts resulting in successful counter marketing strategies that eliminated or diminished the impact of targeted campaigns conducted by the tobacco industry. Pathways to Freedom made it possible for multiple community-based organizations, especially black churches, to engage in tobacco control. Indeed, PTF remains the only cessation guide to acknowledge the helpfulness of prayer in quitting tobacco use; the PTF guide retained a reference to prayer and religion when it was revised in 2003 (Robinson, Sutton, James, & Orleans, 2003)[2]. The black community made the best of these core assets (i.e., PTF, national organization, advocacy campaigns, and community involvement), combined with the benefits accruing from ongoing national policy efforts, to maintain low prevalence rates among black youth and to increase adult quit rates relative to whites. Importantly, this disparity elimination contradicted a review of National Health Interview Study data from 1974 through 1985 that concluded that black smoking prevalence in 2000 would be 25 percent compared to 21 percent for whites (Pierce, Fiore, Novotny, Hatziandreu, & Davis, 1989). In fairness, there was no way to anticipate the emergence of initiatives supportive of black community development post-1990.

---

[2] Pathways to Freedom can be accessed by visiting the CDC's Smoking & Tobacco Use Web site at www.cdc .gov/tobacco and clicking on " Publications and Products" then "Publications Catalog." Individuals can download and print PDFs; there is no charge for this publication as long as the quantity does not exceed 500 copies.

BACKGROUND: EPIDEMIOLOGICAL TRENDS

Health Consequences

The negative health consequences of smoking are undeniable. Smoking is associated with a myriad of diseases that increase mortality rates and reduce quality of life, including cancer (lung, oral cavity, pharynx, larynx, esophagus, pancreas, bladder, and kidney), cardiovascular disease, and respiratory diseases (Armour, Woollery, Malarcher, Pechacek, & Husten, 2005). Between 1997 and 2001, 438,000 premature deaths, 5.5 million years of potential life lost (YPLL), and $92 billion dollars in lost productivity could be attributed to cigarette smoking and exposure to tobacco products (Armour et al., 2005). There has historically been a disparity in the black-white death rate in cancer, particularly in smoking-related cancers, with black males bearing the brunt of the disparity. Between 1975 and 2002 age-adjusted incidence and mortality rates were higher among black males for oral and pharyngeal cancer (Morse & Kerr, 2006). Although the incidence and mortality rates for these cancers began to decline in the mid-1980s, disparities were still evident. Between 1998 and 2002 incidence rates were 20 percent higher for black males than for white males, while mortality rates were 82 percent higher. Black males had the lowest five-year survival rate among all ethnic groups for those diagnosed, between 1995 and 2001, with oral or pharyngeal cancer (Morse & Kerr, 2006). Examining cancer death rates reveals a recent trend toward reduction in the overall cancer death rate disparity. From the early 1990s through 2004, the black-white disparity in overall cancer death rates gradually narrowed, especially among men. A major reason for the narrowing of this disparity was a more pronounced decrease in mortality from smoking-related cancers in black men as compared with white men (Oliver, DeLancey, Thun, Jemal, & Ward, 2008). Perhaps the emergence of smoking cessation programs targeted specifically toward the black community was effective in reducing the black-white cancer death rate disparity.

Youth and Smoking

Research has demonstrated that people who start smoking at younger ages are more likely than other smokers to exhibit a high level of tobacco dependence, a low number of quit attempts, a long-term smoking history, and tobacco-related health harm (Moolchan et al., 2007). However, this relationship does not seem to hold true for African Americans. Blacks typically begin smoking at a later age, but evidence the same or greater deleterious effects of smoking (Moolchan et al., 2007). Approximately 40 percent of blacks who are current smokers initiated the behavior between the ages of 18 and 21 (Trinidad, Gilpin, Lee, & Pierce, 2004). Various research studies among students attending historically black colleges and universities have demonstrated low levels of smoking, varying from 7.5 percent to 14 percent of the students surveyed (Laws, Holliday, & Huang, 2007; Laws, Huang, Brown, Richmond, & Conerly, 2006; Hestick, Perrino, Rhodes, Sydnor, 2001; Powe, Ross, & Cooper, 2007; Wang, Browne, Storr, Wagner, 2005). These findings are not surprising, given the fact that there exists an association between educational level and smoking.

Additional evidence that smoking initiation begins later for African Americans is demonstrated by smoking rates among middle and high school students. Smoking among black, non-Hispanic middle school students decreased from 9.0 percent in 2002 to 7.6 percent in 2004, and the use of any tobacco products decreased from 13.5 percent to 12.4 percent among black non-Hispanics (Bloch et al., 2005). The rates of any tobacco use were slightly higher for black, non-Hispanic students than for white non-Hispanic students in 2002 (13.5% versus 13.2%) and 2004 (12.4% versus 11.3%), while the rates of cigarette use were slightly lower in 2002 (9.0%) versus 10.1%) and 2004 (7.6% versus 8.5%) (Bloch et al., 2005). The rates of any tobacco use may have been higher for black, non-Hispanic students due to the higher use of cigars and bidis (flavored cigarettes).

Among high school students, the rates of any tobacco use and cigarette smoking were higher in 2002 and 2004 compared with middle school students. Approximately 21.7 percent of black non-Hispanic high school students reported using any tobacco in 2002 compared with 16.8 percent in 2004, a significant decrease from 2002 to 2004 (Bloch et al., 2005). There was also a decline in cigarette use during the same time period, from 13.8 percent in 2002 to 10.9 percent in 2004 (Bloch et al., 2005). The use of any tobacco products and the use of cigarettes were higher among white non-Hispanic high school students during the same time period. In contrast with the black non-Hispanic students, the decrease in both categories over the same time period was minimal (30.9% in 2002 and 30.8% in 2004 for any tobacco products and 25.2% in 2002 and 24.8% in 2004 for cigarette use) (Bloch et al., 2005). While there was a decrease in any tobacco use and cigarette use by both black and white non-Hispanic high school students, the decrease was more pronounced among the black non-Hispanic students (Bloch et al., 2005).

Secondhand Smoke

Distinct from the positive trends associated with tobacco use are disparities related to exposure to secondhand smoke (Pirkle, Bernert, Caudill, Sosnoff, & Pechacek, 2006). If serum cotinine is used as a marker for exposure to secondhand smoke, the 70 percent overall decline suggests a decrease in exposure over this 14-year time period. Yet, cotinine concentrations for blacks remained significantly higher than for other population groups, and levels in children were significantly higher than in adults. These higher levels for black children persisted even though the Healthy People 2010 goal that no more than 45 percent of nonsmokers should have cotinine levels >0.1 ng/mL was met in 2000—a strong indicator that these youth remain at higher risk from exposure to secondhand smoke.

The best explanation for the overall decline in cotinine levels is the success of regulatory efforts in the workplace, public settings, and additional efforts in the home (Pirkle et al., 2006). It is reasonable to conclude that blacks, and especially children, are not receiving the full benefit of these regulations. It is possible that excessive smoking in the home explains the higher cotinine levels for black youth. However, metabolic differences may also explain these concentrations of cotinine. For example, black smokers have higher concentrations of cotinine per cigarette smoked than whites do (Caraballo et al., 1998). One possible explanation is black-white differences in the metabolism of nicotine, cotinine, and their glucuronides (Benowitz et al., 1999). It is possible that metabolic differences could also explain the higher cotinine levels found in nonsmoking black children (Pirkle et al., 2006). However, the most salient conclusion, pending more conclusive findings in regard to metabolism, remains greater exposure levels of black adults and children to secondhand smoke. Pirkle et al. (2006) conclude that blacks, as well as children in general, should receive increased intervention efforts, including encouragement of smoking restrictions in the home, automobiles, and other locations. Preliminary work in Harlem (NYC), though lacking specific recommendations, has initiated a foundation upon which to build scientific support of home-based interventions (Northridge et al., 2009).

Menthol

Menthol cigarettes were introduced in the 1930s but did not exceed three percent of the total market until 1949 (Hebert & Kabat, 1989). The introduction of Penguin by Brown and Williamson in 1931, replaced by Kool in 1933, set the standard for the early menthol market (Gardiner, 2004). Increasing gradually, the menthol market share reached 16 percent in 1963 and 28 percent in 1976 (U.S. Surgeon General's Report, 1989). Over the years market leadership fluctuated between Salem, Kool, and the current leader Newport; however, the defining feature remains the overwhelming preference for menthol cigarettes among black smokers (Gardiner, 2004). By 1986, 75.5 percent of black smokers reported use of menthol cigarettes compared with 23.1 percent of white smokers (U.S. Surgeon General's Report, 1989). The menthol cigarette preferred by black smokers in 1988 was Newport (22%), followed by Kool (16%) and Salem (15%) (Ramirez, 1990).

Menthol has emerged as a particularly salient and controversial issue. Multiple hypotheses exist regarding the potential greater harm of menthol cigarettes including greater exposure to toxins facilitated by deeper inhalation because the harshness is diminished, increased puff volumes, the higher carbon monoxide (CO) content of mainstream smoke from menthol cigarettes, and higher cotinine concentrations; however, the evidence for increased risk of disease is inconclusive (Gardiner, 2004). In regard to cessation, in a cohort of 1,688 patients, black menthol smokers were found to have significantly lower quit rates than non-menthol smokers, despite the fact that they smoked fewer cigarettes (Gandhi, Foulds, Steinberg, Lu, & Williams, 2009). In addition, menthol smokers were significantly more likely to awaken in the middle of the night to smoke. Other evidence has also demonstrated an attenuation of cessation efforts for black menthol smokers (Okuyemi, Faseru, Sanderson, Bronars, & Ahluwalia, 2007). Evidence indicates increased use of menthol products by youth and suggests that adolescents get more enjoyment from mentholated cigarettes and make fewer quit attempts (Hebert, 2004; Hersey et al., 2006). Research has found increased risks of some cancers, perhaps due to increased rates of metabolism of some carcinogens, but no studies have investigated menthol's relationship to cardiovascular or other non-cancer diseases (Hebert, 2004). Research has also concluded that tobacco companies manipulate the sensory characteristics of cigarettes, including menthol content, which in turn affects initiation and addiction. Most significant, menthol brands using this strategy have had the greatest success in attracting youth and young adult smokers (Kreslake et al., 2008).

Increased scrutiny of the impact of menthol on health risks resulted in the first national conference devoted to menthol and cigarette use (Clark, Gardiner, Djordjevic, Leischow, & Robinson, 2004). Plans are underway for a second conference in 2010, in part spurred by unanswered questions and by the controversy associated with legislation giving the Food and Drug Administration (FDA) greater regulatory control over tobacco-related products. In the legislation, despite inclusion of flavored cigarettes such as strawberry and mocha, a deal was struck with Philip Morris to exempt menthol (Saul, 2008b). In debate prior to the passing of the legislation, the role of the Center for Tobacco Free Kids (CTFK) in forging this compromise, as well as the substantive exclusion of black representation, were highlighted. The issue of menthol remains unresolved, and the goal of inclusion representative of the diversity of the movement continues to be elusive within mainstream tobacco prevention and control organizations.

ELIMINATING THE BLACK-WHITE DISPARITY: A CASE STUDY

Epidemiological Data[3]

The graph in Figure 19.1 shows the overall trend in black-white cigarette tobacco use from 1965–2001. Evident is a steady decrease among blacks and whites with a significant dip for blacks occurring in 1990. There are no published studies explaining this "dip" in prevalence, but it is possible that the extraordinary publicity and mobilization that occurred in concert with the Uptown Coalition during the same time period was an important contributing factor. An increased rate of decrease continues after 1990, resulting in the 2001 disparity elimination.

A closer examination of age-specific prevalence rates provides additional insight into this phenomenon. Figures 19.2 through 19.5 show black-white prevalence rates for four specific age cohorts: 19–24, 25–44, 45–64, and 65+.

Not evident in those aged 19–24 years but consistent in each of the other age cohorts is the sharp dip in prevalence that occurred around 1990. The disparity elimination for the 19-to-24-year-old cohort occurred around 1978 and remained constant to 2001. The disparity elimination for the 25-to-44-year-old cohort occurred around 1995 and continued at an accelerated rate to 2001. The 44-to-64-year-old cohort did not demonstrate a disparity elimination, but the reduction from 1997 to 2001 is accelerated and indicates a disparity elimination in the near future. Similarly, the cohort aged 65 and up does not demonstrate a disparity elimination, but an accelerated

---

[3] Special thanks to Jamie P. Morano and Angela Trosclair of the Office on Smoking and Health, Centers for Disease Control (CDC), for their contributions to the data analysis.

FIGURE 19.1 *Prevalence of Current Cigarette Smoking Overall by Race—United States, 1965–2001.*

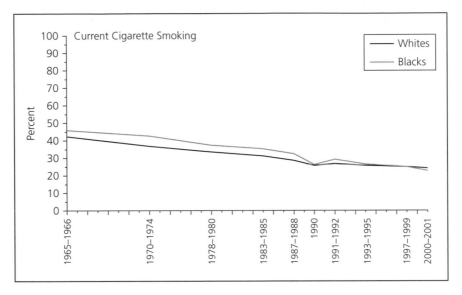

Source: National Health Interview Survey, United States, 1965–2001, aggregate data.

FIGURE 19.2 *Prevalence of Current Cigarette Smoking Among Persons Aged 19–24 by Race—United States, 1965–2001.*

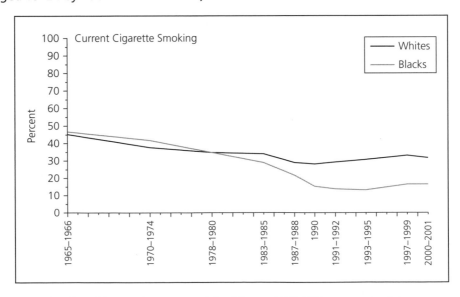

Source: National Health Interview Survey, United States, 1965–2001, aggregate data.

FIGURE 19.3 *Prevalence of Current Cigarette Smoking Among Persons Aged 25–44 by Race—United States, 1965–2001.*

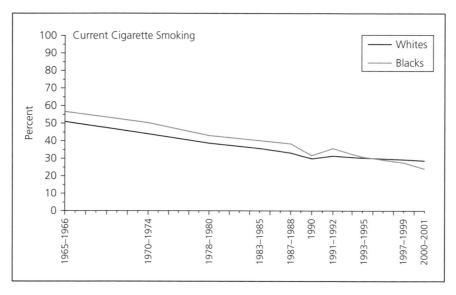

Source: National Health Interview Survey, United States, 1965–2001, aggregate data.

FIGURE 19.4 *Prevalence of Current Cigarette Smoking Among Persons Aged 45–64 by Race—United States, 1965–2001.*

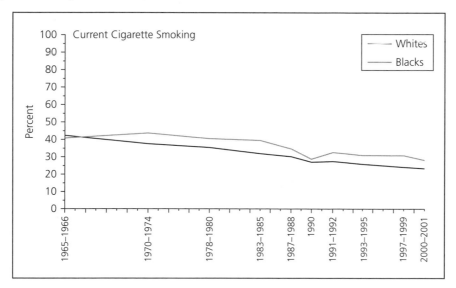

Source: National Health Interview Survey, United States, 1965–2001, aggregate data.

FIGURE 19.5 *Prevalence of Current Cigarette Smoking Among Persons Aged 65 and Older by Race—United States, 1965–2001.*

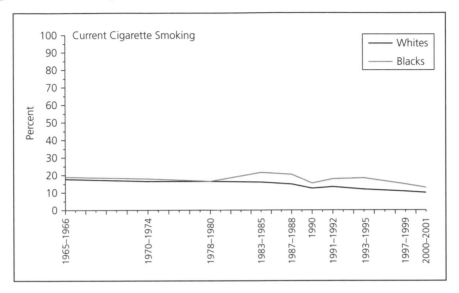

Source: National Health Interview Survey, United States, 1965–2001, aggregate data.

decrease is indicated from 1993 to 2001, making it plausible that one will occur in the near future.

Table 19.1 assesses the age-specific prevalence rates from 1965 to 2001. Most important, for purposes of this analysis, are the age-specific prevalence rates and the average change in prevalence rates from 1990 to 2001.

Focusing only on the aggregate data for blacks and whites and the average change, one observes a two-fold difference between blacks (-0.32) and whites (-0.16). This indicates that the rate of change for blacks was twice that of whites from 1990 to 2001.

If the rate of change between 1990 and 2001 had remained equal to whites, how many more black smokers would we have in 2001? The answer is 368,285 additional smokers. There are certain caveats associated with this number. It assumes no persons were lost to death, and there were no relapses. Regardless of the absence of precision, the aggregate number is significant when measured in potential lives saved and the improved well-being of the population. It is a public health indicator of profound impact.

INTERVENTIONS: 1990–2001

What happened during this time period that might contribute to an explanation of this two-fold rate of decrease in prevalence among black smokers compared with white

TABLE 19.1 Prevalence of Current Smoking by Race and Age— United States, 1965–2001.

Whites	1965–1966	1980	1990	2000–2001	Average Change 1965/1966–1980	Average Change 1980–1990	Average Change 1990–2000/2001
Total	42.2	33.4	25.9	24.1	−0.59	−0.75	−0.16
18–24	45.0	36.3	28.1	31.6	−0.58	−0.82	0.32
25–44	50.8	37.8	30.1	28.9	−0.87	−0.77	−0.11
45–64	42.3	35.5	27.2	23.7	−0.45	−0.83	−0.32
65+	17.8	17.1	12.5	9.8	−0.05	−0.46	−0.24
Blacks							
Total	45.8	37.4	26.2	22.7	−0.56	−1.12	−0.32
18–24	46.6	39.0	15.1	16.3	−0.51	−2.39	0.11
25–44	56.7	41.1	31.9	24.3	−1.04	−0.92	−0.69
45–64	40.8	40.4	29.0	28.2	−0.03	−1.14	−0.07
65+	18.9	17.5	15.4	12.9	−0.09	−0.21	−0.23

Source: National Health Interview Survey, United States, 1965–2001, aggregate data.

smokers? The explanation can be found in a comprehensive approach to eliminating population disparities.

Pathways to Freedom (PTF) and Communication Campaigns

In 1993, PTF was adopted by OSH and became available for national distribution. CDC data indicate that 1,054,464 copies of PTF were distributed between 1993 and 2002. Distribution was aided by a national evaluation sponsored by the ACS, increased interest on the part of community organizations, and efforts by State Health Departments to be responsive to high smoking rates and existing disparities.

PTF was integral to a nationwide communications campaign through a partnership with OSH and the National Medical Association (Skolnick, 1993). The 1993 Legends Campaign consisted of 30-second TV spots on all major commercial and cable outlets. There were live-announcer radio spots for stations with high black audience ratings. An 800 number was included for callers to request a free copy of PTF. Media messages stressed that (1) smoking causes the greatest number of deaths in the black community, (2) the deaths of black leaders were tragedies but not a waste (the imagery of Martin Luther King, Malcolm X, and James Chaney were used), and (3) it is never too late to stop smoking and receive health benefits.

Communication Infrastructure

The Community of Color Tobacco Control listserv (COCTCN) was developed as part of OSH's disparity reduction efforts in the mid-1990s. It provides the only open vehicle through which tobacco prevention and control professionals can communicate. COCTCN serves the tobacco control movement by allowing dissemination and discussion of scientific papers, review of policy initiatives, shared observations of tobacco industry strategies, critical assessments of relevant activities in the tobacco prevention and control movement, and a forum for organizing and agenda setting. Since 2006 COCTCN has been independently managed.[4]

Community Development and Mobilization Campaigns

The national organization initiative implemented by OSH in 1993 gave additional impetus to earlier advocacy efforts that originated in 1985 with counter alcohol and tobacco advertising campaigns in Detroit. The greatest impact, however, was achieved by the successful Uptown Coalition in 1990. The Uptown Coalition provided the model for success in subsequent counter marketing campaigns: community empowerment, tobacco industry demonization, and unity of smokers and nonsmokers. Leadership from the Uptown Coalition created NAAAPI, which received, along with the NMA, the first awards emanating from OSH's national organization initiative.

During the mid-1990s, it almost seemed as if a new cigarette emerged targeting the black community every year. In 1995, Stowecraft Distributors in Boston began marketing a red, black, and green–packaged menthol cigarette named "X." The cigarette was an attempt to capitalize on the mystique of Malcolm X, who is an icon in the black community, and the colors are considered the community's liberation flag. Stowecraft Distributors denied any knowledge of these associations. Leadership from the Boston-based organization Churches Organized to Stop Tobacco (COST) contacted other black leaders in Philadelphia and California. A national protest was launched, producing the second major defeat of the tobacco industry in the 1990s. This achievement underscored the importance of organized protest, but strategically the critical

---

[4]Persons interested in subscribing to COCTCN can contact Vernellia Randall at Vernellia.Randall@notes .udayton.edu or Robert Robinson at rgrbob@earthlink.net.

issue remained the ability (i.e., capacity and infrastructure and social capital) of the black community to engage in self-determined mobilization.

In 1996, R. J. Reynolds introduced a menthol version of Camel. NAAAPI began tracking Camel Menthols and organized the "Say No to Menthol Joe Community Crusade." A news conference at the Washington Press Club was held, and letter-writing campaigns began in St. Louis decrying advertising in black magazines. Stealth efforts emerged, defacing Camel menthol billboards in inner cities, and a one-day protest of calls to Camel Menthol's 800 number was held on St. Patrick's Day. Sit-ins occurred at Walgreens drugstores, resulting in a public announcement that the stores would stop selling Camel menthols. NAAAPI provided documentation to the Federal Trade Commission (FTC) in support of advertising regulations, and within weeks R. J. Reynolds withdrew all Camel menthol advertising. Camel menthols continue to be sold, but without the Camel Joe logo (Headen & Robinson, 2001).

In 1999, Philip Morris introduced Marlboro Milds, a menthol version of Marlboro. They had not succeeded in marketing a menthol brand to the black community. Atlanta and Pittsburgh were chosen as test market sites and simultaneous press conferences by ad hoc coalitions (i.e., The Atlanta Campaign Against Marlboro Milds and The Greater Pittsburgh Coalition Against Marlboro Milds) were held. Philip Morris chose not to roll out an advertising campaign with overt targeting to blacks. Although Atlanta merchants were persuaded to remove Marlboro Milds from shelves, the impact of this mobilization effort was less than previous campaigns. In summary, however, black-led anti-tobacco campaigns facilitated a coherent stream of media advocacy emanating from the black community that resonated across the nation, with special efforts arising in Baltimore (MD), Chicago (IL), California, Dallas (TX), Harlem (NYC), and Philadelphia (PA).

Faith-based and Community Organization Initiatives

The involvement of black churches in tobacco control was an emergent theme throughout the 1990s. Organizing efforts that received funding from the ALA resulted in the formation of Black Clergy for Substance Abuse Prevention (BCSAP). BCSAP was instrumental in promoting PTF and encouraging the engagement of the faith community. Significant faith-based initiatives arose in Alabama, California, Kansas, Maryland, Massachusetts, Michigan, Missouri, and Wyoming. However, also important were some efforts that remained out of public view. For example, in the Eastern Shore region of Maryland, because of proactive engagement and funding from the State Health Department, black churches engaged in tobacco control with activities such as the sponsoring of marches on the Great American Smokeout.

Specific progress was made with respect to adoption of the PTF guide in church-based cessation protocols. In addition, evaluations of other initiatives, such as the Heart, Body, and Soul program in Baltimore, demonstrated the great impact of culturally based approaches in church settings (Voorhees et al., 1996).

Multiple community-based initiatives arose across the nation (Headen & Robinson, 2001). One example, The Ujima! African American Youth Initiative in North Carolina, chose to empower the black community by targeting youth organizations to serve as tobacco control advocates and community activists. Other initiatives utilized PTF, resulting in the development of the PTF Community-Based Smoking Cessation Protocol that provided a blueprint for implementing smoking cessation activities by community volunteers that helped individual smokers to quit and provided support for tobacco-free lifestyles (Headen & Robinson, 2001).

The last important initiative developed during this period was the development in 1999 of Not in Mama's Kitchen (Caffee, 2001). This program targeted secondhand smoke in the household and focused on the theme of the power of the black female in her "kitchen." The initiative collaborated with churches, schools, and community-based organizations to attain commitments from mothers to enforce home regulations. In unpublished survey data, 96 percent of participants indicated they would continue to maintain a smoke-free home and car. In 2005, 75,000 families in more than 50 cities participated, and over 25,000 pledges to establish smoke-free policies were received.

Congressional Black Caucus

In 1998, there was a groundswell of activity aimed towards the creation of comprehensive national legislation regulating tobacco marketing and providing the FDA with a mandate to regulate cigarettes as a nicotine delivery device (Robinson & Headen, 1999). These efforts, though unsuccessful, demonstrated the unprecedented joining of the Congressional Minority Caucuses in support of this legislation that was also seen as a means to limit smoking in communities of color. A press release was provided on June 25, 1998, which stated "The Legislation was developed to address the absence of minority concerns in national tobacco legislation and to reverse the disturbing effects of the tobacco industry's targeting of minorities" (Robinson & Headen, 1999, p. 94). Organizing of the Congressional Minority Caucuses was a symbolic victory, given the historic pattern of support of the tobacco industry to the Congressional Black Caucus. Indeed, since 2002 Altria, parent company of Philip Morris, had provided $1.45 million to the Congressional Black Caucus (Young, 2008).

Ongoing support by the tobacco industry raises concerns about future collaborations with the Congressional Black Caucus, a situation made all the more dire because of the present controversy regarding new FDA legislation and the exclusion of menthol in the proposed regulations. This is a concern despite the heartening response of Representative Donna Christensen, Chair of the Caucus, who stated in an e-mail response to a reporter's query that "We are aware and gravely concerned about the disproportionate incidence of lung cancer in the African American community and, along with so many minority health experts, have long been concerned about the role menthol may play" (Saul, 2008a). The pressure from the tobacco industry will be immense and the disposition of Congressman Henry Waxman, who is the House bill's sponsor, not overly compelling, particularly given his possible acceptance of the thesis that smokers will turn to illicit (i.e., contraband) avenues of procurement if menthol is banned. This notion, not grounded in science, is unfortunately advocated by the Center for Tobacco Free Kids (CTFK) and, in addition, is explicitly pejorative in its connotations regarding the collective class of black menthol smokers.

Population-based Applications

A major theme of this analysis is the importance of comprehensiveness and the essential need for "both/and" approaches in theory, analysis, and applications when addressing the complexity inherent in population disparities (Robinson, 2005). Thus, though greater efficacy is attributed to efforts involving community development and community-competent applications, population-based efforts also have value. Table 19.2 shows the trend in excise tax increases between 1995 and 2001.

It is clear that dramatic increases in excise taxes occurred across the nation, rising from nine states with >50 cents tax per pack of cigarettes in 1995 to nineteen states with >50 cents tax in 2001. Yet, any assessment of the effectiveness of excise taxes must address the issue of regressivity, particularly given the higher risk of smoking among persons living in poverty and those of lower socioeconomic status (Ahrens, 2009). Ahrens (2009) argues that, given the inherent regressivity of excise taxes, they must be offset with targeted funding for low-income populations. The problem is that nowhere does this occur with significance, substance or systemically. The arguments supporting acceptance of excise taxes despite their regressivity is the trade-off with the benefits accruing from lower risks for health consequences. However, because there is no equity in the distribution of tobacco prevention and control resources, the choice between regressivity and improved health offers little consolation to those who express equal concerns for both. Ironically, the impoverishment associated with regressive taxation results in increased disparity independent of the tobacco-related benefits.

Regulation of secondhand smoke is the second most successful population-based intervention after excise taxes. Table 19.3 shows state-based regulatory patterns promoting clean indoor air from 1995 to 2001.

Apart from excise taxes, there was little movement in any of the respective categories of tobacco regulations from 1995 to 2001. Thus, of the two major interventions, excise taxes provided a greater boost to the elimination of the black-white disparity in prevalence of cigarette use during this period. Progress in the regulation of secondhand smoke accelerated after 2001 at the local level but not at the state level because of the

TABLE 19.2 Excise Taxes in States, 1995 and 2001.

Cigarette Excise Taxes	1995	2001
< 25 cents	20	20
25–49 cents	22	12
50+ cents	9	19

Source: Centers for Disease Control and Prevention. State Tobacco Activities Tracking and Evaluation (STATE) System. Available at http://www.cdc.gov/tobacco/statesystem

TABLE 19.3   **Clean Indoor Air Regulations in States, 1995 and 2001.**

	Year	Banned	Designated Areas*	None
Government	1995	8	33	10
	2001	12	31	8
Private Worksites	1995	1	21	29
	2001	1	21	29
Restaurants	1995	2	27	22
	2001	2	28	21
Commercial Day Care	1995	21	8	22
	2001	24	10	17
Bars	1995	0	1	50
	2001	0	2	49

*Includes states with Separate Ventilated Areas restrictions.
Source: Centers for Disease Control and Prevention. State Tobacco Activities Tracking and Evaluation (STATE) System. Available at http://www.cdc.gov/tobacco/statesystem

ability of the tobacco industry to influence state legislatures (Skeer, George, Hamilton, Cheng, & Siegel, 2004). Ironically, with respect to disparities, a consequence analogous to that associated with excise taxes is found. Because such determinants as high educational attainment and higher per capita income are important in achieving outcomes, those geographic areas lacking these attributes experience increased disparities relative to the more advantaged areas (Skeer et al., 2004; Shelley et al., 2007). This same pattern occurred with billboard advertising when it was allowed. In part because zoning laws in higher-income neighborhoods did not allow billboards, the remaining billboards were located in poorer neighborhoods; thus, the higher rate of tobacco advertising in the black community is partially explained by this association. The synergy of targeted marketing, community adaptation to policy interventions, and disenfranchised communities serves to create and reinforce existing disparities.

Summary

The breadth and depth of antismoking interventions reflects one of the most important principles of an effective approach to the elimination of disparities: comprehensiveness. The interventions encompass media efforts, counter marketing, smoking cessation programs, legislation to reduce secondhand smoke, policy initiatives, capacity and infrastructure development, communication infrastructure, social capital, community competence, community organization and mobilization, and involvement of national, state, and local legislative representatives. Comprehensiveness also encompasses interventions that reach people in multiple contextual settings, whether as individuals, groups, social strata, communities, or population-wide. Not all of these efforts were necessarily rooted in evidence-based science; rather, their success depended on a combination of proven and unproven initiatives. In essence, science, especially if narrowly defined as dependent on evaluated work, will not solve the nation's problem of population disparities. The social justice underpinnings of population disparities will necessitate deliberate appreciation for "out of the box" thinking and action. Bottom-up initiatives will emerge whose roots will not be found in the ethos of randomly controlled trials. Advocating for a both/and principle in these circumstances is not without personal cost. Organizations are inherently conservative, and those who dance on the edges of advocacy and science may place their own professional advancement and careers at risk.

POST-2001 INITIATIVES

The focus of this chapter has been to explain the disparity elimination that occurred in 2001, but multiple efforts on this front have continued through the first decade of the twenty-first century. The most important effort was the counter marketing Kool Mixx campaign organized by the American Legacy Foundation and RWJ-funded National African American Tobacco Prevention Network (NAATPN). Brown and Williamson, makers of Kool cigarettes, launched a Kool Mixx campaign composed of advertising and sponsorship of hip-hop DJ competitions across the nation. In response, NAATPN developed the FightKool Operation Storefront Activity, which encouraged youth to take a closer look through monitoring at tobacco advertising and promotions in stores. In addition, protests were organized in concert with the Kool Mixx competitions. NAATPN developed counter marketing imagery and other media tools to assist their campaign. The resulting publicity led to New York's Attorney General sending a letter on behalf of more than two dozen states to Brown and Williamson indicating plans to sue because the company was in violation of the tobacco Master Settlement Agreement's proscriptions regarding the targeting of youth. Brown and Williamson eventually settled and a portion of these monies accrued to NAATPN to support outreach efforts to black youth. Related efforts were the community coalition efforts against the marketing of candy products containing hemp oil (Chronic Candy) and flavored tobacco products that included the taste of marijuana (Crawford, 2007).

The National African American Tobacco Education Network (NAATEN) received the award for OSH's National Organization initiative in 2003. One of NAATEN's major initiatives was an evaluation of the National QuitLine program (Brieon et al., 2007). The evaluation highlighted the QuitLine's failure to systematically track black callers, utilize community-based referral resources, and send targeted materials such as PTF to black callers seeking help in smoking cessation. Indeed, only 47 percent of the sample used targeted strategies, and none of these included sending community-specific materials. NAATPN received the National Organization award in 2008. NAATPN's work since 2000 reflects the advantage of being an independent organization, not embedded in a parent agency, which provides greater freedom to carry out advocacy and community development efforts.

Other important initiatives include the Tobacco-Related Disease Research Program (TRDRP, www.trdrp.org) in California, which remains the state-of-the-art statewide initiative pursuing a focused research program encompassing disparities, community-based partnerships, and participatory models. Minnesota (www.clearwaymn.org), Washington (www.doh.wa.gov/tobacco/disparities/disparity.htm), and Ohio (www.aacoh.org, www.ohiocctca.org) have provided ongoing financial support for targeted program initiatives.

Research is ongoing regarding cessation protocols of benefit to African Americans (Webb, 2008a; Webb, 2008b). The general findings indicate that smoking cessation interventions increased the odds of cessation by 40 percent at posttest and 30 percent at follow-up (Webb, 2008b), and that black smokers prefer community-specific smoking cessation materials. This preference was particularly apparent among those who were considered to be less acculturated (Webb, 2008a). In this study, less-acculturated blacks also had a greater willingness to quit smoking. A cautionary note must be added with respect to the protocol. The study compared PTF and a modified version of PTF minus references specific to the black community. Thus, this was not a comparison between PTF and mainstream materials. Bias is a concern because the comparison material, though absent specific references, still maintained the overall design and literacy levels that had been previously tested and evaluated for competency. Thus, the comparison guide met competency criteria not necessarily accounted for in the study's design. In general, evaluation protocols do not measure community-related impact measures such as generalizability, increased engagement by community organizations, and increased efficacy of media that could result in greater engagement by black smokers and thus, from a public health perspective, increased numbers of quitters (a number distinct from quit rates). For example, Pathways to Freedom continues to be promoted in black media (Walker, 2007); used in community programs such as Morehouse Medical Associates (Essien, personal communication, January 21, 2009) and Atlanta's ZAP Asthma Program (Essien, personal communication, December 15, 2008); and promoted by nationally disseminated newsletters (Goodwin & Robinson, 2009). Consonant with a public health perspective in a review of cessation protocols were recommendations that cessation efforts should use broadcast media, tailoring, and community networks (Stotts, Glynn, & Baquet, 1991). It is the public health impact, which when evaluating requires criteria that distinguishes it from clinical models or interventions that primarily engage individuals, that ultimately is significant for eliminating population disparities. A critical challenge in this regard is an absence of rigor in public health science when dealing with units of analysis larger than the individual. The problem is made more complicated by the dominant tendency towards reductionism. This is especially critical because a community rather than an individual focus is far more important when addressing the problem of population disparities.

Public health science is handicapped by the underdevelopment of analytic models responsive to community-focused interventions.

Theoretical and Conceptual Models

A review of selected publications regarding conceptual approaches to the problem of eliminating population disparities reveals a combination of strengths and weaknesses. Braveman (2003) provides a useful cornerstone for approaching the problem of population disparities. This approach is action oriented, with a primary purpose of assessing programs or policies in relation to achievement of their short-term objectives. Emphasis is placed on policy relevance, simplicity, affordability, sustainability, and timeliness; providing Braveman's approach with the requisites for usefulness in an action-oriented system whose aim is to eliminate, not necessarily study, population disparities. Indicators are generally consistent with social determinant modeling, with a tendency to describe populations either at the aggregate level of the nation or selected comparison groups, with little emphasis or orientation to community. Nevertheless, the value orientation is rooted in the perspective of social injustice with an understanding of conflict between the disenfranchised and the more powerful.

Baquet, Carter-Pokras, & Bengen-Seltzer (2004) emphasize the importance of partnerships, federal-state collaborations with respect to the integration of patient care, improved technology and patient care management, and leveraging of funds at the community level. Limited treatment of cultural competency reflects the analytic paucity of this approach. Emphasis is on the importance of translation services and health literacy, with no analysis that attempts to move this core construct beyond the limited parameters in which it has been historically grounded.

Murray et al. (2006) provide an elaborate model for investigating disparities. The aim of the study was to develop a method whereby population groups in the United States could be divided based on a small number of characteristics that would best demonstrate disparities in life expectancy. The characteristics used were race, county of residence, population density, race-specific county-level per capita income, and cumulative homicide rate. This largely statistical model is highly suitable for highlighting and broadcasting a problem typically submerged by other priorities, but is less useful as a problem-solving method. The aggregate level of analysis, in which specific communities are not readily accessible, makes the model less useful for problem solving but very useful for problem identification. The authors of the study conclude that in the absence of policies aimed at reducing fundamental socioeconomic inequalities, partial solutions will have to be found to reduce risk factors for chronic diseases and injuries.

Kilbourne, Switzer, Hyman, Crowley-Matoka, & Fine (2006) provide a framework that is fully grounded in health systems delivery and research that "outlines a research trajectory from basic detection of disparities in health and health care to understanding the factors that underlie those disparities to ultimately developing and implementing interventions designed to reduce and eliminate those disparities" (Kilbourne et al., 2006, p. 2113). The model derives from epidemiologic methods and proposes three critical phases: detection, understanding, and development/implementation/evaluation of interventions. In fairness, the authors do not propose parameters beyond research in health care delivery settings. It can legitimately be argued that a sole focus on research is insufficient to address a problem rooted in injustice and preventable morbidity and mortality outcomes, particularly if interventions are conducted within a setting that by itself will only have limited impact on population disparities.

A concerted effort is made to describe a robust definition of vulnerability—one that encompasses both race/ethnicity (i.e., historical patterns of discrimination), other populations that could also experience historical patterns of discrimination, and groups more easily identified in terms of the inequitable distribution of social determinants. This is a compelling component of the model. Yet, race/ethnicity is ascribed to the individual and not to the community, reflecting the generic weakness of health systems research that focuses on either health care delivery or the problems of the individual rather than targeting the community as the unit of analysis. The authors do note the importance of researcher-community collaborations and recognize that the absence of such collaborations could impede problem solving. Collaborative efforts of this nature can occur in community-based participatory research programs. But users of this model must recognize the limits of participatory research protocols and understand they are necessary tools that will enhance competency but are insufficient to directly solve disparity problems, with the exception perhaps of those involving diversity and inclusion.

Moolchan et al. (2007) focus on the importance of data collection and monitoring of events across the life cycle with the critical focus remaining on the individual unit of analysis. This approach is heavily reductionist, given the recommendation to generate sub-models that relate to discrete segments of the life cycle for specific population groups, with the likely result being the assessment of social determinant variables such as SES (i.e., education, income, wealth, and occupation). The analysis leads to a prioritization of challenges in research related to measurement and the ability to better characterize groups or individuals across the life cycle. The enhanced ability to measure and describe population groups are a strength, but the result is likely to be an iteration of additional research questions responsive to life cycle issues rather than a clearer focus on reducing disparities at the critical level of community.

Warnecke et al. (2008) describe a comprehensive population-based model for research in concert with NIH-sponsored Centers for Population Health and Health Disparities for understanding and conducting disparity-related research. They provide a comprehensive overview of determinants that are defined through a matrix moving from distal or population-based determinants (i.e., social conditions and policies), through intermediate or second-level determinants (i.e., community, social and physical contexts, and social relationships), and finally through individual determinants (i.e., SES, race/ethnicity, gender, and acculturation). A weakness of this perspective is the absence of a substantive definition of community. But the model is sufficiently robust that if such a definition were available and accepted by the respective Center investigators, a community focus could be included in proposed research initiatives.

Thomas and Quinn (2008) reiterate the problem with respect to insufficient method and theory. The authors outline a hierarchy of research described as "first generation" (disparities are documented), "second generation" (disparities are explained) and "third generation" (solutions are offered). Their focus is the third generation, which rests on three pillars: (1) transdisciplinary research, (2) community engagement, and (3) translation of evidence-based practices. Strengths of this approach include its explicit engagement with the overarching complexity of the problem of disparities; recognition of intersectional partnerships; reliance on community participatory models; and an explicit emphasis on competency, inclusion, and trust building. The weaknesses remain an absence of a conceptual framework for engaging the "community variable" in the research paradigm beyond interactive processes that create social capital without moving beyond the individual unit of analysis. Nevertheless, the importance of using race/ethnicity as context, particularly with respect to a social justice paradigm, is made explicit. Both the empirical example provided and the values and ideas articulated provide bridges to community-focused and comprehensive initiatives to eliminate population disparities.

Summary

This overview of recent analyses of conceptual models pertinent to the elimination of population disparities reveals a fundamental weakness. The importance of community, while implied and in some cases made explicit, is never engaged with particular rigor. The context of these analyses is essentially on research rather than application, which explains the focus on individual dimensions, albeit disguised in population-based paradigms, because of the paucity of community-oriented theory and research. However, this emphasis also suggests that a failure to, at a minimum, integrate a substantive conceptual framework of community into proposed research models will lead not to a deeper understanding but a continued absence of in-depth treatment of community as the unit of analysis, whether as process, outcome, or impact.

Syme (2004) commented that evaluations of large-scale community interventions fail to provide examples of successful or significant impacts. In a response to this assessment, Robinson (2004) suggested that a critical weakness explaining this conclusion is the absence of a rigorous approach to community. This problem is entwined with a reliance on population-based models that create the illusion of penetrating needed segments of society but in fact facilitate inattention to community-focused approaches. A critical flaw of population-based approaches is that they bypass community parameters in exchange for macrolevel variables, be they census tracts or shared hopes and beliefs.

Communities are too complex to be encompassed by a simplistic attribution to cultural characteristics or singular geographic boundaries and defy methods whereby a group is designated as a community just because its members are a cohesive unit, such as when research on bus drivers is related to as a "community" or a school system is referenced as a "community." Indeed, these formulas suggest that any "group" can be arbitrarily defined as a community. In the absence of adequate theory and practice, there is no reason to assume that interventions based on less than rigorous assumptions will be effective.

COMMUNITY DEVELOPMENT MODEL TO ELIMINATE POPULATION DISPARITIES

The review of research models underscores the absence of a clear focus on community as the critical reference point for either research or practice. The concept of community is consistently referenced but not substantively explained. In addition, none of the research models explains the black-white disparity elimination in tobacco prevalence described in this chapter. The community development model provides the most substantive vehicle for explanation and points the way for both research and practice relevant to eliminating other disparities (Robinson, 2005). This model was first developed in 1995 (Robinson et al., 1995). It was further explicated in 2001, suggesting both barriers and steps needed for implementation (Headen & Robinson, 2001). It was published in its current form in 2005 (Robinson, 2005).

The three core constructs of the community development model are community competence, community development, and community prevention. Community prevention represents the sum and/or synergistic intersection of community competence and community development.

There are fourteen reasons why the community development model serves as an explanation for the elimination of the black-white disparity in tobacco prevalence. The first reason is that the model resolves but does not end the ongoing debate regarding race/ethnicity. The model is premised on recognition of the critical importance of race/ethnicity as a viable scientific variable. In this sense it reflects the assertion by Thomas and Quinn (2008) that a social justice imperative exists mandating an appreciation of race as "context." Refuted is the thesis that because the historical biological-focused treatment of the race construct is racist, it is imperative to do away with the notion of race as a viable scientific entity. Indeed, the perceived solution of focusing instead on racism is viewed as insufficient. More importantly, the focus on the problem of racism as a substitute for substantive respect for race is problematic because it ignores the scientific imperative of constructing a rigorous variable of race that can be readily articulated in research protocols, in a manner more substantial than descriptors of self or perceived identity. Indeed, a reliance on identity reinforces a focus on the individual as the unit of analysis and facilitates the population-based error of aggregating individuals into a mass and calling them a "community" without providing any additional explication of what is meant by "community."

In addition, a primary focus on racism centers one firmly on identifying the problem but not necessarily the locus of the solution. Not accepted is the idea that ethnicity is an adequate substitute for race. Indeed, both race and ethnicity are viewed as social constructs, with race being meta to ethnicity, allowing for an array of different groupings (i.e., tribes, nationalities) within the larger category of race. Similarly rejected are the reductionist tendency to denote race as culture (Freeman, 1998); the linguistic reconstruction of replacing race/ethnicity with "racially classified social group" (King, Polednak, Bendel, Milsain, & Hahata, 2004), and the use of such terms as "macroethnicity" (Jackson, 2006). Race remains a social construct, but one with parameters more explicitly defined. Finally, the idea of race only as "context" or a social construct without further elaboration is insufficient. Social scientists have rested on this minimalist definition and have not assumed the responsibility of bringing a deeper level of substance and complexity to our understanding of race as a scientific variable or integrating it more fully into social theory.

Reason two is that the community development model views community and race as synonymous. Indeed, when approached in terms of public health applications that address disparities, race is most viable when directly linked with community. The determinants of community and race are equivalent: history, culture, context, and geography. To fully understand a particular community or race/ethnicity, whether within narrowly defined parameters of science or broader applications of public health theory and practice, is to be grounded in these determinants.

Third, the community development model places primary importance on the principle of heterogeneity. It allows for defined differences in terms of distinct ethnic or tribal affiliations, as well as geographical location, that occur within the meta categories of race/ethnicity including Native American/American Indian.

Homogeneity, the fourth reason, is a core consideration when distinguishing between a community, group, stratum, or family/individual. For example, a degree of homogeneity is implied in relation to the black community. Implicit are the common denominators of history, culture, context, and geography, all forming the ties that bond. We need to know less about a stratum that is inherently fragmented by different race/ethnicities, each with varying kinds of history, culture, and geography. Actually, it is not so much that we need to know less, but rather that one is unable to know more because strata typically do not benefit from the associated characteristics of homogeneity. Homogeneity means that more can be known about race/ethnic communities precisely because their identity is shaped by a collective social experience, made visible through the lens of history, culture, context, and geography. Homogeneity and heterogeneity are dynamic concepts that require consideration in the context of research or intervention development.

Reason five: the model incorporates complexity as a principle, both in relation to a specific problem or a population group. For example, it does not assume that every problem requires an understanding of history, only that a historical perspective may sometimes be necessary. Understanding the role of tobacco in the lives of blacks requires a grasp of the institution of slavery; the evolution of slave labor into sharecropping, farming, and factory work; the role of the tobacco industry with regard to employment as well as targeted marketing; and the pattern of the menthol cigarette advance over time to its current status as the preferred choice of black smokers.

Reason six is the model's explicit integration of complexity which allows for a more nuanced appreciation of race/ethnic differences. For example, it is not necessary for the Latino community to self-define as a race. African Americans more easily ascribe to a racial categorization because they resonate with the historical experience of slavery; a compelling common denominator. Alternatively, there are nations in South America that have no history of enslaving Africans. When Latinos search for a unifying theme of community they are more likely to attend to the community determinant of culture rather than history. And even though there are multiple ethnic communities within the broader rubric of Latino, when they draw together in environments such as the United States to mobilize or organize for the collective good, they do so within the meta rubric of Latinos and/or Hispanics, depending largely on the unifying construct of culture. A reliance on culture is not a panacea. Latinos, similar to other communities, struggle with fragmentation.

The seventh reason is that complexity is also expressed by explicit attention to the relative and dynamic nature of the determinants. Because every community is unique with regard to the impact of history, culture, context, and geography, it cannot be assumed that each determinant must be treated as equally important. A given determinant will have varying levels of importance in different communities. With respect to African and African American communities, history is likely to be more important than it would be for immigrants who may have left their "history" behind. In this case, when responding to immigrants in U.S. settings, the culture of the respective immigrant community may be most critical or they may rely on geography or place of residence as the bonding agent. Similarly, because the determinants are dynamic, it cannot be assumed that they remain the same over time A community's understanding of its own history can change; and consequently, the role of history in shaping the collective can become more or less important over time. In essence, none of the determinants (i.e., history, culture, context, geography) are static.

The eighth reason is a broader appreciation of competency than is available by relying on cultural competence. Community Competence provides a more substantive basis for assessing competency. Appreciation of the relative and dynamic qualities associated with the community determinants of history, culture, context and geography allows one to also understand how each of these must be singularly assessed in respect to different population groups and selected problems when developing competent interventions. In essence, communities are more than the sum of culture. If only culture is relied on to ensure competency then we risk the error of leaving out other important influences. Alternatively, if everything of importance is defined as "culture" then we risk transforming the construct into a multiplicity of unrelated content. It is a theoretical approach. In addition to the four determinants, other constructs ensuring competency are consideration of positive imagery, salient imagery, literacy, language, multi-generational needs, and diversity. The important principle is not that each must be included to achieve competency; rather, each must be considered. The protocol is one of quality control.

In the ninth reason, interventions related to community development are categorized as (a) capacity and infrastructure and (b) social capital. This distinction serves an important purpose. The public health literature is dominated by an elaborate, often confused, discussion of social capital (Robinson, 2005). The model defines capacity and infrastructure as research, programs, leaders, organizations, and networks. Social capital is defined as cooperation, collaboration, reciprocity, and trust. Why the distinction? The dominance of social capital in the literature, composed largely of process-related variables, expresses levels of cohesion and the quality of interactions that occur. This reliance on process has meant that the fundamental task of building the bricks and mortar needed by a community have either been neglected or transferred to other non-health sectors in terms of responsibility. Who is responsible for building the capacity and infrastructure necessary for any struggle or problem-solving endeavor? Typically, the answer is "the other person or entity." By making the distinction between capacity and infrastructure and social capital, the model brings into full focus not only the "needs" that need to be addressed or the "variables" that need to be studied, but the underlying theme of comprehensiveness and the "both/and" paradigm inherent in every aspect of the model and its underlying constructs. Community development involves both capacity/infrastructure and social capital. The questions to be asked are: (i) what and how much is needed? (ii) what is critically missing? (iii) where are the core strengths upon which to build so as to avoid the error of a "deficit model"? and (iv) what is critically important with regard to history, culture, context, and geography, including the other components of community competency, that will help to achieve the goal, be it research or intervention development?

Tenth, the model implies prioritization of capacity and infrastructure over social capital. The metaphor is that of a car with or without gas. The car is the capacity/infrastructure and the gas is social capital. Without the car one can have all the gas in the world but still go nowhere. Alternatively, a car without gas can be pushed. Yet there is a danger if the importance of social capital is ignored. Social capital is focused on creating alliances and collaborations. However, if the larger aim is ignored (community development), the result is not social capital of the collective but a fragmented array of micro social capital entities that lead to disorganization, dysfunctionality, and absence of unity.

Reason eleven is that complexity and heterogeneity also govern community competence and community development. The higher the order of complexity, the more inputs of community competence or development are likely to be needed. The model proposes an order of complexity as follows: community, group, stratum, individual/family. A population aggregate may disguise underlying heterogeneity; for example, a Vietnamese community may exist within a geographical area dominated by Chinese or Korean residents. The needs of the larger Asian community could be significantly less than that of the Vietnamese. Indeed, not only may the "needs" or "resources" be disguised, but a disparity experienced not by the larger but by the smaller community may become invisible. This disparity could surface if diversity is highlighted in the assessment protocol. Similarly, solutions will likely require greater attention to components of community competence and community development because of the greater need and greater degree of homogeneity within the Vietnamese community in contrast with the larger Asian community within which it resides. It does not mean that history is unimportant when dealing with an individual or family, a group such as bus drivers, or a stratum such as persons of low income; rather, the model assumes that the nature of the history of a community is more layered and robust than that of other aggregations. In other words, there is more to miss (increasing the possibility for error) if history is ignored as a possible important consideration when addressing a community than would be the case in the treatment of less complex aggregations. However, rigor requires a thorough consideration of each determinant regardless of the target audience. This problem underscores the nature of the commitment that must be made by scientists or practitioners when addressing the problem of population disparities. There must be a willingness to accept the rigors of complexity, and challenge the resource efficiency often associated with reductionism.

The twelfth reason is that the model sharply criticizes the tendency of reductionism in science. This is considered the major weakness of attention to the social determinants of health. A core problem with focusing on social determinants is that fundamentally it remains an effort to improve measurement. Intervention efforts fall prey to the assumption that if we can measure something we can understand it. Actually, the mistake is the illusion that to measure is to understand. The focus on measurement grounds the construct in reductionism. This approach will always be etiological in nature, which is not the same as creating problem-solving interventions. Many advocates of social determinant constructs have no reference point for community and no sensibility for the importance of race. The reductionist reliance on income or education, and the inherent tendency of measurement to predict an outcome rather than resolve the outcome, facilitates inattention to a cohesive construct of race/ethnicity. Personal identity more often than not suffices. Alternatively, ethnicity replaces race, ignoring the fundamental truth that both are social constructs. Indeed, the concept of ethnicity arose in the early twentieth century as a means of defining the European populations immigrating into the United States (Steinberg, 1995; Glaser, 1997; Feagin & Feagin 2003). It is ironic how a failure to understand history facilitates the borrowing of Eurocentric constructs as a solution to race theory.[5]

The limits of the approach of looking solely at social determinants are its (a) focus on measurement, (b) inherent reductionism, (c) constraints of etiologic models, (d) challenges to transitioning to intervention models, (e) inattention to community as the unit of analysis, and (f) tendencies to reject race based on ideological assumptions. If we focus on the issue of interventions, it offers a useful way to distinguish social determinants from the community model. Because the concerns are primarily measurement and, relatedly, prediction, social determinant analyses will describe the locus of problems: where and who.

The community development model focuses on competency and development and prevention: how and what. In other words, the distinction is one of etiology and prediction in contrast with intervention development and dissemination. However, there is movement on the part of social determinant adherents toward designating indicators such as poverty not as cause but as the objects of change; not as predictors but as the outcome that needs to be transformed. Yet, as social determinant theory evolves to capture this end of the continuum, it effectively morphs into the community development model. It does not, however, necessarily overcome its reluctance to accept the

---

[5] Special thanks to Drs. Michael Byrd and Linda Clayton for their contributions regarding the historical evolution of the construct of ethnicity.

role of race, and implicitly embedded racial/ethnic communities. Social determinant theory would do well to adopt a "both/and" paradigm.

Reason thirteen is that the model's emphasis on diversity and heterogeneity make it completely compatible with participatory models of research, recognition of the importance of disaggregating data to pursue hidden relationships or ethnic-based phenomena, acknowledgment of the need for transdisciplinary research and inter-agency collaboration and partnerships, and explicit promotion of the values of transparency and inclusiveness.

The fourteenth and final reason for adoption of the community development model is that its emphasis on community prevention, or the combined synergy of community competence and community development, enhances the prevention and control continuum. Control strategies typically focus on disease or behavior, are clinical in nature, and emphasize the individual as the unit of analysis. Prevention strategies, though upstream with regard to treatment and medical practice, are inclusive of ecological and environmental paradigms capable of a national and global perspective, but may disregard targeted interventions and a community focus. Community prevention makes explicit the importance of community as a focus and a unit of analysis that is differentiated from prevention and control protocols. The problem of methodology (i.e., measurement, analytic models) is not solved, but the model provides conceptual underpinnings that advance the theory of community and understanding of its relationship to the science and practice of eliminating population disparities.

Logic of the Community Development Model[6]

Figure 19.6 demonstrates that the core components of the community development model are foundations upon which intervention development and elimination of population disparities can be addressed. Outputs include intermediate outcomes, facilitating both data collection efforts that can be considered needs assessments and more traditional epidemiological exercises that help describe the problem more accurately while also speaking directly to the importance of disaggregation of racial/ethnic profiles. It is critically important that the intervention planning process be both inclusive and transparent, with a guiding question being "Who is missing from the table?" Intervention development will be influenced by the existing state-of-the-art theories; but given the nature of disparities and the absence of attention to both the problem and the communities in which they are experienced, it is not surprising that many interventions will have to be developed and not merely translated from what is available. This is an uncomfortable position for scientists and policy makers, who are influenced by professional values of rigor and the more mundane realities of scarce resources. Nevertheless, it remains the garden in which we dig. And rose gardens were promised to none.

---

[6] Special thanks to the Program Services Branch at the Office on Smoking and Health at CDC, especially Sharon Kohout, who now works in Texas. Development of the logic model was a collective exercise in commitment and vision of the work that needed to be done.

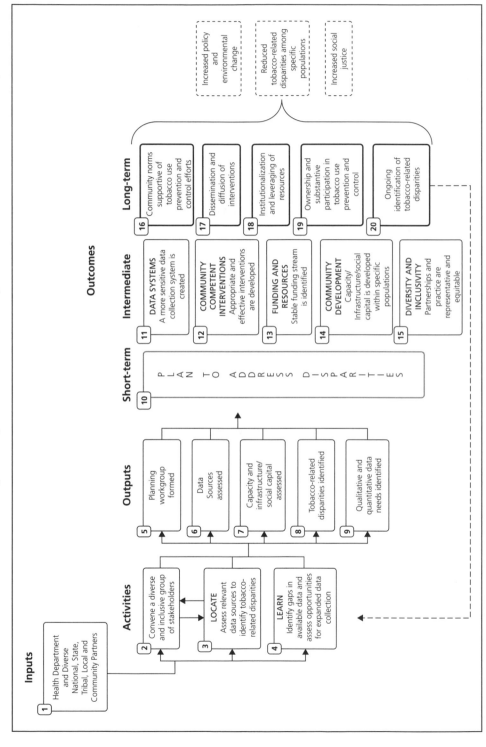

FIGURE 19.6 *Use of the Community Development Model to Identify and Eliminate Tobacco-Related Disparities.*

A useful way to assess the comprehensiveness of the community development model relative to the problem of eliminating population disparities is to examine it in relation to a definition of tobacco-related disparities, which can be described as

> . . . differences in the patterns, prevention, and treatment of tobacco use; the risk, incidence, morbidity, mortality, and burden of tobacco-related illness that exist among specific population groups in the United States; and related differences in capacity and infrastructure, access to resources, and environmental tobacco smoke exposure. (Fagan et al., 2004, p. 211)

The inclusion of capacity and infrastructure is deemed critical and should guide other public health arenas when defining the problem. They would do well to include a part of the solution into the problem definition to better arm those engaged with the purpose of finding the solutions.

RECOMMENDATIONS TO PUBLIC HEALTH SCIENTISTS AND PRACTITIONERS

Examining the disparity elimination of black-white prevalence in 2001 has relied on a tri-angulizaton of theory, data, and practice. The conclusions drawn are not based on a rigorous evaluation design. Indeed, the observed outcome emerged from an unplanned set of events that were both top down and bottom up. The level of intensity of work in the African American community reflected both breadth and depth. It serves as a demarcation of what is traditionally viewed as community-based and what is better explained by community-focused. *Community-based* is a more limited construct and requires only that interventions are placed within a community milieu. *Community-focused* raises the ante and requires a level of comprehensiveness, founded on competency and development, in which the process of creating is as important as achieving the outcomes of change. What lessons can we discern from this example? What recommendations can be provided to public health scientists and practitioners?

Recommendation one: Transparency and inclusiveness should be the gold standard, otherwise thought of as "best practices," of all processes regarding the development of legislation, policy, research, and program priorities at the federal, state and local levels.

Recommendation two: The American Legacy Foundation and Centers for Tobacco Free Kids, founded on funds from the Masters Settlement, should recommit to transparent and inclusive processes, organize community-based advisory committees, and engage these committees fully.

Recommendation three: Research is a critical component of any national strategy regarding the elimination of population disparities; but a note of caution is imperative because if the black community had waited until all the research and the evaluations necessary for coherent translation of the research were completed, the nation would still be facing the crisis of extraordinary high tobacco-use prevalence levels among black smokers.

Recommendation four: Proactive use of "promising practices" will help provide a platform for ongoing work independent of a focus on "best practices," which as regards initiatives responsive to communities of color, is more often than not a barrier to progress. Best practices evolves from a body of work that is primarily mainstream, focused on randomized control trials governed by a reductionist model of research, and consequently less relevant to the social context in which communities of color are embedded. Looking for "promising practices" will provide a proactive environment in which competent work can advance relative to defining and eliminating population disparities.

Recommendation five: Policy, research, and program initiatives responsive to community competence and community development are critical for the elimination of population disparities. Community prevention provides synthesis while highlighting the ongoing importance of the "community construct" in policy, research, and program initiatives.

Recommendation six: Public health models must hold supremacy over research-specific agendas with regard to the elimination of population disparities, especially in a research environment in which race and community are inadequately defined. Communities experiencing disparities should not be held hostage to the state-of-the-art status of science. The tendency in research is to disaggregate in order to evaluate, often resulting in interactions whereby the community is sliced into distinct strata such as high or low income or education and the conclusion is that one or the other will be affected by a given intervention. A public health model emphasizes the total community and results in the greatest possible impact with regard to eliminating population disparities.

Recommendation seven: Research must be conducted to advance the measurement and evaluation tools related to race, community, competency and development. A paradigm shift away from the focus on the individual as the unit of analysis to "units of the collective" must occur. Research, to have more impact in regard to population disparities, requires an enhanced methodology capable of assessing community-level outcomes.

Recommendation eight: The CDC requires enhanced funding and authority for disparity-related initiatives, including a mandate to target community competency and community development initiatives. In addition, the CDC must have authority to require performance standards of state health departments that will ensure that eliminating disparities is a top priority and that a sufficient funding stream is provided to communities experiencing population disparities.

Recommendation nine: State health departments must evaluate their disparity initiatives, including allocation of resources, according to criteria of equity and need, and based on core values that highlight the social justice underpinnings of population disparities. The present status of inequitable funding streams cannot be maintained.

Recommendation ten: National QuitLine programs, under federal and state auspices, should include PTF as part of the materials they send to black smokers who call for help in quitting, and to members of their social networks who are seeking ways to help family, friends, or colleagues quit. This provides a public health benefit to the QuitLine program estimated to reach up to 4.28 percent of all U.S. smokers (NAQC, 2005, 2006). The QuitLines justify their failure to distribute PTF on the assumption that targeting is not effective, despite PTF's proven efficacy in a telephone cessation counseling environment. This rationale is analogous to the infamous Tuskegee Experiment in which black men with syphilis were refused penicillin treatment (Jones, 1981). The assumption regarding the ineffectiveness of targeting, reinforced by related issues such as expense or lack of prioritization, is analogous to the conseqences associated with the ill-defined assumption in the early twentieth century that there was something different about blacks that required observation of untreated victims of syphilis. Black smokers deserve the benefit of PTF in the same way that black men in Alabama deserved to be cured of "bad blood." Denying dissemination of PTF is equivalent to withholding treatment of an effective intervention.

Recommendation eleven: Population disparities must be defined comprehensively and not according to reductionist tendencies that focus on available data such as prevalence, morbidity, and mortality, resulting in inattention to the capacity and infrastructure needs of communities experiencing disparities.

Recommendation twelve: Menthol requires priority status in regard to research, policy, and applications. The evaluation of menthol must be comprehensive and not reduced to morbidity and mortality outcomes. The role of menthol in regard to increased rates of smoking by youth and adults, addiction, and barriers to quitting should be regarded as equally important. In addition, these indicators should be the core foundation in determining federal policy regarding regulation of tobacco products and support for needed interventions.

Recommendation thirteen: A critical research priority, receiving almost no attention to date, is the problem of secondhand exposure caused by smoking in the home. Black children are at greater risk than the general population for exposure to secondhand smoke, and little is known with respect to intervention approaches.

Recommendation fourteen: Sustainable resources for support of national networks must be found, independent of the federal government.

Recommendation fifteen: The Office on Smoking and Health, in recognition of its responsibility as the sole source for PTF, should support and promote communication campaigns to increase the availability and dissemination of PTF at levels comparable to or greater than those of the period from 1993 to 2002 (more than a million copies).

Recommendation sixteen: Given the likelihood of advances with regard to FDA legislation, inclusion of menthol, and the development of a more effective national tobacco prevention and control infrastructure, evaluation of the cessation needs of black smokers should be carried out. A plan of action should be developed that includes utilization of organizations such as the National African American Tobacco Prevention Network (NAATPN) to support communication and training initiatives that will aid in meeting anticipated cessation needs.

CONCLUSION

The disparity elimination described in this chapter represents a phenomenal public health success story. It was made possible by the engagement of multiple interagency and intercommunity coalitions along with intracommunity cohesion replicated across the nation. It reflected an unimagined level of commitment from dedicated professionals and community representatives. We have learned that the same compelling argument that is the guidepost for tobacco prevention and control applies to the problem of disparities: the best strategy or the best practice is an approach that incorporates media, policy, individual behavior change, counter marketing, communication mechanisms, community mobilization, community competence, and community development, ultimately leading to interventions that encompass the best of each factor at the community level of analysis and engagement. Research and evaluation are not distinct activities that must occur before any other activity can begin; rather, they are integral at every level of activity, never impeding and always helping the process to move forward.

Tobacco prevention and control were advantaged by what is termed a "mature" public health problem. There is much that is known regarding individual behavior change, communication strategies, and policy applications in tobacco prevention and control. Tobacco control advocates have an extremely rich and powerful enemy, but one that makes an easy target: the tobacco industry. When considering other behavioral-based public health problems, one would do well to ask "Where are the easy targets, and what is known of the array of activities needed to form a comprehensive package of interventions?" Public health practitioners in obesity would love to have a policy application as simple as an excise tax, an enemy as clear as the tobacco industry, or even a self-help behavior guide as effective as Pathway to Freedom.

Yet, as rich as the assets available to tobacco control advocates happen to be, we cannot forget an essential part of the history. We knew very little, apart from epidemiological trends, in 1990 about tobacco control and the black community. We confronted a tobacco control movement that had at best one or two national African American advocates. The movement itself was, perhaps, the least diverse of any public health movement in the nation. There were no self-help guides, networks, or cadre of researchers and senior managers of major institutions directly responsive to the black community. So how did tobacco control advocates succeed? We honored community. We honored race. We honored competency. We fought like hell for development.[7]

---

[7] The success of the black community would not have been possible without the dedicated work of Charyn Sutton, who transitioned to the ancestors in 2004. Charyn's brilliance left a mark on every aspect of the community's efforts: Pathways to Freedom, Uptown Coalition, National Networks, counter marketing campaigns, marketing behavior of blacks, the distinct role of excise taxes in the black community, and the constant need for advocacy and development. To say that we would not have gotten where we are today without her is not an exercise in idolization; it is a simple statement of fact and a testimonial to power.

REFERENCES

Ahrens, D. (2009). Tobacco taxes and cigarette consumption in low income populations. *American Journal of Public Health, 99*, 6.

Armour, B. S., Woollery, T., Malarcher, A., Pechacek, T. F., & Husten, C. (2005). Annual smoking-attributable mortality, years of potential life lost, and productivity losses—United States, 1997–2001. *Morbidity and Mortality Weekly Report, 54*, 625–628.

Baquet, C. R., Carter-Pokras, O., & Bengen-Seltzer, B. (2004). Healthcare disparities and models for change. *American Journal of Managed Care, 10*, SP5–11.

Barg, J. (2007, April 25–May 1). Puff daddies: Smoking ban be damned, tobacco companies are still targeting blacks in the city's poorest neighborhoods. *Philadelphia Weekly*, pp. 26–32.

Benowitz, N. L., Perez-Stable, J., Fong, I., Modin, G., Herrera, B., & Jacob, P. (1999). Ethnic differences in N-glucuronidation of nicotine and cotinine, *Journal of Pharmacology and Experimental Therapeutics, 291*, 1195–1203.

Bloch, A. B., Mowery, P. D., Caraballo, R. S., Malarcher, A. M., Pechacek, T., & Husten, C. G. (2005). Tobacco use, access, and exposure to tobacco among middle and high school students—United States, 2004. *Morbidity and Mortality Weekly Report, 54*, 297–301.

Boyd, N. R., Sutton, C., Orleans, C.T., et al. (1998). Quit today! A targeted communications campaign to increase the use of the cancer information service by African American smokers. *Preventive Medicine, 27*, S50–S60.

Braveman, P. A. (2003). Monitoring equity in health and healthcare: A conceptual framework. *Journal of Health, Population and Nutrition, 21(3)*, 181–192.

Brieon, A., Kiburi, A.L., Morris, D., Oto-Kent, D.S., Robinson, C.M., Robinson, R., et al. (2007). *Black folks don't use quitlines: Exploring the true story* (pp. 1–16). Sacramento, CA: Health Education Council.

Caffee, B. (2001). *Not in Mama's kitchen* (2nd ed.) Hattiesburg, MS: Caffee and Associates Public Health Foundation, Inc.

Caraballo, R. S., Giovino, G. A., Pechacek, T. F., Mowery, P. D., Richter, P. A., Strauss, W. J., et al. (1998). Racial and ethnic differences in serum cotinine levels of cigarette smokers. Third national health and nutrition examination survey. *Journal of the American Medical Association, 280*, 35–139.

Centers for Disease Control and Prevention (CDC). (1999). *Best practices for comprehensive tobacco control programs—August 1999*. Atlanta, GA: USDHHS, CDC, NCCDPHP, OSH.

Clark, P. I., Gardiner, P. S., Djordjevic, M. V., Leischow, S. J., & Robinson, R. G. (2004). Menthol cigarettes: Setting the research agenda. *Nicotine & Tobacco Research, 6* (S1), S5–9.

Crawford, G. E. (2007). Flavoured tobacco products with marijuana names. *Tobacco Control, 16*, 70.

Fagan, P., King, G., Lawrence, D., Petucci, S.A., Robinson, R.G., Banks, D., et al. (2004). Eliminating tobacco-related health disparities: Directions for future research. *American Journal of Public Health, 92(2)*, 211–217.

Feagin, J. R., & Feagin, C. B. (2003). *Racial and ethnic relations* (7th ed.). Upper Saddle River, NJ: Prentice Hall.

Freeman, H. P. (1998). The meaning of race in science—considerations for cancer research: Concerns of special populations in the national cancer program. *Cancer, 82(1)*, 219–225.

Gandhi, K. K., Foulds, J., Steinberg, M. B., Lu, S. E., & Williams, J. M. (2009). Lower quit rates among African American and Latino menthol cigarette smokers at a tobacco treatment clinic. *The International Journal of Clinical Practice, 63*, 360–367.

Gardiner, P. S. (2004). The African Americanization of menthol cigarette use in the United States. *Nicotine & Tobacco Research, 6* (S1), S55–65.

Glaser, N. (1997). *We are all multiculturalists now*. Cambridge, MA: Harvard University Press.

Goodwin, N. J., & Robinson, R. (2009). Pathways to Freedom: A guide to help African Americans quit smoking, and Health power quit smoking tip sheets. *Health Power News, 6(1)*.

Headen, S. W., & Robinson, R. G. (2001). Tobacco: From slavery to addiction. In R. L. Braithwaite and S. E. Taylor (Eds.), *Health issues in the black community* (pp. 347–383). San Francisco: Jossey-Bass Publishers.

Hebert, J. R. (2004). What's new in nicotine and tobacco research. *Nicotine & Tobacco Research, 6(S1)*, S1–4.

Hebert, J. R., & Kabat, G. C. (1989). Menthol cigarettes and esophageal cancer. *International Journal of Epidemiology, 18*, 37–44.

Hersey, J. C., Ng, S. W., Nonmemake, J. M., Mowary, P., Thomas, K. Y., & Vilsaint, M. C., et al. (2006). Are menthol cigarettes a starter product for youth? *Nicotine &Tobacco Research, 8,* 403–413.

Hestick, H., Perrino, S. C., Rhodes, W. A., & Sydnor, K. D. (2001). Trial and lifetime smoking risks among African American college students. *Journal of American College Health, 49*(5), 213–219.

Jackson, F. (2006). Lecture presented at the Fourth Annual Summer Workshop, Disparities in Health in America: Working toward Social Justice, Houston, TX, June 28, 2006.

Jones, J. H. (1981). *Bad blood: The Tuskegee syphilis experiment.* New York: Free Press.

Kilbourne, A. M., Switzer, G., Hyman, K., Crowley-Matoka, M., & Fine, M. J. (2006). Advancing health disparities research within the health care system: A conceptual framework. *American Journal of Public Health, 96*(12), 2113–2121.

King, G., Gebreselassie, T., Mallett, R. K., Kozlowski, L., & Bendel, R.B. (2007). Opinions of African Americans about tobacco industry philanthropy. *Preventive Medicine, 45,* 464–470.

King, G., Polednak, A., Bendel, R. B., Milsain, M. C., & Hahata, S. B. (2004). Disparities in smoking cessation between African Americans and Whites: 1990–2000. *American Journal of Public Health, 94*(11), 1965–1971.

Kreslake, J. M., Wayner, G. F., Alpert, H. R., Koh, H. K., & Connolly, G. N. (2008). Tobacco industry control of menthol in cigarettes and targeting of adolescents and young adults. *American Journal of Public Health, 98*(9), 1–8.

Laws, M. A., Holliday, R. C, & Huang, C. J. (2007). Prevalence and social norms associated with cigarette smoking among college students attending historically black colleges and universities. *American Journal of Health Studies, 22,* 96–104.

Laws, M. A., Huang, C. J., Brown, R. F., Richmond, A., & Conerly, R. C. (2006). Cigarette smoking among college students attending a historically black college and university. *Journal of Health Care for the Poor and Underserved, 16,* 143–156.

Moolchan, E. T, Fagan, P., Fernander, A. F., Velicer, W. F., Hayward, M. D., King, G., et al. (2007). Addressing tobacco-related health disparities. *Addiction, 102,* 30–42.

Morse, D. E., & Kerr, A. R. (2006). Disparities in oral and pharyngeal cancer incidence, mortality and survival among black and white Americans. *Journal of the American Dental Association, 137*(2), 203–212.

Murray, C. J. L., Kulkarni, S. C., Michaud, C., Tomijima, N., Bulzacchelli, M. T., Landiorlo, T. J., et al. (2006). Eight Americas: Investigating mortality disparities across races, counties, and race-counties in the United States. *PLoS Medicine, 3*(9), 1513–1524.

North American Quitline Consortium. (2005, 2006). *Annual Survey of Quitlines in North America.* Available at http://www.naquitline.org/?page=survey2008

Northridge, M. R, Scott, G., Swaner, R., Northridge, J. I., Jean-Louis, B., Klihr-Beall, S., et al. (2009). Toward a smoke-free Harlem: Engaging families, agencies, and community-based programs. *Journal of Health Care for the Poor and Underserved, 20,* 107–121.

Okuyemi, K. S., Faseru, B., Sanderson, C. L., Bronars, C. A., & Ahluwalia, J. S. (2007). Relationship between menthol cigarettes and smoking cessation among African American light smokers. *Addiction, 102,* 1978–1986.

Oliver, J., DeLancey, L., Thun, M. J., Jemal, A., & Ward, E. M. (2008). Recent trends in black-white disparities in cancer mortality. *Cancer Epidemiology Biomarkers & Prevention, 17,* 2908–2912.

Orleans, C. T., Boyd, N. R., Bingler, R., et al. (1998). A self-help intervention for African American smokers: Tailoring cancer information service counseling for a special population. *Preventive Medicine, 27,* S61–S69.

Pierce, J. P., Fiore, M. C., Novotny, T. E., Hatziandreu, E. J., & Davis, R. M. (1989). Trends in cigarette smoking in the United States: Projections to the year 2000. *Journal of the American Medical Association, 261*(1), 61–65.

Pirkle, J. L., Bernert, J. T., Caudill, S. P., Sosnoff, C. S., & Pechacek, T. F. (2006). Trends in the exposure of nonsmokers in the U.S. population to secondhand smoke: 1988–2002. *Environmental Health Perspectives, 114*(6), 853–858.

Powe, B. D., Ross, L., & Cooper, D. L. (2007). Attitudes and beliefs about smoking among African-American college students at historically black colleges and universities. *Journal of the National Medical Association, 99*(4), 338–344.

Ramirez, A. (1990, January 20). Reynolds, after protests, cancels cigarette aimed at black smokers. *New York Times.*

Robinson, R. (1998). African American farmers and workers in the tobacco industry. *Tobacco farming: Current challenges and future alternatives.* Southern Research Report #10, Academic Affairs Library, Center for the Study of the American South, Southern Historical Collection.

Robinson, R. (2004). Response to S. Leonard Syme's essay. Preventing chronic disease [serial online]. Retrieved February 15, 2009, from http://www.cdc.gov/pcd/issues/2004/apr/04_0005.htm

Robinson, R. G. (2005). Community development model for public health applications: Overview of a model to eliminate population disparities. *Journal of Health Education Practice, 6*(3), 338–346.

Robinson, R. G., & Headen, S. W. (1999). Tobacco use and the African American community: A conceptual framework for the year 2000 and beyond. In Martin L. Forst (Ed.), *Planning and implementing effective tobacco education and prevention programs* (pp. 83–111). Springfield, IL: Charles C. Thomas.

Robinson, R. G., Orleans, C. T., James, D., & Sutton, C. (1992). *Pathways to freedom: Winning the fight against tobacco.* Fox Chase Cancer Institute.

Robinson, R. G., Pertschuk, M., & Sutton, C. (1992). Smoking and African Americans: Spotlighting the effects of smoking and tobacco promotion in the African American community. In S. E. Samuels & M. D. Smith (Eds.), *Improving the health of the poor.* Menlo Park, CA: The Henry J. Kaiser Family Foundation.

Robinson, R. G., Shelton, D., Hodge, F., Lew, R., Lopes, E., Toy, P., et al. (1995). Tobacco control capacity index for communities of color in the United States. In K. Slama (Ed.), *Tobacco and health* (pp. 359–365). New York: Plenum Press.

Robinson, R. G., & Sutton, C. (1994). The coalition against Uptown cigarettes. In D. Jernigan and P. A. Wright (Eds.), *Making news, changing policy: Case studies of media advocacy on alcohol and tobacco issues.* Center for Substance Abuse Prevention Monograph. University Research Corporation and the Marin Institute for the Prevention of Alcohol and Other Drug Problems.

Robinson, R. G., Sutton, C., James, D., & Orleans, T. (2003). *Pathways to freedom: Winning the fight against tobacco* (rev. ed.). Atlanta: CDC.

Saul, S. (2008a, July 1). Cigarette bill treats menthol with leniency. *New York Times,* pp. A1, 15.

Saul, S. (2008b, May 13). Black lawmakers seek restrictions on menthol cigarettes. *New York Times.*

Shelley, D., Cantrell, J., Moon-Howard, J., et al. (2007). The $5 man: The underground economic response to a large cigarette tax increase in New York City. *American Journal of Public Health, 97*(8), 1483–1488.

Skeer, M., George, S., Hamilton, W. L., Cheng, D. M., & Siegel, M. (2004). Town-level characteristics and smoking policy adoption in Massachusetts: Are local restaurant smoking regulations fostering disparities in health protection? *American Journal of Public Health, 94*(2), 286–293.

Skolnick, A. A. (1993). National medical association unveils billboard campaign to promote health in black communities. *Journal of the American Medical Association, 270*(10), 1166–1168.

Steinberg, S. (1995). *Turning back: Retreat from racial justice in American thought and policy.* Boston: Beacon Press.

Stotts, R. C., Glynn, T. J., & Baquet, C. R. (1991). Smoking cessation among blacks. *Journal of Health Care for the Poor and Underserved, 2*(2), 307–319.

Syme, S. L. (2004). Social determinants of health: The community as an empowered partner. *Preventing chronic disease* [serial online]. Retrieved February 15, 2009, from http://www.cdc.gov/pcd/issues/2004/jan/03_0001.htm

Thomas, S. B., & Quinn, S. C. (2008). Poverty and elimination of urban health disparities: Challenge and opportunity. *Annals of the New York Academy of Science, 1136,* 111–125.

Trinidad, D. R., Gilpin, E. A., Lee, L., & Pierce, J. P. (2004). Do the majority of Asian-American and African-American smokers start as adults? *American Journal of Preventive Medicine, 26*(2),156–158.

United States Department of Health and Human Services. (1998). Tobacco use among U.S. racial/ethnic minority groups—African Americans, American Indians and Alaska Natives, Asian Americans and Pacific Islanders, and Hispanics: A report of the surgeon general. Atlanta: U.S. Department of Health and Human Services, Centers for Disease Control and Prevention, National Center for Chronic Disease Prevention and Health Promotion, Office on Smoking and Health.

U. S. Surgeon General's Report (1989). *Reducing the health consequences of smoking: 25 years of progress.* USDHHS, PHS, CDC, OSH, Publication No. (CDC) 89-8411.

Voorhees, C. C., Stillman, F. A., Swank, R. T., Heagerty, P. J., Levine, D. M., & Becker, D. M. (1996). Heart, body, and soul: Impact of church-based smoking cessation interventions on readiness to quit. *Preventive Medicine, 25,* 277–285.

Walker, T. C. (2007). What is it worth to you? Blacks pay the consequences for smoking in more ways than one. *Black Enterprise, 38*(2), 34.

Wang, Y., Browne, D. C., Storr, C. L., & Wagner, F. A. (2005). Gender and the tobacco-depression relationship: A sample of African American college students at a historically black college or university (HBCU). *Addictive Behaviors, 30*(7), 1437–1441.

Warnecke, R. B., Breen, N., Gehlert, S., Paskett, E., Tucker, K. L., Lurie, N., et al. (2008). Approaching health disparities from a population perspective: The national institutes of health centers for population and health disparities. *American Journal of Public Health, 98*(9),1608–1615.

Webb, M. S. (2008a). Does one size fit all African American smokers? The moderating role of acculturation in culturally specific interventions. *Psychology of Addictive Behaviors, 22*(4), 592–596.

Webb, M. S. (2008b). Treating tobacco dependence among African Americans: A meta-analytic review. *Health Psychology, 27*(3S), S271–S282.

Yerger, V. B., Przewonznik, J., & Malone, R. I. (2007). Racialized geography, corporate activity, and health disparities: Tobacco industry targeting of inner cities. *Journal of Health Care for the Poor and Underserved, 18*, 10–38.

Young, Y. (2008, September 26). Black caucus should end big tobacco ties. *USA Today*, p. 15A.

20

ALCOHOL USE AND CONSEQUENCES FOR BLACKS

DIONNE C. GODETTE

This chapter provides an overview of the history, epidemiology, and consequences of alcohol use among blacks in the United States. The chapter will also highlight disparities in alcohol use and related consequences that blacks experience and review common approaches to intervention. Limitations of standard approaches to intervention on the inequities that blacks experience related to alcohol use are reviewed, and suggestions for developing interventions that may be more effective and efficacious for all subpopulations of blacks living in this country are provided.

BACKGROUND: A HISTORICAL CONTEXT

Much like other racial or ethnic groups, blacks in the United States have a long history with the use of alcoholic beverages. In pre-colonial times, the use of alcohol in African society was not for the purpose of producing intoxication; instead, it was for the purpose of participation in religious and cultural traditions within families and communities (Christmon, 1995). However, when blacks were brought to the United States as slaves, their more conservative traditions concerning the use of alcohol diminished. Alcohol use became increasingly more prevalent in the social context among blacks, and young people began to have increased access to this substance (Christmon, 1995). These factors represent a major departure from the more protective African traditions and marked the beginning of U.S.-based blacks' more negative trajectory with alcohol use and related problems.

Although the epidemiology of alcohol use among racial and ethnic groups was not well documented prior to the 1970s, we know that, for various reasons, drinking and drunkenness were more common occurrences among both enslaved and freed blacks than it had been for those in pre-colonial Africa (Christmon, 1995; Welte & Barnes, 1987). However, during the early nineteenth century, American blacks embraced the Colored Temperance Movement (Herd, 1985). This movement discouraged blacks from the use of all alcoholic beverages. The temperance movement was well diffused and supported by the press, faith-based organizations, and self-improvement organizations (Herd, 1985). It was also instrumental in bringing rates of drinking, drunkenness, and other alcohol-related problems down throughout the nineteenth century (Herd, 1985). Nevertheless, by the twentieth century black participation in the temperance movement saw a decline, mostly attributed to the support that the overall temperance movement gave to the Jim Crow laws and other policies and organizations that discriminated against people of color (Herd, 1985). As a result, the rates of alcohol use began to rise again in the black community.

In spite of the increased involvement of blacks with alcohol, black drinking rates never surpassed those of whites and several other racial/ethnic groups (Herd, 1985). Today, the rates of black involvement in health-compromising alcohol use are low compared to the rates of many other U.S.-based groups (Substance Abuse and Mental Health Services Administration, 2008). Lighter patterns of drinking (abstention to moderate) tend to be the most prevalent patterns of drinking for blacks overall (Caetano, Clark, & Tam, 1998); however, the problems that they experience as a result of alcohol use are disproportionately high (Caetano, 1997; Ellickson et al., 1996; Herd, 1985; Wallace, 1999). This constitutes the major inequity that blacks experience related to alcohol and it will be the primary focus of this chapter.

The following sections provide an analysis of the problem of alcohol use among blacks across the life span. This discussion provides (1) a review of the epidemiology of alcohol use among blacks in the United States and the health, social, and physical consequences that they experience related to use; (2) a review of several social determinants of alcohol use known to compromise the health and social welfare of many within this population; and (3) a description of innovative methods for developing a multilevel understanding of these social and contextual determinants over the life course. Finally, throughout history, we have observed that the social and environmental context have influenced patterns of drinking and related problems among U.S.-based blacks. This chapter provides suggestions for developing interventions that may prove to be more relevant for populations of blacks living in the variety of rural, urban, and suburban contexts offered by the United States at this point in the country's sociopolitical history.

EPIDEMIOLOGY

Alcohol Use

Alcohol use in the United States rarely occurs prior to age 12 regardless of the racial or ethnic group of the target population. Most report their age of first use as being between the ages of 15 and 17 years (Substance Abuse and Mental Health Services Administration, 2004). In general, persons who report initiation of alcohol use prior to age 15 are at significantly increased risk of experiencing alcohol abuse or dependence compared to those who initiate at older ages (Chen, Dufour, & Yi, 2004/2005; Grant, Stinson, & Harford, 2001; Hawkins et al., 1997; Substance Abuse and Mental Health Services Administration, 2004).

Blacks have some of the lowest rates of drinking, relative to other racial groups, for all patterns of drinking. These patterns include past month alcohol use ($\geq$ 1 drink in the past month), binge or heavy episodic alcohol use ($\geq$ 5 drinks on the same occasion in past month) and frequent heavy episodic alcohol use ($\geq$ 5 drinks on the same occasion on $\geq$ 5 days in the past month) (Substance Abuse and Mental Health Services Administration, 2008). In a recent study of young adult drinkers, black young adults reported the oldest average age of drinking onset (18 years old), lowest estimates of heavy episodic drinking (approximately 23 days), lowest frequency of intoxication (13 days), lowest drinking quantity (approximately three drinks/drinking day) and lowest tolerance (approximately four drinks) in the past year compared to other groups (Chen et al., 2004/2005).

Table 20.1 illustrates the 2007 estimates of alcohol use for persons aged 12 and older. It shows that blacks reported the third lowest prevalence of drinking for past month/current drinking and second lowest for binge drinking. This tells us that although blacks are not the most problematic drinkers, they are certainly engaging in alcohol use behaviors.

Although the prevalence for heavy alcohol use was not reported in Table 20.1, we show the prevalence of this behavior among persons aged 12–20 in Table 20.2. During this period of the life course, blacks display the lowest prevalence of heavy drinking behavior. In fact, according to results of the 2007 National Survey of Drug Use and Health, all race/ethnicities exhibit the highest prevalence of heavy drinking between the ages of 18 and 30 and then decrease at later points in the life span. It is unlikely that blacks surpass other groups in their prevalence of heavy drinking between the ages of 18 and 30 (young adulthood), but these results were not reported for 2007 so that cannot be stated as a matter of fact.

However, if we look back at past surveillance data, when young adult data was reported (Table 20.3), we find that blacks report the lowest prevalence of drinking for all categories of drinking. The differences between blacks and all groups except Asians are quite large for binge and heavy alcohol use compared to past month/current use. These comparisons are displayed to emphasize, again, the lighter and less prevalent patterns of drinking by blacks relative to other groups in the United States.

TABLE 20.1 **2007 Prevalence of Past Month/Current and Binge Alcohol Use Among Persons Aged 12 or Older by Category of Drinking by Race/Ethnicity.**

Race	Past Month Alcohol Use*	Binge Alcohol Use*
White	56.1	24.6
Black/African American	39.3	19.1
Hispanic	23.4	23.4
Native American/Alaska Native	44.7	28.2
Asian	35.2	12.6
≥ 2 Races	47.7	23.2

*No estimates for past month or binge alcohol use for Native Hawaiians/Other Pacific Islanders.
Source: SAMHSA, Office of Applied Studies, National Survey on Drug Use and Health, 2008.

TABLE 20.2 **2007 Prevalence of Heavy Alcohol Use Among Persons Aged 12 to 20 by Race/Ethnicity.**

Race	Heavy Alcohol Use*
White	8.0
Black/African American	1.5
Hispanic	4.1
Native Hawaiian/Other Pacific Islander	4.7
Asian	1.9
≥ 2 Races	5.0

*No estimates reported for heavy alcohol use for Native American/Alaska Native.
Source: SAMHSA, Office of Applied Studies, National Survey on Drug Use and Health, 2008.

TABLE 20.3 **2003 Prevalence of Alcohol Use Among Persons Aged 18 to 25 by Category of Drinking.**

Race	Past Month Alcohol Use	Binge Alcohol Use	Heavy Alcohol Use
White	68.0	47.8	19.0
Black/African American	47.2	24.2	5.4
Native American/Alaska Native	52.3	41.6	13.0
Asian	48.9	27.8	7.8
≥ 2 Races	66.6	40.0	16.6

*No estimates reported for Hawaiian/Pacific Islanders.
Source: SAMHSA, Office of Applied Studies, National Survey on Drug Use and Health, 2004.

Alcohol-related Consequences

In spite of blacks' relative moderation in the use of alcohol, they suffer disproportionately from the physical and social consequences of drinking (Jones-Webb, 1998; National Institute on Alcohol Abuse and Alcoholism, 2001; Wallace et al., 1999). These consequences include, but are not limited to, problems at school or work, problems with friends or spouses (Bailey & Rachal, 1993; Caetano & Clark, 1998), family instability (Caetano et al., 2005; Ramisetty-Mikler & Caetano, 2004), drinking and driving, problems with the police, emotional problems (Caetano, 1993, 1997; Caetano & Clark, 1998; Caetano & McGrath, 2005), and physical problems such as liver disease, alcoholic cardiomyopathy, pancreatitis, and fetal alcohol syndrome (National Institute on Alcohol Abuse and Alcoholism, 2001). Prior research has also revealed that blacks are disproportionately affected by consequences such as intimate partner violence (Caetano et al., 2000). Rates of alcohol-related mortality due to alcohol-related car crashes are also consistently higher among blacks than among those in majority populations, after controlling for age, income, education, employment status, and levels of alcohol use (Jones-Webb, 1998). Blacks have also been found to have a higher incidence and chronicity of the social consequences of alcohol use than do majority groups (Caetano, 1997).

Some studies suggest that one reason why blacks experience higher numbers of alcohol-related problems than non-minorities is related to the greater density of alcohol outlets in minority communities than in non-minority communities (Alaniz, 1998; LaVeist & Wallace, 2000). The neighborhoods with high alcohol outlet densities are associated with higher rates of alcohol-related problems such as public drunkenness, drunken driving, violence, and homicide (Alaniz, 1998). These problems may occur because social restrictions are relaxed and monitoring is limited in areas where alcohol outlets are highly concentrated (Alaniz, 1998). This is just one of several reasons why the level of alcohol use is not a sufficient explanation for disparate alcohol-related problems in minority communities.

The Focus on Young People

Historically, the majority of attention in the area of alcohol prevention and treatment has been on adolescents aged 12–17 years or adults aged 18 years and older. However, very little focus has been placed on understanding drinking behavior within the sub-group of emerging adults aged 18–25 other than those enrolled in colleges and universities. The focus on adolescence is clear because it is the period when most initiate alcohol use. The age of alcohol use onset and the patterns of use in adolescence also influence alcohol use outcomes later in life (Grant et al., 2001; Wagner, Lloyd, & Gil, 2002).

The studies focused on populations aged 18 years and older tend to track trends in alcohol use and examine alcohol treatment and treatment outcomes. With the exception of college populations, there is relatively little in the alcohol literature focused on young adults aged 18–25 years. Prior studies of young adults draw primarily from in-school college populations and focus on campus drinking (Quigley & Marlatt, 1996). Yet, college-bound high school seniors of all races, including blacks, are less likely to report occasions of heavy drinking than high school seniors not bound for college (Johnston, O'Malley, & Bachman, 2000). Additionally, since 1980, college students have reported daily drinking rates that are lower than their non-college peers (Johnston, O'Malley, & Bachman, 2000). College campuses constitute a limited setting for black young adults; and relative to whites, blacks constitute the minority of enrollment in degree-granting institutions (US Department of Education, 2001).

As previously noted, blacks are more likely to initiate alcohol use in late adolescence or young adulthood. As a result, young adulthood may serve as a critical period in the trajectory of alcohol use and related problems for blacks.

SOCIAL DETERMINANTS OF ALCOHOL USE AND RELATED PROBLEMS

Alcohol use and related problems experienced by young blacks stem from several determinants. The preponderance of evidence on the etiology of alcohol use among young people derives from studies focused on the relationship between psychosocial factors (parents, family, peers, personality, behaviors, and gender) (Donovan, 2004) and alcohol use. The majority of evidence on the etiology of alcohol-related problems derives from studies focused on the relationship between levels of alcohol use and related problems. A minority of studies on alcohol-related problems has focused on investigating determinants, other than alcohol use. In the cases where studies focus on other determinants of alcohol-related problems, they are often psychosocial determinants that contribute to the etiology of these problems within the population in general, but not among blacks specifically.

A select few psychosocial determinants of alcohol use and related problems are briefly reviewed below. This is by no means a comprehensive list, but they are determinants that have been found to influence alcohol use and related outcomes in young people, and are believed to be salient for young blacks.

THEORETICAL PERSPECTIVES ON THE ISSUE

Prior investigations of minority substance use have attempted to use social and behavioral science theory to understand how alcohol problems develop. One such theory is primary socialization theory, which attempts to explain how the social environment may influence trajectories of problem drinking. Primary socialization theory posits that normative and deviant behaviors, such as problem drinking, are learned (Oetting & Donnermmeyer, 1998). The theory's fundamental tenets are that there are specific sources for learning social norms in every society, and that family, peers, and school serve as the primary socialization sources for adolescents in Western society (Oetting & Donnermmeyer, 1998). The theory also identifies secondary sources of socialization, with religion as one of those secondary sources.

NORMS ABOUT ALCOHOL USE

Friends/Peers

According to primary socialization theory, bonds with peers dominate when bonds with other primary socialization sources such as parents are weak. Although peer bonds are not always negative, peers are the socialization source with the highest probability of transmitting deviant norms (Nurco & Lerner, 1999; Oetting & Donnermmeyer, 1998; Octting et al., 1998). This happens when peer groups consist of adolescents with high potential for deviance (Oetting & Donnermmeyer, 1998).

The transmission of behavioral norms from friends and peers in early to middle adolescence has been demonstrated and widely documented in studies of adolescent alcohol and other substance use behaviors. One study demonstrated associations between peer attitudes toward adolescent drinking and initiation of adolescent alcohol use in a study of African American middle school students (Sullivan & Farrell, 1999). The study found that peer approval was significantly and positively related to adolescent use of beer and wine (Sullivan & Farrell, 1999). In another study of adolescent drinking, investigators also found that perceived peer norms and perceived friend use, along with other social influences and problem behaviors, were associated with adolescent alcohol use in a sample of black and Hispanic seventh graders (Epstein et al., 1999).

Parental/Family

Evidence for the transmission of alcohol use norms by parents is provided by studies of parent alcohol use behavior (Chassin et al., 1996; Jackson et al., 1997; McNeal & Amato, 2000), parental attitudes toward adolescent alcohol use (approval/disapproval)

(Li, Duncan, & Hops, 2001), and parent communication about alcohol use (Ennett et al., 2001). Only one study was found to have investigated parent/family approval of adolescent alcohol and other drug use in a population of young blacks. In contrast to studies based on predominantly white samples, Sullivan and Farrell (1999) found that parent/family approval of alcohol and other drug use was not significantly related to the prevalence of alcohol use in a population of eighth graders in a southeastern U.S. city.

There is also a growing body of literature on the influence of parental communication on adolescent behavior, but the findings concerning these influences on risky adolescent behaviors are somewhat equivocal. In one study, mother communication with adolescent males about delinquent behaviors was not a deterrent to delinquent behaviors, including the use of alcohol (Paschall, Ringwalt, & Flewelling, 2003). Other studies have found that parental communication may have a protective effect on adolescent alcohol use and its absence may be deleterious. A cross-sectional study of adolescent substance use (including alcohol) revealed that parent-child communication was inversely related to substance use in late adolescence (Kafka & London, 1991). Additionally, findings from a longitudinal study of parental communication showed that infrequent parent-child communication was associated with the highest rates of alcohol use among a racially mixed sample of young people in early to middle adolescence (Cohen, Richardson, & LaBree, 1994).

Religion

Black youth are embedded in the primary socialization network of family, peers, and religion. Although the theory identifies religion as a secondary socialization source, religion, religiosity, and faith are central to the culture and lives of most blacks in the United States. It may actually be a primary socialization source in the lives of blacks.

Data on the level of involvement of U.S. blacks in religion and religious institutions suggest that by the time members of this group reach adolescence, religious identification may serve as a primary socialization source. Due to the black church's embrace of the Colored Temperance Movement in the early nineteenth century, religious norms are more likely to influence problem drinking (Herd, 1985). The Colored Temperance Movement discouraged blacks from using alcoholic beverages. Although the black church is no longer affiliated with this movement, its norms and values may still operate through the church to discourage drinking in the black community today.

Studies have shown that 95 percent of all U.S. adolescents seventeen years and younger believe in God or a Universal Spirit/Higher Power; the percentage of adults that believe in God or a Universal Spirit/Higher Power is approximately the same (Gallup & Lindsay, 1999; Wallace & Forman, 1998). A higher proportion of blacks in the United States practice religion ardently relative to other major U.S. racial groups (Benson, Donahue, & Erickson, 1989). Most blacks consider religion to be very important in their lives (82%) (Benson, Donahue, & Erickson, 1989). They think religion can answer all or most of today's problems (86%), and most are formal members of churches (82%) (Gallup & Lindsay, 1999). The majority of U.S. blacks are Christians: 75 percent are Protestant (mostly Southern Baptist and many of the other Baptist conventions) and 10 percent are Roman Catholic (Gallup & Lindsay, 1999). Black adolescents have the highest rates of church attendance and are more likely to be involved in religious youth groups than adolescents of other racial backgrounds (Smith et al., 2002).

Additionally, a nationally representative, cross-sectional study of high school seniors provides evidence of religious identification as a determinant of pro-social behavior. The study demonstrated that seniors who attended religious services weekly, those for whom religion was very important, and those who participated in religious youth groups for at least six years were more likely to have never gotten drunk or to delay getting drunk significantly longer than were non-religious youth (Smith & Faris, 2002). These youth were also less likely to go to bars and drink to get drunk than non-religious youth (Smith & Faris, 2002).

Religion and religiosity have also been shown to be determinants of pro-social and normative behaviors in young adults. In a cross-sectional study conducted by Patock-Peckham, Hutchinson, Cheong, and Nagoshi (1998), college students with no religious affiliation reported significantly higher levels of drinking frequency, quantity, and drunkenness than those with religious affiliations. These students were also more likely to drink for celebratory reasons and to perceive that a variety of social influences indicate higher amounts of alcohol as being appropriate for consumption (Patock-Peckham et al., 1998). In a review of the literature on adult religiosity and drinking, and other drug use, investigators found that adult populations who were religious/spiritually involved or who had high religious identification tended to be less likely to engage in alcohol and other drug use than those who were not (Miller, 1998). The Miller (1998) review also revealed that individuals who were currently suffering from alcohol and other drug involvement were found to have low religious involvement or identification.

SALIENT THEORY FOR YOUNG ADULTS

Though primary socialization theory is certainly relevant to the lives of young adults (particularly those on the younger end of this period of the life span), as this population ages, more macrolevel theories of the etiology of alcohol use and related problems may take precedence. Sociological theories about race, social networks, social capital, or social position may better explain alcohol use behavior and its consequences as black adolescents age into young adults (Godette, Headen, & Ford, 2006). Additionally, theories that account for multiple levels of influence across the life span, such as ecosocial theory (Krieger, 1994), may be more relevant than psychosocial theories for black young adults. The more macrolevel theories are also more likely to explain the development of alcohol-related problems than are psychosocial theories. The inequities that blacks experience related to alcohol-related problems mostly stem from racism and discrimination, lower levels of social position, reduced access to care and services, and relatively worse employment, housing, and neighborhood conditions than majority populations face in this country.

INTERVENING ON ALCOHOL USE AND RELATED PROBLEMS IN THE BLACK COMMUNITY

The primary mode of intervention for young blacks is through school-based universal alcohol prevention programs. These programs do not address the needs of specific subpopulations of adolescents. Rather, they are designed to address determinants believed to be common among all groups of young people. But these determinants are often psychosocial in nature, and the development of such programs is often based on data from etiological studies of majority populations. There are many small, selective prevention programs developed to target young blacks, but many of these programs have not been rigorously evaluated, and they are not well disseminated. Additional work on the evaluation and dissemination of promising and proven programs that target young blacks is indicated.

The programs targeting young adults, often considered secondary prevention programs because they are designed for those who have tried alcohol and are at risk for progression to problematic use, are primarily based in college and university settings. At this level, selective prevention programs that target specific groups within the population are more prevalent than the selective programs available for adolescents. Groups commonly targeted for these interventions are athletes and sports fans and members of Greek letter organizations.

Most black young adults who do attend college attend historically black colleges and universities (HBCUs). These settings are very different from predominantly white institutions (PWIs). In fact, there is evidence that there may be something protective about HBCUs relative to PWIs (Weitzman, Nelson, & Wechsler, 2003); however, the mechanism by which HBCUs protect against alcohol problems is still not well understood.

Unfortunately, colleges and universities are still not the usual setting for most black young adults, and this larger segment of black young adults, not attending colleges or universities, is often overlooked in prevention programming. The lack of programming for this population becomes fertile ground for progression to problematic alcohol use. This group is particularly vulnerable because, during young adulthood, young people experience many transitions that may induce stress. The transitions include, but are not limited to, leaving home, joining the labor force as full- or part-time employees, establishing long-term relationships such as marriage, and childbearing (Arnett, 2000, 2001). These transitions are especially stressful for black young adults because they occupy minority status in the United States. Blacks are more vulnerable to societal inequities as young adults than they are at earlier points in the life course.

When out-of-school black young adults are fortunate enough to participate in an alcohol intervention, they have often already progressed to the point of needing tertiary-level interventions (treatment). This type of intervention is the most costly to both the individual and society, and there are still concerns about whether or not blacks receive appropriate alcohol treatment in terms of the match to treatment modality (e.g., inpatient vs. outpatient), type of treatment (e.g., cognitive behavioral therapy, self-help), and treatment provider (e.g., clinician's experience and orientation toward working with young black clients). These areas of alcohol treatment research warrant further study in conjunction with the studies on disparities in treatment access.

THE NEXT GENERATION OF ALCOHOL INTERVENTIONS

We have now moved into the era of the next generation of alcohol interventions that are most likely to have significant impact on the health and social well-being of blacks. These interventions focus less on individuals and more on physical environments and social context. Earlier in the chapter, we proposed that young adulthood might be a critical period in the development of alcohol-related disparities experienced by blacks. We also proposed that multilevel and macrolevel theories that account for the individual as well as the physical and social environments are most relevant to this population. As a result, interventions that focus on the modifiable potential of characteristics of the physical and social environment are indicated (Furr-Holden et al., 2008).

Neighborhoods and communities play an important role in determining health outcomes. Vandalism, vacant houses, vacant lots, alcohol billboards, transit placards and other advertisements, lack of green space, noise pollution, densely populated neighborhoods, and high densities of alcohol outlets all contribute to risk for alcohol-related problems. These determinants serve as indicators of decay and low levels of social cohesion within neighborhoods. There is no evidence that these environments contribute to increases in alcohol use within black communities but there is evidence that they contribute to alcohol-related problems for those that do drink (Alaniz, 1998).

Future interventions that focus on modifying neighborhood blight, low social cohesion, and targeted alcohol advertisements will do much to change the prevalence of alcohol problems within the black community. We have both the ability to tailor these multilevel interventions by individual community and the methods for evaluating their efficacy (Furr-Holden et al., 2008).

POLICY IMPLICATIONS

Federal, state, or local programs that encourage collaborative efforts with faith-based institutions may play an important role in interventions that target blacks from adolescence and beyond. We have established that the church is an important part of the life of most black Americans so it may serve as a ready base for community-based alcohol interventions. Churches and other faith-based institutions are often landmark establishments in neighborhoods. They prove to be good neighbors and positive prosocial influences on young people.

Local policymakers should focus on eliminating alcohol advertisements (billboards, transportation placards, and events where alcohol sponsors might advertise) in areas where residential housing, elementary and secondary schools, or colleges and universities exist. The presence and density of alcohol advertisements is indicative of the accessibility of alcohol in the area. In conjunction with reductions in alcohol advertising, local policymakers should more critically evaluate the locations where businesses are allowed to sell and/or serve alcohol. The guidelines for the areas where these businesses can operate must be consistent with the guidelines for where alcohol can be advertised.

Taxation has also proved to be a very effective intervention with other health behaviors such as tobacco use. The higher the taxes on alcohol products, the less likely individuals are to use them. Young people are particularly sensitive to pricing.

Finally, policies that facilitate mental health parity will increase access to alcohol treatment. Mental health parity guarantees dollar-for-dollar benefits for issues such as addictions treatment as compared with other medical services. It guarantees rights to a more reasonable number of treatment visits than has been guaranteed in the past. It also stops the practice of differential co-pays for addictions services as compared with medical services.

CONCLUSIONS

Blacks are less likely to drink and have lighter patterns of drinking when they do drink than many other U.S.-based racial and ethnic groups. However, from birth to death, they suffer disproportionately from the health and social consequences of drinking. This chapter identifies adolescence and young adulthood as important periods in the trajectory of black drinking. Adolescence is important because it is when most initiate drinking. Young adulthood is important because it is a time when young people experience transitions and societal factors that may leave them more prone to drinking and related problems. It is also a period when the prevalence of drinking is highest for all patterns of drinking and in all racial and ethnic groups (including blacks).

When we think about what period of the life course is most important to intervene on the progression of alcohol-related problems, we must look to young adulthood. We must also think more broadly than the long-time standard one-dimensional interventions that address psychosocial factors. Public health practitioners and researchers must develop interventions that move past the individual and help us to even the playing field for blacks as a group. These interventions are multilevel in nature and developed in the context of the physical and social environment of the target community. Future research on alcohol-related problems and blacks should also further probe social position, based on the black experience, and policy interventions that may reduce related risks for blacks.

REFERENCES

Alaniz, M. (1998). Alcohol availability and targeted advertising in racial/ethnic minority communities. *Alcohol Health & Research World, 22*(4), 286–289.

Arnett, J. (2000). Emerging adulthood: A theory of development from the late teens through the twenties. *American Psychologist, 55*(5), 469–480.

Arnett, J. (2001). Conceptions of the transition to adulthood: Perspectives from adolescence through midlife. *Journal of Adult Development, 8*(2), 133–143.

Bailey, S., & Rachal, J. (1993). Dimensions of adolescent problem drinking. *Journal of Studies on Alcohol, 54,* 555–565.

Benson, P., Donahue, M., & Erickson, J. (1989). Adolescence and religion: A review of the literature from 1970 to 1986. *Social Scientific Study of Religion, 1*, 153–181.

Caetano, R. (1993). The association between severity of DSM-III-R alcohol dependence and medical and social consequences. *Addiction, 88*, 631–642.

Caetano, R. (1997). Prevalence, incidence, and stability of drinking problems among whites, blacks and Hispanics: 1984–1992. *Journal of Studies on Alcohol, 58*, 565–572.

Caetano, R., & Clark, C. (1998). Trends in alcohol-related problems among whites, blacks, and Hispanics: 1984–1995. *Alcoholism: Clinical and Experimental Research, 22*(2), 534–538.

Caetano, R., Clark, C., & Tam, T. (1998). Alcohol consumption among racial/ethnic minorities: Theory and research. *Alcohol World: Health & Research, 22*(4), 233–241.

Caetano, R., Cunradi, C. B., Clark, C. L., & Schafer, J. (2000). Intimate partner violence and drinking patterns among white, black, and Hispanic couples in the U.S. *Journal of Substance Abuse, 11*(2), 123–138.

Caetano, R., & McGrath, C. (2005). Driving under the influence (DUI) among U.S. ethnic groups. *Accident Analysis & Prevention, 37*(2), 217–224.

Caetano, R., McGrath, C., Ramisetty-Mikler, S., & Field, C. (2005). Drinking, alcohol problems and the five-year recurrence and incidence of male to female and female to male partner violence. *Alcohol: Clinical and Experimental Research, 29*(1), 98–106.

Chassin, L., Curran, P., Hussong, A., & Colder, C. (1996). The relation of parent alcoholism to adolescent substance use: A longitudinal follow-up study. *Journal of Abnormal Psychology, 105*(1).

Chen, C., Dufour, M., & Yi, H. (2004/2005). Alcohol consumption among young adults 18–24 in the United States: Results from the 2001–2002 NESARC survey. *Alcohol Research & Health, 28*(4), 269–280.

Christmon, K. (1995). Historical overview of alcohol in the African American community. *Journal of Black Studies, 25*(3), 318–330.

Cohen, D., Richardson, J., & LaBree, L. (1994). Parenting behaviors and the onset of smoking and alcohol use: A longitudinal study. *Pediatrics, 94*(3), 368–375.

Donovan, J. (2004). Adolescent alcohol initiation: A review of psychosocial risk factors. *Journal of Adolescent Health, 35*, 529.e7–529.e18.

Ellickson, P., McGuigan, K., Adams, V., Bell, R., & Hays, R. (1996). Teenagers and alcohol misuse in the United States: By any definition, it's a big problem. *Addiction, 91*(10), 1489–1503.

Ennett, S., Bauman, K., Foshee, V., Pemberton, M., & Hicks, K. (2001). Parent-child communication about adolescent tobacco and alcohol use: What do parents say and does it affect youth behavior? *Journal of Marriage and the Family, 63*, 48–62.

Epstein, J., Botvin, G., Baker, E., & Diaz, T. (1999). Impact of social influences and problem behavior on alcohol use among inner-city Hispanic and black adolescents. *Journal of Studies on Alcohol, 60*, 595–604.

Furr-Holden, C., Smart, M., Pokorni, J., Ialongo, N., Leaf, P., Holder, H., et al. (2008). The NIfETy method for environmental assessment of neighborhood-level indicators of violence, alcohol and other drug exposure. *Prevention Science, 9*(4), 245–255.

Gallup, G., & Lindsay, D. (1999). *Surveying the Religious Landscape: Trends in U.S. Beliefs*. Harrisburg, PA: Morehouse Publishing.

Godette, D., Headen, S., & Ford, C. (2006). Windows of opportunity: Fundamental concepts for understanding alcohol-related disparities experienced by young blacks in the United States. *Prevention Science, 7*, 377–387.

Grant, B., Stinson, F., & Harford, T. (2001). Age of onset of alcohol use and DSM-IV alcohol abuse and dependence. *Journal of Substance Abuse, 13*, 493–504.

Hawkins, J. D., Graham, J. W., Maguin, E., Abbott, R., Hill, K. G., & Catalano, R. F. (1997). Exploring the effects of age of alcohol use initiation and psychosocial risk factors on subsequent alcohol misuse. *Journal of Studies on Alcohol, 58*, 280–290.

Herd, D. (1985). The epidemiology of drinking patterns and alcohol-related problems among US blacks. In D. Spiegler, D. Tate, S. Aitken, C. Christian (eds.), *Alcohol Use Among U.S. Ethnic Minorities* (Vol. 18, pp. 3–45). Rockville, MD: U.S. Department of Health and Human Services.

Jackson, C., Henriksen, L., Dickinson, D., & Levine, D. (1997). The early use of alcohol and tobacco: Its relation to children's competence and parents' behavior. *American Journal of Public Health, 87*(3), 359–364.

Johnston, L., O'Malley, P., & Bachman, J. (2000). *Monitoring the Future National Survey Results on Drug Use, 1975–1999, Volume II: College Students & Adults Ages 19–40*. Rockville, MD: U.S. Department of Health and Human Services, Public Health Service, National Institute of Health, National Institute on Drug Abuse.

Jones-Webb, R. (1998). Drinking patterns and problems among African-Americans: Recent findings. *Alcohol World: Health & Research, 22*(4), 260–264.

Kafka, R. R., & London, P. (1991). Communication in relationships and adolescent substance use: The influence of parents and friends. *Adolescence, 26*(103), 587–597.

Krieger, N. (1994). Epidemiology and the web of causation: Has anyone seen the spider? *Social Science & Medicine, 39*(7), 887–903.

LaVeist, T., & Wallace, J. (2000). Health risk and inequitable distribution of liquor stores in African American neighborhoods. *Social Science & Medicine, 51*, 613–617.

Li, F., Duncan, T., & Hops, H. (2001). Examining developmental trajectories in adolescent alcohol use using piecewise growth mixture modeling analysis. *Journal of Studies on Alcohol, 62*, 199–210.

McNeal, C., & Amato, P. (2000). Parental alcohol use: Effects on African American and White adults. *Race & Society, 3*, 61–74.

Miller, W. (1998). Researching the spiritual dimensions of alcohol and other drug problems. *Addiction, 93*(7), 979–990.

National Institute on Alcohol Abuse and Alcoholism. (2001). Strategic Plan to Address Health Disparities. Retrieved October 9, 2004, from http://www.niaaa.nih.gov/Publications

Nurco, D., & Lerner, M. (1999). A complementary perspective to primary socialization theory. *Substance Use & Misuse, 34*(7), 993–1003.

Oetting, E., & Donnermmeyer, J. (1998). Primary socialization theory: The etiology of drug use and deviance. I. *Substance Use & Misuse, 33*(4), 995–1026.

Oetting, E., Donnermmeyer, J., Trimble, J., & Beavais, F. (1998). Primary socialization theory: Culture, ethnicity, and cultural identification. The links between culture and substance use. IV. *Substance Use & Misuse, 33*(10), 2075–2107.

Paschall, M., Ringwalt, C., & Flewelling, R. (2003). Effects of parenting, father absence, and affiliation with delinquent peers on delinquent behavior among African-American male adolescents. *Adolescence, 38*(149), 16–34.

Patock-Peckham, J., Hutchinson, G., Cheong, J., & Nagoshi, C. (1998). Effect of religion and religiosity on alcohol use in a college student sample. *Drug and Alcohol Dependence, 49*, 81–88.

Quigley, L., & Marlatt, G. (1996). Drinking among young adults. *Alcohol World: Health & Research, 20*(3), 185–191.

Ramisetty-Mikler, S., & Caetano, R. (2004). Ethnic differences in the estimates of children exposed to alcohol problems and alcohol dependence in the United States. *Journal of Studies on Alcohol, 65*(5), 593–599.

Smith, C., Denton, M., Faris, R., & Regnerus, M. (2002). Mapping American adolescent religious participation. *Journal for the Scientific Study of Religion, 41*(4), 597–612.

Smith, C., & Faris, R. (2002). *Religion and American adolescent delinquency, risk behaviors and constructive social activities* (No. 1). Chapel Hill: The University of North Carolina at Chapel Hill.

Substance Abuse and Mental Health Services Administration. (2004). *Alcohol dependence or abuse and age at first use*. Rockville, MD: Author.

Substance Abuse and Mental Health Services Administration. (2008). Results from the National Survey on Drug Use and Health: National Findings. In Office of Applied Studies (Ed.), *NSDUH Series H-32* (pp. 31–40). Rockville, MD.

Sullivan, T., & Farrell, A. (1999). Identification and impact of risk and protective factors for drug use among urban African American adolescents. *Journal of Clinical Child Psychology, 28*(2), 122–136.

U.S. Department of Education, National Center for Education Statistics. (2001). Digest of Education Statistics, 2001. Retrieved May 1, 2002, from http://nces.ed.gov/pubs2002/digest2001/tables/dt207.asp

Wagner, E., Lloyd, D., & Gil, A. (2002). Racial/ethnic and gender differences in the incidence and onset of DSM-IV alcohol use disorder symptoms among adolescents. *Journal of Studies on Alcohol, 63*, 609–619.

Wallace, J. (1999). Explaining race differences in adolescent and young adult drug use: The role of racialized social systems. *Drugs and Society, 14*(1–2), 21–36.

Wallace, J., & Forman, T. (1998). Religion's role in promoting health and reducing risk among American youth. *Health Education & Behavior, 25*(6), 721–741.

Wallace, J., Forman, T., Guthrie, B., Bachman, J., O'Malley, P., & Johnston, L. (1999). The epidemiology of alcohol, tobacco, and other drug use among black youth. *Journal of Studies on Alcohol, 60*, 800–809.

Weitzman, E. R., Nelson, T. F., & Wechsler, H. (2003). Taking up binge drinking in college: The influences of person, social group, and environment. *Journal of Adolescent Health, 32*(1), 26–35.

Welte, J., & Barnes, G. (1987). Alcohol use among adolescent minority groups. *Journal of Studies on Alcohol, 48*(4), 329–366.

CHAPTER

21

NUTRITION AND OBESITY ISSUES FOR AFRICAN AMERICANS

MONICA L. BASKIN
ANGELA M. ODOMS-YOUNG
SHIRIKI K. KUMANYIKA
JAMY D. ARD

A large body of evidence has emphasized the role of nutrition and dietary intake in growth, development, and the sustaining of life, as well in the prevention and management of chronic diseases (World Health Organization, 2003). Higher or lower than optimal intake of certain dietary constituents is associated with cardiovascular diseases, obesity, diabetes, and certain cancers (Dietary Guidelines Advisory Committee, 2005; World Health Organization, 2003). Differences in dietary intake between black Americans and white Americans have been documented (Kant et al., 2007) and are parallel to disproportionately high rates of morbidity and mortality among black Americans (Arab et al., 2003; Kumanyika & Krebs-Smith, 2001).

Addressing the issue of food and dietary intake among black Americans is quite complex. Food insecurity (i.e., the sense of not having enough to eat) among black households is nearly three times the rate of white households (22.2% vs. 7.9%, respectively) (Nord et al., 2008). At the same time, rates of overweight and obesity (which for most people is a function of overconsumption of calories and/or inadequate physical activity) are also significantly higher among blacks than whites (Ogden et al., 2006). Further, even if overconsumption of calories is a large culprit in obesity among blacks, the quality of this food may be inadequate as the intakes of essential nutrients are still below recommended levels (Kumanyika & Krebs-Smith, 2001; Reis et al., 2008). As a result, efforts to restrict and/or modify the diets of blacks may be especially challenging.

In this chapter, we describe some of the primary aspects of dietary behaviors and obesity as they relate to the health of black Americans, discussing relevant social, cultural, and environmental factors. We include implications for population health promotion, research, and policy, and conclude by offering recommendations for improving the health of the black community and reducing the disparity relative to whites.

WHAT DO AFRICAN AMERICANS EAT?

Historical and Social Influences

As with all ethnic groups, cultural food patterns of blacks reflect their social and historical experiences. The culinary heritage of foods commonly eaten in the black community has roots in Africa, the Caribbean, and U.S. slavery (Dirks & Duran, 2001; Hess, 1992). African slaves brought traditional West African cooking methods and foods such as black-eyed peas, okra, and watermelon. West African food traditions were modified based on food available to slaves in the South. Plants indigenous to North America were substituted for traditional West African ingredients (Poe, 1999). For the most part, food availability was largely contingent on provisions from slave owners and, as a result, varied from plantation to plantation. Common foods included salt pork and corn with rice, salted fish, and molasses used to a lesser extent based on availability (Sucher & Kittler, 2008). Some slaves supplemented their diets with vegetables grown in "their" gardens. Slaves also caught and ate small animals (e.g., opossums, rabbits, and raccoons) and fish (e.g.., catfish) in addition to food received. In the fall, hog slaughtering sometimes provided slaves with a variety of pork cuts including ham hocks and intestines or chitterlings.

Women were primarily responsible for food preparation on most plantations (Poe, 1999). Meal patterns and cooking techniques were adapted to plantation work schedules and available resources for cooking. Field work was done from dawn to dusk, yielding 12-to-14-hour work days for slaves. This allowed only a small amount of time to procure and prepare meals. Breakfast was the largest meal to sustain slaves during work in the fields, with lunch or the afternoon meal consisting of leftovers or one-dish vegetable stews (Sucher & Kittler, 2008). Evening meals were also commonly one-pot dishes that were prepared in the morning and cooked throughout the day (Poe, 1999). One-pot meals and stewing were preferred due to a dearth of cooking utensils and the need to prepare multiple items at once. Frying was used as a means of quick preparation for meats and breads because the time-consuming alternatives of roasting or baking were not options (Seemes, 1996). Sundays and holidays were times when extended family and friends came together to share larger meals, reflecting communal patterns and gatherings common in African societies (Poe, 1999).

These food patterns continued after emancipation from slavery and were further shaped by the employment and economic situation of black Americans. For example, during sharecropping, blacks focused on cash crops and continued to acquire foods similar to those during slavery (Whitehead, 1992). A significant amount of food was obtained from white landowners using cash or on credit. The diets of blacks remaining in the South typically included staples such as fat salt pork, molasses, cornmeal, flour, sweet potatoes, and greens. Secondary food items such as fish, ham, eggs, rice, fruit, etc. were occasionally present, but dependent on seasonal variation in crops planted. In general, energy intake was lower in the winter months when food sources were more limited (Dirks & Duran, 2001).

Northern migration by freed blacks brought new challenges of having to adapt from agricultural to urban lifestyles. Although many dietary patterns continued, new work habits and food availability changed several aspects of the traditional meal patterns. The diets of northern blacks were more likely to include beef, wheat, and white potatoes, unlike blacks residing in the South (Dirks & Duran, 2001). In addition, northern migration saw daily meals become lighter, whereas communal meals on Sunday and holidays continued to be large and included extended kinship groups and traditional favorites (Jerome, 1969).

Food habits among blacks in the United States are often described as reflecting a "Southern diet" (American Dietetic Association, 1998; Veale-Jones & Darling, 1996). This may reflect both the high proportion of blacks who live or were raised in the South (Pollard & O'Hare, 1999) as well as the difficulty of labeling any other set of eating or food preparation practices common to African Americans. Others have characterized the diet of blacks as "soul food." For some the term represents the connection between the black diet and its roots in Africa and the Southern United States (Dirks & Duran, 2001). For others, it takes on a more spiritual meaning reflecting the struggles, sacrifices, and ingenuity taken to prepare the food (Liburd, 2003). As shown in Table 21.1, typical black core foods continue to reflect many of the foods and preparation methods brought from West Africa and foods available in the South. Characteristic preparation styles also continue to be popular, including frying meats in pork fat or other fat, stewing or boiling vegetables using pork as seasoning, and using excess sugars in desserts and drinks (Airhihenbuwa et al., 1996; Sucher & Kittler, 2008).

Healthful aspects of the traditional diet of blacks in the United States include the core position of certain plant foods such as legumes, dark green leafy vegetables, and yellow vegetables. These foods are inherently low in fat and salt and high in dietary fiber, and are also good sources of several protective nutrients. However, there is less habitual use of fresh fruits and vegetables, which are underconsumed by Americans in general. The traditional southern practice of cooking vegetables for long periods, and the addition of salted meat or fat as a seasoning for legumes or vegetables, adds significant sodium and calories from fat, detracting from their potential positive health benefits. The emphasis on rice, grits, and breads is consistent with the recommendation to

TABLE 21.1 Typical Characterization of the Southern African American Diet.

Core	Secondary	Infrequent
Rice	Bought (light) breads	
Corn bread	Spaghetti, meat	
Biscuits	Macaroni and cheese	
Grits		
Meat (pork and chicken)	Fish	
Meat; variety cuts		
Cooked green leafy vegetables	White potatoes	Fresh vegetables
Okra, tomatoes, legumes, corn, yams	Other vegetables	Fruits
	Desserts	Dairy

Source: Veale-Jones, D., & Darling, M. (1996). Ethnic Foodways in Minneosta. St. Paul, MN: University of Minnesota.

eat several servings of grain products daily, but if prepared in the traditional manner, high consumption of these foods may not be consistent with recommendations to decrease fat and salt intake. The intake of these grains is often in the refined format, where the husk containing the bulk of the fiber and key phytochemicals has been removed in the processing of the grain. White rice, processed grits, and white bread or flour may dominate the grain intake of blacks, displacing whole-grain alternatives that are more nutrient dense (Sucher & Kittler, 2008).

Having meat as part of a meal is a core value in black food habits that may have been protective historically, when meat was relatively unavailable or expensive and could only be obtained in small quantities. With meat now widely available and more affordable, blacks may be predisposed to overconsumption of meat and poultry (major sources of total and saturated fat) and disinclined to follow advice to consume fewer servings, substitute plant-based protein sources, and to have some meatless meals (Smit et al., 1999).

Dietary Intake and Quality

High intakes of calories, total fat and saturated fat, and salt, and low intakes of fiber and complex carbohydrates are associated with atherosclerosis, cancer, and diabetes. High salt intake is associated with low potassium intake, and this ratio may be a predisposing factor to high blood pressure and stroke (Dietary Guidelines Advisory Committee, 2005). Other diet–disease associations of current public health interest include the relationship of calcium intake to osteoporosis and, potentially, to colon cancer; the association of cataracts with low intakes of antioxidants; and the association of folic acid and other nutrients with birth outcomes and immune function (Bendich & Deckelbaum, 1997). These associations give rise to general recommendations to increase the proportion of caloric intake from plant foods in relation to animal foods (USDHHS & USDA, 2005). Increased intakes of fruits, vegetables, whole grains, and legumes (such as dried beans and peas) are recommended as plant sources of dietary fiber and protein, with a commensurate decrease in the consumption of meat and poultry (USDHHS and USDA, 2005). Fish (other than fried fish) is recommended because it is lower in either total fat or saturated fat than a portion of meat with the equivalent amount of protein. Fish such as salmon, tuna, and mackerel contain a type of fat (omega-3 fatty acids) that may have protective effects in relation to chronic disease development. A high intake of foods containing antioxidant substances (e.g., phytochemicals—certain vitamins or minerals or other constituents of plant foods with antioxidant activity) has also been associated with protection from chronic diseases, specifically cancer (Deckelbaum et al., 1999).

Food consumption patterns of Americans in general are inconsistent with recommendations for chronic disease prevention (USDHHS & USDA, 2005). The average consumption of grains and whole grains, fruits, vegetables, fiber, and dairy products tends to be lower than recommended, whereas total calorie consumption, total and saturated fat, cholesterol, and sugar-sweetened beverage intakes are higher than recommended (Nielsen et al., 2002).

With respect to current dietary recommendations, black food habits are a mixture of positives and negatives. Multiple studies indicate that blacks have lower energy intake from saturated fat and higher vitamin C intake relative to their white counterparts. At the same time, blacks have lower intakes of vegetables, potassium, and calcium (Kant et al., 2007). Such differences in dietary intake between blacks and whites have remained relatively stable over the past three decades (Kant et al., 2007) and may contribute to the persistence of disparities in chronic diseases (Arab et al., 2003; Kumanyika & Krebs-Smith, 2001).

The Healthy Eating Index (HEI) is a measure of diet quality developed by the U.S. Department of Agriculture to help with evaluating American diets in relation to current dietary guidance (Kennedy et al., 1995). The original HEI, released in 1995, was based on servings following the original Food Guide Pyramid: fruit, vegetables, grains, milk, and meat (USDA, 1996). More recently the HEI was updated to be consistent with the Dietary Guidelines for Americans, 2005 (Guenther et al., 2007). The HEI-2005 is based on twelve components: Total Fruit (includes 100% juice); Whole Fruit (forms other than juice); Total Vegetables; Dark Green and Orange Vegetables and Legumes (dry peas and beans); Total Grains; Whole Grains; Milk (includes all milk products and soy beverages); Meat and Beans (includes meat, poultry, fish, eggs, soybean products other than beverages, nuts, and seeds); Oils (includes nonhydrogenated vegetable oils and oils in fish, nuts, and seeds); Saturated Fat; Sodium; and Calories from Solid Fats, Alcoholic Beverages, and Added Sugars (SoFAAS).

An evaluation of national data using HEI-2005 to examine diet quality among racial/ethnic subgroups has yet to be published. However, the most recent review of diet quality by racial subgroup presents deficits in black American dietary quality relative to both dietary recommendations and their white peers. Relative to whites, black Americans score lower in overall diet quality, vegetable intake, and milk intake (all differences statistically significant) (Basiotis et al., 2002).

Is it possible that these dietary data overstate or understate dietary problems among black Americans? Dietary data, as such, are inherently error prone because of the day-to-day variability in what people eat, because people have difficulty in remembering and describing what they eat, and because self-reports of eating behavior may be biased for psychosocial reasons. In addition, because of the considerable intraperson variation in nutrient requirements and other factors such as food fortification, use of vitamin and mineral supplements, and physiological adaptability to varying levels of daily nutrient intakes, an individual with below-average or below-recommended intake might actually be meeting his or her nutritional needs. On the other hand, in populations where diagnoses of diet-related conditions such as high blood pressure or diabetes are common, people might have either modified their diets based on medical advice or might report their dietary intakes differently on this basis.

Another note of caution with respect to what we know about the diets of black Americans relates to the fallacy that black Americans are a homogenous group. We recognize that blacks in the United States represent a diverse group, with cultural variation including ethnicity (Hispanic vs. non-Hispanic) and country of birth (e.g., Caribbean). For example, some evidence suggests that Caribbean islanders maintain many aspects of their dietary patterns after migration to the United States. In a study comparing dietary risk factors among blacks in central Harlem, Caribbean-born respondents reported higher fruit and vegetable consumption compared to their Southern-born counterparts (Greenberg et al., 1998). Similarly, the analysis of national survey data by Lancaster and colleagues (2006) suggests blacks born outside of the United States consumed more healthful diets including higher fruit and vegetable intake, increased fiber and whole grains, and lower levels of total and saturated fat than their U.S.-born black counterparts (2006). Healthier dietary profiles for immigrants was also consistent with a more positive coronary heart disease (CHD) risk profile, reduced ten-year risk of CHD, and fewer CHD-related conditions (e.g., metabolic syndrome) than U.S.-born blacks (2006).

The issue of within-group variation in the black community is further underscored with a recent analysis of dietary patterns among black men and women (James, 2009). This study identified six clusters of black men with thirteen distinctive patterns of food consumption and six clusters of black women with fifteen distinctive patterns of food consumption. The clusters differed with respect to how closely they resembled national recommendations on dietary intake (James, 2009). Clearly, there is no such thing as "the black diet."

OVERWEIGHT AND OBESITY AMONG BLACKS IN THE UNITED STATES

The terms overweight and obesity reflect a range of weights that are believed to be heavier than is considered healthy for a particular height and that may increase the risk of certain diseases and health conditions (CDC, n.d.). Weight status is typically evaluated using the body mass index (BMI), a calculation comparing one's weight and height that is highly correlated with measures of body fatness for most people (NHLBI, 1998; Pietrobelli et al., 1998). Though there are myriad factors considered to contribute to overweight and obesity, energy imbalance, in which too many calories are consumed (diet) and not enough calories are burned (energy expenditure), is commonly considered the root cause (CDC, n.d.).

Obesity is a major public health issue in the United States (Kumanyika et al., 2008). Data from the National Health and Nutrition Examination Surveys (NHANES), the U.S. system for collecting measured heights and weights and tracking the prevalence of overweight and obesity, indicate that rates of overweight (BMI of 25 kg/m^2–29.9 kg/m^2) and obesity (BMI $\geq$ 30 kg/m^2) have increased significantly over the past three decades (Flegal et al., 1998; Hedley et al., 2004; Strauss & Pollack, 2001). As seen in Table 21.2, the prevalence of obesity among adults doubled between 1980 and 2006 (Flegal et al., 2002; National Center for Health Statistics, 2009; Ogden et al., 2006). Similarly, youth rates of obesity ($\geq$ 95th percentile of sex-specific, BMI-for-age growth charts) have tripled in this same time period (Hedley et al., 2004; National Center for Health Statistics, 2009; Ogden et al., 2008; Troiano et al., 1995). Currently, about one in three adults and one in five children and adolescents are obese (NCHS, 2009).

Although obesity has increased in all racial/ethnic groups, blacks and other populations of color are disproportionately affected (Ogden et al., 2006). Over 80 percent of non-Hispanic black women are either overweight or obese (BMI $\geq$ 25 kg/m^2), compared to 58 percent of non-Hispanic white women. About 54 percent of black women are classified as obese (BMI $\geq$ 30 kg/m^2; about 35 lbs of excess weight), compared to 30 percent of white women. Further, 15 percent of black women are considered "extremely obese" (BMI $\geq$ 40 kg/m^2; about 100 lbs of excess weight) compared to about 6 percent of their white counterparts. Non-Hispanic black men are as likely as non-Hispanic white men to be overweight or obese (69% and 70%, respectively). An estimated 34 percent of black men and 31 percent of white men are obese. However, non-Hispanic black men are nearly twice as likely to be classified as "extremely obese" (5.4% vs. 2.8%) compared to non-Hispanic white men (Ogden et al., 2006).

The prevalence of overweight and obesity among youth mirrors trends seen in the adult population. Disparities in childhood overweight between blacks and whites emerge as early as the preschool years and widen as children increase in age (Ogden et al., 2006). Non-Hispanic black girls have a higher prevalence of overweight or obesity (BMI for age $\geq$ 85th percentile) than non-Hispanic white girls. An estimated 40 percent of black girls fall into this category compared to 31 percent of white girls. About 16 percent of black girls age two to five, 27 percent age six to eleven, and 25 percent

TABLE 21.2 **U.S. Prevalence of Obesity* by Sex, Age, and Race/ Ethnicity: 1976–2006.**

	1976–1980 (NHANES ii)		1988–1994 (NHANES iii)		1999–2002 (NHANES)		2003–2006 (NHANES)	
	White	Black	Non-Hispanic White	Non-Hispanic Black	Non-Hispanic White	Non-Hispanic Black	Non-Hispanic White	Non-Hispanic Black
Males								
6–11y	6.1	6.8	10.7	12.3	14.0	17.0	15.5	18.6
12–19y	3.8	6.1	11.6	10.7	14.6	18.7	17.3	18.5
≥20y[a]	12.4	16.5	20.3	20.9	28.0	27.8	32.4	35.7
Female								
6–11y	5.2	11.2	9.8[a]	17.0	13.1	22.8	14.4	24.0
12–19y	4.6	10.7	8.9	16.3	12.6	23.5	14.5	27.7
≥20y[a]	15.4	31.0	22.9	38.3	30.7	48.6	31.6	53.4

* For children and adolescents (6–19y), obesity = ≥ 95th age-sex-specific BMI percentile cutoff based on CDC growth charts. For adults (≥ 20y), obesity = BMI ≥ 30 kg/m².
[a] Estimate is considered unreliable (standard error of 20 to 30%).
Source: National Center for Health Statistics (2009).

age 12 to 19 are obese (BMI for age ≥ 95th percentile) compared to white girls, whose prevalence is 10, 17, and 15 percent, respectively (Ogden et al., 2006). Black girls are also disproportionately represented among youth with BMI-for-age ≥ 97th percentile. Among 2- to 19-year-old black girls, 18 percent are estimated to have the higher BMI classification compared to 9 percent of white girls this age (Ogden et al., 2008). For boys, overweight or obesity prevalence among non-Hispanic blacks and non-Hispanic whites is similar. An estimated 30 percent of black boys fall into this category compared to 35 percent of white boys. About 10 percent of black boys age two to five, 18 percent age six to eleven, and 19 percent age 12 to 19 are obese (BMI for age ≥ 95th percentile) compared to white boys, whose prevalence is 13, 19, and 19 percent, respectively (Ogden et al., 2006). Black boys are slightly more likely to have a BMI for age at or about the 97th percentile, with 14 percent of youth falling into this category compared with 11 percent of white boys (Ogden et al., 2008).

The high rates of excess weight in the black community are particularly troubling given the link between obesity and chronic conditions such as hypertension, cardiovascular disease, diabetes, and certain cancers (U.S. Department of Health and Human Services, 2000) and the evidence that the health consequences of obesity apply to all ethnic groups (NHLBI, 1998; Smith et al., 2005). The health implications of the high prevalence of extreme obesity among black women are particularly troubling (McTigue et al., 2006).

MULTIPLE INFLUENCES ON DIET AND OBESITY

Health behavior may be seen as a function of the interaction between multiple subsystems (Bronfenbrenner, 1979). Consistent with this perspective, contributors to the excess risk for obesity in blacks exist at multiple levels, including the individual, interpersonal, institutional, environmental, and political (IOM, 2004). The following paragraphs describe how biology, demographics, social relationships, culture, and the environment influence dietary intake and obesity prevalence in the black community.

Biological Influences

Genetic and biological factors are certain to influence diet and weight status to some extent (Fernández et al., 2008; Galgani & Ravussin, 2008). There is biological evidence that blacks have a higher preference for high-fat and high-calorie foods (Troiano et al., 2000), a greater predilection for sweets (Bacon et al., 1994; Pepino & Mennella, 2005; Schiffman et al., 2000), and a lower preference for vegetables (Granner et al., 2004) than their white counterparts. These patterns of food preference may influence overall dietary quality and may predispose blacks to overconsumption of calories due to higher dietary energy density (at least one part of the energy balance equation for obesity).

With respect to energy expenditure, metabolic differences between blacks and whites have been observed, raising the question of whether such differences confer a particular type of susceptibility to weight gain among blacks. For example, studies examining racial/ethnic differences in energy metabolism suggest lower resting metabolic rate among black adults (Gannon et al., 2000). Similar studies with pediatric populations indicate inconsistent findings. Several studies found lower resting energy expenditure (REE) among black prepubertal children compared to their white counterparts (Treuth et al., 2000; Wong et al., 1999; Yanovski et al., 1997); however, others have found no such group differences (Nagy et al., 1997; Sun et al., 1999; Sun et al., 1998; Trowbridge et al., 1997). A longitudinal study tracked REE from childhood through puberty among African American and white youth and found lower REE among black youth after adjusting for age, Tanner stage, fat mass, and lean mass (Sun et al., 2001). Lower REE combined with higher intakes of energy-dense foods, particularly if not compensated by increased physical activity, will promote a positive energy balance. Overall, no conclusions can yet be drawn about excess risk of obesity in blacks on the basis of metabolic profiles.

Socioeconomic Status

Socioeconomic status (SES) is a major predictor of dietary intake. Blacks are dispro-portionately represented among the low-income segment of the population, and low SES has been linked to a variety of dietary or nutritional problems (FASEB, 1995; Levedahl & Oliveira, 1999). In 2006, the majority of black persons (55%) lived in families that could be classified as poor or near poor, representing 100 or 125 percent of their poverty threshold (DeNavas-Walt et al., 2007). In addition, poverty rates for non-Hispanic blacks (24%) are three times that for non-Hispanic whites (8%) (DeNavas-Walt et al., 2007). Families with limited financial resources are at great risk for food insecurity. In 2006, approximately 12.6 million households could be classi-fied as food insecure (i.e., not always having access to enough food to meet basic needs, or experiencing hunger), with a greater proportion of those affected being households with children (Nord et al., 2007; Nord & Hopwood, 2007). Black house-holds with children were over twice as likely to be classified as experiencing hunger as their white counterparts (26.4% vs. 11.3%) (Nord et al., 2007).

Higher levels of food insecurity may lead to poorer diet quality and increased cal-orie consumption. Energy-dense but nutrient-poor foods and beverages may be less expensive and therefore more likely to be available in households with limited finan-cial resources (Drewnowski, 2003). In addition, persons who are food insecure may overeat during periods when food is available, to compensate for periods when food may be scarce (Polivy, 1996).

Dietary quality generally improves with increasing income or education. However, disparities in dietary quality and nutritional status between African Americans and whites appear to persist regardless of income. For example, analyses of national dietary data indicate that diet quality scores were lower for blacks com-pared to whites even after controlling for family income (Forshee & Storey, 2006). In addition, multivariate analyses of diet quality scores in models that included mea-sures of nutrition knowledge and awareness suggest limited levels of nutrition infor-mation among blacks, perhaps explaining some of the residual race effect (Variyam et al., 1998).

The association between socioeconomic status (SES) and obesity is complex. National data in the U.S. population suggests an association between SES and risk for obesity (Troiano & Flegal, 1998); however, the strength and direction of the associa-tion may vary. Among non-Hispanic white women, an inverse relationship between SES and weight has been noted, but this pattern was not found among non-Hispanic black women (Ogden et al., 2007). Among men, evidence of a linear relationship between SES and obesity was noted for Mexican American men only (Ogden et al., 2007). In young people, an inverse association between SES and risk of obesity was found for white girls only (Wang & Zhang, 2006). Though obesity prevalence for black youth is higher than for white youth across nearly all SES categories (Wang & Zhang, 2006), SES factors do not reliably predict overweight for non-Hispanic black children and adolescents (Gordon-Larsen et al., 2003).

Family Influences

Overweight children are more likely to have at least one parent who is also overweight (Whitaker et al., 1997). Genetic influences notwithstanding, certain behaviors may partially explain the familial link. Families provide the context for learning about food and eating (Birch & Fisher, 1988). Food preferences are learned through early and repeated exposures to foods (Birch, 1999; Hill, 2002) and norms about meal size and frequency of eating are often learned at home (Campbell et al., 2006). Unhealthy family eating patterns may be passed from generation to generation (Peters et al., 2006). Food availability and accessibility are linked with dietary intake and weight status (Pearson et al., 2009), and black households are more likely to contain foods with higher amounts of fat (Befort et al., 2006).

As fewer meals are being prepared at home (Sturm & Datar, 2005), food availability from other sources is also important to consider. Black adolescent girls are more likely to consume food from fast-food restaurants (which are associated with higher caloric intake) than are white teen girls (Schmidt et al., 2005). Some evidence suggests that black youth may be more likely to eat at all-you-can-eat or buffet-type restaurants as compared to whites (Befort et al., 2006).

Parent feeding styles have also been linked with dietary intake and weight status (Faith et al., 2004). Both restrictive feeding (i.e., limiting access to select foods by setting limits on the quantity and/or imposing standards on quality of food) and indulgent feeding (i.e., not controlling or setting limits on food quality or quantity) have been associated with child overweight (Faith et al., 2004; Hughes et al., 2008). Both feeding styles are apparent among black mothers, though a slightly higher use of controlling (i.e., restrictive) versus indulgent feeding styles has been noted (Hughes et al., 2005; Sacco et al., 2007). Black mothers are also more likely to monitor child intake and pressure the child to eat than are white mothers (Spruijt-Metz et al., 2006; Spruijt-Metz et al., 2002).

Consuming meals together as a family is another practice that is associated with better dietary intake (Boutelle et al., 2003; Neumark-Sztainer et al., 2003). On the other hand, eating in front of the television is associated with both poor dietary quality (e.g., higher caloric intake, greater intake of fat, lower fruit and vegetable intake) (Boynton-Jarrett et al., 2003) and overweight (Coon & Tucker, 2002). Findings from these studies are based on multi-ethnic samples; however, separate analyses by race/ethnicity are not described. Further, data on the prevalence of this eating behavior among black households relative to other groups is lacking.

Families also influence the physical activity of their members. Residing in a single-parent household (of which 58% are black) is associated with less physical activity among youth (Lindquist et al., 1999). In general, parental activity, parental support, and sibling activity are among the variables associated with physical activity in youth (Sallis et al., 2000; van der Horst et al., 2007). Inconsistency in the role of parents and black youth activity is noted. Earlier studies found no relationship between parent modeling and youth physical activity among black girls (Nichols-English et al., 2006;

Polley et al., 2005; Trost et al., 1999); however, a recent longitudinal study (Madsen et al., 2009) found that black girls' perception of parent activity predicts physical activity throughout adolescence.

Parent evaluation of child weight status may also be important to consider. It is reasonable to propose that a necessary precursor to improved dietary quality and weight management is a recognition that the child's diet and/or weight status is outside of the normal realm and problematic. This often may not be the case. Studies with parents of overweight black girls suggested that parents were not particularly concerned about their daughter's weight status as they believed that "she'll grow out of it" (Baskin et al., 2001). Other researchers note that there may be a discrepancy between parent and health provider perceptions of obesity and its relationship with the child's health (Burnet et al., 2008; Katz et al., 2004; Skelton, Busey, et al., 2006). In addition, overweight black adults in general are more likely to misperceive their weight status as within normal limits or underweight compared to their white counterparts (Bennett & Wolin, 2006).

Cultural Influence

Religious Influences Religion has played a major role in the lives of blacks. The majority of blacks participate in Christianity, specifically Baptist and Methodist denominations, with a large percentage active in religious worship (Chatters et al., 1998; Lincoln & Mamiya, 1990). A significant number of blacks are involved in religious groups that advocate dietary practices that depart in various degrees from traditional food patterns, including Seventh Day Adventist, Islam, Mormonism, and Judaism/Hebrew Israelite (Lincoln, 1999). It has been estimated that 35 percent of Muslim Americans are black (Pew Research Center, 2007), and consumption of pork, one of the cornerstones of the traditional African American diet, is taboo for Muslims. However, many black Muslims continue to use other traditional black foods and preparation methods (Odoms, 1999). Members of the Nation of Islam, an exclusively black Muslim group, are required to abstain from eating most traditional foods, including pork, cornbread, black-eyed peas, and sweet potatoes (McCloud, 1995; Muhammad, 1972), because traditional dietary habits are believed to be associated with slavery and thus a "fast road to death" (Muhammad, 1972). Other religious communities, including Seventh Day Adventists and Hebrew Israelites, advocate vegetarian lifestyles (Markowitz, 1996; Murphy et al., 1997).

An increasing body of literature illustrates that dietary behaviors valued by some religious communities are consistent with lifestyle recommendations for reducing the risk of chronic disease (Jarvis & Northcott, 1987; Levin & Vanderpool, 1989; Phillips & Snowdon, 1985). Black Seventh Day Adventists who adhered to religious recommendations of a vegetarian lifestyle had lower serum cholesterol and triglyceride levels compared to those who did not (Melby et al., 1994). The Adventist Health Study, a California-based prospective study, analyzed the association of food consumption in 1976 with all-cause mortality ascertained through 1985 in approximately 1,700 black men and women (Fraser et al., 1997). Even within this highly-educated population (nearly half were college graduates) with lower than average meat consumption, a protective effect of certain dietary patterns was evident: frequent consumption of nuts, fruits, and green salads was significantly associated with a lower risk of death during the follow-up period.

Although black membership in religious communities with health-promoting dietary practices may be increasing, their numbers are probably still too small to influence the data collected from national samples of blacks. Furthermore, the traditional black churches maintain a practice of providing highly favored, but not necessarily healthful, meals during many of their services. However, the Muslim communities and the Seventh Day Adventists can provide insights into the diversity issues in food choice and health-related dietary habits within the black community (Fraser et al., 1997; Odoms, 1999).

Social/Cultural Norms   Individual attitudes and beliefs about healthy eating, physical activity, and weight status are influenced by peers and social/cultural norms. In general, there may be limited social norms to encourage healthy eating and activity in the black community. Black adults and youth appear to exhibit less shame about what they eat and impose fewer restrictions on their eating than do their white counterparts (Becker et al., 1999; Desmond et al., 1989; Kumanyika et al., 1991; Parnell et al., 1996; Stevens et al., 1994). In addition, specific dietary habits and physical activity behaviors may be closely connected to one's racial or ethnic identity (Liburd, 2003; Malpede et al., 2007; Sucher & Kittler, 1991).

Eating in the black community has been considered a ritual, as it involves people who perform a particular action that is repetitive, translates information about cultural traditions, and communicates a collection of meanings to participants (Liburd, 2003). Specific connotations of the link between being black and dietary intake suggest a social relevance of food. Food preparation may be considered a labor of love, with generous portions offered to friends and family as a symbol of affection. As such, significantly modifying dietary practices may be particularly challenging as some may believe that removing traditional foods or cooking practices would represent a devaluing of their identity as an African American (Liburd, 2003).

An expanded list of social cultural beliefs may also be salient for understanding the lower levels of physical activity noted among black youth (Crespo et al., 2001; Gordon-Larsen et al., 2004; McGarvey et al., 2006) and adults (Whitt-Glover et al., 2007). For example, valuing automobiles as a sign of economic attainment and/or purchasing multiple televisions (including for children's bedrooms) may support sedentary behaviors (Kumanyika, 2008b). Further, physical activity may be seen as "work" and thus competing with desires for rest and relaxation (Airhihenbuwa et al., 1995). When blacks do participate in physical activities, they may prefer activities that are different than those preferred by whites (Hooker et al., 2005; Resnicow, Jackson, et al., 2002). For example, blacks may view physical activities such as basketball and jump rope/double dutch as "mostly black" activities, attributing other activities such as hiking and ice skating as being "mostly white" (Resnicow, Jackson, et al., 2002). Water sports and activities that generally exert more energy may be seen as less favorable for black girls and women, who often express hairstyle-related barriers to participation in physical activity (Barnes et al., 2007; Baskin et al., 2001). In addition, black youth and adults have higher levels of TV watching and other sedentary behaviors (Crespo et al., 2001; Marshall et al., 2007). Increased television viewing is particularly problematic, given findings that more advertisements of unhealthy foods (e.g., desserts, soda, candy, and fast food) are found in commercials for programs with large African American audiences (Outley & Taddese, 2006). In fact, findings from a recent review indicated that advertising and other forms of targeted marketing to blacks are more likely to predispose them to excess calorie consumption and poor dietary quality (Grier & Kumanyika, 2008).

Culturally based body image perceptions are important to consider (Kumanyika & Obarzanek, 2003). For example, blacks appear to possess a different standard of physical beauty and ideal body image than whites. Both adult and adolescent blacks prefer fuller body types than whites. Black women report a higher ideal body weight, and are more likely to be satisfied with their weight, even when they are statistically overweight than white women (Gipson et al., 2005). Black youth are more likely to report that their ideal weight is determined by adults in their lives (e.g., immediate family members, athletic coaches, and teachers/administrators) whereas the body image of whites is more influenced by their peers (Desmond et al., 1989; Parnell et al., 1996). Because adults tend to be larger than children, de facto, blacks may be basing their ideal body image on a larger adult standard, compared to their white counterparts, who may be using a younger, leaner ideal.

Neighborhood Influences

An increasing body of literature is exploring the links between healthy eating, active living, obesity, and neighborhood environments. Studies have explored associations between obesity and dietary patterns, physical activity, and neighborhood deprivation, minority composition, and population density (Chang, 2006; Robert & Reither, 2004; Stimpson et al., 2007). In general, findings suggest that individuals residing in neighborhoods with better access to supermarkets, limited access to convenience stores, and limited access to fast-food restaurants are more likely to have healthier diets and lower levels of obesity (Larson et al., 2009). However, across multiple national and local studies, residents of predominantly black neighborhoods have relatively poor access to healthy foods (Baker et al., 2006; Block & Kouba, 2006; Casagrande et al., 2009; Galvez et al., 2008; Moore & Diez Roux, 2006; Morland & Filomena, 2007; Morland et al., 2002; Powell et al., 2007). Based on a study in New Orleans, predominantly black neighborhoods had 2.4 fast-food restaurants per square mile compared to 1.5 restaurants in predominantly white neighborhoods (Block et al., 2004). Supermarkets are also less prevalent in low-income and predominantly black communities (Morland et al., 2002), and when present, they are associated with higher diet quality (Casagrande et al., 2009; Morland et al., 2002).

With respect to physical activity and neighborhood environments, poorer neighborhoods offer few affordable exercise opportunities for residents (Moore et al., 2008). Low-income and minority neighborhoods are likely to lack adequate sidewalks (Griffin et al., 2008), which may discourage walking to destinations. They also offer few free or inexpensive places to actively participate in sports/recreation or other physical activity (Moore et al., 2008) and are characterized by nonexistent or dilapidated parks and recreation facilities (Powell et al., 2006).

Perceptions of neighborhood environments are also relevant. Parents who believe their neighborhoods are unsafe are less likely to send their kids out to play (Gordon-Larsen et al., 2004). Similarly, the perceptions of access to healthy foods preferred by blacks may differ from objective measures of food availability. Food stores may carry foods that are considered "healthy" with respect to dietary guidelines, but if those items are not among the foods that are commonly preferred by blacks, there may be a perception of limited healthy food access (Casagrande et al., 2009).

NUTRITION AND OBESITY INTERVENTIONS

Behavioral Interventions

Achieving long-term dietary changes and healthy weight to meet health objectives is a daunting proposition (Kumanyika et al., 2005; Kumanyika et al., 2000). The assumptions underlying nutrition and weight management counseling approaches are that health motivations can support the effort needed to learn the new behaviors, that the new behaviors will eventually become habitual (and therefore less onerous), and that the health benefits of the new behavior will help to sustain behavior over time. However, as described in this chapter, food and activity preferences and patterns are strongly anchored by cultural, psychosocial, and lifestyle influences that do not necessarily yield to behavioral changes, even among highly motivated individuals. People attempting to make changes in the composition of their diet or the amount of food they eat may feel deprived of the pleasures of eating. The taste and cost of food are stronger influences on food choices than are nutrition or weight control issues, even among those for whom health is a primary lifestyle focus (Glanz et al., 1998). Further, individuals looking to increase their physical activity may feel cheated out of time that could otherwise be spent resting or see additional costs such as hairstyle maintenance as too great to overcome.

A review of behavioral interventions aimed at preventing weight gain or weight reduction among U.S. multiethnic and minority populations of adults identified twenty-four controlled studies (Seo & Sa, 2008). Among those reviewed, only nine involved only minority participants and multiple studies did not report separate results for minority subgroups when more than one minority group was included (Kumanyika, 2008a). There was also variability in treatment length (2.75 to 58 months) and setting (clinical vs. community) (Seo & Sa, 2008). Weight loss ranged from 0.4 kg to 8.6 kg, with a mean weight loss of 3.5 kg. Effect sizes ranged from -0.07 to 1.01, with only four of twenty-four studies with an effect size near or above 0.50. Despite these limitations, the meta-analyses revealed intervention characteristics associated with successful behavioral change. Three-component interventions (addressing three of four strategies such as nutrition, physical activity, counseling, and medication) revealed a greater effect size ($d = .52$) than two-component ($d = .22$) or one-component interventions ($d = .08$). Higher effect sizes were also noted for individual session interventions ($d = .40$) rather than group session interventions ($d = .08$) (Seo & Sa, 2008).

Given the complexity of factors contributing to dietary intake and excessive weight, focusing on multiple behaviors (e.g., multi-component programs) seems reasonable and appropriate. It is also logical that individual sessions might lead to increased behavior change as intervention materials may be more specific to the unique barriers to change of the participant. In fact, there has been an increasing appreciation of the potential improvement in the effectiveness of behavioral change interventions when they are tailored to participant motivations and, with respect to minority populations, cultural contexts. For example, a recent study by Resnicow and colleagues (2008) examined the impact of tailoring a print-based fruit and vegetable intervention on constructs from self-determination theory (SDT) and motivational interviewing (MI) among African Americans. Intervention materials for the control group included tailoring on age, gender, medical history, food preferences, outcome expectancies, social support, and barriers to eating fruit and vegetables. The experimental group materials received most of the tailoring of the control group, but also included text and graphic designed to increase autonomous motivation to eat more fruit and vegetables. Study participants who at baseline preferred a style of communication that acknowledged and supported their ability to make choices (i.e., autonomy-supportive) and were randomly assigned to the experimental condition evidenced higher increases in fruit and vegetable consumption than did their counterparts in the control condition. They were also more likely to highly rate the relevance of the intervention materials than were control participants (Resnicow et al., 2008). These findings underscore the potential importance of tailoring health promotion interventions to individual differences even within an exclusively black population.

Cultural targeting—tailoring to a group rather than at the individual level (Kreuter et al., 2003)—has also been employed to enhance nutrition and weight management interventions. An example is *Sister Talk*, a cable TV–delivered weight control program for black women (Gans et al., 2003). This intervention featured twelve one-hour weekly broadcasts including a live call-in segment, written educational materials corresponding to the shows' content, motivational phone calls from peer educators, and videotaped booster sessions. An extensive description of formative work to design the intervention can be found elsewhere (Gans et al., 2003). Key elements of the cultural targeting included matching program materials and messages to preferences of the target population (i.e., surface structure) as well as incorporating core cultural values, social norms, and historical factors into program components (Resnicow et al., 1999; Resnicow, Braithwaite, et al., 2002). Targeted elements included the use of an African-inspired logo and related art, incorporation of black poetry and literature, testimonies from national and local black health authorities (e.g., Dr. David Satcher, the former surgeon general; local physicians), inclusion of commonly eaten African American and Caribbean dishes, and demonstrations of African dance and funk aerobics. In addition, the program incorporated key contextual issues: helping black women understand how taking better care of themselves is relevant to their roles and personal identities as caregivers; motivating weight control within the framework of culturally influenced body image issues; directly addressing emotional eating; providing peer role models; addressing certain food-related social and cultural traditions; and using presentation styles that convey authenticity and respect (Gans et al., 2003).

Descriptive reviews underscore the dearth of published studies targeting black children and adolescents (Baskin et al., 2001; Hudson, 2008). A recent review (Hudson, 2008) found twenty-eight experimental and non-experimental studies that focused on obesity prevention in African American youth. Of the six randomized control trials in the review, only two (Fitzgibbon et al., 2005; Gortmaker et al., 1999) showed significant improvements in weight status. The remaining were pilot studies, (Baranowski et al., 2003; Beech et al., 2003; Robinson et al., 2003; Story et al., 2003) not powered to detect an effect on BMI, though three of the four showed trends in the direction of improved dietary intake and/or increased physical activity.

Environment/Policy Interventions

Given the noted complexity of following recommended guidelines for dietary intake and weight status while living in environments that promote the opposite, there has been a recent surge in interest for environmental and policy interventions to help address nutrition and obesity among subgroups at greatest risk. Efforts aimed at food industry regulation have been proposed. Some suggest that high-calorie/low-nutrient foods should be treated as environmental toxins and thus regulated by federal agencies (Henderson & Brownell, 2004; Jeffrey, 2002). Others have suggested the standardization of portion sizes in restaurants such that consumers are aware of the number of servings that they are consuming with each meal purchased. Similarly, products can be sold in single serving units or at least large containers can be packaged in such a way as to partition off for the consumer the amount equivalent to one serving (Wansink, 2003). Similar to tobacco and alcohol, there has been a call for warning labels on foods that are high in calories and low in nutrients.

Restrictions on targeted food and beverage marketing, particularly to children, have also been suggested (Ebbeling et al., 2002; Henderson & Brownell, 2004; IOM, 2004). Yet another approach to target marketing has been the counterbalancing of advertisement of unhealthy foods and behaviors with healthier foods and physical activity promotion, particularly as a strategy to address racial/ethnic disparities. Grier and Kumanyika (2008) suggest that we engage food marketers, social marketers, policy-makers, and the public health community in a collaboration to apply a marketing framework to promoting healthy eating among blacks and other groups who may be specifically targeted with unhealthy food choices. Similarly, large-scale media campaigns designed to educate the public about healthy eating and physical activity can help combat the negative behaviors associated with excess weight (Bauman et al., 2008; Center for Science in the Public Interest, 2003).

Food taxation proposals represent another line of policy interventions. Taxation of unhealthy foods includes at least two lines of thinking. First, there would be a higher tax on food items that were high in calories and low in nutrient content (Ebbeling et al., 2002). Advocates suggest that the revenue generated from this increased tax be used to subsidize costs of healthier foods, thus making it less expensive to purchase the healthier food alternative than the less nutritious product (Henderson & Brownell, 2004). Second, there is a call to tax unhealthy food advertising. This proposal calls for an additional tax on those corporations choosing to advertise their unhealthy or non-nutritious foods. Again, revenue generated would be used to promote healthier alternatives and potentially address the relationship between poverty and obesity (Henderson & Brownell, 2004).

Further efforts to curb unhealthy food advertisement include the elimination of the selling and/or advertising of unhealthy foods in schools. Children spend a substantial part of their young lives in school. As such, the selling and marketing of products to this captive audience has been very lucrative. The food industry gains by familiarizing the youngest consumers with their products in an effort to establish brand loyalty that may last a lifetime. Not only will children purchase these items during the school day, but they are also likely to pester their parents to select these same products at home (CSPI, 2003). Schools also benefit from partnering with food and beverage companies. In exchange for advertising and selling rights (often an exclusive contract with a single vendor for multiple years), schools often receive significant revenue to assist with ever-shrinking budgets. Contracts with vendors who supply unhealthy items could be restricted and other types of incentives to school systems could be provided to address real difficulties in growing financial demands on schools with limited resources.

Changes to the built environment to increase access to healthy food choices and physical activity have been proposed. Efforts to increase the presence of supermarkets in low-income and communities of color have been called for as the presence of each additional supermarket has been shown to significantly increase the likelihood of meeting dietary recommendations, particularly among blacks (Morland et al., 2002). Other options include the development of urban farms, community gardens, and other options for communities in which there is little or no access to foods needed to maintain a healthy diet (i.e., food deserts) (Larson et al., 2009). Restrictions on the total number per capita and location (e.g., minimum distance from schools, playgrounds) of fast-food restaurants, lower pricing of healthier items, and improved availability and identification of healthier options on menus have been identified as other strategies to improve access to healthier foods from restaurants (Glanz & Hoelscher, 2004).

Policy efforts aimed at the built environment include efforts to increase easy access to physical activity. Specific strategies include the development and maintenance of walking and bicycling trails, funding of public parks and recreational facilities, zoning and land use regulations to promote activity, and required physical education in schools (Brownson et al., 2006; Kahn et al., 2002; Sallis et al., 1998). In the general population, consistent associations between access to recreational facilities, opportunities to be active, and aesthetic qualities of environments (e.g., attractiveness) and physical activity have been found (Humpel et al., 2002). Findings suggest that residents are more inclined to walk or cycle when living in neighborhoods with high residential density, mixed land use (e.g., retail outlets in walking distance of residence), and street connectivity (e.g., system of streets with multiple routes to a given location) (Saelens et al., 2003). However, the evidence for associations between the built environment and physical activity among black populations is less consistent (Casagrande et al., 2009).

Recently enacted school wellness policies resulting from The Child Nutrition and WIC Reauthorization Act of 2004 have encouraged the development and implementation of policies to increase physical activity among youth. A number of states have implemented school physical education components as well as state-specific standards for PE participation (81% of a national sample of school districts surveyed), and some have established a specified number of minutes for physical activity per day (68% of a national sample of school districts surveyed) (Longley & Sneed, 2009). The impact of state physical education requirements on child physical activity and obesity is supported by evidence suggesting that additional time in PE increases the number of days that girls spend engaged in vigorous activity and/or strength training (Cawley et al., 2007). However, neither activity-related benefits for boys nor decreases in BMI for boys or girls were associated with these policies (Cawley et al., 2007).

Research Implications

The formulation of relevant research and translation of the resulting data into meaningful strategies and programs can benefit from cultural knowledge that may be unique to black researchers and will require collaboration among investigators trained in both social science and biomedical fields and community partners. The African American Collaborative Obesity Research Network (AACORN; www.aacorn.org) proposes an expanded paradigm for research related to nutrition, physical activity, and obesity with African Americans (see Kumanyika et al., 2005; Kumanyika et al., 2007 for detailed discussion of the development of this paradigm). As illustrated in Figure 21.1, we suggest that the design and implementation of obesity-related interventions should be viewed through three different lenses: (1) African Americans in communities where research is conducted, (2) African American researchers, and (3) other researchers (including those engaged in academic-community partnerships) and sponsors of research. The perspectives of African American researchers are depicted as interacting with community perspectives and linked to, but also distinct in some ways from, those of researchers in general (i.e., researchers who are not also members of the African American community). The dual (and perhaps competing) perspectives that may apply when researchers are members (with respect to ethnic identity and shared history and experiences) of the communities they study while also being members of the academic community and accountable to research sponsors should be recognized. Most researchers have competing perspectives to some extent, but for historical and sociopolitical reasons, African American researchers may have to resolve intense social dichotomies inherent in their duality.

At the center of the expanded paradigm is the positioning of the traditional focus on energy balance and weight control at the intersection of three knowledge domains

FIGURE 21.1 *Expanded Paradigm for Research Related to Nutrition, Physical Activity, and Obesity with African Americans.*

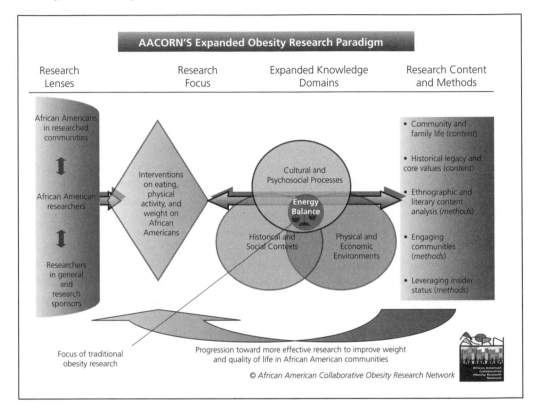

that are highly relevant to understanding eating and physical activity behaviors and weight issues in African American communities ("expanded knowledge domains")—historical and social contexts; cultural and psychosocial processes; and physical and economic environments. As discussed in this chapter, these contexts are fundamental to the worlds within which African Americans live and function. To explore these knowledge domains through the three different perspectives (the "research lenses") requires attention to relevant content and the use of methods that can facilitate accessing this content. Important content themes relate to community and family life, historical legacy, and core values. Methods must include qualitative approaches, such as ethnography, and can also include more novel approaches, such as content analysis of literary works. Engaging communities is essential and in so doing African American researchers must find ways to leverage their insider status to benefit both communities and the research endeavor. This expanded paradigm poses new challenges for those who study nutrition and obesity-related health disparities but also offers to reveal new directions that will lead to new solutions.

CONCLUSIONS AND RECOMMENDATIONS

Although the published literature on diet and obesity-related health issues for blacks is far from adequate, the consistency of the evidence suggesting important, modifiable health behaviors in the black community is undeniable. Current African American eating patterns reflect historical factors, such as the evolution of dietary practices and traditions under conditions of slavery as well as current societal conditions such as disparities in access to healthy foods and opportunities for physical activity. The persistence of food insecurity and nutritional inadequacies in the black population alongside an excess of "over nutrition" related health problems means that the goals of nutrition and obesity interventions must be carefully formulated to address both problems. Both clinical and community-based approaches are indicated, as well as general communication strategies (e.g, social marketing) that facilitate the understanding and adoption of health-promoting behaviors. Several areas have been noted where a more complete picture is needed to understand the variation in nutrition and obesity-related attitudes and practices of black Americans. Among these gaps is the need to further study variations within subgroups of blacks (e.g., geographic residence, country of origin, socioeconomic status). Though we have made broad statements about issues relevant to the black community in this chapter, we do not embrace the fallacy that black Americans are a homogeneous group. We recognize that blacks in the United States represent a diverse group with cultural variation, and encourage future research to consider this variation in the design and execution of studies with blacks. This research can benefit from an expanded research paradigm to draw on the unique insights obtained through a combination of insider and outsider perspectives and on knowledge domains that extend well beyond biomedical or biochemical constructions of food and eating.

This paradigm expansion is based on the premise that the behaviors that determine weight status are embedded in the core social and cultural processes and environments of day-to-day life. Therefore, identifying effective solutions to obesity requires an ecological model that is inclusive of relevant contextual variables, which include variables influenced by race, ethnicity, and social position.

Center The traditional focus on caloric intake and output is depicted in the intersection of knowledge domains potentially informative for developing interventions on eating, physical activity, and weight. This representation conveys the utility of factoring in knowledge of historical and social contexts, cultural and psychosocial processes, and the physical and economic environments that influence preferences, perceived and actual choices related to food and activity, and the relative ease or difficulty of exercising these choices. Such knowledge is fundamental to understanding the perspectives and day-to-day experiences that are the backdrop for weight control efforts. Accessing relevant knowledge from these expanded domains is enhanced by interactions with scholars in fields such as family sociology, literature, philosophy, transcultural psychology, economics, marketing, and urban planning.

Left What is seen, asked, and heard depends on who is looking and listening. Important eyes and ears for understanding weight issues include those of lay members of the communities of interest (e.g., African Americans in researched communities) and researchers in relevant fields whose expertise incorporates insights based on lived experiences and shared identity with the community of interest (e.g., African American researchers in nutrition, physical activity, public health, and other areas), in addition to other researchers with relevant interests and expertise, and research sponsors.

Right Content and methodological themes emanating from this inclusive, integrative paradigm applied to African Americans highlight 1) the importance of considering family and community interactions related to food acquisition, food- and activity-related social interactions, the structure and organization of community processes, women's roles, and differences by generation, social position, and other demographic variables; 2) the potential influence of the collective historical legacy of slavery and its derivatives on core values such as trust and loyalty and on interactions with the health care system, media, and other social institutions; 3) the potential value of qualitative investigations that include direct observations, eliciting and analyzing narratives, and exploring the content of literary expressions to yield different or richer insights than obtained from more typical biomedical approaches; 4) the essential need to fully incorporate the views, expertise, and agency of community partners in the research process; and 5) the potential benefits and challenges of encouraging African American researchers to leverage their insider status in ways that benefit the communities they study, the research endeavor, and their own academic careers.

REFERENCES

Airhihenbuwa, C. O., Kumanyika, S., Agurs, T. D., & Lowe, A. (1995). Perceptions and beliefs about exercise, rest, and health among African-Americans. *American Journal of Health Promotion, 9*(6), 426–429.

Airhihenbuwa, C. O., Kumanyika, S., Agurs, T. D., Lowe, A., Saunders, D., & Morssink, C. B. (1996). Cultural aspects of African American eating patterns. *Ethnicity and Health, 3*, 245–260.

American Dietetic Association. (1998). *Food guide pyramid with popular southern fare.* Chicago, IL: National Center for Nutrition and Dietetics.

Arab, L., Carriquiry, A., Steck-Scott, S., & Gaudet, M. M. (2003). Ethnic differences in the nutrient intake adequacy of premenopausal US women: Results from the third national health examination survey. *Journal of the American Dietetic Association, 103*(8), 1008.

Bacon, A. W., Miles, J. S., & Schiffman, S. S. (1994). Effect of race on perception of fat alone and in combination with sugar. *Physiology & Behavior, 55*(3), 603.

Baker, E. A., Kelly, C., Barnidge, E., Strayhorn, J., Schootman, M., Struthers, J., et al. (2006). The garden of eden: Acknowledging the impact of race and class in efforts to decrease obesity rates. *American Journal of Public Health, 96*(7), 1170–1174.

Baranowski, T., Baranowski, J. C., Cullen, K. W., Thompson, D. I., Nicklas, T., Zakeri, I. E., et al. (2003). The fun, food, and fitness project (FFFP): The Baylor gems pilot study. *Ethnicity & Disease, 13*(1 (Suppl 1), S30–39.

Barnes, A., Goodrick, G., Pavlik, V., Markesino, J., Laws, D., & Taylor, W. (2007). Weight loss maintenance in African-American women: Focus group results and questionnaire development. *Journal of General Internal Medicine, 22*(7), 915.

Basiotis, P., Carlson, A., Gerrior, S., Juan, W., & Lino, M. (2002). The Healthy Eating Index 1999–2000. Washington, DC: U. S. Department of Agriculture.

Baskin, M. L., Ahluwalia, H. K., & Resnicow, K. (2001). Obesity intervention among African-American children and adolescents. *Pediatric Clinics of North America, 48*(4), 1027–1039.

Bauman, A., Bowles, H. R., Huhman, M., Heitzler, C. D., Owen, N., Smith, B. J., et al. (2008). Testing a hierarchy-of-effects model: Pathways from awareness to outcomes in the VERB campaign 2002–2003. *American Journal of Preventive Medicine, 34*(6 (Suppl), S249–256.

Becker, D. M., Yanek, L. R., Koffman, D. M., & Bronner, Y. C. (1999). Body image preferences among urban African Americans and whites from low income communities. *Ethnicity & Disease, 9*, 377–386.

Beech, B. M., Klesges, R. C., Kumanyika, S., Murray, D., Klesges, L., McClanahan, B., et al. (2003). Child- and parent-targeted interventions: The Memphis gems pilot study. *Ethnicity and Disease, 13*(Supplement 1), S40–53.

Befort, C., Kaur, H., Nollen, N., Sullivan, D. K., Nazir, N., Choi, W. S., et al. (2006). Fruit, vegetable, and fat intake among non-Hispanic black and non-Hispanic white adolescents: Associations with home availability and food consumption settings. *Journal of the American Dietetic Association, 106*(3), 367.

Bendich, A., & Deckelbaum, R. (1997). *Preventive nutrition: The comprehensive guide for health professionals.* Totowa, NJ: Humana Press.

Bennett, G., & Wolin, K. (2006). Satisfied or unaware? Racial differences in perceived weight status. *International Journal of Behavioral Nutrition and Physical Activity, 3*(1), 40.

Birch, L. L. (1999). Development of food preferences. *Annual Review of Nutrition, 19*, 41–62.

Birch, L. L., & Fisher, J. O. (1988). Development of eating behaviors among children and adolescents. *Pediatrics, 101*, 539–559.

Block, D., & Kouba, J. (2006). A comparison of the availability and affordability of a market basket in two communities in the Chicago area. *Public Health Nutrition, 9*(07), 837–845.

Block, J. P., Scribner, R. A., & DeSalvo, K. B. (2004). Fast food, race/ethnicity, and income: A geographic analysis. *American Journal of Preventive Medicine, 27*(3), 211.

Boutelle, K. N., Birnbaum, A. S., Lytle, L. A., Murray, D. M., & Story, M. (2003). Associations between perceived family meal environment and parent intake of fruit, vegetables, and fat. *Journal of Nutritional Education Behavior, 35*(1), 24–29.

Boynton-Jarrett, R., Thomas, T. N., Peterson, K. E., Wiecha, J., Sobol, A. M., & Gortmaker, S. L. (2003). Impact of television viewing patterns on fruit and vegetable consumption among adolescents. *Pediatrics, 112*(6 Pt 1), 1321–1326.

Bronfenbrenner, U. (1979). *The ecology of human development.* Cambridge, MA: Harvard University Press.

Brownson, R. C., Haire-Joshu, D., & Luke, D. A. (2006). Shaping the context of health: A review of environmental and policy approaches in the prevention of chronic diseases. *Annual Review of Public Health, 27*(1), 341–370.

Burnet, D. L., Plaut, A. J., Ossowski, K., Ahmad, A., Quinn, M. T., Radovick, S., et al. (2008). Community and family perspectives on addressing overweight in urban, African-American youth. *Journal of General Internal Medicine, 23*(2), 175–179.

Campbell, K. J., Crawford, D. A., & Ball, K. (2006). Family food environment and dietary behaviors likely to promote fatness in 5–6 year-old children. *International Journal of Obesity, 30*(8), 1272.

Casagrande, S. S., Whitt-Glover, M. C., Lancaster, K. J., Odoms-Young, A. M., & Gary, T. L. (2009). Built environment and health behaviors among African Americans: A systematic review. *American Journal of Preventive Medicine, 36*(2), 174.

Cawley, J., Meyerhoefer, C., & Newhouse, D. (2007). The impact of state physical education requirements on youth physical activity and overweight. *Health Economics, 16*(12), 1287–1301.

Center for Science in the Public Interest. (2003). *Pestering parents: How food companies market obesity to children.* Washington, DC: Author.

Centers for Disease Control and Prevention. (January 28, 2009). Obesity and overweight. Retrieved March 5, 2009, from http://www.cdc.gov/nccdphp/dnpa/obesity/index.htm

Centers for Disease Control and Prevention. (n.d.). Obesity and Overweight. In: *Division of Nutrition, Physical Activity, and Obesity: National Center for Chronic Disease Prevention and Health Promotion.* Retrieved June 24, 2009, from http://www.cdc.gov/obesity/defining.html

Chang, V. W. (2006). Racial residential segregation and weight status among US adults. *Social Science & Medicine, 63*(5), 1289.

Chatters, L. M., Levin, J. S., & Ellison, C. G. (1998). Public health and health education in faith communities. *Health Education & Behavior, 25*, 689.

Coon, K. A., & Tucker, K. L. (2002). Television and children's consumption patterns. A review of the literature. *Minerva Pediatrica, 54*(5), 423–436.

Crespo, C. J., Smit, E., Troiano, R. P., Bartlett, S. J., Macera, C. A., & Andersen, R. E. (2001). Television watching, energy intake, and obesity in US children: Results from the third National Health and Nutrition Examination Survey, 1988–1994. *Arch Pediatric Adolescent Medicine, 155*(3), 360–365.

Deckelbaum, R. J., Fisher, E. A., Winston, M., Kumanyika, S., Lauer, R. M., Pi-Sunyer, F. X., et al. (1999). Summary of a scientific conference on preventive nutrition: Pediatrics to geriatrics. *Circulation, 100*(4), 450–456.

DeNavas-Walt, C., Proctor, B. D., & Smith, J. (2007). Income, poverty, and health insurance coverage in the United States: 2006. U. S. Census Bureau, Current Population Reports, P60-233. Washington, DC: U.S. Government Printing Office.

Desmond, S., Price, J., Hallinan, C., & Smith, D. (1989). Black and white adolescents' perceptions of their weight. *Journal of School Health, 59*, 353–358.

Dietary Guidelines Advisory Committee. (2005). The report of the dietary guidelines advisory committee on Dietary Guidelines for Americans, 2005. Retrieved from http://www.health.gov/dietaryguidelines/dga2005/

Dirks, R. T., & Duran, N. (2001). African American dietary patterns at the beginning of the 20th century. *Journal of Nutrition, 131*(7), 1881–1889.

Drewnowski, A. (2003). Fat and sugar: An economic analysis. *Journal of Nutrition, 133*(3), 838S-840.

Ebbeling, C. B., Pawlak, D. B., & Ludwig, D. S. (2002). Childhood obesity: Public health crisis, common sense cure. *The Lancet, 360*, 473–482.

Faith, M. S., Scanlon, K. S., Birch, L. L., Francis, L. A., & Sherry, B. (2004). Parent-child feeding strategies and their relationships to child eating and weight status. *Obesity, 12*(11), 1711.

Federation of American Societies for Experimental Biology, & Life Science Research Office. (1995). *Third report on nutrition monitoring in the United States* (vol 1, prepared for the inter-agency board for nutrition monitoring and related research). Washington, DC: U. S. Government Printing Office.

Fernández, J. R., Casazza, K., Divers, J., & López-Alarcón, M. (2008). Disruptions in energy balance: Does nature overcome nurture? *Physiology & Behavior, 94*(1), 105.

Fitzgibbon, M. L., Stolley, M. R., Schiffer, L., Van Horn, L., & KauferChristoffel, K. (2005). Two-year follow-up results for Hip-Hop to Health Jr.: A randomized controlled trial for overweight prevention in preschool minority children. *Journal of Pediatrics, 146*, 618–625.

Flegal, K. M., Carroll, M. D., Kuczmarski, R. J., & Johnson, C. L. (1998). Overweight and obesity in the United States: Prevalence and trends, 1960–1994. *International Journal of Obesity, 22*, 39–47.

Flegal, K. M., Carroll, M. D., Ogden, C. L., & Johnson, C. L. (2002). Prevalence and trends in obesity among US adults, 1999–2000. *Journal of American Medical Association, 288*, 1723–1727.

Forshee, R. A., & Storey, M. L. (2006). Demographics, not beverage consumption, is associated with diet quality. *International Journal of Food Sciences and Nutrition, 57*(7), 494.

Fraser, G. E., Sumbureru, D., Pribis, P., Neil, R. L., Frankson, M., & Anthony, C. (1997). Association among health habits, risk factors, and all-cause mortality in a black California population. *Epidemiology, 8*(2), 168–174.

Galgani, J., & Ravussin, E. (2008). Energy metabolism, fuel selection and body weight regulation. *International Journal of Obesity, 32*(S7), S109–S119.

Galvez, M. P., Morland, K., Raines, C., Kobil, J., Siskind, J., Godbold, J., et al. (2008). Race and food store availability in an inner-city neighbourhood. *Public Health Nutrition, 11*(06), 624–631.

Gannon, B., DiPietro, D., & Poehlman, E. T. (2000). Do African Americans have lower energy expenditure than Caucasians? *International Journal of Obesity Related Metabolic Disorders, 24*, 4–13.

Gans, K. M., Kumanyika, S., Lovell, H. J., Risica, P. M., Goldman, R., Odoms-Young, A., et al. (2003). The development of SisterTalk: A cable TV-delivered weight control program for black women. *Preventive Medicine, 37*, 654–667.

Gipson, G. W., Reese, S., Vieweg, V. R., Anum, E. A., Pandurangi, A. K., Olbrisch, M. E., et al. (2005). Body image and attitude toward obesity in an historically black university. *Journal of the National Medical Association, 97*(2), 225–236.

Glanz, K., Basil, M., Maibach, E., Goldberg, J., & Snyder, D. (1998). Why Americans eat what they do: Taste, nutrition, cost, convenience, and weight control concerns as influences on food consumption. *Journal of the American Dietetic Association, 98*(10), 1118–1126.

Glanz, K., & Hoelscher, D. (2004). Increasing fruit and vegetable intake by changing environments, policy and pricing: Restaurant-based research, strategies, and recommendations. *Preventive Medicine, 39*(Suppl 2), S88–93.

Gordon-Larsen, P., Adair, L. S., & Popkin, B. M. (2003). The relationship of ethnicity, socioeconomic factors, and overweight in US adolescents. *Obesity Research, 11*(1), 121–129.

Gordon-Larsen, P., Griffiths, P., Bentley, M. E., Ward, D. S., Kelsey, K., Shields, K., et al. (2004). Barriers to physical activity: Qualitative data on caregiver-daughter perceptions and practices. *American Journal of Preventive Medicine, 27*(3), 218.

Gortmaker, S. L., Peterson, K., Wiecha, J., Sobol, A. M., Dixit, S., Fox, M. K., et al. (1999). Reducing obesity via a school-based interdisciplinary intervention among youth. *Archives of Pediatric Adolescent Medicine, 153*, 409–418.

Granner, M. L., Sargent, R. G., Calderon, K. S., Hussey, J. R., Evans, A. E., & Watkins, K. W. (2004). Factors of fruit and vegetable intake by race, gender, and age among young adolescents. *Journal of Nutrition Education & Behavior, 36*(4), 173.

Greenberg, M. R., Schneider, D., Northridge, M. E., & Ganz, M. L. (1998). Region of birth and black diets: The Harlem household survey. *American Journal of Public Health, 88*(8), 1199–1202.

Grier, S. A., & Kumanyika, S. K. (2008). The context for choice: Health implications of targeted food and beverage marketing to African Americans. *American Journal of Public Health, 98*(9), 1616–1629.

Griffin, S. F., Wilson, D. K., Wilcox, S., Buck, J., & Ainsworth, B. E. (2008). Physical activity influences in a disadvantaged African American community and the communities' proposed solutions. *Health Promotion Practices, 9*(2), 180–190.

Guenther, P. M., Reedy, J., Krebs-Smith, S. M., Reeve, B. B., & Basiotis, P. P. (2007). Development and evaluation of the healthy eating index-2005: Technical report. Center for Nutrition Policy and Promotion, U. S. Department of Agriculture. Available at http://www.cnpp.usda.gov/HealthyEatingIndex.htm

Hedley, A. A., Ogden, C. L., Johnson, C. L., Carroll, M. D., Curtin, L. R., & Flegal, K. M. (2004). Prevalence of overweight and obesity among US children, adolescents, and adults, 1999–2002. *Journal of the American Medical Association, 291*(23), 2847–2850.

Henderson, K. E., & Brownell, K. D. (2004). The toxic environment and obesity: Contribution and cure. In J. K. Thompson (Ed.), *Handbook of eating disorders and obesity*. Hoboken, NJ: John Wiley & Sons, pp. 339–348.

Hess, K. (1992). *The Carolina rice kitchen: The African connection*. Columbia, SC: University of South Carolina Press.

Hill, A. J. (2002). Developmental issues in attitudes to food and diet. *The Proceedings of the Nutrition Society, 61*(2), 259–266.

Hooker, S. P., Wilson, D. K., Griffin, S. F., & Ainsworth, B. E. (2005). Perceptions of environmental supports for physical activity in African American and white adults in a rural county in South Carolina. The Proceedings of the Nutrition Society, *Prev chronic dis., 2*(4), A11. Retrieved from http://www.cdc.gov/pcd/issues/2005/oct/05_0048.htm

Hudson, C. E. (2008). An integrative review of obesity prevention in African American children. *Issues in Comprehensive Pediatric Nursing, 31*(4), 147.

Hughes, S. O., Power, T. G., Orlet Fisher, J., Mueller, S., & Nicklas, T. A. (2005). Revisiting a neglected construct: Parenting styles in a child-feeding context. *Appetite, 44*(1), 83.

Hughes, S. O., Shewchuk, R. M., Baskin, M. L., Nicklas, T. A., & Qu, H. (2008). Indulgent feeding style and children's weight status in preschool. *Journal of Developmental Behavior Pediatrics, 29*(5), 403–410.

Humpel, N., Owen, N., & Leslie, E. (2002). Environmental factors associated with adults' participation in physical activity: A review. *American Journal of Preventive Medicine, 22*(3), 188–199.

Institute of Medicine. (2004). *Preventing childhood obesity: Health in the balance*. Washington, DC: The National Academies Press.

James, D. C. S. (2009). Cluster analysis defines distinct dietary patterns for African-American men and women. *Journal of the American Dietetic Association, 109*(2), 255.

Jarvis, G. K., & Northcott, H. C. (1987). Religion and differences in morbidity and mortality. *Social Science & Medicine, 25*(7), 813–824.

Jeffrey, R. W. (2002). Public health approaches to the management of obesity. In C. G. Fairburn & K. D. Brownell (Eds.), *Eating disorders and obesity* (2nd ed.,). New York: Guilford Press, pp. 613–618.

Jerome, N. (1969). Northern urbanization and food consumption patterns of southern-born Negroes. *American Journal of Clinical Nutrition, 22*, 1667–1669.

Kahn, E. B., Ramsey, L. T., Brownson, R. C., Heath, G. W., Howze, E. H., Powell, K. E., et al. (2002). The effectiveness of interventions to increase physical activity: A systematic review. *American Journal of Preventive Medicine, 22*(4, Supplement 1), 73.

Kant, A. K., Graubard, B. I., & Kumanyika, S. K. (2007). Trends in black-white differentials in dietary intakes of U.S. Adults, 1971–2002. *American Journal of Preventive Medicine, 32*(4), 264.

Katz, D. L., Gordon-Larsen, P., Bentley, M. E., Kelsey, K., Shields, K., & Ammerman, A. (2004). "Does skinny mean healthy?" Perceived ideal, current, and healthy body sizes among African-American girls and their female caregivers. *Ethnic Disease, 14*(4), 533–541.

Kennedy, E. T., Ohls, J., Carlson, S., & Fleming, K. (1995). The healthy eating index: Design and applications. *Journal of the American Dietetic Association, 95*(10), 1103.

Kreuter, M. W., Lukwago, S. N., Bucholtz, D. C., Clark, E. M., & Sanders-Thompson, V. (2003). Achieving cultural appropriateness in health promotion programs: Targeted and tailored approaches. *Health Education Behavior, 30*(2), 133–146.

Kumanyika, S. (2008a). Ethnic minorities and weight control research priorities: Where are we now and where do we need to be? *Preventive Medicine, 47*(6), 583.

Kumanyika, S. K. (2008b). Environmental influences on childhood obesity: Ethnic and cultural influences in context. *Physiology & Behavior, 94*(1), 61.

Kumanyika, S. K., Gary, T. L., Lancaster, K. J., Samuel-Hodge, C. D., Banks-Wallace, J., Beech, B. M., et al. (2005). Achieving healthy weight in African-American communities: Research perspectives and priorities. *Obesity Res, 13*(12), 2037–2047.

Kumanyika, S. K., & Krebs-Smith, S. M. (2001). Preventive nutrition issues in ethnic and socioeconomic groups in the United States. In A. Bendich & R. J. Deckelbaum (Eds.), *Primary and secondary prevention nutrition*. Totawa, NJ: Humana Press, Inc., pp. 325–355

Kumanyika, S. K., & Obarzanek, E. (2003). Pathways to obesity prevention: Report of a National Institutes of Health workshop. *Obesity Research, 11*(10), 1263–1274.

Kumanyika, S. K., Obarzanek, E., Stettler, N., Bell, R., Field, A. E., Fortmann, S. P., et al. (2008). Population-based prevention of obesity: The need for comprehensive promotion of healthful eating, physical activity, and energy balance: A scientific statement from American Heart Association Council on Epidemiology and Prevention, Interdisciplinary Committee for Prevention (formerly the Expert Panel on Population and Prevention Science). *Circulation, 118*(4), 428–464.

Kumanyika, S. K., Obarzanek, E., Stevens, V. J., Herbert, P. R., & Whelton, P. K. (1991). Weight-loss experience of black and white participants in NHLBI-sponsored clinical trials. *American Journal of Clinical Nursing, 53*(supplement), 1631S-1638S.

Kumanyika, S. K., Van Horn, L., Bowen, D., Perri, M. G., Rolls, B. J., Czajkowski, S. M., et al. (2000). Maintenance of dietary behavior change. *Health Psychology, 19*(Suppl), 42–56.

Kumanyika, S. K., Whitt-Glover, M. C., Gary, T. L., Prewitt, T. E., Odoms-Young, A. M., Banks-Wallace, J., et al. (2007). Expanding the obesity research paradigm to reach African American communities. *Preventing Chronic Disease, 4*(4), A112.

Lancaster, K. J., Watts, S. O., & Dixon, L. B. (2006). Dietary intake and risk of coronary heart disease differ among ethnic subgroups of black Americans. *Journal of Nutrition, 136*(2), 446–451.

Larson, N. I., Story, M. T., & Nelson, M. C. (2009). Neighborhood environments: Disparities in access to healthy foods in the U.S. *American Journal of Preventive Medicine, 36*(1), 74.

Levedahl, J. W., & Oliveira, V. (1999). Dietary impacts of food assistance and programs. In E. Frazao (Ed.), *America's eating habits: Changes and consequences* (agricultural information bulletin no. 750). Washington, DC: U.S. Department of Agriculture, Economic Research Service, Food and Rural Economics Division.

Levin, J., & Vanderpool, Y. (1989). Is religion therapeutically significant for hypertension? *Social Science & Medicine, 29*, 69–78.

Liburd, L. C. (2003). Food, identity, and African-American women with type 2 diabetes: An anthropological perspective. *Diabetes Spectrum, 16*(3), 160–165.

Lincoln, C. E. (1999). *Race, religion, & the continuing American dilemma*. New York: Hill & Wang.

Lincoln, C. E., & Mamiya, L. H. (1990). The black church in the African American experience. *Gerontologist, 33*, 16–23.

Lindquist, C. H., Reynolds, K. D., & Goran, M. I. (1999). Sociocultural determinants of physical activity among children. *Preventive Medicine, 29*(4), 305.

Longley, C. H., & Sneed, J. (2009). Effects of federal legislation on wellness policy formation in school districts in the United States. *Journal of the American Dietetic Association, 109*(1), 95.

Madsen, K. A., McCulloch, C. E., & Crawford, P. B. (2009). Parent modeling: Perceptions of parents' physical activity predict girls' activity throughout adolescence. *The Journal of Pediatrics, 154*(2), 278.

Malpede, C. Z., Faulk, L. E., Fitzpatrick, S. L., Jefferson, W. K., Shewchuk, R. M., Baskin, M. L., et al. (2007). Racial influences associated with weight related beliefs in African American and Caucasian women. *Ethnicity and Disease, 17*(1), 1–5.

Markowitz, F. (1996). Israel as Africa, Africa as Israel: Divine geography in the personal narratives and community identity of the black Hebrew Israelites. *Anthropological Quarterly, 69*, 193–205.

Marshall, S. J., Jones, D. A., Ainsworth, B. E., Reis, J. P., Levy, S. S., & Macera, C. A. (2007). Race/ethnicity, social class, and leisure-time physical inactivity. *Medicine and Science in Sports and Exercise 39*(1), 44–51.

McCloud, A. (1995). *African-American Islam*. Great Britain: Routledge.

McGarvey, E. L., Collie, K. R., Fraser, G., Shufflebarger, C., Lloyd, B., & Oliver, M. N. (2006). Using focus group results to inform preschool childhood obesity prevention programming. *Ethnicity & Health, 11*(3), 265.

McTigue, K., Larson, J. C., Valoski, A., Burke, G., Kotchen, J., Lewis, C. E., et al. (2006). Mortality and cardiac and vascular outcomes in extremely obese women. *Journal of the American Medical Association, 296*(1), 79–86.

Melby, C. L., Toohey, M. L., & Cebrick, J. (1994). Blood pressure and blood lipids among vegetarian, semivegetarian, and nonvegetarian African Americans. *American Journal of Clinical Nutrition, 59*(1), 103–109.

Moore, L. V., & Diez Roux, A. V. (2006). Associations of neighborhood characteristics with the location and type of food stores. *American Journal of Public Health, 96*(2), 325–331.

Moore, L. V., Diez Roux, A. V., Evenson, K. R., McGinn, A. P., & Brines, S. J. (2008). Availability of recreational resources in minority and low socioeconomic status areas. *American Journal of Preventive Medicine, 34*(1), 16.

Morland, K., & Filomena, S. (2007). Disparities in the availability of fruits and vegetables between racially segregated urban neighbourhoods. *Public Health Nutrition, 10*(12), 1481–1489.

Morland, K., Wing, S., Diez Roux, A., & Poole, C. (2002). Neighborhood characteristics associated with the location of food stores and food service places. *American Journal of Preventive Medicine, 22*(1), 23–29.

Muhammad, E. (1972). *How to eat to live, volume 1*. Chicago, IL: Muhammad's Temple of Islam No 2.

Murphy, F., Gwebu, E., Braithwaite, R., Green-Goodman, D., & Brown, L. (1997). Health values and practices among Seventh-day Adventists. *American Journal of Health Behavior, 21*, 43–50.

Nagy, T. R., Gower, B. A., Shewchuk, R. M., & Goran, M. I. (1997). Serum leptin and energy expenditure in children. *Journal of Clinical Endocrinology and Metabolism, 82*, 4149–4153.

National Center for Health Statistics. (2009). Health, United States, 2008, with chartbook. Retrieved from http://www.cdc.gov/nchs/hus.htm

Neumark-Sztainer, D., Wall, M., Perry, C., & Story, M. (2003). Correlates of fruit and vegetable intake among adolescents: Findings from project eat. *Preventive Medicine, 37*(3), 198.

NHLBI Obesity Education Initiative. (1998). *Clinical guidelines on the identification, evaluation, and treatment of overweight and obesity in adults: The evidence report* (No. 98–4083). Bethesda, MD: U.S. Department of Health and Human Services, Public Health Service, National Institutes of Health, National Heart, Lung, and Blood Institute.

Nichols-English, G. J., Lemmon, C. R., Litaker, M. S., Cartee, S. G., Yin, Z., Gutin, B., et al. (2006). Relations of black mothers' and daughters' body fatness, physical activity beliefs and behavior. *Ethnicity & Disease, 16*, 172–179.

Nielsen, S. J., Siega-Riz, A. M., & Popkin, B. M. (2002). Trends in energy intake in U.S. between 1977 and 1996: Similar shifts across age groups. *Obesity Research, 10*, 370–378.

Nord, M., Andrews, M., & Carlson, S. (2007). *Household food security in the United States, 2006*. Washington, DC: U.S. Department of Agriculture, Economic Research Service.

Nord, M., Andrews, M., & Carlson, S. (2008). *Household food security in the United States, 2007*. Washington, DC: U.S. Department of Agriculture, Economic Research Service.

Nord, M., & Hopwood, H. (2007). Recent advances provide improved tools for measuring children's food security. *Journal of Nutrition, 137*(3), 533–536.

Odoms, A. (1999). The role of religion in the dietary and food choice practices of African-American Muslim women (unpublished doctoral dissertation): Cornell University.

Ogden, C. L., Carroll, M. D., Curtin, L. R., McDowell, M. A., Tabak, C. J., & Flegal, K. M. (2006). Prevalence of overweight and obesity in the United States, 1999–2004. *Journal of the American Medical Association, 295*(13), 1549–1555.

Ogden, C. L., Carroll, M. D., & Flegal, K. M. (2008). High body mass index for age among US children and adolescents, 2003–2006. *Journal of the American Medical Association, 299*(20), 2401–2405.

Ogden, C. L., Yanovski, S. Z., Carroll, M. D., & Flegal, K. M. (2007). The epidemiology of obesity. *Gastroenterology, 132*(6), 2087.

Outley, C. W., & Taddese, A. (2006). A content analysis of health and physical activity messages marketed to African American children during after-school television programming. *Archives of Pediatrics & Adolescent Medicine, 160*(4), 432–435.

Parnell, K., Sargent, R., Thompson, S. H., Duhe, S. F., Valois, R. F., & Kemper, R. C. (1996). Black and white adolescent females' perceptions of ideal body size. *Journal of School Health, 66,* 112–118.

Pearson, N., Biddle, S. J. H., & Gorely, T. (2009). Family correlates of fruit and vegetable consumption in children and adolescents: A systematic review. *Public Health Nutrition, 12*(02), 267–283.

Pepino, M. Y., & Mennella, J. A. (2005). Factors contributing to individual differences in sucrose preference. *Chemical Senses, 30*(suppl_1), 319–320.

Peters, R. M., Aroian, K. J., & Flack, J. M. (2006). African American culture and hypertension prevention. *The Journal of Nursing Research 28*(7), 831–854.

Pew Research Center. (2007). Muslim Americans: Middle class and mostly mainstream. Retrieved from http://www.pewresearch.org/assets/pdf/muslim-americans.pdf

Phillips, R. L., & Snowdon, D. A. (1985). Dietary relationships with fatal colorectal cancer among Seventh Day Adventists. *Journal of the National Cancer Institute, 74*(2), 307–317.

Pietrobelli, A., Faith, M. S., Allison, D. B., Gallagher, D., Chiumello, G., & Heymsfield, S. B. (1998). Body mass index as a measure of adiposity among children and adolescents: A validation study. *Journal of Pediatrics, 132,* 204–210.

Poe, T. (1999). The origins of soul food in the black urban identity: Chicago, 1915–1947. *American Studies International, 37,* 4–33.

Polivy, J. (1996). Psychological consequences of food restriction. *Journal of the American Dietetic Association, 96*(6), 589.

Pollard, K., & O'Hare, W. (1999). America's racial and ethnic minorities. *Population Bulletin, 54,* 1–34.

Polley, D. C., Spicer, M. T., Knight, A. P., & Hartley, B. L. (2005). Intrafamilial correlates of overweight and obesity in African-American and Native-American grandparents, parents, and children in rural Oklahoma. *Journal of the American Dietetic Association, 105*(2), 262.

Powell, L. M., Slater, S., Chaloupka, F. J., & Harper, D. (2006). Availability of physical activity-related facilities and neighborhood demographic and socioeconomic characteristics: A national study. *American Journal of Public Health, 96*(9), 1676–1680.

Powell, L. M., Slater, S., Mirtcheva, D., Bao, Y., & Chaloupka, F. J. (2007). Food store availability and neighborhood characteristics in the United States. *Preventive Medicine, 44*(3), 189.

Reis, J. P., Michos, E. D., von Muhlen, D., & Miller, E. R., III. (2008). Differences in vitamin D status as a possible contributor to the racial disparity in peripheral arterial disease. *American Journal of Clinical Nutrition, 88*(6), 1469–1477.

Resnicow, K., Baranowski, T., Ahluwalia, J. S., & Braithwaite, R. L. (1999). Cultural sensitivity in public health: Defined and demystified. *Ethnicity & Disease, 9,* 10.

Resnicow, K., Braithwaite, R., DiIorio, C., & Glanz, K. (2002). Applying theory to culturally diverse and unique populations. In K. Glanz, F. M. Lewis, & B. K. Rimer (Eds.), *Health behavior and health education: Theory, research and practice.* San Francisco: Jossey-Bass, pp. 485–509.

Resnicow, K., Davis, R., Zhang, G., Konkel, J., Strecher, V., Shaikh, A., et al. (2008). Tailoring a fruit and vegetable intervention on novel motivational constructs: Results of a randomized study. *Annals of Behavioral Medicine, 35*(2), 159.

Resnicow, K., Jackson, A., Braithwaite, R., DiIorio, C., Blissett, D., Rahotep, S., et al. (2002). Healthy Body/Healthy Spirit: A church-based nutrition and physical activity intervention. *Health Education Research, 17*(5), 562–573.

Robert, S. A., & Reither, E. N. (2004). A multilevel analysis of race, community disadvantage, and body mass index among adults in the US. *Social Science & Medicine, 59*(12), 2421.

Robinson, T. N., Killen, J. D., Kraemer, H. C., Wilson, D. M., Matheson, D. M., Haskell, W. L., et al. (2003). Dance and reducing television viewing to prevent weight gain in African-American girls: The Stanford GEMS pilot study. *Ethnicity and Disease, 13*(Supplement 1), 65–77.

Sacco, L. M., Bentley, M. E., Carby-Shields, K., Borja, J. B., & Goldman, B. D. (2007). Assessment of infant feeding styles among low-income African-American mothers: Comparing reported and observed behaviors. *Appetite, 49*(1), 131.

Saelens, B. E., Sallis, J. F., & Frank, L. D. (2003). Environmental correlates of walking and cycling: Findings from the transportation, urban design, and planning literatures. *Annals of Behavioral Medicine, 25*(2), 80–91.

Sallis, J., Prochaska, J. J., & Taylor, W. C. (2000). A review of correlates of physical activity of children and adolescents. *Medicine and Science in Sports and Exercise, 32*(2), 963–975.

Sallis, J. F., Bauman, A., & Pratt, M. (1998). Environmental and policy interventions to promote physical activity. *American Journal of Preventive Medicine, 15*(4), 379–397.

Schiffman, S. S., Graham, B. G., Sattely-Miller, E. A., & Peterson-Dancy, M. (2000). Elevated and sustained desire for sweet taste in African-Americans: A potential factor in the development of obesity. *Nutrition, 16*(10), 886.

Schmidt, M., Affenito, S. G., Striegel-Moore, R., Khoury, P. R., Barton, B., Crawford, P., et al. (2005). Fast-food intake and diet quality in black and white girls: The National Heart, Lung, and Blood Institute Growth and Health study. *Archives of pediatrics & adolescent medicine, 159*(7), 626–631.

Seemes, C. E. (1996). *Racism, health, and post-industrialism: A theory of African-American health.* Westport, CT: Praeger Publishers.

Seo, D.-C., & Sa, J. (2008). A meta-analysis of psycho-behavioral obesity interventions among US multiethnic and minority adults. *Preventive Medicine, 47*(6), 573–582.

Skelton, J. A., Busey, S. L., & Havens, P. L. (2006). Weight and health status of inner city african american children: Perceptions of children and their parents. *Body Image, 3*(3), 289–293.

Smit, E., Nieto, F. J., Crespo, C. J., & Mitchell, P. (1999). Estimates of animal and plant protein intake in U.S. adults. Results from the third national health examination survey, 1988–1991. *Journal of the American Dietetic Association, 99*, 813–820.

Smith, S. C., Jr., Clark, L. T., Cooper, R. S., Daniels, S. R., Kumanyika, S. K., Ofili, E., et al. (2005). Discovering the full spectrum of cardiovascular disease: Minority health summit 2003: Report of the obesity, metabolic syndrome, and hypertension writing group. *Circulation, 111*(10), e134–139.

Spruijt-Metz, D., Li, C., Cohen, E., Birch, L., & Goran, M. (2006). Longitudinal influence of mother's child-feeding practices on adiposity in children. *The Journal of Pediatrics, 148*(3), 314.

Spruijt-Metz, D., Lindquist, C. H., Birch, L. L., Fisher, J. O., & Goran, M. I. (2002). Relation between mothers' child-feeding practices and children's adiposity. *American Journal of Clinical Nutrition, 75*(3), 581–586.

Stevens, J., Kumanyika, S., & Keil, J. (1994). Attitudes toward body size and dieting: Differences between elderly black and white women. *American Journal of Public Health, 84*, 1322–1325.

Stimpson, J. P., Nash, A. C., Ju, H., & Eschbach, K. (2007). Neighborhood deprivation is associated with lower levels of serum carotenoids among adults participating in the third National Health and Nutrition Examination Survey. *Journal of the American Dietetic Association, 107*(11), 1895.

Story, M., Sherwood, N. E., Himes, J. H., Davis, M., Jacobs, D. R. J., Cartwright, Y., et al. (2003). An after-school obesity prevention program for African-American girls: The Minnesota GEMS pilot study. *Ethnicity & Disease, 13*(Suppl 1), S54–64.

Strauss, R. S., & Pollack, H. A. (2001). Epidemic increase in childhood overweight, 1986–1998. *Journal of American Medical Association, 286*, 2845–2848.

Sturm, R., & Datar, A. (2005). Body mass index in elementary school children, metropolitan area food prices and food outlet density. *Public Health, 119*(12), 1059.

Sucher, K. P., & Kittler, P. G. (1991). Nutrition isn't color blind. *Journal of the American Dietetic Association, 91*(3), 297–299.

Sucher, K. P., & Kittler, P. G. (2008). *Food and culture.* Belmont, CA: Wadsworth Publishing Co.

Sun, M., Gower, B. A., Bartolucci, A. A., Hunter, G. R., Figueroa-Colon, R., & Goran, M. I. (2001). A longitudinal study of resting energy expenditure relative to body composition during puberty in African American and white children. *American Journal of Clinical Nutrition, 73*, 308–315.

Sun, M., Gower, B. A., Nagy, T. R., Bartolucci, A. A., & Goran, M. I. (1999). Do hormonal indices of maturation explain energy expenditure differences in African American and Caucasian prepubertal children? *International Journal of Obesity Relted Metabolic Disorders, 23*, 1320–1226.

Sun, M., Gower, B. A., Nagy, T. R., Trowbridge, C. A., Dezenberg, C., & Goran, M. I. (1998). Total, resting, and activity-related energy expenditures are similar in caucasian and African-American children. *American Journal of Physiology, 274*, E232–237.

Treuth, M. S., Butte, N. F., & Wong, W. W. (2000). Effects of familial predisposition to obesity on energy expenditure in multiethnic prepubertal girls. *American Journal of Clinical Nutrition, 71*, 893–900.

Troiano, R., Flegal, K. M., Kuczmarski, R. J., Campbell, S. M., & Johnson, C. L. (1995). Overweight prevalence and trends for children and adolescents: The National Health and Nutrition Examination Surveys 1963 to 1991. *Archives of Pediatric Adolescent Medicine, 149*, 1085–1091.

Troiano, R. P., Briefel, R. R., Carroll, M. D., & Bialostosky, K. (2000). Energy and fat intakes of children and adolescents in the United States: Data from the national health and nutrition examination surveys. *American Journal of Clinical Nutrition, 72*(5), 1343S-1353.

Troiano, R. P., & Flegal, K. M. (1998). Overweight children and adolescents: Description, epidemiology, and demographics. *Pediatrics, 101*, 497–504.

Trost, S. G., Pate, R. R., Ward, D. S., Saunders, R., & Riner, W. (1999). Correlates of objectively measured physical activity in preadolescent youth. *American Journal of Preventive Medicine, 17*(2), 120.

Trowbridge, C. A., Gower, B. A., Nagy, T. R., Hunter, G. R., Treuth, M. S., & Goran, M. I. (1997). Maximal aerobic capacity in African-American and Caucasian prepubertal children. *American Journal of Physiology, 273*, E809–814.

U.S. Department of Agriculture & Center for Nutrition Policy and Promotion. (1996 sl.rev.). *The food guide pyramid*. Washington, DC: U.S. Government Printing Office.

U.S. Department of Health and Human Services and U.S. Department of Agriculture. (2005). *Dietary Guidelines for Americans, 2005*. (6th ed.). Washington, DC: U.S. Government Printing Office.

U.S. Department of Health and Human Services. (2000). *Healthy people 2010: Nutrition and Overweight*. Washington, DC: U.S. Government Printing Office.

van der Horst, K., Oenema, A., Ferreira, I., Wendel-Vos, W., Giskes, K., van Lenthe, F., et al. (2007). A systematic review of environmental correlates of obesity-related dietary behaviors in youth. *Health Education Research, 22*(2), 203–226.

Variyam, J. N., Blaylock, J., Smallwood, D., & Basiotis, P. P. (1998). *USDA's healthy eating index and nutrition information. Technical bull. no. 1866*. Washington, DC: U.S. Department of Agriculture.

Veale-Jones, D., & Darling, M. (1996). *Ethnic foodways in Minnesota: Handbook of food and wellness across cultures*. St Paul, MN: University of Minnesota Press.

Wang, Y., & Zhang, Q. (2006). Are American children and adolescents of low socioeconomic status at increased risk of obesity? Changes in the association between overweight and family income between 1971 and 2002. *American Journal of Clinical Nutrition, 84*(4), 707–716.

Wansink, B. (2003, July 30). *The de-marketing of obesity*. Paper presented at the National Academy of Sciences Food and Nutrition Division, Washington, DC.

Whitaker, R. C., Wright, J. A., Pepe, M. S., Seidel, K. D., & Dietz, W. H. (1997). Predicting obesity in young adulthood from childhood and parental obesity. *New England Journal of Medicine, 337*, 869–873.

Whitehead, T. L. (1992). In search of soul food and meaning: Culture, food and health. In J. A. Baer & Y. Jones (Eds.), *African americans in the south: Issues of race, class, and gender*. Athens, GA: University of Georgia Press, pp. 94–110.

Whitt-Glover, M. C., Taylor, W. C., Heath, G. W., & Macera, C. A. (2007). Self-reported physical activity among blacks: Estimates from national surveys. *American Journal of Preventive Medicine, 33*(5), 412.

Wong, W. W., Butte, N. F., Ellis, J. K., Hergenroeder, A. C., Hill, R. B., Stuff, J. E., et al. (1999). Pubertal African-American girls expend less energy at rest and during physical activity than Caucasian girls. *Journal of Clinical Endocrinology and Metabolism, 84*, 906–911.

World Health Organization. (2003). Diet, nutrition, and prevention of chronic diseases. A report of the joint WHO/FAO expert consultation (Vol. WHO Technical Report Series, No. 916). Geneva: World Health Organization.

Yanovski, S. Z., Reynolds, J. C., Boyle, A. J., & Yanovski, J. A. (1997). Resting metabolic rate in African-American and Caucasian girls. *Obesity Research, 5*, 321–325.

CHAPTER

22

PHYSICAL ACTIVITY

ANTRONETTE K. YANCEY
MELICIA C. WHITT-GLOVER
MONA AUYOUNG

Physical activity is a critical element of a health promotion agenda. The purpose of this chapter is to present a synthesis of the public health literature on physical activity among African Americans. The chapter begins by defining physical activity–related terms and concepts. Commonly used measures, their limitations, and measurement challenges in research involving African American populations are then identified. We present a broad picture of the distribution of physical activity participation among African Americans, as gleaned from the epidemiology literature. Physical activity intervention research and practice issues and challenges are followed by a discussion of the implications, completing the chapter.

Physical Activity Challenges and Opportunities Among African Americans

Physical inactivity is an important contributor to the risk profiles for many chronic diseases (Physical Activity Guidelines Advisory Committee [PAGAC], 2008). Physical inactivity is considered an independent primary risk factor for cardiovascular disease, comparable to smoking and hyperlipidemia (Bull, Armstrong, et al., 2003).

In October 2008, the first-ever Physical Activity Guidelines for Americans were released by the federal government, recommending a minimum of 30 minutes of moderate to vigorous physical activity every day for adults, and 60 minutes for children (PAGAC, 2008). Physical activity levels among African Americans are generally lower than among whites. Health outcomes that could be prevented or ameliorated by physical activity occur at above-average prevalence rates among racial/ethnic minorities. African Americans have higher rates of most chronic conditions associated with low levels of physical activity and high levels of sedentary behaviors, including coronary artery disease, stroke, hypertension, and type 2 diabetes mellitus. In addition, a recent study identified physical inactivity as one of two health behaviors for which relative inequalities are increasing among those with less formal education (Harper & Lynch, 2007). This underscores the central role of physical inactivity as a contributor to the health disparities facing the African American community (Yancey, Wold, et al. 2004; Smith, Clark, et al., 2005).

Physical inactivity also contributes to the energy imbalance that produces obesity (Hill, Thompson, et al., 2005). Many studies have implicated reduction in energy expenditure or physical activity (through increasing occupational sedentariness and growing reliance on labor-saving devices, motorized transportation, and sedentary entertainment) as a key driver of the obesity epidemic during the past several decades (Sturm, 2004; Brownson, Boehmer, et al., 2005). The health and economic costs imposed on society by people with a sedentary lifestyle may be greater than those imposed by smokers (Keeler, Manning, et al., 1989; Sturm, 2002), and are similar to lifetime external costs imposed by overweight and obesity (Finkelstein, Fiebelkorn, et al., 2003). Socioeconomic status–related obesity disparities are also increasing in women and among African Americans (Truong & Sturm, 2005), and African American women and girls already have among the highest obesity rates of any demographic population segment.

Paucity of Physical Activity Research in African American Populations

Physical activity represents a burgeoning area of public health investigation, and epidemiologic surveillance and determinants research studies have documented the many disparities and their antecedents (e.g., Day, 2006; Kelly, Baker, et al., 2007; Van Duyn, McCrae, et al., 2007). However, African Americans are poorly represented in physical activity intervention research. Many trials have been conducted during the past several decades, but relatively few have targeted African Americans. Studies have not generally succeeded in engaging representative samples of community residents or staff members of the geographic areas and organizations from which they recruit (Gibson, Kirk, et al., 2005). Reviews of the intervention research literature (Story, 1999; Marcus, Williams, et al., 2006; Sharma, 2006) have identified a number of recurrent challenges encountered in promoting physical activity. First, an active lifestyle typically competes for time and financial resources with other sedentary but socially valued leisure activities such as personal care (e.g., manicures and hair maintenance). Second, most obligatory physical activity (e.g., for transportation, household chores) has been engineered out of daily life (Stone, McKenzie, et al., 1998; Marcus, Dubbert, et al., 2000; Biddle, Gorely, et al., 2004; Timperio, Salmon, et al., 2004; Marcus, Williams, et al., 2006). Third, intervention approaches have not successfully prompted generalization of physical activity to situations outside of the immediate intervention (Marcus, Williams, et al., 2006).

In addition, it has been difficult to disentangle effects of an intervention approach, particularly in interpreting null findings—was the approach truly unacceptable or was the marketing of that approach ineffective or inappropriate (Yancey, Ortega, et al., 2006; Yancey & Tomiyama, 2007)? For example, a study of the utilization of stair prompts (point-of-decision posters or stair riser banners) to encourage stair use conducted subgroup analyses by race/ethnicity (Andersen, Franckowiak, et al., 1998) and found that the intervention did not work in African Americans. The same research group repeated the study with a poster featuring an African American, and the intervention was effective in both African Americans and whites (Andersen, Franckowiak et al., 2006). Finally, physical activity intervention studies have not been strongly rooted in applicable theory or designed to test relevant constructs. However, theoretical models have been fairly anemic in this area, explaining relatively little of the variance in physical activity adoption, or especially maintenance and discontinuation/resumption.

Definitions of Terminology Used in Physical Activity Research and Practice

Physical activity is defined as bodily movement that is produced by the contraction of skeletal muscle and that substantially increases energy expenditure. The majority of energy is expended through muscular activity during daily pursuits such as occupation, transportation, recreation, and home care. Physical activity is further categorized by intensity, with most researchers focused on moderate and vigorous physical activity. Moderate physical activity is defined as activity that uses large muscle groups (such as the legs and arms) and is at least equivalent to brisk walking. Moderate physical activities may also include swimming, cycling, dancing, gardening and yard work, and various domestic and occupational activities.

Vigorous physical activity is defined as rhythmic, repetitive physical activities that use large muscle groups at 70 percent or more of maximum heart rate (roughly equal to 220 beats per minute minus one's age). Examples of vigorous physical activities include jogging or running, lap swimming, race cycling, aerobic dancing, skating, rowing, jumping rope, cross-country skiing, hiking or backpacking, racquet sports, and competitive group sports such as soccer and basketball (USDHHS, 1996). Most exercise science studies seek to characterize physical activity in terms of frequency, intensity, type, and time (FITT). Physical activity measurement issues are discussed in the following section.

Sedentary behavior does not have a standard definition, but typically describes a state of physical inactivity and low energy expenditure, classically characterized by excessive time spent sitting in front of a television, computer, or video game (Ricciardi, 2005). Studies have attempted to define sedentary lifestyle in a number of ways, such as expending less than 10 percent of one's daily energy in moderate to vigorous activity (in which the metabolic rate increases at least four times from baseline (Bernstein, Morabia, et al., 1999), or performing physical activities such as walking or biking less than

10 minutes continuously per week (Yancey, Wold, et al., 2004). A current dialogue in physical activity research centers on the association between physical activity and sedentary behaviors. Correlation analyses demonstrate that a negligible amount of the variance in leisure-time physical activity is explained by indices of sedentariness (Kronenberg, Pereira, et al., 2000; Gustat, Srinivasan, et al., 2002). The physiology of inactivity is a burgeoning area of inquiry, distinct from exercise physiology. Some researchers argue that the risk of prolonged periods of sitting is independent of and equal to the risk of insufficient moderate to vigorous physical activity (Hamilton, Hamilton, et al., 2007). However, the terms sedentariness and physical inactivity are often used interchangeably in the literature and such use is unavoidable in this chapter. Whether the risks are independent or related, both increase an individual's risk for chronic disease.

Fitness is that set of physical attributes associated with the ability to perform exercise. Five components are generally included: aerobic or cardiorespiratory fitness, muscular strength, muscular endurance, flexibility, and body composition. Obesity, the most widely used indicator of body composition, is defined as a Body Mass Index (BMI) $\geq$ 30 kg/m^2. Overweight is a BMI of 25 to 29.9 kg/m^2. BMI is a ratio that compares a person's height to their weight and is measured as weight in kg divided by the square of height in meters.

MEASURES AND MEASUREMENT CHALLENGES

Surveys

Surveys were first used in physical activity epidemiology research in the 1950s to measure physical activity participation and were based on job title and job classification. Most recent versions of physical activity surveys have included activities performed at work and in the home (Ainsworth, Jacobs, et al., 1993), as well as participation in leisure-time sports and recreational activities. The three types of surveys used to measure physical activity are global surveys, recall surveys, and quantitative history surveys (Ainsworth, 1998). Global surveys limit the number of questions to three or four that ask about overall physical activity participation habits. Recall surveys measure physical activity during the past one to four weeks and generally include no more than thirty questions. Quantitative history surveys are the most comprehensive, measuring physical activity participation patterns over long periods of time, which may vary from the past year to one's lifetime.

Three national surveillance systems—the Behavioral Risk Factor Surveillance System (BRFSS), the National Health Interview Survey (NHIS), and the National Health and Nutrition Examination Survey (NHANES)—provide population-level estimates of physical activity participation among adults in the United States. These surveys provide information about physical activity type, frequency, intensity, duration, and achievement of national physical activity objectives overall and by population subgroup. The BRFSS assesses moderate- and vigorous-intensity physical activity during a usual week in bouts lasting at least ten minutes at a time among adults

($\geq$ 18 years) (Centers for Disease Control and Prevention [CDC], 1998). The NHIS has a major emphasis on national-level estimates to track progress toward *Healthy People 2010* objectives (USDHHS, 2000; CDC and USDHHS, 2003; USDHHS Office of Disease Prevention and Health Promotion, 2003) and assesses light/moderate and vigorous-intensity physical activity during leisure time, in bouts lasting at least ten minutes. The NHANES assesses the frequency and duration per session of moderate- and vigorous-intensity physical activity, during leisure time, over the previous thirty days from a list of forty-seven activities, and up to three additional unlisted activities (CDC and National Center for Health Statistics [NCHS], 2005; CDC and National Center for Chronic Disease Prevention and Health Promotion, 2005). Intensity of each activity is classified based on the Compendium of Physical Activities (Ainsworth, Haskell, et al., 2000). In addition, NHANES assesses participation in television viewing and computer use on a typical day (outside of work hours), which provides an estimate of sedentary behaviors.

Other surveys have been developed for use in specific population subgroups among adults (e.g., CHAMPS for older adults) and for specific studies (e.g., Cross-Cultural Activity Participation, MESA). Many of these surveys have been tested for validity and reliability. In 1997, "A Collection of Physical Activity Questionnaires for Health-Related Research" was published in *Medicine and Science in Sports and Exercise* (Kriska, 1997). The collection of surveys was further updated recently and made publicly available via the Physical Activity Assessment Tools website. The website is an online repository of physical activity assessment tools, along with validity and reliability information for each tool as available.

Surveys are an attractive method of assessment because they may be interviewer- or self-administered, are less costly and time consuming to administer than other methods, and are less likely than direct methods of measurement to alter typical physical activity behavior patterns. However, surveys are susceptible to two important forms of bias—recall bias and error in classification. Recall bias is the result of a dependence on the survey participants to accurately recall past physical activities, which can lead to over- or underestimation of actual activity levels. Errors in classification are those in which individuals are inappropriately placed into a category to which they should not be assigned. It has also been hypothesized that current physical activity surveys may not accurately assess activity in all population groups (e.g., racial/ethnic minority groups; women) (McGinnis, 1992) because they do not always include occupational, household, volunteer, or other activities that are relevant to these populations (Mayer, Alderman, et al. 1991; Whitt, Levin, et al., 2003).

Objective Electronic Monitoring

The two most common forms of electronic monitoring of physical activity are pedometers, which measure daily locomotion, and accelerometers or motion detectors, which measure physical activity intensity. One of the most common methods for assessing physical activity energy expenditure is the use of accelerometers. The accelerometer, which can be worn on the belt, ankle, or wrist, is designed to measure the occurrence and intensity of motion from the body each minute over a twenty-four-hour period, storing information for up to a four-week period. In general, the monitors utilize an electronic sensor and digital signaling to record numerical values to represent each time the body accelerates past a baseline reference value. Using pre-determined activity count values to identify intensity level, these accelerometer data can then be used to calculate total daily energy expenditure through physical activity, total daily participation in different levels of activity (inactivity, light, moderate, and vigorous-intensity activity), and the average length of each bout of activity at a given intensity level.

Accelerometers have been compared to objective measures of energy expenditure such as indirect calorimetry or doubly labeled water (Bouten, Verboeket-van de Venne, et al., 1996; Jakicic, Winters, et al., 1999; Levine, Baukol, et al., 2001), but these comparisons only provide an estimate of the accuracy of the device regarding total energy expenditure. Some of the limitations in using accelerometers to collect physical activity data are the inability of accelerometers to accurately assess activities that are not locomotive (e.g., cycling) or to accurately detect changes in activity intensity level unrelated to speed (e.g., walking on an incline or while carrying a load). Other limitations include the lack of accelerometer testing with diverse populations or field settings, validity of the data, and the overall relationship of activity patterns to specific health or performance outcomes, although this area of research is currently growing.

Studies have demonstrated the feasibility of the pedometer, also known as a step counter, both as an objective measure of physical activity and as a potential motivator to increase activity levels (Tudor-Locke & Myers, 2001a; Tudor-Locke & Myers, 2001b). Pedometers, usually worn clipped to the belt or waistband or worn on the ankle, are used to count the number of steps taken during a specified period of time to estimate distance walked. Vertical acceleration of the body through walking or running causes a lever arm in the pedometer to move vertically and a ratchet to rotate (Ainsworth, Montoye, et al., 1994).

Pedometers are more widely available than accelerometers to the general public because they are relatively inexpensive and sold in various types of retail stores. Although there are a variety of pedometers available on the market, some pedometers are more accurate than others because simpler models are more sensitive to different positioning or placement on different body types (Bassett, Ainsworth, et al., 1996; Schneider, Crouter, et al., 2004). New pedometer models are equipped with a seven-day memory or longer, to aid in physical activity data collection. Criteria from Tudor-Locke and Bassett have been established to determine physical activity levels among adults based on steps taken per day: <5,000 steps/day (sedentary), 5,000–7,499 (low active), 7,500–9,999 (somewhat active), ≥10,000 (active), and ≥12,500 (highly active) (Tudor-Locke & Bassett, 2004).

Observed Engagement

Observed engagement (behavioral observation) is one of the earliest methods for assessing physical activity, involving real-time observation and recording of physical activity participation. Observation may involve pen and paper recording, video recording, or an event-counting digital recording system. These types of observations can be as simple as logging the total amount of time the participant spends engaging in particular activities (e.g., reclining, walking) or as complex as recording each activity as it is performed by the participant. Behavioral observation is beneficial when studying groups such as children or elderly adults who may have trouble recording activities and using other measurement tools. In addition, the investigator is able to measure all variables of interest using relatively inexpensive equipment. However, behavioral observation has disadvantages—it takes considerable time, and it may not be possible to measure normal daily behaviors. Plus, constant observation may also alter the normal behavior of the participants under observation, resulting in biased estimates of physical activity and computed energy expenditure. Examples of observed engagement tools include the System for Observing Play and Leisure in Youth (SOPLAY), System for Observing Fitness Instruction Time (SOFIT), and System for Observing Play and Recreation in Communities (SOPARC). The aforementioned instruments and instructions for their use may be downloaded at www.activelivingresearch.org.

Physical activity records and physical activity logs can serve as a direct measure of physical activity among adults. Generally, physical activity records require participants to record all physical activity as it is being performed. The information that is recorded includes the time the activity began, body position while performing the activity, a description of the activity, and the perceived intensity level of the activity (Figure 22.1). The Compendium of Physical Activities (Ainsworth, Haskell, et al. 2000) is used to

FIGURE 22.1 *Sample Physical Activity Record.*

Physical Activity Records			
Time Began	**Position**	**Description**	**How Hard**
2.00	Recline Sit Stand (Walk)	Mowing lawn	Light Moderate (Heavy)
3.45	Recline (Sit) Stand Walk	Riding unicycle	Light (Moderate) Heavy
4.15	Recline Sit Stand (Walk)	Walking into house	Light (Moderate) Heavy

FIGURE 22.2 *Sample Physical Activity Log.*

			Amount of Time	
			Hours	Minutes
Household (Indoors)				
Cooking	Yes	No	_____	_____
Cleaning up	Yes	No	_____	_____
Laundry	Yes	No	_____	_____
Shopping	Yes	No	_____	_____
Dusting	Yes	No	_____	_____
Scrubbing	Yes	No	_____	_____
Vacuuming	Yes	No	_____	_____
Home Repair	Yes	No	_____	_____
Mopping	Yes	No	_____	_____
Washing Car	Yes	No	_____	_____
Other	Yes	No	_____	_____
Household (Outdoors)				
Mowing lawn	Yes	No	_____	_____
Raking lawn	Yes	No	_____	_____
Weeding	Yes	No	_____	_____
Sweeping	Yes	No	_____	_____
Shoveling	Yes	No	_____	_____
Pruning	Yes	No	_____	_____
Chopping wood	Yes	No	_____	_____
Other	Yes	No	_____	_____
Care of Others				
Bathing	Yes	No	_____	_____
Feeding	Yes	No	_____	_____
Playing	Yes	No	_____	_____
Lifting	Yes	No	_____	_____
Pushing wheelchair	Yes	No	_____	_____
Transportation				
Drive/ride in car/bus/subway	Yes	No	_____	_____
Walking				
To get to places	Yes	No	_____	_____
For exercise	Yes	No	_____	_____
With the dog	Yes	No	_____	_____
Work breaks/pleasure	Yes	No	_____	_____

determine the actual intensity level of each activity and to calculate energy expenditure. This process is extremely time consuming, however, because recording every activity a person performs (as it is being performed) per twenty-four-hour period could result in thousands of entries that must be coded using the Compendium of Physical Activities. Physical activity logs are less time consuming because activities are recorded at the end of a specified period of time (generally twenty-four hours) using a checklist (Figure 22.2). Respondents are required to estimate the amount of time they engaged in the activities marked "yes" in the physical activity log.

EPIDEMIOLOGY OF PHYSICAL ACTIVITY

As mentioned previously, three national surveillance systems—BRFSS, NHIS, and NHANES—provide population-level estimates of physical activity participation among adults in the United States. Each survey uses different questions to assess physical activity, and estimates derived from each survey differ slightly; however, patterns observed across each survey are similar. Two published papers describe physical activity participation specifically among African American adults and children using national surveillance data (Whitt-Glover, Taylor, et al., 2007; Whitt-Glover, Taylor, et al., 2009). In general, these data show that physical activity participation among African American adults in the United States is low and that most African American adults are not meeting current physical activity recommendations (24 to 36% meet recommendations, depending on the survey used) (Whitt-Glover, Taylor, et al., 2007).

In 2003, the NHANES began using accelerometers to collect population-level estimates of objectively monitored physical activity (Troiano, Berrigan, et al., 2008). Participants wore an Actigraph model 7164 accelerometer (Actigraph, LLC, Ft. Walton Beach, FL) for seven days. These data showed that African American men aged 20 to 59 years participated for an average of forty minutes per day in moderate-to-vigorous physical activity and African American men aged 60+ participated in eleven minutes of moderate-to-vigorous physical activity. When analyses were restricted to bouts of moderate-to-vigorous physical activity lasting at least ten minutes, estimates decreased to eleven and three minutes per day for 20–59 and 60+ African American men. Participation rates in African American women were much lower. African American women aged 20 to 59 years and 60+ years participated for twenty and six minutes per day in moderate-to-vigorous physical activity, when all data were counted. They participated in only seven and one minute(s) per day when data were restricted to ten minute bouts. These participation levels contrast starkly with the national recommendations for physical activity—a minimum of 30 minutes of moderate-to-vigorous physical activity daily for adults in continuous bouts of at least ten minutes, including resistance and flexibility exercises (PAGAC, 2008).

Among children and adolescents, sixty minutes are recommended, covering a range of pursuits to optimize physical, cognitive, and emotional development (PAGAC, 2008). However, data from NHANES 2003–2004 showed minutes per day in moderate-to-vigorous physical activity ranged from 42 to 114 in African American boys and 18 to 87 in African American girls (Troiano, Berrigan, et al., 2008). However, when examining only those physically active for ten-minute bouts or longer, participation decreased to 17 minutes in 16-to-19-year-old African American boys and 4 minutes in African American girls in the same age group.

Sedentary behavior is most commonly examined through a proxy measure, based on television viewing and computer/sedentary video game use (sometimes combined to represent "screen time"). Although there are currently no recommendations in place for television viewing for adults, several studies have suggested that increased television viewing/computer usage ($>$1 hour/day) has been associated with increased risk for overweight and sedentary behavior among adults (Hu, Li, et al., 2003; Yancey, Wold, et al., 2004; Bowman, 2006). The American Academy of Pediatrics recommends that children participate in less than two hours of screen time/sedentary behavior daily. NHANES 2003–2004 data showed that the number of waking hours spent, per day, in sedentary behaviors among African American $\geq$6 years of age ranged from 6 to 9 (Matthews, Chen, et al., 2008).

Correlates and Determinants

An understanding of behavioral correlates (e.g., demographic, cultural, environmental) is important for explaining disparities in physical activity participation and for understanding the most effective methods for increasing physical activity in targeted subgroups (e.g., what works for men may not work for women; what works for whites may not work for African Americans). The data previously described tend to report greater physical activity participation among men than women. Among men, the proportion who reported meeting physical activity recommendations decreased with age and increased with greater education, income, and among those who were employed and married. Interestingly, physical activity participation appeared to be higher among overweight and obese men compared to normal-weight men (weight status was based on self-reported BMI for NHIS and BRFSS and on measured BMI for NHANES). Among women, physical activity participation was highest among those in younger age groups, those with higher education and income, those who were married, and those with a lower body mass index. Among both men and women, physical activity participation was lowest in the Southern region of the United States compared to the Northwest, Midwest, and West. Data on sedentary behaviors showed similar patterns—women engaged in greater levels of sedentary behavior than men, and engagement in sedentary behavior increased with age (Matthews, Chen, et al., 2008). Patterns among African American children and adolescents are similar—boys are more physically active than girls, normal-weight children and adolescents are more physically active than overweight or obese children and adolescents, and physical activity participation tends to decrease with age (Whitt-Glover, Taylor, et al., 2009).

There are also strong cultural influences on physical activity, serving both as barriers and facilitators. Different cultures have different ideas and norms surrounding physical activity. For example, African American girls and women may not wish to perspire because of arduous hair styling maintenance (Kumanyika, 2002; Day, 2006; Yancey, Ory, et al., 2006). Data from Airhihenbuwa and colleagues suggest that certain segments of the African American population may view rest as more important for maintaining health than participation in physical activity (Airhihenbuwa, Kumanyika, et al., 1995). African Americans may also hold cultural beliefs related to physical activity stemming from prior life experiences that may have been influenced by race (Henderson & Ainsworth, 2000a; Henderson & Ainsworth, 2000b; Henderson & Ainsworth, 2003). For example, African Americans who were forced to walk for transportation because of racial discrimination or poverty may be reluctant to walk for exercise. On the other hand, sports are imbedded in African American culture as an opportunity for success denied them in so many other arenas. Disproportionate military involvement similarly increases fitness. Correlates, determinants, constraints, facilitators, and barriers must be carefully considered when attempting to increase physical activity participation in population subgroups.

Links to Disease Outcomes

The preventive and therapeutic benefits of physical activity are well-established. Physical fitness is an independent protective factor against all-cause and cardiovascular disease mortality (Blair, Kohl, et al. 1995; Haapanen-Niemi, Miilunpalo, et al., 2000), and the metabolic syndrome (Kriska, Saremi, et al., 2003; Lee, Kuk, et al., 2005). Studies have shown that regular physical activity is associated with a decreased incidence of chronic diseases including type 2 diabetes mellitus, cardiovascular disease, hypertension, stroke, as well as cancer (breast and colon), obesity, osteoporosis, and anxiety and depression (Haskell, Lee, et al., 2007).

Physical activity may also protect mental (Singh-Manoux, Hillsdon, et al., 2005) and physical agility (Fox 1999; Gass & Dawson-Hughes 2006), improve sleep quality (King, Oman et al., 1997; de Jong, Lemmink, et al., 2006), elevate mood (Fox, 1999; Wise, Adams-Campbell, et al., 2006), improve affect and energy (Ekkekakis, Hall, et al., 2000; Bixby, Spalding, et al., 2001), enhance sexual enjoyment (USDHHS, 2001), serve as a relative appetite suppressant (Prentice & Jebb, 2000), and decrease preference for highly sweetened beverages (Westerterp-Plantenga, Verwegen, et al., 1997; Passe, Horn, et al., 2000). In children, physical activity also fosters optimal growth and development, both physical and cognitive (Institute of Medicine, 2005). Physical activity is important in weight loss, especially for long-term maintenance (Miller, Koceja, et al., 1997; Jeffery, Drewnowski, et al., 2000), and in the prevention of weight gain (Jeffery, Wing, et al., 2003; Donnelly, Smith, et al., 2004; Sternfeld, Wang, et al., 2004; Hill, Thompson, et al., 2005; Jakicic & Otto 2005; Parsons, Manor, et al., 2006). Physical activity is an essential element of cardiac and musculoskeletal injury rehabilitation (Jolly, Taylor, et al., 2005; Bellelli, Guerini, et al., 2006) and of long-term breast cancer and depression treatment (Pinto & Maruyama 1999; Singh, Clements, et al., 2001; Pickett, Mock, et al., 2002).

Though most studies have been prospective and observational, Haskell and colleagues (Haskell, Lee, et al., 2007) emphasize that these circumstances are comparable to looking at the role of smoking in coronary heart disease. Despite the modest evidence from randomized controlled trials, the evidence is compelling enough to establish public health guidelines to reduce smoking to prevent coronary heart disease.

This inverse relationship between regular physical activity and disease outcomes (and complications from these diseases) is even more important when considering the disproportionate rate at which these diseases affect the African American population. Diabetic African Americans also suffer higher rates of kidney disease and blindness, and are more likely to have lower-leg amputations (Two Feathers, Kieffer et al., 2005). The disproportionate number of disease outcomes and complications from these diseases among African Americans underscores the importance of prevention, treatment, and rehabilitation through the promotion of physical activity in both healthy African American populations as well as those with the chronic conditions.

PHYSICAL ACTIVITY INTERVENTION RESEARCH

Research on physical activity interventions in underserved populations is central to population health. As noted above, such research is critical for the generalizability of study results and to inform public health policy and practice, given the increasingly diverse U.S. population (NCHS, 2000). Empirical results must guide the development of relevant theoretical models or adaptation of existing models to identify appropriate constructs to examine (e.g., Kumanyika & Ewart, 1990). In particular, the "behavioral economics" of physical activity must be recognized and accommodated (Yancey, in press-a, in press-b)—our evolutionary "hard-wiring" to avoid energy expenditure in adulthood (Sturm 2004; Zimring, Joseph, et al., 2005; Levine, Vander Weg, et al., 2006), stress/mood responses to discrimination and other forms of socioeconomic marginalization (Krieger, 2005), and culturally influenced affective/emotional appeal or distaste for certain environmental cues and activities (Day, 2006; Yancey, Ory, et al., 2006).

Despite the critical nature of programmatic and policy interventions to increase physical activity in addressing disparities in obesity and chronic disease in African Americans, very few data are available. Most large-scale physical activity intervention studies do not have large numbers of African American participants and thus do not allow for further analysis of subgroups. The use of homogeneous (usually white/European-American) samples is especially problematic in prevention trials because relatively advantaged populations may already be functioning at a high level, with little "room for improvement." This ceiling effect may lead to underestimation of the influence of the intervention. In addition, subgroup-specific patterns of intervention response may be uncovered in ethnically inclusive studies. The number of studies specifically targeting and enrolling only African American participants is growing, but still quite limited. To provide a more quantitative understanding of these limitations, as of 2003, fewer than 5,000 people of color in individual-level interventions of obesity prevention, and fewer than 14,000 in population-based interventions, had been studied to address the needs of more than 100 million people (Yancey, Kumanyika, et al., 2004).

Individual Level

At the individual level, several review articles capture the state of the science of physical activity promotion in African American adults, but this gap in the literature represents a major obstacle in developing effective policies and programs. In examining physical activity interventions targeting people of color and other "special populations," Taylor et al. (1998) identified only six studies of African Americans. The only physical activity interventions found in a review by Kumanyika (2002) were those documented by Taylor et al. (1998). A review of physical activity interventions studies in women, conducted between 1984 and 2000, found only eighteen studies with at least 35 percent African Americans comprising the sample (Banks-Wallace & Conn, 2002). Further, these studies were low in scientific rigor and had high attrition rates with little reliable long-term data (Banks-Wallace & Conn, 2002; Yancey, McCarthy, et al., 2006). Prior to 1996, most had small sample sizes and enrolled only low-income segments of the population. Of those that did provide long-term (≥6 months) follow-up data, none was able to retain more than 60 percent of the participants (Yancey, McCarthy, et al., 2006).

The more recent contributions to the literature have more than doubled the numbers of studies of this nature, most with larger samples and more rigorous designs (Appel, Champagne, et al., 2003; Will, Farris, et al., 2004; Wadden, West, et al., 2006; Grier & Kumanyika, 2008). However, most target weight and involve dietary as well as physical activity components, making it difficult to disentangle the independent physical activity–related process or outcome effects. What data are available suggest that physical activity interventions are modestly successful, but generally only in the short-term, similar to findings for whites (Marcus, Dubbert et al., 2000; Banks-Wallace & Conn 2002; Kumanyika 2002; Yancey, McCarthy et al., 2006). For example, the African American Women *Fight Cancer with Fitness* (FCF) intervention (Yancey, McCarthy et al., 2006), which had over a 70 percent retention rate at one year follow-up, found significant increases in fitness and decreases in BMI at two months post-intervention compared to control participants. The intervention effects disappeared at the six- and twelve-month follow-up assessments, although fitness improvements remained relative to baseline.

Organizational Level

The social environment has received considerably less emphasis than physical surroundings in population-level physical activity promotion (Stahl, Rutten, et al., 2001; Giles-Corti & Donovan, 2002; Matson-Koffman, Brownstein, et al., 2005; McNeill, Kreuter, et al., 2006), despite the emergence of social support and social norms as key factors in behavioral change in many areas (McNeill, Wyrwich, et al., 2006; Christakis & Fowler, 2007; Maibach, 2007; Van Duyn, McCrae, et al., 2007; Christakis & Fowler, 2008). Diffusion of active living practices in socioeconomically and ethnically diverse populations is more likely to occur at work than in other settings (Sorensen, Barbeau, et al., 2005), although the church is emerging as a target for intervention (Wilcox, Laken, et al., 2007a; Wilcox, Laken, et al., 2007b). The workplace is a particularly important venue for physical activity promotion, given the obstacle of lack of discretionary time among less affluent workers (longer work hours and commutes, less decisional latitude, and less flexible time schedules) (Wolin & Bennett, 2008; Yancey, Pronk, et al., 2007), along with fewer resources for active leisure in terms of free public recreational facilities and money for equipment and paid-use active leisure options (Marcus, Williams, et al., 2006; Yancey, Ory, et al., 2006; Yancey & Kumanyika, 2007).

There is a dearth of literature, however, in evaluations of specific practices and policies designed to change the organizational fabric of the workplace to reduce sedentary behaviors and increase the level of physical activity (Yancey, Pronk, et al., 2007). Even recently published worksite wellness studies still promote the use of individually targeted activities rather than addressing the organizational infrastructure (Beresford, Locke, et al., 2007), though a growing (but still small) number of such studies endeavor to improve environmental influences on dietary intake (French, Jeffery, et al., 2001; Matson-Koffman, Brownstein, et al., 2005). As the sociocultural environment is at least as important as the physical setting in producing sustainable lifestyle change, culturally targeted group interventions such as short dance breaks on paid time that rely *less* on individual initiative and motivation may have greater organizational impact than past efforts, such as walking groups during lunchtime or exercise classes after work hours.

Needless to say, very few studies of worksite physical activity promotion using an environmental approach have focused on the particular needs and barriers of the substantial numbers of workers of ethnic minority or lower socioeconomic status backgrounds, those further down in the organizational hierarchy, and those employed in government or private/non-profit settings (Aldana & Pronk, 2001; Peltomaki, Johansson, et al., 2003; Yancey, Pronk, et al., in press). This gap is particularly apparent, and addressing the gap is especially pressing, in these populations. Nonetheless, some models are beginning to emerge (Linenger, Chesson, et al., 1991; Pronk, Pronk, et al., 1995; Kerr, Eves, et al., 2001; Pohjonen & Ranta 2001; Crawford, Gosliner, et al., 2004; Stewart, Dennison, et al., 2004; Yancey, Kumanyika, et al., 2004). Promising environmental physical activity promotion interventions in the workplace include peer-led physical activity intervention with factory blue-collar workers delivered during regularly-scheduled safety meetings (Elbel, Aldana, et al., 2003), twenty-minute exercise sessions three times weekly during paid time for convalescent home aides (Pohjonen & Ranta, 2001), installation of slowed hydraulic or skip-stop elevators (which only stop at designated floors, requiring employees to either go up or down a flight of stairs to get to other floors), and requiring able-bodied employees to park in distant parking lots (Sinaiko, Donahue, et al., 1999; Zernike, 2003).

Interventions utilizing exercise to reduce injury reflect growing recognition of the opportunity to link fitness promotion and occupational safety interests (Sorensen, et al., 2008). These policies, practices, and programs may also reduce fatigue and anger, and improve mood state (Pronk, Pronk, et al., 1995). Co-worker-led, five-minute mandatory stretch breaks three times each day at sporting goods manufacturer L. L. Bean have been shown to increase productivity, and reduce injuries and sick days (California Nutrition Network [CNN] and California Department of Health Service [CDHS], 2004). Important elements of effective interventions include supportive group dynamics (Fox, Rejeski, et al., 2000), inclusion of performance or skills practice, and visible commitment of organizational leaders on-site (Englberger, 1999; Yancey, Miles, et al., 1999; Hammond, Leonard et al., 2000; Yancey, Jordan, et al., 2003; Crawford, Gosliner, et al., 2004; Yancey, Lewis, et al., 2004).

Structural integration of group physical activity within work and leisure time appears to be particularly valued and salient in communities of color (Englberger, 1999; McKeever, Faddis et al., 2004). For example, dance traditions (dancing to culturally grounded music at parties and holiday celebrations) are normative behavior, even among middle-aged and older adults of color. Structured, five- to ten-minute group exercise breaks, utilizing music and sports moves or dance steps, integrated into organizational routine have been embraced in government and community-based human services agencies (Yancey, 2004; Yancey, Kumanyika, et al., 2004; Yancey, Lewis, et al., 2004; Yancey, McCarthy, et al., 2004; Lara, Yancey, et al., 2008), schools (Stewart, Dennison, et al., 2004; Gibson, Smith, et al., 2008; Honas, Washburn, et al., 2008; Donnelly et al., in press), churches (Wilcox, Laken, et al., 2007), corporations (Pronk, Pronk, et al., 1995; CNN and CDHS, 2004; Heinen & Darling, 2009), and professional sports organizations (Yancey, Winfield, et al. In press, 2009). There is some evidence of spill-over into leisure time as active recreation (Yancey, Lewis, et al., 2006; Donnelly et al., in press). Although an emerging body of evidence has shown the feasibility and potential benefits of this strategy through service-oriented local and state health department program evaluations and federal demonstration projects, there are as yet only a few rigorous studies of intervention effects such as those of Pronk and colleagues (1995) and Donnelly and colleagues (in press).

Population Level

Yancey, Kumanyika, and colleagues (2004) completed a review of studies of population-based interventions targeting communities of color or including sufficient samples to permit subgroup analyses by ethnicity. Twenty-three studies conducted between January 1970 and May 2003 were identified, nineteen of which included physical activity as a target. Eight of these focused on or included substantial numbers of African Americans. As in many individual-level interventions targeting underserved and understudied groups, characteristics of the community-level interventions included: building coalitions and involving communities from study inception; targeting "captive audiences" already congregated for other purposes; mobilizing social networks; and tailoring culturally specific messages and messengers. Fewer than half of the studies presented outcome evaluation data, and statistically significant effects were few and modest. While the best available data address how to engage and retain African Americans in these interventions, they do not focus on how to achieve and sustain regular engagement in physical activity.

Since 2003, several community-level studies including physical activity outcomes targeting African Americans have been published, mostly funded by the CDC Racial and Ethnic Approaches to Community Health initiative (Yancey, Lewis, et al., 2004; Plescia, Herrick, et al., 2008). Some promising evidence is emerging. For example, Plescia and colleagues (2008) demonstrated a significant increase in physical activity among middle-aged African American adults in Charlotte, NC, utilizing lay health advisors and a community coalition to expand YWCA fitness programs into community settings and organize walking groups. However, these studies are too few in number and short in duration to permit conclusions beyond those drawn here.

The only published community-level physical activity promotion intervention for children (teens or 9-to-13-year-olds) that broke out findings by race/ethnicity and included substantial numbers of African Americans was the VERB™ campaign (Huhman, Potter, et al., 2007; Huhman, Berkowitz, et al., 2008). In fact, van Sluijs and colleagues (2007), in a review of youth-focused physical activity interventions, identified no such studies. VERB's huge budget by public health standards (in excess of $150 million by a direct Congressional appropriation) was spent mostly on commercial ads targeting different population segments (Huhman, Berkowitz, et al., 2008). During the first year, the campaign was most effective among girls, children with previously low activity levels, those from urban areas, and those whose parents had less than a high school education—demographic segments that are disproportionately African American (Huhman, Potter, et al., 2005). These subgroup differences disappeared over time, with equal effectiveness population-wide. Unfortunately, VERB™ funding was withdrawn, despite these successful outcomes, after only three years.

Overall Issues and Challenges

Conducting physical activity intervention research in African American populations presents many challenges. These challenges, including issues pertaining to recruitment, implementation, and evaluation (Yancey & Tomiyama, 2007), are presented only briefly here. *Recruitment* refers to the phase of enrolling participants into a research study. *Implementation* refers to how well an intervention is actually carried out or delivered. This includes the *retention* and *adherence* of participants, meaning they have remained in the study through the end and have completed all intervention protocols and assessments, respectively. Implementation also includes the use of *cultural targeting*, meaning that content conveyed (including the language used, and the people and settings depicted) is culturally salient and compatible (Kreuter, Lukwago, et al., 2003). *Evaluation* is the process of measuring outcomes in order to draw conclusions about the results of the intervention, although care must be taken in selecting measures that account for socio-cultural factors within the population (McCarthy, Yancey, et al., 2008).

The challenges in studying African American populations are similar across all of these phases of intervention research. First and foremost, members of underserved populations are often reluctant to participate in scientific trials for many reasons (see Yancey, Ortega, et al., 2006, for a comprehensive review). These obstacles include negative perceptions of the scientific community; inadequate community involvement, particularly in the early decision-making process; and sampling approaches that either net inadequate numbers or lack external validity. Study designs that involve randomization have also been problematic because motivation to participate in research in underserved communities is strongly driven by the desire to take action to address entrenched disparities.

Additionally, there are psychosocial barriers (increased risk of depression, low self-efficacy, increased hostility, increased distress, limited social support, and low quality of life), socioeconomic barriers (lack of financial resources, time, transportation, access to childcare, and education), and other sociodemographic factors (immigration status, religious restrictions, cultural barriers). Feelings of discomfort during data collection might interfere with honesty in self-report measures, and may negatively affect future study retention and intervention adherence. For example, in the *Fight Cancer with Fitness* intervention mentioned earlier, problems arose when young white female college student interns assisted staff in measuring the waist and hip circumference of obese older African American women (Yancey, McCarthy, et al., 2006). Participants felt that the students' facial expressions and comments conveyed disdain for their body size and shape. Interns were quickly reassigned to other study tasks.

These may be overcome by providing logistical support, adequate and appropriate incentives for participation, and study design alternatives. Some of the more successful approaches include reducing these barriers to participation (providing transportation, flexible scheduling, or childcare) and providing timely incentive payments (Yancey, Miles, et al., 2001; Yancey, McCarthy, et al., 2006). The consistent use of the same staff (preferably from the community from which the sample is recruited) to provide social support who are accessible to and familiar with the participants and their families has also been shown to improve retention (Yancey, Ortega, et al., 2006). Alternative approaches for conducting randomized controlled trials have also been successfully utilized such as delayed intervention (i.e., the control group receives the active intervention after comparisons between intervention and control groups are completed) or attention control conditions (an alternative treatment that is also considered valuable). For example, cancer screening education has been used as a control for primary cancer prevention studies promoting physical activity (Yancey, McCarthy et al., 2006), just as physical activity has been used as a control in cancer screening studies (Maxwell, Bastani, et al., 2002). Using physical activity promotion as an attention control condition for randomized trials in other content areas is a "two-fer," a capacity building opportunity in this understudied area to capitalize on existing research infrastructure and establish collaborations between investigators involved in other areas of disparities prevention and physical activity researchers, particularly mentoring junior colleagues.

PHYSICAL ACTIVITY PRACTICE

Public Sector

Physical activity promotion did not explicitly appear among the core functions of public health until 1993 (Novick, 2001). Nutrition, on the other hand, has been a part of the public health practice infrastructure since its inception in the mid-1800s, because of the necessity to assure food and water safety, and to promote maternal and child health. For this reason, chronic disease and obesity prevention efforts at the federal, state, and local levels are markedly skewed toward improving eating habits and nutrient-rich food choices. Public health practice in physical activity is in its infancy.

The 1996 surgeon general's report represents a landmark in the recognition of physical activity as central to public health protection and improvement (Pratt, Epping & Dietz, In press, 2009). This document summarized the health benefits and surveillance data, and signaled the recognition of physical activity as a public health policy issue worthy of widespread attention. The creation of the Physical Activity and Health Branch at the CDC provided a national infrastructure for building public health capacity for physical activity, through training courses in physical activity and public health (Brown, Pate, et al., 2001), modest block grant funding for state health departments (Yee, Williams-Piehota, et al., 2006), and, in 2006, networking and communications support in the formation of a National Society of Physical Activity Practitioners in Public Health.

As chronic disease rates have escalated, numerous and substantial benefits of physical activity have increasingly been documented, and modest funding streams have become available. In this climate, addressing physical activity has often been assigned by default to nutrition staff with few additional resources and often little training or interest (Yancey, Fielding, et al., 2007). CDC-funded physical activity promotion programs, at varying stages of development, exist in at least twenty-eight state health departments (Yee, Williams-Piehota, et al., 2006). However, the California Department of Public Health, for example, only recently increased its physical activity staff from two positions to fourteen, to handle the more than 30 million residents of the state (Dorfman & Yancey, In press, 2009). Local health departments rarely have dedicated physical activity staff, although a few models for developing such programs in areas with large African American populations are emerging (Yancey, Jordan, et al., 2003; Jilcott, Macon, et al., 2004; Yancey, 2004; Yancey, Kumanyika, et al., 2004; Yancey, Ory, et al., 2006; Brownson, Ballew, et al., 2007; Slater, Powell, et al., 2007).

Private Sector

The promotion of physical activity in the private sector through both nonprofit and commercial entities has been on the rise in recent decades. Commercial gyms that were formerly considered the domain of adult males now include franchises marketed toward specific segments of the population such as women, secondary school youth, and young children. Although the relative abundance of health clubs would seem to address many obstacles to finding safe places to exercise, the populations that would most benefit from these gyms often face additional barriers in the form of high membership fees, as well as transportation and childcare issues.

There are, however, nonprofit organizations, such as faith-based organizations or senior centers, that provide physical activity classes for their local communities. These organizations often target low-income or elderly populations that otherwise would not have access to a place to be physically active.

Some workplaces are becoming more aware of their employees' health needs, particularly because healthy employees mean reduced health care costs and improved productivity. Larger companies are able to provide on-site gyms, often with a wellness consultant or other similar health professional, and others subsidize memberships to a local gym. However, smaller organizations are usually not able to afford the costs of either of these options. As a result, there are ongoing studies of alternative interventions or environmental changes to promote physical activity in the workplace, from structurally integrated activity breaks to skip-stop elevators. Importantly, at least some of these studies have accounted for a diverse workforce and the need to find interventions that appeal to all segments of the population.

Ironically, the commercial promotion of physical activity has also included the providers of sedentary entertainment. Recent video games such as Dance Dance Revolution and the Wii Fit have offered the sedentary population a more active option for their lifestyle. Preliminary research to date has indicated that these new types of active video games require more energy expenditure than sedentary games, although not enough to meet daily requirements and less than would be expended when playing the actual sports (Graves, Stratton, et al., 2008). However, this option of active video games does present an alternative for parents whose concerns about neighborhood safety routinely preclude their allowing their children to play outdoors.

CONCLUSIONS AND RECOMMENDATIONS

African Americans are at high risk for living and working in environments hostile to physical activity participation, and, especially among girls and women, for failing to meet federally recommended levels of regular daily physical activity. Consequently, disproportionate numbers of African Americans suffer from physical activity–related diseases and conditions, such as hypertension, stroke, and diabetes. The irony is inescapable that the racial/ethnic group boasting the most elite and celebrated athletes in the world is saddled with a disproportionate burden of physical inactivity, sedentariness, and their co-morbidities.

Despite such concentrations of disease risk and burden, this population remains extremely understudied and underserved with respect to the development of effective policy and programmatic interventions to increase physical inactivity and reduce sedentariness. Attention to this population in terms of research and service is indicated, and should be directed to:

- Enhanced epidemiologic surveillance to permit a greater understanding of microtrends, demographic characteristics, and environmental factors influencing physical activity,

- Increased research funding targeted to ethnic-specific and ethnically inclusive studies,

- Increased recruitment and support for undergraduate and graduate research in physical activity and public health, particularly mentoring opportunities for junior investigators,

- Creation of incentive programs to encourage collaboration between public health physical activity professionals and their counterparts in public education, urban planning and community design, transportation and social services, and

■ Investment in public health education to create degree and certificate programs with a concentration in physical activity and physical activity specialist credentialing programs for public health professionals.

Physical activity is one of the most effective and underutilized tools for disease prevention and health promotion in the public health arsenal. If it could be packaged in pill form, it would likely be the most widely prescribed pharmaceutical product in the world. Like consuming a plant-based, nutrient-rich diet of whole foods, however, regularly engaging for sufficient periods of time in a range of aerobic, resistance, and flexibility activities is a monumental task in our obesogenic (obesity-producing) postmodern society. In accordance with the dictates of the 1986 Ottawa Charter, the world's first health promotion conference, the active choice must be the easy choice in order to achieve widespread population participation. To that end, an emphasis on "push" or "opt-out" interventions is needed: those that take into account human nature's sedentary programming to make the active choice the default choice, the path of least resistance (Yancey, in press-a, in press-b). In order to gain the political will and traction that will permit investment in public transportation at the expense of cars, and active recreation at the expense of revenue sports, the population must be mobilized through incremental changes, such as regulatory and organizational practices and policies that re-integrate brief bouts of physical activity into normal daily routine. Intervening to make the built, organizational, and sociocultural environments activity conducive and *activity-inducing* must become a national public health priority.

REFERENCES

Ainsworth, B. A. (1998). Practical assessment of physical activity. In K. A. Tritschler (Ed.), *Barrow and McGee's practical measurement and assessment*. Baltimore, MD: Williams and Wilkins.

Ainsworth, B. E., Haskell, W. L., et al. (2000). Compendium of physical activities: An update of activity codes and MET intensities. *Medicine & Science in Sports & Exercise, 32*(9 Suppl), S498–504.

Ainsworth, B. E., Jacobs, D. R., Jr., et al. (1993). Assessment of the accuracy of physical activity questionnaire occupational data. *Journal of Occupational Medicine 35*(10), 1017–1027.

Ainsworth, B. E., Montoye, H. J., et al. (1994). Methods of assessing physical activity during leisure and work. In C. Bouchard, R. Shepherd, & T. Stephens (Eds.), *Physical activity, fitness, and health: International proceedings and consensus statement*. Champaign, IL: Human Kinetics Publishers, Inc., pp. 146–159.

Airhihenbuwa, C. O., Kumanyika, S., et al. (1995). Perceptions and beliefs about exercise, rest, and health among African-Americans. *American Journal of Health Promotion, 9*(6), 426–429.

Aldana, S. G., & Pronk, N. P. (2001). Health promotion programs, modifiable health risks, and employee absenteeism. *Journal of Occupational Environment Medicine, 43*(1), 36–46.

Andersen, R. E., Franckowiak, S. C., et al. (1998). Can inexpensive signs encourage the use of stairs? Results from a community intervention. *Annals of Internal Medicine, 129*(5), 363–369.

Andersen, R. E., Franckowiak, S. C., et al. (2006). Effects of a culturally sensitive sign on the use of stairs in African American commuters. *Sozial-und Präventivmedizin, 51*(6), 373–380.

Appel, L. J., Champagne, C. M., et al. (2003). Effects of comprehensive lifestyle modification on blood pressure control: Main results of the PREMIER clinical trial. *Journal of the American Medical Association, 289*(16), 2083–2093.

Banks-Wallace, J., & Conn, V. (2002). Interventions to promote physical activity among African American women. *Public Health Nursing, 19*(5), 321–335.

Bassett, D. R., Jr., Ainsworth, B. E., et al. (1996). Accuracy of five electronic pedometers for measuring distance walked. *Medicine & Science in Sports & Exercise, 28*(8), 1071–1077.

Bellelli, G., Guerini, F., et al. (2006). Body weight-supported treadmill in the physical rehabilitation of severely demented subjects after hip fracture: A case report. *Journal of American Geriatrics & Society, 54*(4), 717–718.

Beresford, S. A., Locke, E., et al. (2007). Worksite study promoting activity and changes in eating (PACE): Design and baseline results. *Obesity* (Silver Spring) (15 Suppl 1), 4S–15S.

Bernstein, M. S., Morabia, A., et al. (1999). Definition and prevalence of sedentarism in an urban population. *American Journal of Public Health, 89*(6): 862–867.

Biddle, S. J., Gorely, T., et al. (2004). Health-enhancing physical activity and sedentary behaviour in children and adolescents. *Journal of Sports Science, 22*(8), 679–701.

Bixby, W. R., Spalding, T. W., et al. (2001). Temporal dynamics and dimensional specificity of the affective response to exercise of varying intensity: Differing pathways to a common outcome. *Journal of Sport & Exercise Psychology, 23*(3), 171–190.

Blair, S. N., Kohl, H. W., 3rd, et al. (1995). Changes in physical fitness and all-cause mortality. A prospective study of healthy and unhealthy men. *Journal of American Merical Association, 273*(14), 1093–1098.

Bouten, C. V., Verboeket-van de Venne, W. P., et al. (1996). Daily physical activity assessment: Comparison between movement registration and doubly labeled water. *Journal of Applied Physiology, 81*(2), 1019–1026.

Bowman, S. A. (2006). Television-viewing characteristics of adults: Correlations to eating practices and overweight and health status. *Preview of Chronic Disease, 3*(2), A38.

Brown, D. R., Pate, R. R., et al. (2001). Physical activity and public health: Training courses for researchers and practitioners. *Public Health Rep, 116*(3), 197–202.

Brownson, R. C., Ballew, P., et al. (2007). The effect of disseminating evidence-based interventions that promote physical activity to health departments. *American Journal of Public Health, 97*(10), 1900–1907.

Brownson, R. C., Boehmer, T. K., et al. (2005). Declining rates of physical activity in the United States: What are the contributors? *Annual Review of Public Health, 26*, 421–443.

Bull, F. C., Armstrong, T., et al. (2003). Burden attributable to physical inactivity: Examination of the 2002 World Health Report estimates. *Medical Science Sports Exercise, 35*(5 (Suppl 1), S359.

California Nutrition Network and California Department of Health Service (2004). Workplace nutrition and physical activity. *Issue Brief, 1*(1), 1–8.

Centers for Disease Control and Prevention (1998). *Behavioral Risk Factor Surveillance System user's guide.* Atlanta, GA: U.S. Department of Health and Human Services, Centers for Disease Control and Prevention.

Centers for Disease Control and Prevention and National Center for Chronic Disease Prevention and Health Promotion (2005). Chronic Disease Overview. Retrieved from http://www.cdc.gov/nccdphp/overview.htm

Centers for Disease Control and Prevention and National Center for Health Statistics (NCHS). (2005). National Health and Nutrition Examination Survey Questionnaire. Retrieved from http://www.cdc.gov/nchs/nhanes.htm

Centers for Disease Control and Prevention and U.S. Department of Health and Human Services (2003). *NHIS Survey Description.* Hyattsville, MD: Division of Health Interview Statistics, National Center for Health Statistics.

Christakis, N. A., & Fowler, J. H. (2007). The spread of obesity in a large social network over 32 years. *New England Journal of Medicine, 357*(4), 370–379.

Christakis, N. A., & Fowler, J. H. (2008). The collective dynamics of smoking in a large social network. *New England Journal of Medicine, 358*(21), 2249–2258.

Crawford, P. B., Gosliner, W., et al. (2004). Walking the talk: Fit WIC wellness programs improve self-efficacy in pediatric obesity prevention counseling. *American Journal of Public Health, 94*(9), 1480–1485.

Day, K. (2006). Active living and social justice: Planning for physical activity in low-income, black, and Latino communities. *Journal of the American Planning Association, 72*(1), 88–99.

de Jong, J., Lemmink, K. A., et al. (2006). Six-month effects of the Groningen active living model (GALM) on physical activity, health and fitness outcomes in sedentary and underactive older adults aged 55–65. *Patient Education Counseling, 62*(1), 132–141.

Donnelly, J. E., Greene, J. L., Gibson, C. A., Washburn, R. A., Sullivan, D. K., DuBose, K. D., Mayo, M. S., Schmelzle, K. H., Ryan, J. J., Williams, S. L., Jacobsen, D. J., Smith, B. (in press). Physical Activity Across the Curriculum (PAAC): A randomized, controlled trial to promote physical activity and diminish overweight and obesity in elementary school children. *Preventive Medicine.*

Donnelly, J. E., Smith, B., et al. (2004). The role of exercise for weight loss and maintenance. *Best Practice & Research: Clinical Gastroenterology, 18*(6), 1009–1029.

Dorfman, L., & Yancey, A. K. (in press). Promoting physical activity and healthy eating: Convergence in framing the role of industry. *Preventive Medicine*.

Ekkekakis, P., Hall, E. E., et al. (2000). Walking in (affective) circles: Can short walks enhance affect? *Journal of Behavior Medicine, 23*(3), 245–275.

Elbel, R., Aldana, S., et al. (2003). A pilot study evaluating a peer led and professional led physical activity intervention with blue-collar employees. *Work, 21*(3), 199–210.

Englberger, L. (1999). Prizes for weight loss. *Bulletin of the World Health Organization, 77*(1), 50–53.

Finkelstein, E. A., Fiebelkorn, I. C., et al. (2003). National Medical Spending Attributable To Overweight And Obesity: How much, and who's paying?, *Health Affairs*, W3-219–226.

Fox, K. R. (1999). The influence of physical activity on mental well-being. *Public Health & Nutrition, 2*(3A): 411–418.

Fox, L. D., Rejeski, W. J., et al. (2000). Effects of leadership style and group dynamics on enjoyment of physical activity. *American Journal of Health Promotion, 14*(5): 277–283.

French, S. A., Jeffery, R. W., et al. (2001). Pricing and promotion effects on low-fat vending snack purchases: The CHIPS Study. *American Journal of Public Health, 91*(1), 112–117.

Gass, M., & Dawson-Hughes, B. (2006). Preventing osteoporosis-related fractures: An overview. *American Journal of Medicine, 119*(4 Suppl 1), S3–S11.

Gibson, C. A., Kirk, E. P., et al. (2005). Reporting quality of randomized trials in the diet and exercise literature for weight loss. *BMC Medical Research Methodology, 5*(1), 9.

Gibson, C. A., Smith, B. K., et al. (2008). Physical activity across the curriculum: Year one process evaluation results. *The International Journal of Behavioral Nutrition and Physical Activity, 5*, 36.

Giles-Corti, B., & Donovan, R. J. (2002). The relative influence of individual, social and physical environment determinants of physical activity. *Social Science & Medicine, 54*(12), 1793–1812.

Graves, L., Stratton, G., et al. (2008). Energy expenditure in adolescents playing new generation computer games. *British Journal of Sports Medicine, 42*(7), 592–594.

Grier, S. A., & Kumanyika, S. K. (2008). The context for choice: Health implications of targeted food and beverage marketing to African Americans. *American Journal of Public Health, 98*(9), 1616–1629.

Gustat, J., Srinivasan, S. R., et al. (2002). Relation of self-rated measures of physical activity to multiple risk factors of insulin resistance syndrome in young adults: The Bogalusa Heart Study. *Journal of Clinical Epidemiology, 55*(10), 997–1006.

Haapanen-Niemi, N., Miilunpalo, S., et al. (2000). Body mass index, physical inactivity and low level of physical fitness as determinants of all-cause and cardiovascular disease mortality–16 y follow-up of middle-aged and elderly men and women. *International Journal of Obesity & Related Metabolic Disorders, 24*(11), 1465–1474.

Hamilton, M. T., Hamilton, D. G., et al. (2007). Role of low energy expenditure and sitting in obesity, metabolic syndrome, type 2 diabetes, and cardiovascular disease. *Diabetes, 56*(11), 2655–2667.

Hammond, S. L., Leonard, B., et al. (2000). The Centers for Disease Control and Prevention Director's Physical Activity Challenge: An evaluation of a worksite health promotion intervention. *American Journal of Health Promotion, 15*(1), 17–20, ii.

Harper, S., & Lynch, J. (2007). Trends in socioeconomic inequalities in adult health behaviors among U.S. states, 1990–2004. *Public Health Rep, 122*(2), 177–189.

Haskell, W. L., Lee, I. M., et al. (2007). Physical activity and public health: Updated recommendation for adults from the American College of Sports Medicine and the American Heart Association. *Medicine and Science in Sports and Exercise, 39*(8), 1423–1434.

Heinen, L., & Darling, H. (2009, March). Addressing obesity in the workplace: The role of employers. *Milbank Quarterly, 87*(1), 101–122.

Henderson, K. A., & Ainsworth, B. E. (2000a). Enablers and constraints to walking for older African American and American Indian women: The Cultural Activity Participation Study. *Research Quarterly for Exercise and Sport, 71*(4), 313–321.

Henderson, K. A., & Ainsworth, B. E. (2000b). Sociocultural perspectives on physical activity in the lives of older African American and American Indian women: A cross cultural activity participation study. *Women & Health, 31*(1), 1–20.

Henderson, K. A., & Ainsworth, B. E. (2003). A synthesis of perceptions about physical activity among older african american and american Indian women. *American Journal of Public Health, 93*(2), 313–317.

Hill, J. O., Thompson, H., et al. (2005). Weight maintenance: What's missing? *Journal of the American Dietetic Association, 105*(5 Suppl 1), S63–66.

Honas, J. J., Washburn, R. A., et al. (2008). Energy expenditure of the physical activity across the curriculum intervention. *Medicine and Science in Sports and Exercise, 40*(8), 1501–1505.

Hu, F. B., Li, T. Y., et al. (2003). Television watching and other sedentary behaviors in relation to risk of obesity and type 2 diabetes mellitus in women. *Journal of the American Medical Association, 289*(14), 1785–1791.

Huhman, M., Berkowitz, J. M., et al. (2008). The VERB campaign's strategy for reaching African-American, Hispanic, Asian, and American Indian children and parents. *American Journal of Preventive Medicine, 34*(6 Suppl), S194–209.

Huhman, M., Potter, L. D., et al. (2005). Effects of a mass media campaign to increase physical activity among children: Year-1 results of the VERB campaign. *Pediatrics, 116*(2), e277–284.

Huhman, M. E., Potter, L. D., et al. (2007). Evaluation of a national physical activity intervention for children: VERB campaign, 2002–2004. *American Journal of Preventive Medicine, 32*(1): 38–43.

Institute of Medicine (U.S.). Committee on Prevention of Obesity in Children and Youth. (2005). J. Koplan, et al. (Eds.), *Preventing childhood obesity: Health in the balance*. Washington, DC: National Academies Press.

Jakicic, J. M., & Otto, A. D. (2005). Physical activity considerations for the treatment and prevention of obesity. *American Journal of Clinical Nutrition, 82*(1 Suppl), 226S–229S.

Jakicic, J., Winters, M. C., et al. (1999). The accuracy of the TriTrac-R3D accelerometer to estimate energy expenditure. *Medicine & Science in Sports & Exercise, 31*(5), 747–574.

Jeffery, R. W., Drewnowski, A., et al. (2000). Long-term maintenance of weight loss: Current status. *Health Psychology, 19*(1 Suppl), 5–16.

Jeffery, R. W., Wing, R. R., et al. (2003). Physical activity and weight loss: Does prescribing higher physical activity goals improve outcome? *American Journal of Clinical Nutrition, 78*(4), 684–689.

Jilcott, S. B., Macon, M. L., et al. (2004). Implementing the WISEWOMAN program in local health departments: Staff attitudes, beliefs, and perceived barriers. *Journal of Womens Health* (Larchmt), *13*(5), 598–606.

Jolly, K., Taylor, R. S., et al. (2005). Home-based cardiac rehabilitation compared with centre-based rehabilitation and usual care: A systematic review and meta-analysis. *International Journal of Cardiology, 111*(3), 343–351.

Kahn, E. B., Ramsey, L. T., et al. (2002). The effectiveness of interventions to increase physical activity: A systematic review. *American Journal of Preventive Medicine, 22*(4 Suppl), 73–107.

Keeler, E. B., Manning, W. G., et al. (1989). The external costs of a sedentary life-style. *American Journal of Public Health, 79*(8), 975–981.

Kelly, C. M., Baker, E. A., et al. (2007). Translating research into practice: Using concept mapping to determine locally relevant intervention strategies to increase physical activity. *Evaluation and Program Planning, 30*(3), 282–293.

Kerr, J., Eves, F., et al. (2001). Encouraging stair use: Stair-riser banners are better than posters. *American Journal of Public Health, 91*(8), 1192–1193.

King, A. C., Oman, R. F., et al. (1997). Moderate-intensity exercise and self-rated quality of sleep in older adults: A randomized controlled trial. *Journal of the American Medical Association, 277*(1), 32–37.

Kreuter, M. W., Lukwago, S. N., et al. (2003). Achieving cultural appropriateness in health promotion programs: Targeted and tailored approaches. *Health Education & Behavior, 30*(2), 133–146.

Krieger, N. (2005). Stormy weather: Race, gene expression, and the science of health disparities. *American Journal of Public Health, 95*(12), 2155–2160.

Kriska, A. M. (1997). A collection of physical activity questionnaires for health-related research. *Medicine & Science in Sports & Exercise, 29*(6 Supplement).

Kriska, A. M., Saremi, A., et al. (2003). Physical activity, obesity, and the incidence of type 2 diabetes in a high-risk population. *American Journal of Epidemiology, 158*(7), 669–675.

Kronenberg, F., Pereira, M. A., et al. (2000). Influence of leisure time physical activity and television watching on atherosclerosis risk factors in the NHLBI Family Heart Study. *Atherosclerosis, 153*(2), 433–443.

Kumanyika, S. K. (2002). Obesity treatment in minorities. In T. A. Wadden & A. J. Stunkard (Eds.), *Obesity: Theory and Therapy*. New York, NY: Guilford Publications.

Kumanyika, S. K., & Ewart, C. K. (1990). Theoretical and baseline considerations for diet and weight control of diabetes among blacks. *Diabetes Care, 13*(11), 1154–1162.

Lara, A., Yancey, A. K., et al. (2008). Pausa para tu Salud: Reduction of weight and waistlines by integrating exercise breaks into workplace organizational routine. *Preventing Chronic Disease, 5*(1), A12.

Lee, S., Kuk, J. L., et al. (2005). Cardiorespiratory fitness attenuates metabolic risk independent of abdominal subcutaneous and visceral fat in men. *Diabetes Care, 28*(4), 895–901.

Levine, J. A., Baukol, P. A., et al. (2001). Validation of the Tracmor triaxial accelerometer system for walking. *Medicine & Science in Sports & Exercise, 33*(9), 1593–1597.

Levine, J. A., Vander Weg, M. W., et al. (2006). Non-exercise activity thermogenesis: The crouching tiger hidden dragon of societal weight gain. *Arteriosclerosis, Thrombosis, and Vascular Biology, 26*(4), 729–736.

Linenger, J. M., Chesson, C. V., 2nd, et al. (1991). Physical fitness gains following simple environmental change. *American Journal of Preventive Medicine, 7*(5), 298–310.

Maibach, E. (2007). The influence of the media environment on physical activity: Looking for the big picture. *American Journal of Health Promotion, 21*(4 Suppl), 353–362, iii.

Marcus, B. H., Dubbert, P. M., et al. (2000). Physical activity behavior change: Issues in adoption and maintenance. *Health Psychology, 19*(1 Suppl), 32–41.

Marcus, B. H., Williams, D. M., et al. (2006). Physical activity intervention studies: What we know and what we need to know: A scientific statement from the American Heart Association Council on Nutrition, Physical Activity, and Metabolism (Subcommittee on Physical Activity); Council on Cardiovascular Disease in the Young; and the Interdisciplinary Working Group on Quality of Care and Outcomes Research. *Circulation, 114*(24), 2739–2752.

Matson-Koffman, D. M., Brownstein, J. N., et al. (2005). A site-specific literature review of policy and environmental interventions that promote physical activity and nutrition for cardiovascular health: What works? *American Journal of Health Promotion, 19*(3), 167–193.

Matthews, C. E., Chen, K. Y., et al. (2008). Amount of time spent in sedentary behaviors in the United States, 2003–2004. *American Journal of Epidemiology, 167*(7), 875–881.

Maxwell, A. E., Bastani, R., et al. (2002). Physical activity among older Filipino-American women. *Women and Health, 36*(1),67–79.

Mayer, E. J., Alderman, B. W., et al. (1991). Physical-activity-assessment measures compared in a biethnic rural population: The San Luis Valley Diabetes Study. *American Journal of Clinical Nutrition, 53*(4), 812–820.

McCarthy, W. J., Yancey, A. K., et al. (2008). Correlation of obesity with elevated blood pressure among racial/ethnic minority children in two Los Angeles middle schools. *Preventing Chronic Disease, 5*(2), A46.

McGinnis, J. M. (1992). The public health burden of a sedentary lifestyle. *Medicine & Science in Sports & Exercise, 24*(6), s196–s200.

McKeever, C., Faddis, C., et al. (2004). Wellness Within REACH: Mind, body, and soul: A no-cost physical activity program for African Americans in Portland, Oregon, to combat cardiovascular disease. *Ethnicity & Disease, 14*(3 Suppl 1), S93–101.

McNeill, L. H., Kreuter, M. W., et al. (2006). Social environment and physical activity: A review of concepts and evidence. *Social Science & Medicine, 63*(4), 1011–1022.

McNeill, L. H., Wyrwich, K. W., et al. (2006). Individual, social environmental, and physical environmental influences on physical activity among black and white adults: A structural equation analysis. *Annals of Behavioral Medicine, 31*(1): 36–44.

Miller, W. C., Koceja, D. M., et al. (1997). A meta-analysis of the past 25 years of weight loss research using diet, exercise or diet plus exercise intervention. *International Journal of Obesity & Related Metabolic Disorders, 21*(10), 941–947.

National Center for Health Statistics (2000). Methodology and Assumptions for the Population Projections of the United States: 1999–2100. Washington, DC: Population Projections Program, Population Division, U.S. Census Bureau, Department of Commerce.

Novick, L. F. (2001). A framework for public health administration and practice. In L. F. Novick & G. P. Mays (Eds.), *Public health administration: Principles for population-based management*. Gaithersburg, MD: Aspen Publishers, pp. xxv, 806.

Parsons, T. J., Manor, O., et al. (2006). Physical activity and change in body mass index from adolescence to mid-adulthood in the 1958 British cohort. *International Journal of Epidemiology, 35*(1), 197–204.

Passe, D. H., Horn, M., et al. (2000). Impact of beverage acceptability on fluid intake during exercise. *Appetite, 35*(3), 219–229.

Peltomaki, P., Johansson, M., et al. (2003). Social context for workplace health promotion: Feasibility considerations in Costa Rica, Finland, Germany, Spain and Sweden. *Health Promotion International, 18*(2), 115–126.

Physical Activity Guidelines Advisory Committee. (2008). *Physical Activity Guidelines Advisory Committee report, 2008*. Washington, DC: U.S. Department of Health and Human Services, 2008. Retrieved from http://www .health.gov/paguidelines

Pickett, M., Mock, V., et al. (2002). Adherence to moderate-intensity exercise during breast cancer therapy. *Cancer Practice, 10*(6), 284–292.

Pinto, B. M., & Maruyama, N. C. (1999). Exercise in the rehabilitation of breast cancer survivors. *Psychooncology, 8*(3), 191–206.

Plescia, M., Herrick, H., et al. (2008). Improving health behaviors in an African American community: The Charlotte Racial and Ethnic Approaches to Community Health project. *American Journal of Public Health, 98*(9), 1678–1684.

Pohjonen, T., & Ranta, R. (2001). Effects of worksite physical exercise intervention on physical fitness, perceived health status, and work ability among home care workers: Five-year follow-up. *Preventive Medicine, 32*(6), 465–475.

Pratt, M., Epping, J. N., Dietz, W. (in press). Putting Physical Activity into Public Health: A CDC Perspective. *Preventive Medicine.*

Prentice, A. M., & Jebb, S. A. (2000). Physical activity level and weight control in adults. In C. Bouchard (Ed.), *Physical activity and obesity*. Champaign, IL: Human Kinetics, pp. vii, 400.

Pronk, S. J., Pronk, N. P., et al. (1995). Impact of a daily 10-minute strength and flexibility program in a manufacturing plant. *American Journal of Health Promotion, 9*(3), 175–178.

Ricciardi, R. (2005). Sedentarism: A concept analysis. *Nursing Forum, 40*(3), 79–87.

Schneider, P. L., Crouter, S. E., et al. (2004). Pedometer measures of free-living physical activity: Comparison of 13 models. *Medicine & Science in Sports & Exercise, 36*(2), 331–335.

Sharma, M. (2006). School-based interventions for childhood and adolescent obesity. *Obesity Review, 7*(3), 261–269.

Sinaiko, A. R., Donahue, R. P., et al. (1999). Relation of weight and rate of increase in weight during childhood and adolescence to body size, blood pressure, fasting insulin, and lipids in young adults. The Minneapolis Children's Blood Pressure Study. *Circulation, 99*(11), 1471–1476.

Singh, N. A., Clements, K. M., et al. (2001). The efficacy of exercise as a long-term antidepressant in elderly subjects: A randomized, controlled trial. *The Journals of Gerontology, Series A, Biological Sciences and Medical Sciences 56*(8), M497–504.

Singh-Manoux, A., Hillsdon, A. M., et al. (2005). Effects of physical activity on cognitive functioning in middle age: Evidence from the Whitehall II prospective cohort study. *American Journal of Public Health, 95*(12), 2252–2258.

Slater, S. J., Powell, L. M., et al. (2007). Missed opportunities: Local health departments as providers of obesity prevention programs for adolescents. *American Journal of Preventive Medicine, 33*(4 Suppl), S246–250.

Smith, S. C., Jr., Clark, L. T., et al. (2005). Discovering the full spectrum of cardiovascular disease: Minority Health Summit 2003: Report of the Obesity, Metabolic Syndrome, and Hypertension Writing Group. *Circulation, 111*(10), e134–139.

Sorensen, G., Barbeau, E., et al. (2005). Promoting behavior change among working-class, multiethnic workers: Results of the healthy directions—small business study. *American Journal of Public Health, 95*(8), 1389–1395.

Stahl, T., Rutten, A., et al. (2001). The importance of the social environment for physically active lifestyle—results from an international study. *Social Science & Medicine 52*(1), 1–10.

Sternfeld, B., Wang, H., et al. (2004). Physical activity and changes in weight and waist circumference in midlife women: Findings from the Study of Women's Health Across the Nation. *American Journal of Epidemiology, 160*(9), 912–922.

Stewart, J. A., Dennison, D. A., et al. (2004). Exercise level and energy expenditure in the TAKE 10! in-class physical activity program. *Journal of School Health, 74*(10), 397–400.

Stone, E. J., McKenzie, T. L., et al. (1998). Effects of physical activity interventions in youth. Review and synthesis. *American Journal of Preventive Medicine, 15*(4), 298–315.

Story, M. (1999). School-based approaches for preventing and treating obesity. *International Journal of Obesity Related Metabolic Disorders*, *23*(Suppl 2), S43–51.

Sturm, R. (2002). The effects of obesity, smoking, and drinking on medical problems and costs. Obesity outranks both smoking and drinking in its deleterious effects on health and health costs. *Health Affairs (Millwood), 21*(2), 245–253.

Sturm, R. (2004). The economics of physical activity: Societal trends and rationales for interventions. *American Journal of Preventive Medicine, 27*(3 Suppl), 126–135.

Taylor, W. C., Baranowski, T., et al. (1998). Physical activity interventions in low-income, ethnic minority, and populations with disability. *American Journal of Preventive Medicine, 15*(4), 334–343.

Timperio, A., Salmon, J., et al. (2004). Evidence-based strategies to promote physical activity among children, adolescents and young adults: Review and update. *Journal of Science & Medicine in Sports, 7*(1 Suppl), 20–29.

Troiano, R. P., Berrigan, D., et al. (2008). Physical activity in the United States measured by accelerometer. *Medicine & Science in Sports & Exercise, 40*(1), 181–188.

Truong, K. D., & Sturm, R. (2005). Weight gain trends across sociodemographic groups in the United States. *American Journal of Public Health, 95*(9), 1602–1606.

Tudor-Locke, C., & Bassett, D. R., Jr. (2004). How many steps/day are enough? Preliminary pedometer indices for public health. *Sports Medicine, 34*(1), 1–8.

Tudor-Locke, C. E., & Myers, A. M. (2001a). Challenges and opportunities for measuring physical activity in sedentary adults. *Sports Medicine, 31*(2), 91–100.

Tudor-Locke, C. E., & Myers, A. M. (2001b). Methodological considerations for researchers and practitioners using pedometers to measure physical (ambulatory) activity. *Research Quarterly for Exercise and Sport, 72*(1), 1–12.

Two Feathers, J., Kieffer, E. C., et al. (2005). Racial and Ethnic Approaches to Community Health (REACH) Detroit partnership: Improving diabetes-related outcomes among African American and Latino adults. *American Journal of Public Health, 95*(9), 1552–1560.

U.S. Department of Health and Human Services. (1996). *Physical activity and health: A report of the Surgeon General*. Atlanta, GA: U.S. Department of Health and Human Services, Centers for Disease Control and Prevention.

U.S. Department of Health and Human Services. (2000). *Healthy people 2010: Understanding and improving health*. Washington, DC: U.S. Government Printing Office.

U.S. Department of Health and Human Services. (2001). *The Surgeon General's call to action to prevent and decrease overweight and obesity*. Washington, DC: U.S. Department of Health and Human Services, Public Health Service, Office of the Surgeon General.

U.S. Department of Health and Human Services Office of Disease Prevention and Health Promotion. (2003). Data 2010. The Healthy People 2010 Database [online]. Retrieved February 7, 2003 from http://wonder.cdc .gov/data2010/obj.htm

Van Duyn, M. A., McCrae, T., et al. (2007). Adapting evidence-based strategies to increase physical activity among African Americans, Hispanics, Hmong, and Native Hawaiians: A social marketing approach. *Prevention of Chronic Disease, 4*(4), A102.

van Sluijs, E. M., McMinn, A. M., et al. (2007). Effectiveness of interventions to promote physical activity in children and adolescents: Systematic review of controlled trials. *British Medical Journal, 335*(7622), 703.

Wadden, T. A., West, D. S., et al. (2006). The Look AHEAD study: A description of the lifestyle intervention and the evidence supporting it. *Obesity* (Silver Spring), *14*(5), 737–752.

Westerterp-Plantenga, M. S., Verwegen, C. R., et al. (1997). Acute effects of exercise or sauna on appetite in obese and nonobese men. *Physiology & Behavior, 62*(6), 1345–1354.

Whitt, M. C., Levin, S., et al. (2003). Evaluation of a two-part survey item to assess moderate physical activity: The Cross-Cultural Activity Participation Study. *Journal of Women's Health 12*(3), 203–212.

Whitt-Glover, M. C., Taylor, W. C., et al. (2007). Self-reported physical activity among blacks estimates from national surveys. *American Journal of Preventive Medicine 33*(5), 412–417.

Whitt-Glover, M. C., Taylor, W. C., et al. (2009). Disparities in physical activity and sedentary behaviors among U.S. children and adolescents: Prevalence, correlates, and intervention implications. *Journal of Public Health Policy 2009; 30*(Suppl 1), S309–34.

Wilcox, S., Laken, M., et al. (2007a). The health-e-AME faith-based physical activity initiative: Description and baseline findings. *Health Promotion Practices, 8*(1), 69–78.

Wilcox, S., Laken, M., et al. (2007b). Increasing physical activity among church members: Community-based participatory research. *American Journal of Preventive Medicine, 32*(2), 131–138.

Will, J. C., Farris, R. P., et al. (2004). Health promotion interventions for disadvantaged women: Overview of the WISEWOMAN projects. *Journal of Women's Health, 13*(5): 484–502.

Wise, L. A., Adams-Campbell, L. L., et al. (2006). Leisure time physical activity in relation to depressive symptoms in the Black Women's Health Study. *Annals of Behavioral Medicine, 32*(1), 68–76.

Wolin, K. Y., & Bennett, G. G. (2008). Interrelations of socioeconomic position and occupational and leisure-time physical activity in the National Health and Nutrition Examination Survey. *Journal of Physical Activity & Health, 5*(2), 229–241.

Yancey, A., Pronk, N., et al. (2007). Environmental and policy approaches to obesity prevention in the workplace. In S. K. Kumanyika & R. Brownson (Eds.), *Obesity epidemiology & prevention: A Handbook.* New York: Springer.

Yancey, A. K. (2004). Building capacity to prevent and control chronic disease in underserved communities: Expanding the wisdom of WISEWOMAN in intervening at the environmental level. *Journal of Womens Health (Larchmt), 13*(5), 644–649.

Yancey, A. K. (in press-a). *Instant recess: How to build a fit nation for the 21st century.* Berkeley, CA: University of California Press.

Yancey, A. K. (in press-b). The Meta-Motivation Model: Organizational leadership is the key to getting society moving. *Preventive Medicine.*

Yancey, A. K., Fielding, J. E., et al. (2007). Creating a robust public health infrastructure for physical activity promotion. *American Journal of Preventive Medicine, 32*(1), 68–78.

Yancey, A. K., Jordan, A., et al. (2003). Engaging high-risk populations in community-level fitness promotion: ROCK! Richmond. *Health Promotion Practice, 4*(2), 180–188.

Yancey, A. K., & Kumanyika, S. K. (2007). Bridging the gap: Understanding the structure of social inequities in childhood obesity. *American Journal of Preventive Medicine, 33*(4 Suppl), S172–174.

Yancey, A. K., Kumanyika, S. K., et al. (2004). Population-based interventions engaging communities of color in healthy eating and active living: A review. *Preventing Chronic Disease, 1*(1), A09.

Yancey, A. K., Lewis, L. B., et al. (2004). Leading by example: A local health department-community collaboration to incorporate physical activity into organizational practice. *Journal of Public Health Management Practices, 10*(2), 116–123.

Yancey, A. K., Lewis, L. B., et al. (2006). Putting promotion into practice: The African Americans building a legacy of health organizational wellness program. *Health Promotion Practices, 7*(3 Suppl), 233S–246S.

Yancey, A. K., McCarthy, W. J., et al. (2004). The Los Angeles Lift Off: A sociocultural environmental change intervention to integrate physical activity into the workplace. *Preventive Medicine, 38*(6), 848–856.

Yancey, A. K., McCarthy, W. J., et al. (2006). Challenges in improving fitness: Results of a community-based, randomized, controlled lifestyle change intervention. *Journal of Women's Health, 15*(4), 412–429.

Yancey, A. K., Miles, O., et al. (1999). Organizational characteristics facilitating initiation and institutionalization of physical activity programs in a multi-ethnic, urban community. *Journal of Health Education, 30*(2), S44–S51.

Yancey, A. K., Miles, O. L., et al. (2001). Differential response to targeted recruitment strategies to fitness promotion research by African-American women of varying body mass index. *Ethnicity & Disease, 11*(1), 115–23.

Yancey, A. K., Ortega, A. N., et al. (2006). Effective recruitment and retention of minority research participants. *Annual Review of Public Health, 27,* 1–28.

Yancey, A. K., Ory, M. G., et al. (2006). Dissemination of physical activity promotion interventions in underserved populations. *American Journal of Preventive Medicine, 31*(4 Suppl), S82–91.

Yancey, A. K., Pronk, N. P., et al. (in press). Workplace approaches to obesity prevention. In S. K. Kumanyika & R. C. Brownson (Eds.). *Handbook of obesity prevention: A resource for health professionals.* New York: Springer Publishing Company.

Yancey, A. K., & Tomiyama, A. J. (2007). Physical activity as primary prevention to address cancer disparities. *Seminars in Oncology Nursing, 23*(4), 253–263.

Yancey, A. K., Winfield, D., et al. (in press). Live, learn and play: Building strategic alliances between professional sports and public health. *Preventive Medicine.*

Yancey, A. K., Wold, C. M., et al. (2004). Physical inactivity and overweight among Los Angeles County adults. *American Journal of Preventive Medicine, 27*(2), 146–152.

Yee, S. L., Williams-Piehota, P., et al. (2006). The nutrition and physical activity program to prevent obesity and other chronic diseases: Monitoring progress in funded states. *Preventing Chronic Disease, 3*(1), A23.

Zernike, K. (2003). Fight Against Fat Shifting to the Workplace. *New York Times,* A1.

Zimring, C., Joseph, A., et al. (2005). Influences of building design and site design on physical activity: Research and intervention opportunities. *American Journal of Preventive Medicine 28*(2 Suppl 2): 186–193.

PART

5

ALTERNATIVE INTERVENTIONS AND HUMAN RESOURCES DEVELOPMENT

23

CHIROPRACTIC MEDICINE: INTEGRAL TO INTEGRATIVE MEDICINE

MALIKA B. GOODEN
ELTON D. HOLDEN

The U.S. population has become a phantasmagoria of ethnic, cultural, gender, and age groups and the rapidly changing demographics from a less homogeneous to a more heterogeneous society have given rise to growing demands for health care options. Chiropractic, considered a complementary and alternative medicine (CAM) by the National Institutes of Health (NIH), has emerged as a relevant form of health care used to address a litany of health issues facing our communities. As such, it is imperative that an increased awareness of chiropractic and the benefits associated with it are achieved within public health and the broader health care system.

CHIROPRACTIC MEDICINE

Although chiropractic medicine has emerged as a formidable health care option, and is considered the third largest primary health care profession in the United States (NBCE, 2005), there are still those who are misinformed about its underpinnings, benefits, and more broadly how/if it fits within the current U.S. health care system paradigm. Some continue to think of chiropractic as a profession of practitioners who just deal with low back or neck pain, "popping necks" and "cracking backs." This is, to say the least, a misrepresentation and misunderstanding of the true nature of this health field and profession.

Founded in the 1890s by David Daniel (DD) Palmar, in Davenport, Iowa, chiropractic is a distinct field of health care, guided by specific scopes and standards of practice. Educational requirements and clinical training are extensive and in many respects mirror those of allopathic (traditional, and conventional) medicine. As indicated in the National Board of Chiropractic Examiner's (NBCE) report *Job Analysis of Chiropractic 2005: A Project Report, Survey Analysis, and Summary of the Practice of Chiropractic within the United States*, "government inquirers, as well as independent investigations by medical practitioners, have affirmed that today's chiropractic training is of equivalent standard to [conventional] medical training in all preclinical subjects." Contrary to some beliefs, Chiropractic Doctors, also referred to as Chiropractic Physicians or Chiropractors, are primary care practitioners.

Doctors of Chiropractic focus on the relationship between structure (primarily the spine) and function (as coordinated by the nervous system) and how that relationship affects the tissues and organs of the body and overall preservation and restoration of health (ACC, 2008). Although still somewhat controversial, the vertebral subluxation, as defined by many in the chiropractic field and by the Association of Chiropractic Colleges (ACC) in 1996 in an attempt to unify chiropractic terminology, is a complex of functional and/or structural and/or pathological articular changes that compromise neural integrity and may influence organ systems and general health. It is because of the devastating effects of the vertebral subluxation complex (VSC) on human health that the removal of identified vertebral subluxations through varied chiropractic techniques is critical. Specific spinal adjustments are unique to and are the hallmark of chiropractic care. Gentle force introduced into the spine by a chiropractor is used with the intention of releasing a vertebral segment from its abnormal position to decrease the existence of vertebral subluxations and subsequent neural interference.

A chiropractic adjustment can range from a light comfortable dynamic thrust to several ounces of sustained pressure; and there are several adjusting techniques/systems utilized in chiropractic today. Each system has a specific adjusting protocol to restore the spine to normal function. The protocol used reduces the negative neurologic impact, and returns the body to relative normal efficiency. Spinal adjustments, regardless of which technique/system is utilized, are tailored to the patient's age and clinical presentation.

In addition to taking a comprehensive medical/health history, chiropractic analysis incorporates diagnostic imaging for visual assessment of the subluxated spine to detect possible contraindications to spinal adjustments, ruling out bone disease and spinal or other pathologies. Thermographic instrumentation is also used to aid in the detection of subluxations. Because blood flow and subsequent skin temperature are indirect measures of autonomic nervous system function, abnormal temperature patterns palpated or measured externally along the spine can be a sign of autonomic nerve dysfunction. Non-invasive testing, such as surface EMG, is a rising technology that is being utilized in chiropractic to better analyze the impact subluxation has on spinal muscle function. A chiropractor may utilize these technologies in addition to traditional spinal palpation, motion palpation, orthopedic assessment, and muscle, sensory, and neurological examinations. The goal is to restore and maintain optimal health by locating and correcting any interference to the nervous system caused by vertebral subluxations.

Thus, a chiropractic doctor's focus is on finding where distress on a patient's nervous system exists based on dysfunctions (malpositioned vertebra on nerves/subluxation) that may be preventing the body from functioning properly. Removing the cause of neural interferences helps a patient's body to heal naturally without use of medicating drugs. Chiropractors strive to diagnose and correct biomechanical disturbances that cause specific health issues and perform adjustments that influence the body's nervous system and natural defense mechanisms, helping to alleviate pain and improving health in general. Nutritional counseling, therapeutic exercises, physiotherapy, and other rehabilitative approaches may be utilized in conjunction with adjustments.

As an established health care profession used largely for musculoskeletal complaints in the United States, chiropractic has made the largest inroad into private and public health care systems, and is increasingly viewed by many in the medical profession as an effective specialty (Meeker & Haldeman, 2002). Several studies that examine chiropractic utilization indicate that rates vary, but generally fall into a range from about 6 to 12 percent of the U.S. population and often offer lower costs for comparable results when compared to conventional medicine (Lawrence, 2007).

To guide the tenets of chiropractic, the ACC paradigm is currently the most widely accepted among chiropractic associations and individual doctors (see Figure 23.1).

Extraordinary measures continue to be imperative in educating communities at large, medical/health communities, and underserved and marginalized communities in particular about specific and overall health benefits of chiropractic care for the restoration of health and wellness and for the prevention of illness.

INTEGRATIVE MEDICINE

Integrative Medicine, as defined by the Consortium of Academic Health Centers for Integrative Medicine (CAHCIM), is "the practice of medicine that reaffirms the importance of the relationship between practitioner and patient, focuses on the whole person, is informed by evidence, and makes use of all appropriate therapeutic approaches, healthcare professionals and disciplines to achieve optimal health and healing" (CAHCIM, 2005). Basically, it emphasizes a collaborative approach to health care that combines conventional, alternative, and complementary medicine.

CAHCIM currently includes forty-two esteemed academic medical centers (including Harvard University Medical School, Yale University, Stanford University, University of Michigan, and Johns Hopkins University to name a few) and is supported by philanthropic grants and membership dues. The mission of the Consortium is to "help transform medicine and healthcare through rigorous scientific studies, new models of clinical care, and innovative educational programs that integrate biomedicine,

FIGURE 23.1 *The ACC Chiropractic Paradigm.*

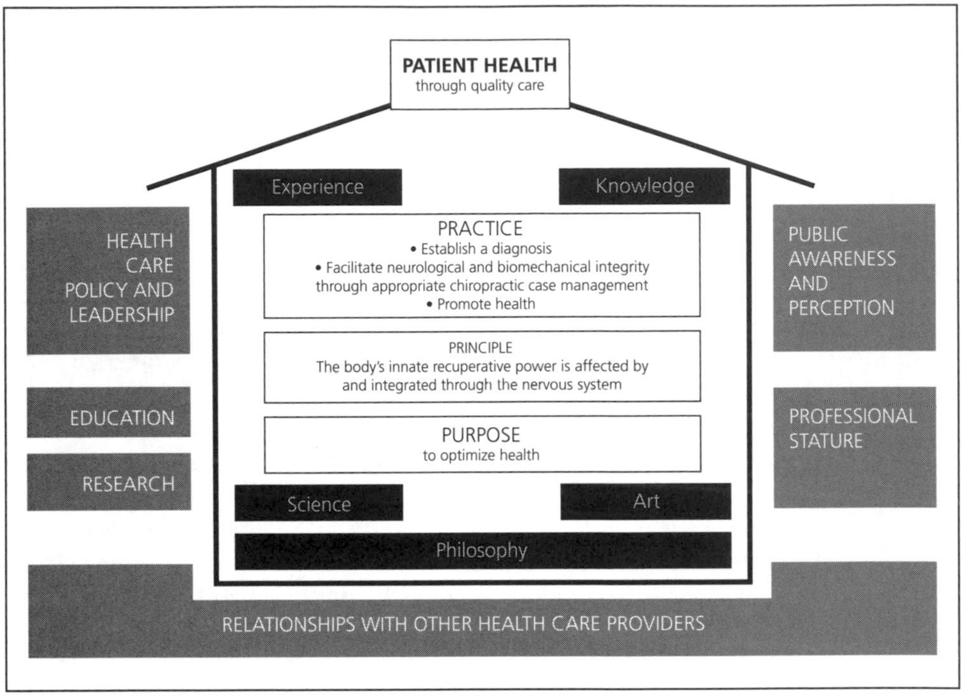

```
                    ┌──────────────────────┐
                    │   PATIENT HEALTH     │
                    │  through quality care │
                    └──────────────────────┘

        ┌────────────┐                    ┌────────────┐
        │ Experience │                    │ Knowledge  │
        └────────────┘                    └────────────┘

HEALTH              PRACTICE                      PUBLIC
CARE            • Establish a diagnosis           AWARENESS
POLICY AND   • Facilitate neurological and        AND
LEADERSHIP   biomechanical integrity through      PERCEPTION
             appropriate chiropractic case
             management
                 • Promote health

                    PRINCIPLE
EDUCATION   The body's innate recuperative        PROFESSIONAL
            power is affected by and              STATURE
            integrated through the nervous
            system

                    PURPOSE
RESEARCH          to optimize health

        ┌────────────┐                    ┌────────────┐
        │  Science   │                    │    Art     │
        └────────────┘                    └────────────┘

                    Philosophy

        RELATIONSHIPS WITH OTHER HEALTH CARE PROVIDERS
```

Source: Association of Chiropractic Colleges, 2008.

the complexity of human beings, the intrinsic nature of healing, and the rich diversity of therapeutic systems" (CAHCIM, 2005).

The relevance of integrated medicine and a consortium is substantiated by the relatively high percentage of adults who use CAM. According to a nationwide survey released May 2004, "36% of U.S. adults aged 18 years and older use[d] some form of CAM" (NIH, NCCAM, 2008). Research has shown that most people who use CAM (which is typically a more personalized and tailored approach to patient care and concerns; valuing prevention and promotion of good health and well-being) combine it with conventional medicine, because they believe the combination to be superior to either alone and seek a strong therapeutic relationship with their providers (McCaffrey et al., 2007). The relationship between allopathic and chiropractic medicine undoubtedly substantiates co-management opportunities and the need for a comprehensive referral system. The ACC chiropractic scope and practice diagram in Figure 23.2 depicts the opportunity for collaborative care.

Use of Complementary and Alternative Medicine (CAM) by the American Public, a report released by the Institute of Medicine of the National Academies (IOM) in

FIGURE 23.2 *ACC Chiropractic Scope and Practice.*

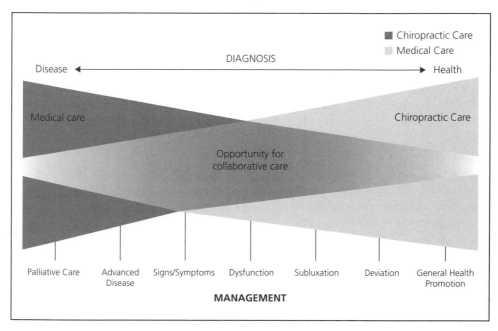

DIAGNOSIS

■ Chiropractic Care
▨ Medical Care

Disease ◄——————————————————————► Health

Medical care

Chiropractic Care

Opportunity for
collaborative care

| Palliative Care | Advanced Disease | Signs/Symptoms | Dysfunction | Subluxation | Deviation | General Health Promotion |

MANAGEMENT

Source: Association of Chiropractic Colleges, 2008.

January 2005, recommended that "health profession schools incorporate sufficient information about complementary and alternative medicine (CAM) into the standard curriculum at all levels to enable licensed professionals to competently advise their patients about CAM" (IOM, 2005). One important reason to inform patients of CAM and/or determine which patients may be using CAM is to determine potential contraindications and decrease the potential for adverse interactions with conventional medicine. Clinical research to support the emergent trends for the benefits of integrated medicine to address several chronic illnesses is also growing.

Chiropractic care for the management of a myriad of chronic illnesses is increasingly being recognized as an important approach and treatment modality, and in some cases, adjunct to traditional medical interventions. Selected illnesses prevalent among ethnic minorities—diabetes, cardiovascular disease, and asthma—warrant further examination into the role of integrative medicine, with an emphasis on chiropractic care's role in improving health outcomes relative to these diseases.

CHRONIC ILLNESSES

Diabetes mellitus, a multi-system disease, is characterized by persistent hyperglycemia that has both acute and chronic biochemical and anatomical sequelae. Ethnic minorities are disproportionately affected by both type I and type II diabetes. African Americans, Hispanic Americans, and Native Americans have rates significantly greater than those for non-Hispanic whites (NCCAM, 2008). Approximately 3.7 million (14.7%) of all non-Hispanic African Americans aged 20 and older in the United States have diabetes, diagnosed or undiagnosed (NIDDKD, 2008). Some research suggests chiropractic is a useful strategy to assist in the management of diabetes, particularly the myriad of neuromusculoskeletal conditions often associated with the disease (Ferrance & Wyatt, 2006). Studies have indicated that chiropractic manipulations and active rehabilitation in addition to dietary modification and exercise have assisted in positively altering glucose levels and physiological changes associated with diabetic patients (Blum, 2006; Valli, 2004; So et al., 2004).

Cardiovascular disease is the leading cause of death and disability in the United States (CDC, 2007). African American adults are less likely to be diagnosed with coronary heart disease, yet are more likely to die from heart disease (OMH, 2007). High blood pressure is one symptom often associated with cardiovascular disease, and chiropractors have utilized techniques to aid in its management. Manual correction of malalignment of the cervical spine at the level of the Atlas vertebra has been associated with reduced arterial pressure. In a randomized, double blind, placebo-controlled study design with fifty hypertensive patients, restoration of Atlas alignment was associated with marked reductions in blood pressure similar to the use of two-drug combination therapy (Bakris et al., 2007). However, larger studies are needed to validate these findings.

Similarly, So et al. (2004) found that the use of a thermomechanical device (a chiropractic rehabilitative modality) with hypertensive and type II diabetic patients exhibited significant decreases in systolic, diastolic, and pulse pressures following treatment regimens. It is suggested that the treatment addressed improvement in the alignment of the pituitary-adrenal cortex axis. A randomized clinical trial indicated that two months of full spine chiropractic care with adjustments delivered at motion segments exhibiting signs of subluxation yielded lower diastolic blood pressure (Long et al., 2002). Chiropractic management was also indicated as an essential component to alleviating discomfort in a case study of a patient with congestive heart failure (Kettner et al., 2005).

Asthma is characterized by inflammation of the air passages, resulting in the temporary narrowing of the airways that transport air from the nose and mouth to the lungs. Asthma symptoms can be caused by allergens or irritants that are inhaled into the lungs, resulting in inflamed, clogged, and constricted airways. Symptoms include difficulty breathing, wheezing, coughing, and tightness in the chest (AAFA, 2008). Asthma is the leading serious chronic illness of children in the United States. In 2006, an estimated 6.8 million children under age 18 (almost 1.2 million under age 5) had asthma, with 4.1 million having had an asthma attack, and many others with "hidden" or undiagnosed asthma (CDC, 2006). Asthma is slightly more prevalent among African Americans than among whites, and ethnic differences in asthma prevalence, morbidity, and mortality are highly correlated with poverty, urban air quality, indoor allergens, lack of patient education, and inadequate medical care (NIAID, 2001).

There is no cure for asthma, but asthma can be managed with proper prevention and treatment. Chiropractic care may be a viable option for individuals and families to consider. Some studies have indicated the benefits of reducing asthma-associated symptoms using a multi-modal chiropractic protocol among patients (Cuthbert, 2008; Fedorchuk, 2007). Gibbs (2005) used chiropractic manipulation administered to the upper thoracic spine of patients as an adjunct to conventional pharmacological treatment and yielded positive outcomes among asthmatic patients. Similarly, Blum (2002) reported that one form of chiropractic, Sacro-occipital Technique, offers some conservative alternatives to the treatment of asthma because it can affect the viscera, vertebra, post and preganglionic reflexes, as well as cranial and sacral influences on the primary respiratory mechanism.

In general, it is suggested that chronic illnesses be managed by a supportive network that includes a chiropractor, medical doctor, and family, promoting a holistic approach to comprehensive care. Such an approach encourages better health outcomes that simultaneously respect multidimensional treatment strategies for achieving optimal health care for patients. Chiropractic is identified as one of the manipulative and body-based practices within the National Center for Complementary and Alternative Medicine (NCCAM) at the National Institutes of Health within the U.S. Department of Health and Human Services, and as an integrative health care method supported by NCCAM's 2005–2009 strategic plan that promotes "the conduct and support of basic and applied research, research training, the dissemination of health information, and other programs with respect to identifying, investigating, and validating complementary and alternative treatment, diagnostic and prevention modalities, disciplines and systems" (NCCAM, 2005). Although chiropractors are traditionally known to primarily treat musculoskeletal issues and associated neural interference that may include common complaints associated with back and neck injury/pain, they should also be strongly considered as viable practitioners for co-managing chronic illnesses.

As stated by Dr. Rashad O. Sanford, Chiropractic Physician and partner of Atlanta Spine Dunwoody in Atlanta, Ga., "taking an integrative approach to healthcare is critical in addressing the various health care needs of individuals who seek chiropractic care." He has "seen the positive benefits chiropractic care has had on treating patients coping with Hypertension—by taking an integrative approach and administering chiropractic care along with working collectively with other treating physicians, patients have been able to have their hypertension medication dosage lowered or they have been able to discontinue use of their hypertension medications altogether" (Sanford, 2008).

COMMUNITY ENGAGEMENT, EDUCATION, AND OUTREACH TO ETHNIC MINORITIES

There is no standard definition of "community." However, the term has been used to describe interactions among people in primarily geographic terms. But it is now accepted that people who live in close proximity to one another do not necessarily constitute a community, because they may differ with respect to value systems and other cultural characteristics more relevant to the social concept of community. Although ethnic minorities are not a homogenous population, there are some commonalities that may be shared among some groups, particularly concerning perceptions about the health care system. For example, Johnson et al. (2004) reported that African Americans, Hispanics, and Asians were more likely than whites to perceive that they would have received better medical care if they belonged to a different race/ethnic group, and medical staff judged them unfairly or treated them with disrespect based on race/ethnicity and how well they were able to speak English.

Diverse communities that include ethnic minorities should be especially targeted by health care professionals, including chiropractors, in an attempt to decrease stigma and mistrust of the health care system and to encourage greater access and utilization of various treatment modalities. To highlight the groups who typically seek chiropractic care, data gleaned from research by the NBCE specifically on the "chiropractic patient" (i.e., people who seek chiropractic care) indicated that in both 2003 and in 1998, based on ethnicity, whites sought more chiropractic care when compared to other groups. This continues to be the trend (shown in Table 23.1).

It is also evident from the table that although use of chiropractic care by whites decreased in 2003 (from 60.4% to 56.7%) and African American use increased (from 12.7% to 14.0%), caucasians still utilized chiropractic care more than African Americans and the other races in both represented years. These trends in use of care (or lack thereof by some groups) continue to underscore why outreach to African American communities and other groups is necessary. Ultimately, "it is the nature

TABLE 23.1 Ethnic Origin of Chiropractic Patients.

Patient Ethnicity	1998	2003
African American	12.7%	14.0%
Asian/Pacific Islander	7.9%	9.0%
Caucasian	60.4%	56.7%
Hispanic	13.6%	14.4%
Native American	4.7%	5.3%
Other	0.7%	0.6%

Source: NBCE, Table 8.1 Ethnic Origin, 2005; re-created copy by M. B. Gooden.

between the doctor and the patient [that] has an important influence on the process and outcome of chiropractic care" (CCE, 2007).

With fewer chiropractors and chiropractic patients in areas identified as ethnic minority neighborhoods (Bluestein, 1998), there is a tremendous need for chiropractic services in the African American community, and it may primarily be the responsibility of African American chiropractors to meet that need (Callender, 2006). Greater recruitment at historically African American colleges and universities should be encouraged at all chiropractic colleges to improve the number of minority chiropractic students and subsequently the field's workforce diversity (Wiese, 2004).

Chiropractic doctors who work with ethnically diverse communities may promote further advancement of the field by making it more culturally sensitive and by enhancing the receptiveness and responsiveness of individuals and families to chiropractic care for their health care needs. Cultural competency training should be provided to chiropractors of all ethnicities through continuing education workshops and to students of chiropractic during their matriculation through school to better equip them with the skills of engaging diverse groups of people. Adopting a culturally responsive framework within the scope of chiropractic can greatly support providers in their ability to establish a better rapport with patients and facilitate more effective treatment. For example, a core set of skills that can be learned by chiropractic professionals to respectfully and efficiently communicate health care information with ethnically diverse patient populations is based on the CRASH conceptual model. This mnemonic highlights the following essential components of culturally competent health care: consider Culture, show Respect, Assess/Affirm differences, show Sensitivity and Self-awareness, and do it all with Humility (Rust et al., 2006).

The concept of community engagement goes beyond community participation. It is the process of working collaboratively with relevant partners who share common goals and interests; this involves building authentic partnerships, including mutual respect and active, inclusive participation; power sharing and equity; and finding the mutual benefit or win-win possibility in collaborative initiatives (Zakus & Lysack, 1998). Using approaches that are culturally responsive is particularly significant when working with ethnic minority communities. Chiropractors can strive to develop partnerships with local stakeholders and involve them in assessing local health problems, determining the value of planning, conducting, and overseeing clinical research, and chiropractic practice approaches that can aid in strengthening an integrated public health care system. Specifically, chiropractors can strengthen their collaboration within communities by

■ Improving community-based participatory research opportunities through the establishment of viable academic (colleges of chiropractic) and community partnerships.

■ Using culturally tailored communication approaches to effectively educate community members about the benefits of chiropractic care and preventive health care strategies.

- Developing and disseminating user-friendly educational materials (i.e, brochures, fact sheets, and newsletters) to communities to increase their knowledge and awareness of chiropractic care.

- Participating in local community and public health events (i.e., health fairs, symposiums, charity walk/runs, etc.).

POLICY ISSUES AND IMPLICATIONS

The field of chiropractic has progressed since its inception but still has a way to go in terms of being fully accepted and integrated into our current mainstream health system, as well as being fully accessible to those who need/want such care. Over the years, there has been key legislation proposed in support of growing the field of chiropractic and more clearly defining its place within the U.S. health care system.

Currently, there are several chiropractic-related legislative issues being considered by Congress (1) H.Res 294: Sense of Congress Legislation Urging the Secretary of Defense to Commission Doctors of Chiropractic as Health Care Officers in the Armed Forces, (2) HR 1470: Chiropractic Available to All Veterans Act, and (3) HR 1471: The Better Access to Chiropractors to Keep Our Veterans Healthy Act.

On February 13, 2008, several congressional members introduced *Joint Resolution 294*, which states, "it is the sense of congress that the secretary of defense should take immediate steps to establish a career path for doctors of chiropractic to be appointed as commissioned officers in all branches of the Armed Forces for the purposes of providing chiropractic services to members of armed forces." Integral to the legislation, chiropractic services would include but not be limited to:

1. Increasing the cost effectiveness of military health care expenditures by making optimal use of conservative, drugless, and nonsurgical care pathway chiropractic offers;

2. Helping to meet the growing demand for chiropractic care in the military;

3. Utilizing a highly skilled and trained pool of health care professionals; and

4. Helping to address a growing wave of back-related work time loss, serious injuries, and career-ending disability outcomes (ICA, 2008).

Introduced by Rep. Bob Filner, *HR 1470* would provide for needed improvements in the availability and timeliness of chiropractic services in the U.S. Dept. of Veterans Affairs. A key component to this legislation is "extending veterans' access to in-facility chiropractic services by requiring the expansion of chiropractic personnel requirements to not fewer than 75 medical centers by not later than December 31, 2008 and at all medical centers by not later than December 31, 2011" (ICA, 2008). Legislation has passed in the House of Representatives and is awaiting action in the Senate.

Also introduced by Rep. Bob Filner, *HR 1471* introduces the need for reforms so veteran beneficiaries of the U.S. Dept. of Veteran Affairs can access chiropractic services. This legislation includes but is not limited to veterans being able to "avoid and prevent the current climate of discrimination in which some DVA medical professionals refuse requests for referral to a doctor of chiropractic [and] provide veterans a greater say in their own health care decision making and opening up a new, safe, and proven clinically effective care pathway" (ICA, 2008).

Other chiropractic policy issues currently at the forefront of many discussions are ways to increase care coverage, particularly in areas that are critically lacking and Medicare, as well as general medical coverage for chiropractic care. A practice-based, non-randomized, comparative study of self-referring patients to both chiropractic doctors and medical doctors in chiropractic and general practice community clinics over a two year period to identify provider costs, clinical outcomes, and patient satisfaction for low back pain (LBP) treatment found that "chiropractic care is relatively cost-effective compared with medical care . . . chiropractic and medical care are comparable in cost effectiveness for acute LBP [and] healthcare organizations and policy makers should consider the appropriateness of chiropractic as a treatment option" (Hass et al., 2005, pp. 555–563). Eisenburg et al. (2002) indicate that to ensure high standards of care and more generalizable clinical research, more nationally uniform credentialing mechanisms are necessary.

Federal and state legislation will not only be instrumental in continuing to move chiropractic forward but will accentuate the need for full integration of the profession into the current health care system. Although still controversial in some respects, chiropractic expansion in federal support has substantiated the need for further scientific developments. Preventive chiropractic care may also prove to be instrumental in decreasing overall medical costs continuing to plague individual consumers/patients within the current U.S. health care system.

HIGHLIGHTS OF CURRENT ISSUES

There are several issues currently faced by the chiropractic field and profession. Some of the most significant include the following:

- Sustainability of chiropractic in the health care marketplace as the primary providers of musculoskeletal issues and related neural interference. There are other health professionals (i.e., physical therapists and the like) who are seeking greater infiltration into the spinal care market.

- Delineation of the multitude of philosophies of chiropractic and how they relate the profession's unity and vision and what effect they have on chiropractic practice. It may yield confusing information for consumers attempting to determine the best approach or provider to address their health care needs.

- Cultural legitimacy and integration into the broader U.S. health care system. There is a need for more research and evidence-based science related to chiropractic to improve the profile of chiropractic to the public.

■ Advancements in technology and how they may help to transform chiropractic. For example, use of digital imaging, electronic medical records, and biomarker identification may aid in more cost-effective strategies for health care providers.

■ Managed care and the lowering of reimbursement rates for many health care professions including chiropractic. There is a need to address this issue from a health policy perspective, and allow chiropractors to determine effective treatment for their patients instead of health insurance companies determining what may be appropriate terms of care.

All of these issues are important considerations for the advancement of the chiropractic profession. Chiropractic doctors, administrators of colleges of chiropractic, leaders of chiropractic professional organizations and societies, chiropractic licensing board officials, health policy advocates and legislators, and consumers each have a unique role and responsibility to positively promote the science and art of the profession.

RECOMMENDATIONS FOR CLOSING THE HEALTH DISPARITY GAP

There undoubtedly exists an opportunity to bridge the gap between allopathic and chiropractic medicine as well as other alternative forms of care. Generally, progressive dialogue, development and dissemination of current and relevant chiropractic information to increase awareness and associated benefits, research initiatives to further substantiate clinical relevance, and a real push to decrease barriers to advancements within chiropractic and the larger U.S. health care system are recommended. Federal legislation as well as state and local directives will also be critical to raising awareness, expanding services, and ultimately leading to a comprehensive and more inclusive referral system.

Furthermore, there are several research, practice, and policy issues that need to be examined and subsequently addressed to reduce health disparities that exist within the field of chiropractic. The health of African Americans and other ethnic minorities is disproportionately affected by fewer high-quality comprehensive health care and chiropractic wellness practices in their communities. They perform fewer help-seeking practices for preventive health care, are recruited less frequently to attend colleges of chiropractic or to serve in faculty positions, and are targeted less for participation in various types of chiropractic clinical research. Specific recommendations are as follows:

■ Increase community involvement in research designed to inform the concepts and best practices for chiropractic care; strategies for the recruitment of ethnic minorities for participation in research studies should be a top priority.

■ Enhance efforts for strengthening the network of integrated health care providers and services, which includes chiropractic and a comprehensive referral system.

■ Develop health policies that tackle disparities relative to health promotion and disease prevention among underrepresented, underserved, disenfranchised, marginalized, and vulnerable populations, including ethnic minorities.

■ Intensify recruitment of minority students into colleges of chiropractic and identify specific strategies to attract and retain minority chiropractors as faculty and practicing doctors that can build institutional infrastructures.

■ Establish better collaborations and partnerships with local and national departments of health and human services, agencies/organizations, and foundations that can facilitate funding and grant support for chiropractic research, integrative medicine, and practices that serve ethnic minority communities.

■ Promote new initiatives such as World Spine Day, currently observed on October 16th annually, as a way to advance national and local awareness about spinal health and wellness.

■ Introduce the concept of Integrative Medicine to chiropractic colleges, schools of medicine, and CAM and medical associations not yet aware of or wed to it; additionally, frame proposed training programs for medical residents with a focus on raising awareness of CAM and the development of resources/products (such as pre/post questionnaires, fact/data sheets, FAQ, and talking points on complementary and alternative medicine/options) that medical practitioners can disseminate and/or use to verbally educate their patients.

■ Encourage the use of culturally sensitive diagnostic and treatment systems that have been tested on ethnically diverse populations, and require chiropractic professionals to undergo cultural competency and/or diversity training as a core requirement of professional practice.

The *Journal of Manipulative and Physiological Therapeutics* article Chiropractic and Public Health: Current State and Future Vision states, "efforts from the chiropractic profession to educate patients about how they can reduce risks and adopt healthy lifestyles have a collective effect of improving the health of the population that is being served" (Johnson, 2008, pp. 397–410). Additionally, the American Medical Association (AMA) reports, in a scope of practice partnership (SOPP), "doctors of chiropractic set the highest standards for patient safety, and numerous studies demonstrate that chiropractors provide safe, high quality care . . . Chiropractors are filling a vital need in this country, . . . with shortages in various areas of health care, and more than 45 million uninsured Americans, chiropractors are the solution to this country's healthcare challenges, not the problem" (ACA, 2006). Undoubtedly, integrative medicine and those entities (especially medical schools and associations) who currently subscribe to its tenets and have IM programs integral to their educational curricula have come to the realization that the health gap between chiropractic and allopathic medicine is closing.

Although polemics have existed not only within the field of chiropractic but also as a dynamic within conventional medical and health disciplines, there remains an unprecedented opportunity for doctors of chiropractic and allopathic medicine to capitalize on the public's interest and their demand for varied health care options.

With the daunting economic and health care challenges that the country currently faces, it is imperative that practitioners of both chiropractic and allopathic medicine better understand the health needs of individuals and families (especially of those who are underserved and marginalized) who comprise our communities, and continue efforts that bring practitioners together with more integrated ideologies. Through a comprehensive and coordinated referral system, when appropriate, chiropractic should become the first course of action in addressing specific health issues, not the last resort when other medical options have been exhausted.

From public establishments to private investments in specialty health care facilities and initiatives, we need to continue to think creatively and comprehensively about new opportunities for health care access and delivery as well as public health services. Now is the time for nationalizing and globalizing social networks. Typifying a shift in attitudes toward health care in the United States, the chiropractic approach to health and wellness continues to be defined, gain acceptance, and be integrated into the U.S. health care system.

REFERENCES

American Chiropractic Association (ACA). (2006). *Statement of the American Chiropractic Association on the AMA scope of practice partnership.* Retrieved September 20, 2008, from http://acatoday.org/pdf/aca-ama.pdf

Association of Chiropractic Colleges (ACC). (2008). *Chiropractic paradigm and scope and practice.* Retrieved September 20, 2008, from http://www.chirocolleges.org

Asthma and Allergy Foundation of America (AAFA). (2008). *Asthma facts and figures.* Retrieved from http://www.aafa.org/display.cfm?id=8&sub=42

Bakris, G., Dickholtz, M., Meyer, P., Kravitz, G. et al. (2007, October). Atlas vertebra realignment and achievement of arterial pressure goal in hypertensive patients. *Journal of Vertebral Subluxation Research*, pp. 1–9. Retrieved from http://www.jvsr.com/abstracts/index.asp?id=311

Bluestein, P. (1998). Minorities and the chiropractic profession in Erie County, New York. *Journal of the American Chiropractic Association, 35*(3), 37–45.

Blum, C. L. (2002, March 1). Role of chiropractic in sacro-occipital technique in the treatment of asthma. *Journal of Chiropractic Medicine*, (1), 16–22.

Blum, C. L. (2006, December). Normalization of blood and urine measures following reduction of vertebral subluxation in a patient diagnosed with early onset diabetes mellitus: A case study. *Journal of Vertebral Subluxation Research*, (7), 6pp. Retrieved from http://www.jvsr.com/abstracts/index.asp?id=278

Callender, A. (2006). Recruiting underrepresented minorities to chiropractic colleges. *Journal of Chiropractic Education, 20*(2), 123–127.

Centers for Disease Control and Prevention. National Center for Health Statistics. (2006). *Asthma's impact on children and adolescents.* Retrieved from http://www.cdc.gov/asthma/children.htm

Centers for Disease Control and Prevention, National Center for Health Statistics. (2007). *Health, United States 2007 with chartbook on trends in the health of Americans.* Retrieved from http://www.cdc.gov/nchs/data/hus/hus07acc.pdf

Consortium of Academic Health Centers for Integrative Medicine (CAHCIM). (2005). *Definition of integrative medicine.* Retrieved October 28, 2008, from http://www.imconsortium.org

Council on Chiropractic Education (CCE). (2007). *Standards for doctors of chiropractic: Programs and requirements for institutional status.* Retrieved October 28, 2008, from http://www.cce-usa.org

Cuthbert, S. C. (2008, March). A multi-modal chiropractic treatment approach for asthma: A 10 patient retrospective case series. *Chiropractic Journal of Australia, 38*(1), 17–27.

Eisenberg, D. M., Cohen, M. H., Horbek, A., & Kaptchuk, T. J. (2002). Credentialing complementary and alternative medical providers. *Annals of Internal Medicine 137*(12), 965–973.

Fedorchuk, C. (2007, November). Correction of subluxation and reduction of dysponesis in a seven year old child suffering from chronic cough and asthma: A case report. *Journal of Vertebral Subluxation Research*, (26), 6 pp. Retrieved from http://www.jvsr.com/abstracts/index.asp?id=319

Ferrance, R. J., & Wyatt, L. H. (2006, March). The musculoskeletal effects of diabetes mellitus. *Journal of the Canadian Chiropractic Association, 50*(1), 43–50.

Gibbs, A. L. (2005). Chiropractic co-management of medically treated asthma. *Clinical Chiropractic, 8*(3), 140–144.

Hass, M., Sharma, R., & Stano, M. (2005). Cost-effectiveness of medical and chiropractic care for acute and chronic low back pain. *Journal of Manipulative and Physiological Therapeutics, 28*(8), 555–563.

Institute of Medicine of the National Academics (IOM). (2005). Use of complementary and alternative medicine (CAM) by the American public. Retrieved September 20, 2008, from http://www.iom.edu

International Chiropractic Association (ICA). (2008). *Legislative Issues:* Military commission for doctors of chiropractic; Improving care for america's military veterans; Direct access to chiropractic services for military veterans. Retrieved November 15, 2008, from http://www.chiropractic.org

Johnson, C., Baird, R., Dougherty, P. E., Globe, G., Green, B. N., Haneline, M. et al. (2008). Chiropractic and public health: Current state and future vision. *Journal of Manipulative and Physiological Therapeutics, 31*(6), 397–410.

Johnson, R. L., Saha, S, Arbelaez, J, Beach, M., & Cooper, L. (2004). Racial and ethnic differences in patient perceptions of bias and cultural competence in health care. *Journal of General Internal Medicine, 19*(2), 101–110.

Kettner, N. W., Osterhouse, M. D., & Boesch, R. J. (2005, June). Congestive heart failure: A review and case report from a chiropractic teaching clinic. *Journal of Manipulative and Physiological Therapeutics, 28*(5), 356–364.

Lawrence, D. J. (2007). Chiropractic and CAM utilization: A descriptive review. *Chiropractic & Osteopathy, 15*(2), 27 pp. Retrieved from http://www.biomedcentral.com/content/pdf/1746-1340-15-2.pdf

Long, C. R., Meeker, W. C., Menke, J. M., et al. (2002, May). Practice-based randomized controlled comparison clinical trial of chiropractic adjustments and brief massage on subluxation in subjects with essential hypertension. *Journal of Manipulative and Physiological Therapeutics, 25*(4), 221–239.

McCaffrey, A. M., Pugh, G. F., & O'Connor, B. B. (2007). Understanding patient preference for integrative medical care: Results from patient focus groups, *Journal of General Internal Medicine, 22*(11), 1500–1505.

Meeker, W. C., & Haldeman, S., (2002). Chiropractic: A profession at the crossroads of mainstream and alternative medicine, *Annals of Internal Medicine, 136*(3), 216–227.

National Board of Chiropractic Examiners (NBCE). (2005). Job analysis of chiropractic 2005: A project report, survey analysis, and summary of the practice of chiropractic within the United States. Greeley, CO: Author.

National Center for Complementary and Alternative Medicine (NCCAM), National Institutes of Health, U.S. Department of Health and Human Services. (2005). *Expanding horizons of health care: Strategic plan 2005–2009*. Retrieved from http://nccam.nih.gov/about/plans/2005/index.htm

National Center for Complementary and Alternative Medicine (NCCAM), National Institutes of Health, U.S. Department of Health and Human Services. (2008). *Strategic Plan to Address Racial and Ethnic Health Disparities*. Retrieved from http://nccam.nih.gov/about/plans/healthdisparities/

National Institute of Allergy and Infectious Diseases (NIAID), National Institute of Health. (2001). *Asthma: A Concern for minority populations facts Sheet*. Retrieved from http://www3.niaid.nih.gov/

National Institute of Diabetes and Digestive Kidney Diseases (NIDDKD), National Institute of Health, U.S. Department of Health and Human Services, National Diabetes Statistics. (2008). *The Diabetes epidemic among African Americans fact sheet*. Retrieved from http://www.ndep.nih.gov/diabetes/pubs/FS_AfricanAm.pdf

National Institutes of Health (NIH), National Center for Complementary and Alternative Medicine-NCCAM. (2008). Backgrounder: An introduction to chiropractic, pub No. D403.

Office of Minority Health (OMH), U.S. Department of Health and Human Services. (2007). *Heart disease and African Americans fact sheet*. Retrieved from http://www.omhrc.gov/templates/content.aspx?ID=3018.

Rust, G., Kondwani, K., Martinez, R., Danise, R., Wong, W., Fry-Johnson, Y., Woody, R., Daniels, E., Herbert-Carter, J., Aponte, L., & Strothers, H. (2006). A crash-course in cultural competence. *Ethnicity & Disease, 16*(2), 29–36.

Sanford, R. O. (2008, November 17). Atlanta Spine Dunwoody, Atlanta, Ga. Interviewed by M. B. Gooden.

So, C. S., Giolli, R., Chang, T., & Bae, H. J. (2004, May). Physiological changes following thermomechanical massage in a population of hypertensive patients and/or type II diabetics. *Journal of Vertebral Subluxation Research*, (3), 9 pp. Retrieved from http://miguncerritos.tripod.com/sitebuildercontent/sitebuilderfiles/jvsr-drso2.pdf

Valli, J. (2004, December). Chiropractic management of a 46 year old type 1 diabetic patient with upper crossed syndrome and adhesive capsulitis: A case report. *Journal of Chiropractic Medicine, 3*(4), 138–144.

Wiese, G. (2004). A qualitative study of 16 African Americans in Chiropractic Education. *Journal of Chiropractic Education, 18*(2), 127–136.

Zakus, J. D., & Lysack, C. L. (1998, March). Revisiting community participation. *Health Policy Plan, 13,* 1–12.

CHAPTER

24

THE ROLE OF BLACK FAITH COMMUNITIES IN FOSTERING HEALTH

SCHNAVIA SMITH HATCHER
KIMBERLY S. CLAY
JERONDA T. BURLEY

Douglas and Hopson (2001) defined the black church as "a multitudinous community of churches, which are diversified by origin, denomination, doctrine, worshipping culture, spiritual expression, class, size, and other less-obvious factors . . . they share a special history, culture, and role in black life, all of which attest to their collective identity as the black church" (p. 96). According to Lincoln and Mamiya (1990), black churches, with an estimated membership of 24 million nationwide, have long been recognized as the most independent, stable, and dominant institution in black communities. Eng, Hatch, and Callan (1985) also maintained the idea that churches have been the institution responsible for setting norms, enforcing community values, providing social networks, and serving as the catalyst for change within the black community. For the aforementioned reasons, along with theories describing the importance of community support in health promotion, black churches are becoming an increasingly important avenue for the prevention efforts of major health conditions.

This chapter will discuss the role of black faith communities in fostering health by providing a description of the role of the black church in the community, presenting a review of church-based health promotion projects, and discussing policy implications. Lessons learned and recommendations for closing health disparity gaps within the community through faith-based services will also be presented.

HISTORY OF THE BLACK CHURCH

During slavery, blacks learned of Christianity by attending religious services with their slave masters. Slaves were not allowed to participate in these services, and eventually established their own underground religious worship where evangelical Christianity was mixed with African beliefs and traditions. In the early 1800s, laws in the South prohibited exclusively black churches, black preachers, and unsupervised assembly of blacks in groups. Despite this, these religious gatherings grew into full-fledged churches with the establishment of the African Methodist Episcopal (AME) and AME Zion churches during this period. In 1870, the Colored Methodist Episcopal (CME) Church was founded, and the National Baptist Convention, USA, Inc., now the largest black religious organization in the United States, was founded in 1894. Several more major religious denominations were established, including the Church of God in Christ, National Baptist Convention of America, National Missionary Baptist Convention, and the Progressive National Baptist Convention. Likewise, a number of nondenominational congregations such as the Full Gospel Baptist Church Fellowship International, founded in 1993, were established and remain independent of any major denominational body. These organizations combined represent over one million churches and more than thirty million congregants (DiIulio, 1998; Thumma, 2001). According to data from the National Survey of Black Americans, 68 percent of black adults are official members of a congregation and 92 percent of the congregants attend a predominantly black church (Neighbors, Musick, & Williams, 1998).

COPING WITH HEALTH DISPARITIES IN THE COMMUNITY

Black Americans are, medically speaking, both significantly at risk and underserved relative to the dominant majority population (Levin, 1986). Blacks also experience increasing amounts of distress and strain as a result of racism, discrimination, health problems, and other stressors. Religion has been found to be a viable coping mechanism (Levin, 1986). Researchers commonly defined religiosity in terms of public behavior (e.g., frequency of church attendance) and private behavior (e.g., devotional or prayer time) (Davidson & Norton, 1995; Davidson, Moore, & Ullstrup, 2004; Fehring, Cheever, German, & Philpot, 1998; Morse et al., 2000). Accordingly, the black church has been the vehicle through which many blacks have expressed their religious faith in response to these obstacles (Jang & Johnson, 2004; Kip, Peters, & Morrison-Rodriguez, 2002; Lincoln & Mamiya, 1990; Taylor, Chatters, & Levin, 2004) and serves as a locus for community-wide health programs.

Black churches prove to be an effective vehicle for health service delivery in an attempt to close the health disparity gap. Whether perceived as negative or positive, religion has been fundamental in the lives of blacks. After centuries, black churches remain as the bedrock of most black communities (Lincoln & Mamiya, 1990; Mattis & Jagers, 2001). Black churches have been central in providing a type of cohesiveness and support rarely found in the mainstream, secular community.

Since its inception, the black church has mobilized resources within the black community, and provided a variety of emotional and learning experiences that enhance group cohesion and promote empowerment and behavior change (McRae, Carey, & Anderson-Scott, 1998). Studies have described strong similarities between public health and church-based settings, and posit that partnering with churches may contribute to public health objectives (Chatters, Ellison, & Levin, 1998) because of church legitimacy in the community and the significant role church plays in the lives of many blacks.

The Black Church Facilitating Health Access in the Community

Health policy and promotion discussions inevitably include the topic of health disparities that still plague the United States. The disparity remains within communities that have low socioeconomic conditions, high rates of poverty, and low insurance enrollment. According to the U.S. Census Bureau (2007), at least 19.5 percent of the black population is uninsured compared to the non-Hispanic white population at 10.4 percent. Though lack of insurance can be an indicator of those who are within the disparity, it is not the only aspect to consider. The Black Report in Great Britain gave evidence that after universal access to health services, health status inequalities between whites and blacks not only persisted, but were increasing (McBeath, 1991; Thomas et al., 1994). Given this, a look at the overall living condition of those in disparity was warranted. Without the knowledge of preventive and diagnostic services available, one would lack the resources needed to improve overall health. This is where the idea of utilizing the church as an agent transpired.

The black community has historically relied to some degree on the black church to provide various types of health-related information or to conduct outreach programs for the community. From the time of slavery through the civil rights movement of the 1950s and 1960s to civic participation and local organizing of the 1990s, the church has been a central institution in the black community. At the organizational level, the black church has, throughout the twentieth century and into the twenty first, promoted education, business, and political activism within the black community. In addition to its contribution through organizational structures and social networks, the black church has also played an important cultural role for the black community (Markens, Fox, Taub, & Gilbert, 2002). Given its historical and ongoing roles within the black community, the church was an ideal setting in which to offer health promotion activities for blacks. Such activities are warranted because blacks have lower life expectancies, are less likely to have health insurance, make fewer primary care visits, and have lower birthweights and higher infant mortality rates compared to whites (Sutherland, Hale, & Harris, 1995). In fact, several studies have found that the church can be an important conduit through which to inform racial/ethnic minorities about preventive care, and that the black church, because of its ethic of service to others, is particularly well suited for health promotion (Chatters, 2000).

Faith-based organizations (FBOs) have a long history of independently and collaboratively hosting health promotion programs in areas such as health education, screening for and management of high blood pressure and diabetes, weight loss and smoking cessation, cancer prevention and awareness, geriatric care, nutritional guidance, and mental health care (DeHaven et al., 2004; Hatcher, Burley, & Lee-Ouga, 2008). In fact, just weeks after his inauguration, President George W. Bush remarked that Americans should acknowledge the growing consensus that successful government social programs work in productive partnership with community-serving and faith-based organizations, regardless of their faith experience (Bush, 2001).This call continued a trend set in motion in 1982 by President Ronald Reagan's general call for Good Samaritan support from faith-based communities, and a more specific appeal by President William Clinton in 1996, made to black church leaders of the National Baptist Convention. To achieve this goal of increased participation of community and faith-based organizations in providing publicly funded social services, several pieces of Charitable Choice legislation have been passed that set the statutory precedent for the government to contract with congregations and other explicitly religious organizations on the same basis as with secular social service providers. The nation's 300,000 to 350,000 congregations are expected to be the new partners assisting the government in providing a variety of social programs (Boddie, 2002).

FAITH-BASED HEALTH PROMOTION POLICIES

Religious-affiliated groups have provided an array of social services to the poor and needy for decades, with limited federal funding to assist service provision. Throughout the history of relief efforts, churches and other charitable organizations have worked tirelessly to assist persons living in poverty, as well as those suffering from the bondage of addiction and other diseases. The faith community has always had as its mandate to care for the poor, as it was considered their moral duty as dictated in biblical teachings. Notwithstanding the debate over the effectiveness of faith-based social service programs, national policies have had a positive impact on the ability of FBOs to continue to provide programs to address social problems affecting those in the faith community, and the community as a whole. Grant funding is now provided via programs such as Charitable Choice and Access to Recovery.

Seemingly, the 1996 introduction of Charitable Choice policy publicly conveyed the government's recognition that faith-based organizations were instrumental in meeting the needs of the nation's poor and destitute (Charitable Choice Project Description, n.d.; The White House, 2001). Previously, no legislation existed to delineate guidelines for religious organizations as they administered government-funded services to the poor. However, in 1996, President Clinton signed the Personal Responsibility and Work Opportunity Reconciliation Act (PRWORA). This welfare reform law contained a provision under Section 104 of H.R. 3734 called Charitable

Choice, which intended to expand the inclusion of faith-based providers in social services (Sherwood, 1998; Sherman, 2000). This provision contained the needed guidelines to direct FBOs in program implementation.

The 1996 Charitable Choice legislation has enabled congregations and other faith-based organizations to overcome the previous barriers to applying for federal funding of social service programs and to maintain their religious integrity during the government's grant application process (Cnaan & Boddie, 2002; Sherwood, 1998). Charitable Choice also affords clients of social service programs, such as persons in need of substance abuse services, the opportunity to choose either a secular or faith-based treatment program.

Access to Recovery is another national policy that increased the opportunity for faith-based organizations to receive federal funding of programs to address social problems. This federal policy was launched in 2003 and is a grant program funded by the Substance Abuse and Mental Health Services Administration (SAMHSA) through its Center for Substance Abuse Treatment (CSAT). Access to Recovery provides vouchers to clients, enabling them to purchase substance abuse treatment and/or recovery support service (SAMHSA, 2007). A main goal of the policy is to increase the number of programs providing substance abuse treatment, with a particular emphasis on increasing the number of FBOs to provide drug treatment. Also at the core of this federal initiative is to allow clients to have a more extensive choice about the type of substance abuse treatment received, while including faith-based providers in the selection pool. Researchers suggest that providing persons a choice in the type of substance abuse treatment may contribute to a reduction in drug use or an elimination of substance abuse altogether (Cloud, Ziegler, & Blondell, 2004). In fact, since Access to Recovery's inception in 2003, clients have reported a 71 percent abstinence rate, with an even higher percent of those no longer involved in the criminal justice system (SAMHSA, 2007).

In the past, governmental grants that provided aid in social service delivery excluded black churches and small congregations, but that is not the case any more. Legislation such as Access to Recovery and Charitable Choice is bridging the gap between the government and the religious community by offering the same financial assistance to FBOs as it does to traditional or non-sectarian organizations, while providing an opportunity for persons to have a choice in the entity that provides services. These initiatives have been specifically targeted to members of the black church (Yanek et al., 2001; Matthews, Berrios, Darnell, & Calhoun, 2006; Davis et al., 1994; Wiist & Flack, 1990).

FAITH-BASED HEALTH PROMOTION STUDIES

In response to the barrage of health problems plaguing the black community, congregational and faith-based programs have emerged to combat issues such as depression, homelessness, hunger, HIV/AIDS, cardiovascular risks, and substance abuse. The recently heightened awareness of faith-based programs, particularly those social service programs conducted by congregations, has generated substantial concern and criticism.

A growing body of literature has examined the effectiveness of these faith-based interventions (Bazargan, Sherkat, & Bazargan, 2004; Califano, 2002; CASA Report, 2001; Chatters, 2000; Hodge, Cardenas, & Montoya, 2001). This debate over the effectiveness of religiously affiliated or faith-based programs has sparked a body of research examining various facets of faith-based social service provision (Boddie, 2004; Cnaan, Sinha, & McGrew, 2004; Ebaugh, Pipes, Chafetz, & Daniels, 2003; Gibelman & Gelman, 2003; Sherwood, 2003). Some proponents of faith-based programs argue that religiously affiliated programs are more effective in combating social problems than their secular counterparts (Ebaugh et al., 2003). In spite of the controversy, faith-based programs continue to emerge and address the issues of the community.

Currently, research on the efficacy of faith-based organization programs appears primarily focused on either health or prisoner recidivism. Dehaven's meta-analysis examined three types of faith-based programming: 1) faith-based, 2) faith-placed, and 3) collaborative. Faith-based programs, developed as part of the congregations' health ministries, typically involved white congregations (Dehaven et al., 2004). These programs focused on heart disease, mental illness, and asthma. Studies investigating the impact of faith-based programs on mental illness found a significant decrease of mental illness symptoms. Faith-placed programs, developed by health professionals rather than members of the congregation, were typically directed at blacks and accounted for 43 percent of the studies analyzed (Dehaven et al., 2004). These programs were generally directed at heart disease, healthy weight/nutrition, breast cancer, and prostate cancer. Results indicated increases in fruit and vegetable consumption; decreases in weight, blood pressure, and cholesterol; increased breast cancer examination; and increased knowledge of prostate cancer (Dehaven et al., 2004). Finally, collaborative programs were defined as a combination of faith-based and faith-placed programs. Directed mostly at blacks (80%), these programs also looked to improve health, reduce weight, and encourage smoking cessation. Significant increases in healthy food consumption and decrease in weight and blood pressure were found (Dehaven et al., 2004).

Cardiovascular and Diabetes Risk Reduction

Church-based programs addressing cardiovascular and diabetes risk factors, such as weight and/or blood pressure control, have received the greatest attention in the church-based health promotion literature (Kumanyika & Charleston, 1992; McNabb, Quinn, Kerver, Cook, & Karrison, 1997; Oexmann, Ascanio, & Egan, 2001; Smith & Merritt, 1997; Turner, Sutherland, Harris, & Barber, 1995). In 1985, the Task Force on Black and Minority Health was formed by the Secretary of Health and Human Services. They set out to increase efforts in place to reduce risk factors among the black population for coronary heart disease (Wiist & Flack, 1990). A six-week nutrition class, conducted in a black church, given one hour each week, educated members on how to lower their cholesterol. Information was also mailed to participants. Six months later, 75 percent of the group that returned for follow-up reported a 10 percent decrease in mean cholesterol level (Wiist & Flack, 1990). Wiist & Flack (1990) determined that the church played a large role in accomplishing the results because the classes were conducted by members of the church who were trained with the information to disseminate.

Integrating cardiovascular education with scripture study, goal setting, and social support, one church-based program, directed toward reducing cardiovascular risk through lifestyle modification, was evaluated (Oexmann et al., 2001). The sample was drawn from Southern churches and composed predominantly of blacks. At post-intervention follow-up, black participants (82% women) exhibited reductions in weight, and at one-year follow-up, blacks with high program attendance exhibited significant reductions in both weight and blood pressure (systolic and diastolic). Notably, demographic and clinical health factors were not the same, which may have confounded the findings (Oexmann et al., 2001). However, ongoing church-based social support, reinforcing program weight reduction goals, could be viewed as a key to the program's success.

Cancer Screening

Church-based health promotion programs have been identified as promising means for maintaining and/or increasing cancer screening rates among blacks (Ammerman et al., 2003; Duan, Fox, Pitkin, & Carson, 2000; Erwin et al., 1996; Mann et al., 2000; Markens et al., 2002; Weinrich et al., 1998). The Wellness for Blacks through Churches (WATCH) Project was a church-based colorectal cancer prevention study (Katz et al., 2004). The project was designed to increase fruit and vegetable consumption, reduce fat intake, increase moderate physical activity, and increase colorectal cancer screening among church members. Findings indicated that good patient-provider communication and colorectal cancer knowledge are important for colorectal cancer screening (Katz et al., 2004). Katz et al. (2004) also mentioned that one of the problems that blacks faced was the lack of trust in their medical provider. Perhaps this is where information disseminated via the church can prove to be influential.

The National Cancer Institute established a national program in 1991 entitled the Five a Day for Better Health Program (Campbell et al., 1999). It encouraged Americans to have five or more servings of fruits and vegetables a day to assist in the prevention of chronic diseases and cancer. The National Cancer Institute funded nine research projects to determine whether or not community intervention programs were effective in delivering the message (Campbell et al., 1999; Potter, 1988). The North Carolina Black Churches United for Better Health Project was one of those funded with the goal of increasing consumption by 0.5 daily servings (Campbell et al., 1999). The results of the study showed a strong association between the frequency of church attendance and increased fruit and vegetable intake (Campbell et al., 1999). It was also determined that one of the strengths of the program was incorporating the pastor into the project by charging him with choosing a coordinator and three to seven members to make up the National Action Team.

Although this topic has not been studied extensively, several investigations have shown that church-based interventions such as the projects described above are particularly effective and essential components of breast and cervical cancer education programs. Other studies have reinforced the claim that church-based interventions are effective in increasing the number of blacks who obtain regular cancer screenings. Mann and colleagues (2000) found that parishioners of three churches of markedly different socioeconomic strata were all more likely than average to receive cancer screenings when activist ministers had previously implemented health interventions within those churches.

Prisoner Recidivism

There has been an increasingly expanded role for the faith community in corrections (Camp, Daggett, Kwon, & Klein-Saffran, 2008; Johnson & Larson, 2003). In reviewing one program, Camp and colleagues (2008) examined the efficacy of the Life Connections Program instituted through the Pennsylvania Bureau of Prisons. Life Connections taught a moral component connected to pro-social values, encouraged inmates to recognize cognitive deficits that led them to incarceration, promoted accepting responsibility for harming victims, and provided a mentor from the local faith community. When comparing program participants to those not in the program, Camp et al. found that LCP inmates were less likely to have instances of misconduct while in prison. The program also offered supplemental services afterward. There have been other model faith-based programs developed to reduce adult and juvenile recidivism, assist juveniles with incarcerated parents, and work with juveniles held over to or in the adult penal system (Benda & Corwyn, 1997; Blank & Davie, 2004; Hodge & Pittman, 2003). Nonetheless, Mears and colleagues (2006) noted that the precise causal relationship, if any, between various measures of faith and crime still remains in question and that few rigorous evaluations of faith-based reentry programs exist.

Substance Abuse Treatment

In addition to extensive research on faith-based programs related to health or prisoner recidivism, there is a substantial amount of research of the impact of faith or religiosity on substance use and substance abuse treatment (Aaron, Levine, & Burstin, 2001; Avants, Marcotte, Arnold, & Margolin, 2003). Several authors explored the relationship between substance abuse and religion as an initial step toward determining the effectiveness of faith-based treatment (Bazargan, Sherkat, & Bazargan, 2004; Califano, 2002; CASA Report, 2001; Chatters, 2000; Hodge, Cardenas, & Montoya, 2001). Research has consistently shown that religious factors do contribute to a reduction in substance use (Brome, Owens, Allen, & Vevaina, 2000; Califano, 2002; CASA Report, 2001; Hodge et al., 2001; Kip, Peters, & Morrison-Rodriguez, 2002) and have a positive impact on sexual behavior and other health-related behavior (Aaron et al., 2001; Avants et al., 2003; Elifson, Klein, & Sterk, 2003).

Researchers surmised that persons who attended church regularly and were heavily involved in religious activity paid closer attention to their health care needs, making faith-based health promotion programs highly effective. Blacks as a group are found to be highly active in organized religion (Aaron et al., 2001; Lewis & Green, 2000). However, although authors found that religiosity reduced high-risk behaviors such as substance abuse and provided a source of support for the sick and afflicted, religiosity or participation in organized religion was also found to be restrictive in some samples (Coleman, 2004; Elifson et al., 2003). These findings suggest that religion is a positive factor in risk reduction, but it also reminds FBOs to be cautious in their use of religion, so that prevention efforts are not inadvertently thwarted.

LESSONS LEARNED, BEST PRACTICES, AND RECOMMENDATIONS FOR FAITH-BASED HEALTH PROMOTION

In recent years, public health practitioners, researchers, and policymakers have recognized the role of the black church in the community and have begun to move from traditional settings of hospitals and clinics to neighborhood churches to deliver health promotion programs. Studies have described the features of successful health promotion programs, partnerships in churches, and the importance of the church as an ally in efforts to provide preventive health and social services to at-risk populations. Factors including church size, leadership and support, and establishing connections should be considered when reviewing program potential and opportunities.

Church Characteristics

Several characteristics have been found to be consistently associated with churches that conduct successful community programs. Significant factors of model programs included: (1) mission of serving the community, especially in regard to health matters; (2) church size; (3) church age; (4) economic class of membership; (5) education level of pastor; and (6) number of paid clergy (Thomas et al., 1994, Matthews et al., 2006, Williams et al., 1999; Taylor et al., 2000).

Church size and education level of the minister were found to be the strongest predictors of success of church-sponsored community health outreach programs (Thomas et al., 1994). Thomas and colleagues (1994) divided size into large (>401 members), medium (176–400), small (71–175), and little (1–70). It was determined that 60.3 percent of churches that are "little" had no outreach, whereas "large" churches only had 11.7 percent with no outreach (Thomas et al., 1994). Lincoln and Mamiya (1990) noted that large churches were more actively involved in their surrounding communities and had more programs. Church size may also make a difference in regard to access to resources such as finances and a larger volunteer base. In addition, larger churches tended to offer a wider range of family support services and health-related programs, as well as more specialized services than do their counterparts (Caldwell, Greene, & Billingsley, 1992; Taylor et al., 2000; Thomas et al., 1994). This is parallel to the argument that larger church sizes have more of an impact on ability to incorporate outreach into their mission.

According to Taylor and colleagues (2000), the education level of the pastor determined the amount of outreach and community activism of the church. It was found that only 16.5 percent of churches who had a minister with a Master's degree or above had no outreach programs (Thomas et al., 1994). On the other hand, 52.3 percent of churches that had a minister with only a high school background had no outreach.

Church age was also considered a factor, in that older churches tend to have a larger membership base and reputation in the community they serve. Churches were categorized into three categories: old (>75 years), mid-age (41–75 years) and young (1–40 years), with 78 percent of "old" churches having outreach programs compared to 61 percent of "young" churches (Thomas et al., 1994).

The economic status of the church members was also reviewed. Thomas and colleagues (1994) found that 80 percent of churches made up of middle-class members had outreach programs, whereas 58.8 percent of those with working-class members had outreach programs. Whether or not a church has paid clergy also made a difference in the amount of outreach programs. Without paid clergy, supervision of community programs is difficult (Lincoln & Mamiya, 1990; Taylor et al., 2000), thus creating challenges in carrying out a long-term health promotion initiative. In fact, it was found that churches with no paid clergy or other paid staff were the least likely to offer elderly support programs and wellness initiatives, despite a need within the congregation (Caldwell et al., 1995).

Though these findings were made in some programs across the country, it does not suggest that churches without the model characteristics would not be effective in establishing and providing health promotion strategies. Aside from potential challenges inherent in developing any new program, collaborations prove to be successful if they are planned correctly.

Church Leadership

Church pastors are respected gatekeepers to the black community (Billingsley, 1992; Chatters, 2000; Richardson, 1989), and are particularly well-suited for organizing and stimulating change among blacks. Pastors have long served as a surrogate and parental figure for many black congregants, often viewed as the "father" or "elder" to the congregation (Johnson & Staples, 2005). Past models of church-based health promotion have relied on the pastor as the conduit for generating interest and involvement in projects, as well as for coordinating routine program activities. However, due to the complexities of their multiple community roles and responsibilities, some pastors may be constrained in their level of engagement in church-based health programs.

Clay, Newlin, and Leeks (2005) have also explored the role of pastors' wives in church-based health promotion and suggested that engagement of and partnership with the pastor's wife may be the appropriate model for church-based health promotion among blacks, particularly black women. Pastors' wives are highly influential, esteemed, and recognized figures in their respective communities. As such, the public modeling of the pastor's wife as the "first lady of the church" is expected to help cultivate healthy relationships and gender bonding, as well as spiritual guidance, with women congregants (Chatters, Taylor, Lincoln, & Schroepfer, 2002).

Major lessons learned from past attempts to combine health prevention and the black church include allowing the church to feel ownership by participating in the design of the project (Hatch & Derthick, 1992; Thomas et al., 1994; Yanek et al., 2001), level of pastor involvement, and allowing the pastor to choose "lay leaders" (Yanek et al., 2001; Davis et al., 1994; Wiist & Flack, 1990). It was also found that pastors who included health promotion efforts into their weekly sermons proved to be highly effective in enhancing the overall goal (Matthews et al., 2006). Additionally, utilizing natural helpers (lay leaders) was a positive tactic in accomplishing outreach programs (Wiist & Flack, 1990). Leaders were described as people to whom others seemed to turn naturally for advice, emotional support, and tangible aid in everyday life. These leaders also seemed to be able to influence others to modify their health behavior (Wiist & Flack, 1990). Programs such as the Eat for Life program and Cholesterol Screening program utilized lay leaders to deliver the message of healthy lifestyles (Resnicow et al., 2001). With projects such as Project Joy, the lay leaders were also incorporated into the participant recruitment strategy design (Yanek et al., 2001). This, perhaps, added to the sense of ownership to make the program a success to the church members. Hence, collaborating with churches as a secular organization proved to be a positive tactic to result in effective programs.

Funding Opportunities and Technical Assistance

Religious organizations and congregations have historically provided social services to the poor and needy. However, FBOs have encountered barriers in the past when attempting to secure federal funding, such as having to sacrifice religious character and integrity, being required to ignore religion in hiring decisions, and enduring complex procurement processes (Bush, 2001; Carlson-Thies, 2000; Charitable Choice Project Description, n.d.). Although a large proportion of nongovernmental providers of assistance to the needy are faith-based, nonprofit organizations, the cumbersome nature of the procurement process and limited staff support has prohibited FBOs from pursuing and acquiring available federal funds. In fact, many FBOs do not have the necessary systems in place to administer a federally funded program, nor the available resources to develop these required systems (Hodge, 2000).

As the federal government continues to utilize the faith community to assist in meeting the needs of the poor, it is likely that additional funding will become available to offer financial support in this effort. However, subsequent funding will not make a difference if FBOs are not aware of the funding opportunities or do not have the resources to prepare a competitive application. It is recommended that efforts be made to educate faith-based organizations about opportunities such as Charitable Choice and Access to Recovery in order to dispel some of the myths about the legislation and to help religious providers determine whether or not their organization is prepared to apply for federal funding. This informative effort could be further enhanced by modifying the provision in a way that mandates states to examine and restructure, if necessary, their procurement processes. Currently, the grant application process is extremely complex and acts as a barrier to many FBOs that might apply for federal funds, but do not have the skills to complete the application, nor the financial resources to hire a grant writer.

Performance Measures

Though the faith community has provided social services to the poor and needy for decades, research on the effectiveness of faith-based programs is still limited

(Carlson-Thies, 2000; Cnaan & Boddie, 2002). The majority of FBOs collect process data, but only meager outcome data, and both are useful to make inferences about program effectiveness (Cnaan & Boddie, 2002; Rogers, Yancey, & Singletary, 2005). It is recommended that faith-based programs consistently employ evaluation measures to capture performance or outcome measures, in addition to process measures. Such evaluation would require the government to provide additional support to faith-based organizations to ensure that evaluations are conducted correctly and that useful data is collected. This support can come in the form of technical assistance and/or funding permitted specifically for evaluation efforts.

Currently, there is no standard definition of faith-based (Charitable Choice Project Description, n.d.; Rogers, Yancey, & Singletary, 2005). Because of the inability to uniformly classify faith-based organizations, it is impossible to develop an accurate account of these organizations in order to determine prevalence of religious social service providers or the effectiveness of the programs. Further, without a standard definition, we are unable to assess the diversity of faiths represented among FBOs. As the government permits, and even encourages, faith-based collaborations, some religious organizations might be overlooked during the grant review process and therefore miss funding opportunities. This oversight makes it difficult to recruit and encourage religious providers to apply for available federal funds for which they might be eligible. Therefore, it is recommended that a standardized definition or faith-based typology be developed to assist in identifying and classifying faith-based organizations.

Public Health Professionals Collaborating with Faith-Based Programs

Though an increase in number of programs is seen, there are aspects of the bond created between the church and public health community that are still being explored (Hatch & Derthick, 1992; Campbell et al., 2007). Some researchers have looked into creating alliances between themselves and black churches to strengthen the possibility of a positive outcome from health initiatives. When working with churches, it is important that those outside or unfamiliar with the faith community educate themselves on the language and cultural aspects of the faith tradition—from general tenets to more specific philosophies. For instance, there are multiple denominations within the black church community and each has variations in how the Christian faith is demonstrated within their church. As such, it would behoove researchers and partnering agencies to be at least generally informed about these denominational differences and their ideas about public health issues such as HIV/AIDS initiatives, mental health programs, and substance abuse treatment. Doing so would ensure the development of programs that demonstrate a true collaborative spirit and full buy-in from all parishioners, while also allowing the church to maintain its religious integrity with respect and without offense. Collaborations between the community, government, and the black church are being expanded and have vast potential for positive impact.

CONCLUSION

Throughout the history of black people in the United States—from slavery through the civil rights movement to the election of the first black U.S. president—the church has been a central institution in the black community. The black church has been the focal point of social change, the single most important political organization for blacks. It is the oldest indigenous black institution, and serves as an enduring pillar of strength in the black community (Billingsley, 1992; Boyd-Franklin, 2003; Chatters, 2000; Hill, 1999; Lincoln & Mamiya, 1990; Taylor, Chatters, & Levin, 2004). The black community has historically relied, in some part, on the black church to provide various types of health-related information or to conduct outreach programs for the community. As a result, black congregations have consistently responded to social issues that disproportionately impact the black community, such as diabetes, cancer, hypertension, HIV/AIDS, and substance abuse (Cnaan, Sinha, & McGrew, 2004; Douglas & Hopson, 2001; Rogers et al., 2005). Church-based health promotion targeting blacks continues to serve as a promising means for promoting positive health care practices or lifestyle modifications, and thereby continues to improve quality-of-life outcomes in the black community at large.

REFERENCES

Aaron, K., Levine, D., & Burstin, H. (2003). African American church participation and health care practice. *Journal of General Internal Medicine, 18*, 908–913.

Ammerman, A., Corbie-Smith, G., St. George, D., Washington, C., Weathers, B., & Jackson-Christian, B. (2003). Research expectations among African American church leaders in the PRAISE project: A randomized trial guided by community-based participatory research. *American Journal of Public Health, 93*(10), 1720–1727.

Avants, S., Marcotte, D., Arnold, R., & Margolin, A. (2003). Spiritual beliefs, world assumptions, and HIV risk behavior among heroin and cocaine users. *Psychology of Addictive Behaviors, 17*(2), 159–162.

Bazargan, S., Sherkat, D., & Bazargan, M. (2004). Religion and alcohol use among African-American and Hispanic inner-city emergency care patients. *Journal for the Scientific Study of Religion, 43*(3), 419–428.

Benda, B. B., & Corwyn, R. F. (1997). Religion and delinquency: The relationship after considering family and peer influences. *Journal for the Scientific Study of Religion 36*, 81–92.

Billingsley, A. (1992). *Climbing Jacob's ladder: The enduring legacy of African American families*. Chicago: Simon Schuster.

Blank, S., & Davie, F. (2004). Faith in their futures: The youth and congregations in partnership program of the King's County (Brooklyn, NY) District Attorney's Office. Philadelphia: Public/Private Ventures.

Boddie, S. C. (2002). Fruitful partnerships in a rural African American community: Important lessons for faith-based initiatives. *The Journal of Applied Behavioral Science, 38*(3), 317–333.

Boddie, S. C. (2004). Social services of African-American congregations in the Welfare Reform Era. *African American Research Perspectives, 10*(1), 36–43.

Boyd-Franklin, N. (2003). *Black families in therapy: Understanding the African American experience*. (2nd ed.). New York: Guilford Press.

Brome, D., Owens, M., Allen, K., & Vevaina, T. (2000). An examination of spirituality among African American women in recovery from substance abuse. *Journal of Black Psychology, 26*(4), 470–486.

Bush, G. W. (2001). *Rallying the armies of compassion*. Washington, DC: Government Printing Office.

Caldwell, C. H., Chatters, L. M., Billingsley, A., & Taylor, R. J. (1995). Church-based support programs for elderly black adults: Congregational and clergy characteristics. In M. A. Kimble, S. H. McFadden, J. W. Ellor, & J. Seeber (Eds.), *Aging, spirituality, and religion: A handbook* (306–324). Minneapolis, MN: Fortress.

Caldwell, C. H., Greene, A. D., & Billingsley, A. (1992) The black church as a family support system: Instrumental and expressive functions. *National Journal of Sociology, 6*(21) 440.

Califano, J. A. (2002). Why priests and psychiatrists should get their acts together: Religion, science, and substance abuse. *America, 186*(4), 8–11.

Camp, S., Daggett, D., Kwon, O., & Klein-Saffran, J. (2008). The effect of faith program participation on prison misconduct: The life connections program. *Journal of Criminal Justice, 36*(5), 389–395.

Campbell, M. K., Demark-Wahnefried, W., Symons, M., Kalsbeek, W. D., Dodds, J., Cowan, A., et al. (1999). Fruit and vegetable consumption and prevention of cancer: The black churches united for better health project. *American Journal of Public Health, 89*(9), 1390–1396.

Campbell, M. K., Resnicow, K., Carr, C., Wang, T., & Williams, A. (2007). Process evaluation of an effective church-based diet intervention: Body & soul. *Journal of Health Education, and Behavior, 34*(6), 864–880.

Carlson-Thies, S. (2000). Charitable Choice for welfare community services: An implementation guide for state, local, and federal officials. Retrieved November 4, 2005, from http://downloads.weblogger.com/gems/cpj/CCImplementationGuide.pdf.

CASA Report (2001). So help me God: Substance abuse, religion, and spirituality. New York: National Center on Addiction and Substance Abuse at Columbia University.

Charitable Choice Project Description. (n.d.). Faith-based social service provision under Charitable Choice: A study of implementation in three states. Retrieved February 1, 2009, from http://ccr.urbancenter.iupui.edu/project_descrip.html.

Chatters, L. M. (2000). Religion and health: Public health research and practice. *Annual Review of Public Health, 21*, 335–367.

Chatters, L. M., Ellison, C. G., & Levin, J. S. (1998). Public health and health education in faith communities. *Health Education and Behavior, 25*(6), 689–700.

Chatters, L. M., Taylor, R. J., Lincoln, K. D., & Schroepfer, T. (2002). Patterns of informal support from family and church members among African Americans. *Journal of Black Studies, 33*, 66–85.

Clay, K. S., Newlin, K., & Leeks, K. D. (2005). Pastors' wives as partners: An appropriate model for church-based health promotion. *Cancer Control, 12*(suppl), 111–115.

Cloud, R., Ziegler, C., & Blondell, R. (2004). What is Alcoholics Anonymous Affiliation? *Substance Use & Misuse, 39*(7), 1117–1136.

Cnaan, R. A., & Boddie, S. C. (2002). Charitable Choice and faith-based welfare: A call for social work. *Social Work, 47*(3), 224–235.

Cnaan, R. A., Sinha, J. W., & McGrew, C. C. (2004). Congregations as social service providers: Services, capacity, culture, and organizational behavior. *Administration in Social Work, 28*(3/4), 47–68.

Coleman, C. (2004). Contribution of religious and existential well-being to depression among African American heterosexuals with HIV infection. *Issues in Mental Health Nursing, 25*, 103–110.

Davidson, C., & Norton, L. (1995). Religiosity and the sexuality of women: Sexual behavior and sexual satisfaction revisited. *Journal of Sex Research, 32*(3), 235–244.

Davidson, J., Moore, N., & Ullstrup, K. (2004). Religiosity and sexual responsibility: Relationships of choice. *American Journal of Health Behavior, 28*(4), 335–346.

Davis, D. T., Bustamante, A., Brown, C. P., Wolde-Tsadik, G., Savage, E. W., Cheng, X., & Howland, L. (1994) The urban church and cancer control: A source of social influence in minority communities. *Public Health Reports, 109*(4), 500–506.

DeHaven, M. J., Hunter, I. B., Wilder, L., Walton, J. W., & Berry, J. (2004). Health programs in faith-based organizations: Are they effective? *American Journal of Public Health, 94*(6), 1030–1036.

DiIulio, J. J. Jr. (1998). Living faith: The black church outreach tradition. In The Jeremiah Project: An initiative of the Center for Civic Innovation (Report No. 98-3) (pp. 1–10) [Online]. Available at http://www.manhattan-institute.org/html/jpr-98-3.htm

Douglas, K. B., & Hopson, R. (2001). Understanding the Black church: The dynamics of change. *Journal of Religious Thought, 56/57*(2/1), 95–113.

Duan, N., Fox, S. A., Pitkin, K., & Carson, S. (2000). Maintaining mammography adherence through telephone counseling in a church-based trial. *American Journal of Public Health, 90*, 1468–1471.

Ebaugh, H. R., Pipes, P. F., Chafetz, J., & Daniels, M. (2003). Where's the religion? Distinguishing faith-based from secular social service agencies. *Journal for the Scientific Study of Religion, 42*(3), 411–426.

Elifson, K., Klein, H., & Sterk, C. (2003). Religiosity and HIV risk behavior involvement among 'at risk' women. *Journal of Religion and Health, 42*(1), 47–66.

Eng, E., Hatch, J., & Callan, A. (1985). Institutionalizing social support through the church and into the community. *Journal of Health Education and Behavior, 12*(1), 81–92.

Erwin, D. O., Spatz, T. S., Stotts, R. C., Hollenberg, J. A., & Deloney, L. A. (1996). Increasing mammography and breast self-examination in African American women using the Witness Project model. *Journal of Cancer Education, 11*, 210–215.

Fehring, R., Cheever, K., German, K., & Philpot, C. (1998). Religiosity and sexual activity among older adolescents. *Journal of Religion and Health, 37*(3), 229–247.

Gibelman, M., & Gelman, S. R. (2003). Promise of faith-based social services: Perception versus reality. *Social Thought, 22*(2), 5–23.

Hatch J., & Derthick, S. (1992) Empowering black churches for health promotion. *Health Values, 16*, 3–9.

Hatcher, S., Burley, J., & Lee-Ouga, W. (2008). HIV prevention programs in the Black church: A viable health promotion resource for African American women? *Journal of Human Behavior in the Social Environment, 17*(3–4), 309–324

Hill, R. (1999). Strong religious orientation. In R. Hill (Ed.), *Strength of black families*. Lanham, MD: University Press of America, pp. 134–147.

Hodge, D. R. (2000). The spiritually committed: An examination of the staff at faith-based substance abuse providers. *Social Work and Christianity, 27*(2), 150–167.

Hodge, D. R., Cardenas, P., & Montoya, H. (2001). Substance use: Spirituality and religious participation as protective factors among rural youths. *Social Work Research, 25*(3), 153–161.

Hodge, D. R., & Pittman, J. (2003). Faith-based drug and alcohol treatment providers: An exploratory study of Texan providers. *Journal of Social Service Research, 30*, 19–40.

Jang, S. J., & Johnson, B. R. (2004). Explaining religious effects on distress among African Americans. *Journal for the Scientific Study of Religion, 43*(2), 239–260.

Johnson, B. R., & Larson, D. B. (2003). The innerchange freedom initiative: A preliminary evaluation of a faith-based prison program. The University of Pennsylvania: Center for Research on Religion and Urban Civil Society.

Johnson, L. B., & Staples, R. (2005). *Black families at the crossroads.* (Rev. 2nd ed.). San Francisco: Jossey-Bass.

Katz, M., James, A., Pignone, M., Hudson, M., Jackson, E., Oates, V., et al. (2004). Colorectal cancer screening among African American church members: A qualitative and quantitative study of patient-provider communication. *BMC Public Health, 4*(1), 62.

Kip, K. E., Peters, R. H., & Morrison-Rodriguez, B. (2002). Commentary on why national epidemiological estimates of substance abuse by race should not be used to estimate prevalence and need for substance abuse services at community and local levels. *American Journal of Drug and Alcohol Abuse, 28*(3), 545–556.

Kumanyika, S. K., & Charleston, J. B. (1992). Lose weight and win: A church-based weight loss program for blood pressure control among black women. *Patient Education and Counseling, 19*, 19–32.

Levin, J. S. (1986). Roles for the Black pastor in preventive medicine. *Pastoral Psychology, 35*(2), 94–103.

Lewis, R., & Green, B. L. (2000). Assessing the health attitudes, beliefs, and behaviors of African Americans attending church: A comparison from two communities. *Journal of Community Health, 25*(3), 211–224.

Lincoln, C., & Mamiya, L. (1990). *The Black Church in the African American Experience*. Durham, NC: Duke University Press.

Mann, B. D., Sherman, L., Clayton, C., Johnson, R. F., Keates, J., Kasenge, R., Streeter, K., Goldberg, L., & Nieman, L. Z. (2000). Screening to the converted: An educational intervention in African American churches. *Journal of Cancer Education, 15*, 46–50.

Markens, S., Fox, S. A., Taub, B., & Gilbert, M. L. (2002). Role of black churches in health promotion programs: Lessons from the Los Angeles mammography promotion in churches program. *American Journal of Public Health, 92*(5), 805–810.

Matthews, A. K., Berrios, N., Darnell, J. S., & Calhoun, E. (2006) A qualitative evaluation of a faith-based breast and cervical cancer screening intervention for African American women. *Journal of Health, Education, and Behavior, 33*(5), 643–663.

Mattis, J. S., & Jagers, R. J. (2001). Relational framework for the study of religiosity and spirituality in the lives of African Americans. *Journal of Community Psychology, 29*(5), 519–539.

McBeath, W. H. (1991). Health for all: A public health vision. *American Journal of Public Health, 81*(12), 1560–1565.

McNabb, W., Quinn, M., Kerver, J., Cook, S., & Karrison, T. (1997). The PATHWAYS church-based weight loss program for urban African-American women at risk for diabetes. *Diabetes Care, 20*(10), 1518–1523.

McRae, M. B., Carey, P. M., & Anderson-Scott, R. (1998). African American churches as therapeutic systems: A group process perspective. *Health Education and Behavior, 25*(6), 778–779.

Mears, D. P., Roman, C. G., Wolff, A., & Buck, J. (2006). Faith-based efforts to improve prisoner reentry: Assessing the logic and evidence. *Journal of Criminal Justice, 34*(4), 351–367.

Morse, E., Morse, P., Klebra, K., Stock, M., Forehand, R., & Panayotova, E. (2000). The use of religion among HIV-infected African American women. *Journal of Religion and Health, 39*(3), 261–276.

Neighbors, H. W., Musick, M. A., & Williams, D. R. (1998). The African American minister as a source of help for serious personal crises: Bridge or barrier to mental health care? *Health Education & Behavior, 25*, 759–777.

Oexmann, M. J., Ascanio, R., & Egan, B. M. (2001). Efficacy of a church-based intervention on cardiovascular risk reduction. *Ethnicity & Disease, 11*(4), 817–822.

Potter, J. (1988) Vegetables, dietary fiber and cancer. *Journal of Nutrition, 118*, 1591–1592.

Resnicow, K., Jackson, A., Wang, T., De, A. K., McCarty, F., Dudley, W. N., et al. (2001). A motivational interviewing intervention to increase fruit and vegetable intake through black churches: Results of the eat for life trial. *American Journal of Public Health, 91*(10), 1686–1693.

Richardson, B. (1989). Attitudes of black clergy toward mental health professionals: Implications for pastoral care. *The Journal of Pastoral Care, XLIII*, 33–39.

Rogers, R. K., Yancey, G., & Singletary, J. (2005). Methodological challenges in identifying promising and exemplary practices in urban faith-based social service programs. *Social Work and Christianity, 32*(3), 189–208.

Sherman, A. (2000). Tracking Charitable Choice: A study of the collaboration between faith-based organizations and the government in providing social services in nine states. *Social Work and Christianity, 27*(2), 112–129.

Sherwood, D. A. (1998). Charitable Choice: Opportunity and challenge for Christians in social work. *Social Work and Christianity, 25*(1), 1–23.

Sherwood, D. A. (2003). Churches as contexts for social work practice: Connecting with the mission and identity of congregations. *Social Work and Christianity, 30*(1), 1–13.

Smith, E. D., & Merritt, S. L. (1997). Church-based education: An outreach program for African-Americans with hypertension. *Ethnicity & Health, 2*(3), 243–254.

Substance Abuse and Mental Health Services Administration (SAMHSA). (2007, May 22). *ATR: Aggregated Data Profile*. Retrieved February 1, 2009, from http://www.atr.samhsa.gov/downloads/aggregate_march07.pdf

Sutherland, M., Hale, C. D., & Harris, G. J. (1995). Community health promotion: The church as partner. *The Journal of Primary Prevention, 16*(2), 201–216.

Taylor, R. J., Chatters, L. M., & Levin, J. (2004). *Religion in the lives of African Americans*. Thousand Oaks: Sage.

Taylor, R. J., Ellison, C. G., Chatters, L. M., Levin, J. S., & Lincoln, K. D. (2000) Mental health services in faith communities: The role of clergy in Black churches. *Social Work, 45*(1), 73–87.

Thomas, S. B., Quinn, S. C., Billingsley, A., & Caldwell, C. (1994). The characteristics of northern black churches with community health outreach programs. *American Journal of Public Health, 84*(4), 575–579.

Thumma, S. (2001) Nondenominational congregations today: A report from the faith communities today project. Retrieved February 2, 2009, from www.hirr.hartsem.edu/cong/nondenom_FACT.html

Turner, L. W., Sutherland, M., Harris, G. J., & Barber, M. (1995). Cardiovascular health promotion in north Florida African-American churches. *Health Values, 19*(2), 3–9.

U.S. Census Bureau. (2007). Current population survey, 2007 and 2008 Annual Social and Economic Supplements. Retrieved February 1, 2009, from www.census.gov/cps

Weinrich, S. P., Boyd, M. D., Bradford, D., Mossa, M. S., & Weinrich, M. (1998). Recruitment of African Americans into prostate cancer screening. *Cancer Practice, 6*, 23–30.

The White House (2001). Executive order: Establishment of White House Office of Faith-Based and Community Initiatives. Retrieved February 1, 2009, from http://www.presidency.ucsb.edu/ws/?pid=61481

Wiist, W. H., & Flack, J. M. (1990) A church-based cholesterol education program. *Public Health Reports, 105*(4), 381–388.

Williams, D. R., Griffith, E. E., Young, J. L., Collins, C., & Dodson, J. (1999) Structure and provision of services in black churches in New Haven, Connecticut. *Cultural Diversity Ethnic Minor Psychology, 5*(2), 118–133.

Yanek, L. R., Becker, D. M., Moy, T. F., Gittelsohn, J., & Koffman, D. M. (2001) Project Joy: Faith based cardiovascular health promotion for African American women. *Public Health Reports, 116*(Suppl 1), 68–81.

25

COMMUNITY HEALTH WORKERS IN THE BLACK COMMUNITY

Building Trust, Alleviating Pain, and Improving Health Access

JACQUELINE MARTINEZ
LAURA JOSLIN FRYE
LEDA M. PEREZ

Community Health Workers (CHWs) are integral members of effective health care teams. They are especially useful in the context of the black community due to their ability to address issues of access, trust, and disparities. CHWs have been successfully used to improve the health outcomes of the black community in the areas of social, mental, and environmental health; chronic diseases; and lifestyle and behavior. Policies should be created to expand the utilization of the CHW model, recognize the contribution of CHWs, and support their professional needs. The black community faces formidable health challenges but CHWs have a unique set of tools to promote positive health outcomes in this population.

SUMMARY OF THE NATURE OF CHWs

Traditional medical systems in the United States used to include home-grown doctors taking care of the citizens in the town in which they resided, making home visits, and sharing life experiences with their patients. However, our current medical system is far from this model due to the geographic mobility of providers and the increasing diversity of patients. This creates a situation in which providers may have different experiences, perspectives, cultures, and even languages than the patients they serve. If the biological body and the pathogen were the extent of modern medicine then these differences would not impede a provider's ability to care for a patient. However, our understanding of the determinants of health has expanded and we understand that illnesses result not just from viruses and bacteria, but from environment and lifestyle. It is challenging for providers to care for their patients when they do not have first-hand experience regarding their environmental exposures and are not privy to the realities of their day-to-day lives. The medical textbooks are insufficient to prepare doctors for maximally interacting with this diverse patient population and for comprehensively addressing these holistic determinants. A translator, advocate, guide, and/or facilitator is necessary. A Community Health Worker (CHW) can fill that role.

In an ecological model of health, the determinants exist at several levels—individual, interpersonal, organizational, community, and public policy. The formal medical system is not currently structured to address many of these levels. However, the addition of community health workers to the health care team can expand the reach of interventions from the individual across the dyad and families, all the way to the community and policy.

The American Public Health Association passed a resolution in 2001 entitled "Recognition and Support for Community Health Workers' Contributions to Meeting Our Nation's Health Care Needs" and the Centers for Disease Control and Prevention released a position statement encouraging the use of CHWs in fighting diabetes. It is clear that the heavyweights in the American medical system are beginning to recognize the vital contribution of Community Health Workers. The special role of CHWs in combating disparities is also being acknowledged. In the seminal document *Unequal Treatment: Confronting Racial and Ethnic Disparities in Healthcare*, the Institute of Medicine recommends the use of Community Health Workers as part of a comprehensive strategy to address racial disparities in health. The report explains that CHWs "offer promise as a community-based resource to increase racial and ethnic minorities' access to healthcare and to serve as a liaison between healthcare providers and the communities they serve" (Institute of Medicine, 2002).

THE ROLE OF CHWs IN THE BLACK COMMUNITY

Whether called Community Health Workers, community outreach workers, lay health advisors, village health workers, or *promotoras*, this group consists of indigenous members of a community, who take on health leadership roles. CHWs originated in isolated communities where there was little access to formal health care or a dearth of culturally appropriate care options. However, CHW programs have proven to be useful even in the presence of the best health technology and the most resource-rich environments. Grown out of necessity, the role of CHWs has evolved and they have proven to be integral members of an effective health care team.

The black community presents a context ripe for the integration of the CHW model. The historical lack of access to care, distrust of the medical system, and entrenched economic and social disparities are the backdrop for disparities in health and health outcomes. CHWs, indigenous to the community, have surfaced as the natural helpers in this context and have persevered and thrived despite this backdrop, thus illustrating that they have the innate tools to close the disparities gap and address the barriers across all ecological levels.

Access

The black community experiences both a literal and figurative gap in access to health care, as the care received may not be culturally relevant or adequately tailored. CHWs as educators provide access to a basic level of health care; as advocates and guides they help their communities gain access to more formal care. However, before the actual acquisition of formal health care, community members must seek it. Care-seeking behavior is largely dependent on the provider-and-patient relationship and patient confidence that the provider has his/her best interests at heart.

Distrust

Distrust of the formal medical system by the black community is based on a sordid history of ethical breaches. From the Tuskegee Syphilis Study that allowed black men to die from syphilis in the face of a known cure to very recent research trials on prisoners, it is clear why trust issues exist between the black and medical communities. Furthermore, confronted with a disproportionate burden of HIV, some members of the black community are distrusting of the government's sincerity in their efforts to curb the epidemic.

These trust issues impair care-seeking, adherence to treatment regimens, and ultimately, health status (Wasserman, Flannery, & Clair, 2007). Community Health Workers enter this structure with a valuable source of credibility. As members of the community, they have an earned "insider" trust from their peers and can help assuage fears of the formal medical system. As advocates, they can facilitate relationships between community members and physicians and they can work with both populations to rebuild trust and make the necessary connections between the two. Given the context of the black community, CHWs are poised to offer viable solutions, helping to demystify the roots of disparities in access to care, health outcomes, and disease burden. From their place in the field, they can address disparities on an individual level, while providing crucial information that can inform approaches to address them on a systems level.

ISSUES UNIQUE TO THE BLACK COMMUNITY THAT CHWs ARE ADDRESSING

You have read in this book the myriad health issues that the black community faces. Through each of the broad categories outlined in this book—social, mental, and environmental challenges; chronic diseases; and lifestyle behaviors—CHWs can (and in many cases do) play a role in working toward better health outcomes.

Social, Mental, and Environmental Challenges

Community Health Workers bring a unique and germane toolkit to the social, mental, and environmental challenges faced in black communities. In addressing social problems, CHWs offer a personal familiarity with the society in which a patient interacts. They are aware of the societal norms, the social support structures, and the quotidian trials and tribulations faced by their communities. For mental health issues, CHWs bring ease of communications, an understanding of cultural underpinnings and stigma, and a source of credibility and trust. Community Health Workers can approach environmental issues with a grasp of the environment in which the patients live, work, and play.

The Community Health Worker Model has also been successfully used to address issues of violence in the black community. The Power for Health Project used CHWs to identify health issues of importance to the community. When violence, originating both from gangs and the police, topped the list, the CHW moved forward to demand changes in the police department, build relationships between community members and law enforcement, and teach nonviolent communication to youth (Farquhar, Michael, & Wiggins, 2005).

In the case of mental health, one must first acknowledge the dearth of black professional providers for mental health services. Only 2 percent of psychiatrists and 2 percent of psychologists are black (Braithwaite, 2006). CHWs can help fill this gap by serving as liaisons between patients and providers from disparate cultural backgrounds. This is particularly important in the black community due to the perception that seeking mental help is a sign of weakness. As trusted leaders, CHWs can help to diminish this stigma of mental illness and encourage patients to seek the care they need. In their role as guides through the health care system they can help patients access that care and can also coordinate care for those who suffer from co-occurring mental health and substance use problems.

For those whose problems with violence, mental health, or substance use are not prevented or addressed in their home communities, a prison system awaits. But even here, CHWs can play a role, easing the adjustment of ex-offenders when they exit prison and helping to prevent the "revolving door" of entry and exit from the prison system.

Former prisoners often face a gap in health care coverage, restrictions on public housing, exclusion from cash assistance and food stamp programs, and unemployment (Community Voices, 2006). Here the role of CHWs as advocates and connections to resources may be especially important. Dr. Henrie Treadwell, the director of Community Voices, explains the role that CHWs can play in the reintegration of prisoners into society. "I think community health workers are probably the only solution here. Because people need a guide, a hand, a friend, a helper to get them reestablished. Someone who really takes the entire portfolio of a person's being and gets them connected again" (Treadwell, 2008). She likens the use of patient navigators for the chronically ill to the use of CHWs for the chronically displaced; prisoners who have left their social fabric for an environment rife with mental health challenges, emotional danger, and infectious diseases. Community Health Workers can smooth the harsh transition from prison life to community life, and all the negative health sequelae, connecting former prisoners to health care and addressing the wider causes of their health problems—some of which might be the very thing that precipitated their incarceration.

As an organic part of the society, with a natural insight into the mind, and with proximity and familiarity with the environment, Community Health Workers are well equipped to help address this category of problem.

Chronic Diseases

Chronic diseases present a formidable challenge not only because of their prevalence in the black community, but also due to the intensity and continuity required in their treatment. Episodic treatment in emergency rooms of hospitals is generally insufficient to prevent and manage chronic conditions. The issues with access to care, provider trust, and continuity of care faced by the black community, particularly subsets such as young black men, are particularly dangerous in the face of chronic disease. CHWs can play a particularly vital role as a consistent and credible connection between patients and the ongoing care they need. They can provide timely access to prevention services, promote adequate follow-up, and develop the necessary relationships to ensure adherence to long-term treatment regimens.

For instance, CHWs can play an important role in the detection, treatment, and control of risk factors for heart disease in the black community, where young black men are the group least likely to be detected with hypertension and to achieve blood pressure control (Brownstein et al., 2005). Through community screenings, CHWs can help to identify those at risk for heart disease and facilitate referrals to treatment. In a study of interventions to combat risk factors in black families with a history of heart disease, CHWs were part of a successful strategy that lowered cholesterol and high blood pressure (Becker et al., 2005). Furthermore, in a study of young black men, CHWs played a crucial role by conducting home visits in an intervention that successfully improved blood pressure control (Dennison et al., 2007).

Black women also experience a disproportionate burden of chronic disease, particularly breast cancer. Black women have the highest breast cancer mortality of any racial group in the United States. Contributing to this high mortality rate are low rates of screening mammography and adherence to follow-up appointments after an abnormal mammogram. Community Health Workers, through in-home education (Sung et al., 1997) and tailored telephone counseling (West et al., 2004), can increase the rate of mammography in black women. CHWs have been shown to improve the rate of follow-up after an abnormal mammogram by providing encouragement and reminders, helping to remove barriers, and accompanying women to appointments (Crump et al., 2008).

Both black men and women face a chronic disease that threatens to be increasingly detrimental in the coming years—diabetes (Batts et al., 2001). The National Center for Chronic Disease Prevention and Health Promotion (2003) has recognized CHWs as an important component of diabetes prevention and education. CHWs have been shown to aid in the retention of participants in diabetes interventions (Gary et al., 2003). In Project Sugar, CHWs sought to identify barriers to management and treatment that might otherwise be overlooked by traditional medical care, such as household factors related to medication adherence or literacy levels and filling out forms. Once identified, the CHWs addressed the problems with the patient through home visits, telephone calls, and community events (Gary et al., 2004).

For black men and women, CHWs can provide an important resource in the long-term health issues they face.

Lifestyle Behaviors

Lifestyle behaviors are notoriously difficult to change and an annual clinical encounter is often insufficient to cause lasting transformations. Community Health Workers are able to provide consistent, persistent, and continuous support to promote these behavior changes. The complexities of behavior—emotional triggers, environmental barriers, points of leverage, sources of support—require a deep and compassionate understanding of the patient. CHWs might be best placed to understand these critical components and be trusted to advise on behavior modifications.

Sexual behaviors happen behind closed doors, are often not freely discussed, and are subject to a wide range of emotional reactions, societal norms, and peer pressures. These characteristics make them particularly difficult to modify. However, CHWs have been used in the prevention of sexually transmitted diseases among black women, with such diverse roles as lending credibility to the communication of information on STIs to escorting friends to local STI clinics (Thomas et al., 2001). CHWs can represent trusted sources of information outside of the formal medical system, where sexual issues may be harder to discuss. Furthermore, their connections in the community make them poised to disseminate accurate and targeted information on a large scale.

Another challenging lifestyle behavior is smoking. Social support and smoking self-efficacy are key components to successful smoking cessation or abstinence. One successful smoking cessation intervention used Community Health Workers to enhance smoking self-efficacy, social support, and spiritual well-being. CHWs provided support to those seeking to quit smoking through empathetic listening, display of concern, and advice and also helped participants to identify positive support systems within their own families and networks (Andrews et al., 2007). A study by Andrews et al. (2007) found those with the support of CHWs to be six times more likely to quit smoking than the comparison group without CHW support.

Theories of behavioral change abound, and CHWs can play an important role in efforts based on many of the most popular theories of behavioral change. In the Theory of Reasoned Action where subjective norms and attitudes affect intentions to change behaviors (Ajzan & Fishbein, 1980), CHWs might help to shape those norms and attitudes through one-on-one or group discussions. In the Social Cognitive Theory, interactions, observations, and experiences with others play a large role in behavior change. An important aspect of this theory is the notion that if the learner identifies strongly with the teacher, they will be more likely to effectively imitate a behavior (Bandura, 1986). The indigenous nature of CHWs as models for behavior and as promoters of self-efficacy make them fit nicely into this theory. In the Health Belief Model, where perception of susceptibility, severity, benefit, and barriers affect behavior (Rosenstock, 1966), CHWs can help to shape those perceptions. There is a role for CHWs in most methods of lifestyle behavior change.

Other Challenges

Though some health challenges in the black community are obvious, it is naïve to think that we can easily enumerate all the obstacles and prescribe solutions. With well-documented disparities as wide and deep as we have read in various academic publications, seen in every geographic locale, and experienced in our own daily lives, there simply must be more at play than the inventory of barriers we have amassed. Here, too, CHWs can assist. They can not only work to address the challenges that we know the black community faces, but also on an individual level can uncover and mitigate the countless unseen impediments. Family issues, transportation difficulty, stigma, misinformation, and countless other real obstructions are unlikely to appear in a short clinical encounter. CHWs, with home visits and community knowledge, are better placed to learn about these subtle barriers and, with their knowledge of community resources, may be best equipped to assist patients in surmounting them.

POLICY IMPLICATIONS

Utilize

Evidence exists that CHWs are successful at addressing a variety of health issues and it is time to continue to collect more evidence and creatively use their services to address an expanding number of health issues. Not only have they produced positive health outcomes, but they have been cost effective (Fedder et al., 2003). In a contracting economy it seems even more prudent to focus on this low-cost intervention. Further, in a health care system that is insufficiently responsive to the growing prevalence of chronic illnesses and the need for continuous and preventive care, CHWs could be at the center of a transformative option to reform our broken health care system. Recognizing their contribution, we should work to institutionalize the use of CHWs as part of a care team.

Recognize

Much of this chapter has focused on the benefit of CHWs to patients, increasing access, improving outcomes, and enhancing awareness. However, it is important not to discount the value that CHWs can add to providers, researchers, policymakers, and funders. Given the perspective of CHWs—built on genuine and deep interactions with underserved communities while enhanced by an understanding of the formal medical system— their voices should be amplified in the health care debate. As providers grapple with frustration from disappointing outcomes among patients, CHWs can offer insight into the root causes of the ailments and strategies that may be more salient for the population. As academics develop and test new interventions based on the latest theories and innovations, CHWs can offer insight into the likely effectiveness of such programs or the relevancy of a particular research question. As politicians debate how best to expand health coverage and reduce costs, CHWs can bring the perspective from the field to their offices in city halls. As foundations decide how to allocate their funds, CHWs can provide insight into the projects that may be most important to their communities. The richness of their experiences should not be underestimated, nor their worth as consultants.

Given their knowledge of the health care needs of their community, we should work to create mechanisms to facilitate the work of CHWs as advocates. Creating connections between CHWs and important health care decision makers can improve the quality of policies and bring voices to those who are otherwise not brought to the table of stakeholders.

Support

Given the integral role that CHWs play in the health care delivery team and the evidence of their ability to reduce costs and promote positive health outcomes, we cannot depend on the traditional volunteer nature of CHWs. They offer great worth to our medical system and should be commensurately compensated. One important step in securing adequate compensation is Medicaid reimbursement. State certification can help to facilitate Medicaid reimbursement; however, there is great variation among states in their support for institutionalizing the CHW model. State policies range from Alaska, where there is a statewide training and certification program for CHWs (who are then able to bill Medicaid), to states where individual agencies conduct programs and the state is not involved in funding or administration (Dower et al., 2006). Promoting state-funded certification programs is an important step in recognizing and affirming the role of CHWs.

CONCLUSION

With the immense resources—financial, human, and time— used to treat chronic diseases, prevention has never been a more important strategy. Prevention often does not live in an examination room or a waiting room or even a classroom, but rather in the streets and homes of the community. Community Health Workers can spread the seeds of prevention by sharing knowledge, healthy practices, and skills to promote disease prevention long before a patient encounters the formal medical system. Many of the health problems we see in the black community today—diabetes, hypertension, and homicide—have their roots not in a pathogen invading a host, but rather in the fabric of society. So it is in society where these problems need to be addressed and it is society itself that is best placed to do it. CHWs can provide that internal stimulus to promote health change; they can be a catalyst for everyday healthy living to keep people out of the hospitals and waiting rooms. They are, in essence, a first line of defense.

The black community faces formidable challenges, but has considerable strengths. One such strength is a robust system of Community Health Workers who have the skills, motivation, and knowledge necessary to combat the underlying causes of negative health outcomes and an understanding of the community capacities and assets available to defeat them.

REFERENCES

Ajzen, I., & Fishbein, M. (1980). *Understanding attitudes and predicting social behavior*. Englewood Cliffs, NJ: Prentice-Hall.

American Public Health Association Resolution. (2001). Recognition and Support for Community Health Workers' Contributions to Meeting Our Nation's Healthcare Needs. Retrieved Nov. 25, 2009, from http://www.apha.org/advocacy/policy/policysearch/

Andrews, J. O., Felton, G., Ellen Wewers, M., Waller, J., & Tingen, M. (2007). The effect of a multi-component smoking cessation intervention in African American women residing in public housing. *Research in Nursing & Health, 30*(1), 45–60.

Batts, M. L., Gary, T. L., Huss, K., Hill, M. N., Bone, L., & Brancati, F. L. (2001). Patient priorities and needs for diabetes care among urban African American adults. *The Diabetes Educator, 27*(3), 405–412.

Bandura, A. (1986). *Social foundations of thought and action: A social cognitive theory*. Englewood Cliffs, NJ: Prentice-Hall.

Becker, D. M., Yanek, L. R., Johnson, W. R., Jr., Garrett, D., Moy, T. F., Reynolds, S. S., et al. (2005). Impact of a community-based multiple risk factor intervention on cardiovascular risk in black families with a history of premature coronary disease. *Circulation, 111*(10), 1298–1304.

Braithwaite, K. (2006). Access to mental health care and substance abuse treatment for men of color in the US: Findings from the National Healthcare Disparities Report. *Challenge: A Journal of Research on African American Men, 12*(2) 65–74.

Brownstein, J. N., Bone, L. R., Dennison, C. R., Hill, M. N., Kim, M. T., & Levine, D. M. (2005). Community health workers as interventionists in the prevention and control of heart disease and stroke. *American Journal of Preventive Medicine, 29*(5 Suppl 1), 128–133.

Community Voices: Healthcare for the Underserved. (2006). *Examining the needs of the incarcerated, soon-to-be-released, and ex-offenders. Reentry Stakeholders Meeting*. National Center for Primary Care. Morehouse School of Medicine.

Crump, S. R., Shipp, M. P., McCray, G. G., Morris, S. J., Okoli, J. A., Caplan, L. S., et al. (2008). Abnormal mammogram follow-up: Do community lay health advocates make a difference? *Health Promotion Practice, 9*(2), 140–148.

Dennison, C. R., Post, W. S., Kim, M. T., Bone, L. R., Cohen, D., Blumenthal, R. S., et al. (2007). Underserved urban African American men: Hypertension trial outcomes and mortality during 5 years. *American Journal of Hypertension: Journal of the American Society of Hypertension, 20*(2), 164–171.

Dower, C., Knox, M., Lindler, V., & O'Neill, E. (2006). *Advancing community health worker practice and utilization: The focus on financing*. San Francisco, CA: National Fund for Medical Education.

Farquhar, S. A., Michael, Y. L., & Wiggins, N. (2005). Building on leadership and social capital to create change in 2 urban communities. *American Journal of Public Health, 95*(4), 596–601.

Fedder, D. O., Chang, R. J., Curry, S., & Nichols, G. (2003). For the patient. The effectiveness of a community health worker outreach program on healthcare utilization of west Baltimore city Medicaid patients with diabetes, with or without hypertension. *Ethnicity & Disease, 13*(1), 146.

Gary, T. L., Batts-Turner, M., Bone, L. R., Yeh, H. C., Wang, N. Y., Hill-Briggs, F., et al. (2004). A randomized controlled trial of the effects of nurse case manager and community health worker team interventions in urban African-Americans with type 2 diabetes. *Controlled Clinical Trials, 25*(1), 53–66.

Gary, T. L., Bone, L. R., Hill, M. N., Levine, D. M., McGuire, M., Saudek, C., et al. (2003). Randomized controlled trial of the effects of nurse case manager and community health worker interventions on risk factors for diabetes-related complications in urban African Americans. *Preventive Medicine, 37*(1), 23–32.

Institute of Medicine. (2002). *Unequal treatment: Confronting racial and ethnic disparities in healthcare.* Washington, DC: Institute of Medicine.

National Center for Chronic Disease Prevention and Health Promotion, Division of Diabetes Translation. (2003). *Community health workers/promotores de salud: Critical connections in communities.* Atlanta, GA: Centers for Disease Control and Prevention.

Rosenstock, I. M. (1966). Why people use health services. *Milbank Memorial Fund Quarterly, 44,* 94–124.

Sung, J. F., Blumenthal, D. S., Coates, R. J., Williams, J. E., Alema-Mensah, E., & Liff, J. M. (1997). Effect of a cancer screening intervention conducted by lay health workers among inner-city women. *American Journal of Preventive Medicine, 13*(1), 51–57.

Thomas, J. C., Eng, E., Earp, J. A., & Ellis, H. (2001). Trust and collaboration in the prevention of sexually transmitted diseases. *Public Health Reports (Washington, D.C.: 1974), 116*(6), 540–547.

Treadwell, H., (2008). Transcript of an interview. An Advocate's Voice: Dr. Henrie Treadwell. *2008 National Conference of State Legislators.* Retrieved from http://www.ncsl.org/programs/health/forum/Dr._Treadwell.htm

Wasserman, J., Flannery, M. A., & Clair, J. M. (2007). Raising the ivory tower: The production of knowledge and distrust of medicine among African Americans. *Journal of Medical Ethics, 33*(3), 177–180.

West, D. S., Greene, P., Pulley, L., Kratt, P., Gore, S., Weiss, H., et al. (2004). Stepped-care, community clinic interventions to promote mammography use among low-income rural African American women. *Health Education & Behavior: The Official Publication of the Society for Public Health Education, 31*(4 Suppl), 29S–44S.

6

ETHICAL, POLITICAL, AND ECOLOGICAL ISSUES

CHAPTER

26

USING SOCIAL MARKETING TO LESSEN HEALTH DISPARITIES

MESHA L. ELLIS
JAMES P. GRIFFIN JR.
KEN RESNICOW

Although African Americans constitute roughly 13 percent of the population of the United States of America, they suffer from a disproportionate number of preventable chronic health conditions as well as elevated morbidity and mortality rates (Hopp & Herring, 1999; Marks, Reed, Colby, & Ibrahim, 2004). Examples of chronic conditions known to affect the overall health status of African Americans are heart and cardiovascular disease, various forms of cancer, stroke, and other lifestyle-related disorders such as obesity. Other behaviorally based health challenges include the use of alcohol and other substances, violence, mental health issues, issues related to sexual health (such as HIV/AIDS), and diabetes. Many of these health issues have their genesis in social determinants such as economic deprivation, transitions and mobility, and the influence of media and popular culture.

Although significant improvements in the diagnosis and treatment of chronic disease have occurred as a result of governmental, research, and public health attention, huge disparities between the health status of African Americans and their counterparts from other ethnic groups still remain. For example, although the gap between the mortality rate for African Americans and that for European Americans has consistently decreased since 1990, the mortality rate for African Americans is 31 percent higher than that for European Americans and is also higher than the mortality rates for every other ethnic minority group (LaVeist, 2005; National Center for Health Statistics, 2007). Heart disease and cancer account for the highest death rates among African Americans, with nearly 48 percent of African American male deaths being attributed to these diseases alone (Fort, 2007; LaVeist, 2005; Marks et al., 2004). The death rates for stroke, heart disease, cancer, and HIV among African Americans consistently exceed the death rates for these conditions among their Caucasian counterparts. Further, the number of African American live births is significantly less than that of any other ethnic group within the United States (Baffour, Jones, & Contreras, 2006; National Center for Health Statistics, 2007).

Undoubtedly, the issues of health promotion and health disparity among African Americans are quite complex and cannot be addressed myopically. Instead, efforts to increase the health functioning of African Americans require a comprehensive under-standing of the factors contributing to the poor health status and outcomes of many African American citizens as well as thoughtful, culturally relevant, and ecologically valid strategies to address and lessen their impact. Utilizing an ecological framework, this chapter discusses the individual contributions African Americans make to their overall health while incorporating and acknowledging the role that the family, community, society at large, and governmental policies and legislative efforts play in the development and amelioration of health issues within the African American community. This chapter highlights the potential for and use of social marketing strategies and media in the fight to reduce health disparity within the African American community.

AN ECOLOGICAL MODEL OF AFRICAN AMERICAN HEALTH

It has long been recognized that individuals do not develop and life does not proceed in a vacuum. Instead, many developmentalists and researchers acknowledge the powerful influence environmental contexts exert on individual development, well-being, and overall health functioning (Benner, Graham, & Mistry, 2008; Bronfenbrenner & Ceci, 1994; Diamond, 2009; Lynch, Smith, Kaplan, & House, 2000; Newacheck, Kim, Blumberg, & Rising, 2008). Research has clearly documented that developmental and health outcomes are the result of an interaction between environmental experience and individual characteristics (Bronfenbrenner & Ceci, 1994; Newacheck, Kim, et al., 2008). Research suggests that health status is determined largely by medical and non-medical factors complexly interacting. Along with modes of exposure and individual susceptibility and resilience, these factors affect health over time; they ultimately have an effect on the health not only of individuals but also of the communities in which they live (Newacheck, Rising, & Kim, 2006). In sum, no one factor acts alone, instead multiple factors (i.e., determinants) interact to cause and maintain disease (Starfield, 2001).

Thus, when considering the African American community, one has to consider a multitude of processes, events, predispositions, and circumstances that have contributed to the health crisis now in evidence. A history of enslavement, institutionalized racism, discriminatory health care practices, educational inequity, limited access to employment opportunities, and substandard housing have historically detrimentally affected health attitudes, access, and behaviors of individuals within the African American community, and they continue to do so (Ashley, 1999). At the same time, understanding the role of genetic vulnerability, coping styles, culture, social support, personal responsibility, health literacy, and proactive health advocacy or the lack thereof in the creation, maintenance, and remediation of poor health status is also crucial to both understanding the phenomenon and charting an effective course of action. Consequently, utilizing an ecological frame to identify and highlight the societal, interpersonal, and individual-level systems influencing African American health may help provide insight into appropriate and cost-effective health-promotion efforts.

Utilizing the knowledge gained from population health research as well as pediatric epidemiological and clinical research, Newacheck, Rising, and Kim (2006) developed an ecological model of health risk for children that we have adapted for use in our exploration of African American health. African American health can be understood as existing within six major health-determinant or risk-factor domains (genetic endowment, predisposing characteristics, social environment, physical environment, health-influencing behavior, and health care system characteristics). Each domain contributes to the development and maintenance of chronic health and mental health conditions.

For definitional clarity, genetic endowment comprises an individual's inherited attributes and biological predisposition as a result of the genetic transmission of traits, characteristics, and vulnerabilities from one's biological parents. Predisposing characteristics are biologically based factors such as one's ethnicity, age, gender, temperament, coping style, learning potential, and educational level, which are known to either increase or decrease one's susceptibility to chronic health difficulties as a result of genetic or environmental insults (or both). The social environment encompasses individuals' social relationships, cultural surroundings, and social roles, as well as the social and cultural institutions within which they interact (Barnett & Casper, 2001). The social environment includes access and exposure to social hierarchies, social resources, and material resources. The physical environment is one's surroundings, physical context, and the conditions to which one is exposed. The physical environment includes access to and quality of housing, electricity, gas, sanitation, transportation, paved roads, parks, schools, and playgrounds. Health-influencing behavior can be conceptualized as the habits and behaviors known to affect one's health. These behaviors include sleep patterns, eating habits, level of physical activity, and participation in recreational activities. The final domain, health care system characteristics, includes access to, availability of, and quality of medical care, health and medical services, and functional health systems.

Each health-determinant domain operates at multiple levels over time within the lives of African Americans (i.e., at the level of the individual, the family, the community, and the society) to either increase or decrease susceptibility to chronic and debilitating physical health and mental health conditions. For example, societal factors such as environmental policy, social policy, economic policy, and health policy all have an impact on the physical environment in which one lives. They can provide, among other amenities, access to parks, safe and clean neighborhoods, adequate sanitation, and grocery stores. Such amenities affect and are affected by community, family, and individual factors like neighborhood safety, educational attainment, food affordability, food choices, exercise patterns, stress levels, and level of income to influence behavioral choices, emotional responsivity, and health outcomes (Newacheck et al., 2008; Newacheck, Rising, & Kim, 2006; Sankofa & Johnson-Taylor, 2007; Starfield, 2001). Correspondingly, the minimal health literacy frequently observed among African Americans (Gazmararian, Curran, Parker, Bernhardt, & DeBuono, 2005; Pfizer Incorporated, 2003) has been suggested as a major contributor to many of the health difficulties experienced within this community (Gazmararian et al., 2005). Health literacy, an individual-level indicator, is likely highly influenced by what has occurred or is occurring at the family level, the community level, and even the societal level. Figure 26.1 presents a multilevel model of the complex nature and influence of the overall environment on health outcomes within the African American community. It also provides room for considering individual differences within this heterogeneous group.

SOCIAL MARKETING AS A TOOL TO ADDRESS HEALTH ISSUES

As previously discussed, a number of pervasive health concerns affect the African American community. From an ecological perspective, these health concerns cut across various domains within and across the sectors of the African American social structure. Further, many of the health challenges seen within this community appear to be deep seated and intractable. As a result, many health-promotion efforts have been undertaken to address health disparities within the African American community over the years. Although many researchers have acknowledged the powerful influence of the environment on health risk as well as the need for adopting an ecological approach to health-promotion program development, only a handful of programs that have been developed since 1996 utilize a multilevel structure to address health-risk behaviors (Kok, Gottlieb, Commers, & Smerecnik, 2008). Instead, many programs intervene primarily at the level of the individual without considering the potential gains from addressing social, occupational, cultural, or developmental needs as well (Vrazel, Saunders, & Wilcox, 2008). Further, the active engagement and targeting of African Americans to participate in health-promotion programs is a relatively recent phenomenon (Icard, Bourjolly, & Siddiqui, 2003). Individuals who are charged with the responsibility of helping to reverse detrimental trends in patterns of diseases and health conditions that affect African Americans must find new tools to counteract the obstacles that many African Americans face in regard to health problems.

One of the emerging tools finding a home in the fight against health disparities in the African American community is *social marketing*. Social marketing is an approach to improving the health of target groups by using marketing campaigns, media outlets, and advertising strategies to promote health-related messages (Icard et al., 2003;

FIGURE 26.1 *Determinants of Health Disparity and Chronic Health Conditions Within the African American Community.*

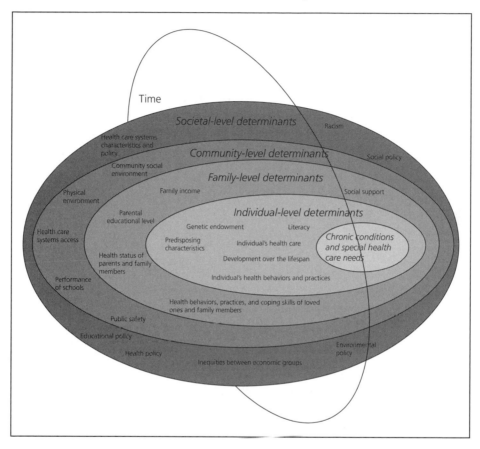

Source: Adapted from work conducted by Newacheck, Rising, and Kim (2006) with permission.

Kotler & Lee, 2008; Stellefson & Eddy, 2008). Social marketing applies commercial marketing tools, technologies, and concepts in the analysis, planning, implementation, and evaluation of programs to improve human welfare (Smith, Tang, & Nutbeam, 2006). Although social marketing is a direct descendent of commercial marketing, unlike its predecessor, social marketing is not product oriented and does not attempt to persuade consumers to purchase tangible goods. Instead, social marketing encourages target audiences to "buy in" to social ideas and engage in voluntary behaviors designed to decrease individual or societal health vulnerability or to increase personal well-being (Icard et al., 2003; Stellefson & Eddy, 2008).

Within the context of social marketing, one party (e.g., welfare agents, health promoters) engages in, develops, and seeks to maintain social relationships with individuals and target population groups. As a result of the developed relationships, it is hoped that the target audience will adopt new behaviors or relinquish old unhealthy behaviors. The focus of social marketing efforts, then, is to address the determinants of a target group's behaviors (Ratzan, 2001). To many health researchers, practitioners, and other decision makers, social marketing may be a foreign concept and not very well recognized as a means for promoting healthy behavior, as it is an offshoot of business and commercial advertising. For this reason, it may be worthwhile to examine in conceptual, theoretical, and practical terms exactly what social marketing is. Therefore, we begin this discussion of social marketing as a behavior-change technology with a formal description of its theoretical foundation.

A Theoretical Context for Social Marketing Activities

The concept of social marketing has its roots in the science of marketing, polling, public opinion, and communication (Ratzan, 2001). Two of the early proponents of social marketing, Kotler and Levy (1969), emphasized that all organizations engage in marketing activities (1) as a means to maintain contact as well as to understand consumer needs, (2) as a way to develop programming or products to satisfy the needs of consumers, and (3) as an avenue for the communication of goals and purposes to consumers. Kotler and Levy encouraged nonbusiness organizations to capitalize on the lessons learned as well as the concepts developed in commercial marketing as guides to help ensure success in socially oriented marketing activities.

Of central importance to marketing efforts and the adoption of business marketing strategies to promote health messages is the concept of *exchange*. Exchange is the transfer of tangible or intangible goods between parties (Bagozzi, 1975). The transfer of goods can occur directly or indirectly. From a marketing perspective, the concept of exchange is central because consumer and organizational needs, goals, and desires can be satisfied only through voluntary, mutually beneficial exchanges of goods, values, social circumstances, or information (Hastings & Haywood, 1991). In general, social marketing seeks to create, maintain, and promote beneficial tangible and intangible exchanges of resources in social relationships (Bagozzi, 1975). Consequently, at the foundation of social marketing activities is social exchange theory.

Social-Exchange Theory

Within his conceptual framework of exchange, Bagozzi (1975) argued that three forms of marketing exchange exist: restricted exchange, generalized exchange, and complex exchange.

Restricted Exchange   Social-exchange theory holds that in restricted exchange, relationships between two parties are formed and maintained as a result of voluntary, mutually negotiated exchanges of resources, benefits, or rewards (Zafirovski, 2003). The value of these benefits, resources, and rewards is individually determined and may be based on factors such as assistance, wealth, power, prestige, status, influence, relational ties, information, access, cultural symbols, or even a sense of well-being.

The exchange of benefits between parties within a restricted-exchange relationship is governed by *rules of reciprocity* that motivate such exchanges (Lester, Meglino, & Korsgaard, 2008). Rules of reciprocity are behavioral norms that suggest that as one individual receives a benefit from a relationship, he or she should also provide some benefit to the relationship.

Decisions regarding whether to remain in relationships are made on the basis of a number of factors, including whether one's actions and the actions of others meet pre-established expectations and moral norms (Lester et al., 2008). Within this theoretical framework, individuals assess the value of relationships by evaluating (1) the balance between what they are required to place into a relationship and what they are able to obtain from the relationship, (2) determinations about the kind of relationship they believe they deserve, and (3) the odds of being able to develop and maintain a better relationship with someone else. Thus, at the center of restricted exchange is an assumption that parties seek to establish mutually beneficial and meaningful bonds with others and that each party is motivated to act based on what it perceives the returns on its effort(s) will be (Bagozzi, 1975; Lester et al., 2008).

Generalized Exchange   Recent social-exchange theorists have expanded the relationship standard to include social networks in an attempt to incorporate and acknowledge the multiple factors known to influence behavioral change. Generalized exchanges are reciprocal relationships that are developed among at least three parties. Unlike restricted exchanges, generalized exchanges among parties do not necessitate that the actions between party members yield direct benefits (Bagozzi, 1975). Instead, benefits may be provided and received indirectly. To illustrate this point, suppose that parties A, B, and C have developed a generalized-exchange relationship. Although party A provides party B with a direct benefit, party A may not receive a direct benefit back from party B. Instead, party B may pass on a benefit to party C, and party C may subsequently provide a benefit to party A.

Complex Exchange   Complex exchanges are formed among at least three parties who establish "a system of mutual relationships" (Bagozzi, 1975). Within complex exchanges, each party maintains at least one direct exchange relationship while being involved in a web of interconnecting, supplementary indirect relationships. To illustrate this point, suppose that parties A, B, and C have developed complex-exchange relationships. Although each party is a member of this web of relationships, parties A and B derive direct benefit from one another and parties B and C derive direct benefit from one another. Although parties A and C are not involved in a direct relationship, they derive an indirect benefit from one another through their relationship with party B. Again, the benefits transferred may be tangible or intangible.

Benefits of Exchanges   Social-exchange theory suggests that parties (individuals and organizations) are compelled to develop social relationships characterized by either general or complex exchanges to satisfy human and societal needs. Bagozzi (1975) provides the following powerful example of the cooperation required in social-exchange relationships. Governmental agencies are provided with authority to develop and implement social-service programs for underserved individuals by members of the larger society. Because the government's efforts are subsidized by society members through the collection and distribution of tax funds, governmental workers charged with implementing programmatic efforts receive a salary and are thus sanctioned to provide services to individuals and families, as well as communities in need. The larger society may receive an indirect benefit from service efforts because the health and well-being of the entire society are dependent, in many ways, on the health and well-being of its individual members. In sum, both general and complex exchanges likely occur in many of our socially sanctioned systems.

The Ecology of Social Exchange in Social Marketing Efforts with African Americans

Social marketing is a viable technique for use within the African American community. Because understanding the needs and preferences of target groups is of utmost importance in social marketing efforts, a full awareness of factors such as the cultural mores, social structures, economic conditions, and community resources that may affect target-group openness and buy-in of presented services, ideas, or products is required for successful implementation (Smith et al., 2006). This is particularly the case within the African American community. The development of effective social-exchange relationships, and thus social marketing efforts, requires buy-in and participation at the level of the individual, family, community, and society. Because of their consumer focus, social marketing efforts are built on three ecologically based tenets that borrow from a number of commercial marketing strategies such as market segmentation, consumer research, product development and testing, directed communication, facilitation, and incentives. These strategies can be used to assess and encourage target-group buy-in of health messages (Kotler & Roberto, 1989). The three primary tenets of social marketing are consumer orientation, the use of an integrated approach, and pursuit of profitability (Buchanan, Reddy, & Hossain, 1994). We provide a brief discussion of each tenet for consideration.

Consumer Orientation Historically, successful social marketing efforts have been characterized by both an understanding of and an ability to relate to the needs, behaviors, perceptions, and motivations of target groups (Buchanan et al., 1994; Hastings & Haywood, 1991; Stellefson & Eddy, 2008). Social marketing recognizes that target-group participation in health-promotion campaign activities is voluntary and is largely a function of target-group interests (Van Duyn, McCrae, Wingrove, Henderson, Penalosa, Boyd, et al., 2007). Target groups regulate their level of exposure to, interest in, comprehension of, and response to social marketing campaign messages. Consequently, empathic understanding of target groups provides the needed foundation for the development of effective health messages. Because target groups (i.e., consumers) lie at the center of any social marketing activity, health-promotion efforts require a thorough knowledge and appreciation of those for whom messages are developed (Stellefson & Eddy, 2008). Otherwise, health promoters risk having their messages fall on deaf ears.

A major issue that has frequently hindered public health campaigns within the African American community has been a lack of knowledge about the diversity represented within that community. As a result, a one-size-fits-all approach has traditionally been taken when working with this group. Social marketing campaigns require that the many contextual factors affecting community health behaviors be assessed and accounted for. As a result, prior to developing and promoting health messages, market research, market segmentation, and the delineation of marketing targets should be undertaken so that health promoters can create individualized campaign activities (Buchanan et al., 1994). These activities encourage optimal responses to the needs and desires of target groups.

An Integrated Approach In order for social marketing efforts to succeed, a comprehensive approach to addressing health issues within a target group must be undertaken. Consequently, those engaged in social marketing must develop the "right product, at the right price, in the right place at [the] right time, presented in such a way as to successfully satisfy the needs of the consumer" (Hastings & Haywood, 1991, p. 140). Social marketers should begin by selecting and articulating campaign goals. Having a general goal of increasing health and well-being will not provide the specificity needed to develop an effective campaign. Instead, social marketers must establish whether the goal is to influence attitudes, behaviors, or values; to increase physical activity or to decrease smoking behavior; to increase safe-sex practices or to increase regular dental visits; and so forth (Kotler & Roberto, 1989).

After determining the goal of the campaign, social marketers must have a realistic idea of the cost to target groups. What will target groups be required to give up in order to accept the challenge presented in the social marketing message? Social marketers are aware that the costs to consumers may fall into one of many categories (e.g., effort, time, change in lifestyle, money, social contacts) (Maibach, 1993). Further, social marketers must determine the most effective channels for promoting their messages. Should community organizations, media outlets, or employment agencies be enlisted? Finally, social marketers must determine the most effective means for communicating their message (i.e., via advertisement, selling, or promotion). Hastings and Haywood (1991) emphasized that each of the four Ps (product, price, place, and promotion) must be addressed in order for marketing efforts to produce their intended effect.

Pursuit of Profitability The pursuit of profitability within the context of social marketing refers to the social marketer's ability to facilitate and encourage voluntary exchanges (of goods, ideas, resources, etc.) among all components of the target group's ecosystem. Social marketing efforts require that health promoters understand, acknowledge, and work within the constraints that environmental influences (e.g., political, cultural, economic, social, and technological factors) place on both the target group's participation and the social marketer's efforts (Hastings & Haywood, 1991). For example, political attitudes and cultural mores may affect the form and avenues for the presentation of health messages. Consequently, successful social marketing campaigns within the African American community must effectively address and work within multiple, if not all, levels of health and community influence.

Potential Benefits of Using Social Marketing Within the African American Community

One of the advantages of using a social marketing approach to fashion an intervention for an African American audience is that program planners can easily focus on instituting a culturally appropriate change mechanism. Researchers and program planners in the past have recognized the importance of including individuals who will be the consumers of an intervention early on in the design process. A social marketing approach incorporates this principle by getting program participants involved in the creation of the campaign through formative research. Formative research and evaluation provide the means by which concept development, message development, message testing, and message reshaping occur.

Another advantage of the social marketing approach is the potential it possesses to foster new ways of conceptualizing and understanding health and well-being within the African American community. Because of their focus on determinants of health behaviors, social marketing efforts provide opportunities to increase health literacy within the African American community. Increased health literacy ultimately provides a foundation for critical thinking, informed decision making, and increased sophistication in the discussion of health information (Ratzan, 2001).

Social marketing additionally provides an effective means to challenge old and promote new behavioral norms. Armed with an awareness of the multiple levels of influence on health and well-being, social marketing campaigns have the potential of opening lines of communication among governmental, organizational, community, and individual-level structures (Maibach, 1993). By targeting communication efforts and engaging government officials, community organizations, corporations, and individuals in campaign development, social marketers become aware of existing behavioral norms and potential challenges to success, and they thereby increase their likelihood of developing appropriate multilevel health-promotion strategies.

Finally, because of technological advances and advances in media forms, social marketing campaigns have the potential to reach more people at faster rates through more means than ever before. Armed with access to print media, radio, the Internet, television, film, and interpersonal communication (e.g., telephones, cell phones, text messaging, instant messaging), social marketers have great potential to exert influence on numerous determinants of health at multiple levels of the African American community's ecological reality (Maibach, 1993).

APPLICATION OF A SOCIAL MARKETING APPROACH TO HEALTH ISSUES AFFECTING THE AFRICAN AMERICAN COMMUNITY

Utilizing the ecological framework for social marketing, we provide here a discussion of the potential use of social marketing strategies and media to address two major chronic health conditions currently affecting the African American community: substance/alcohol abuse and violence.

Substance/Alcohol Abuse and Dependence

Difficulties related to substance and alcohol abuse are major concerns within the African American community. Alcohol and substance use among adolescents is extremely widespread (Johnston, O'Malley, Bachman, & Schulenberg, 2005). Although statistics specifically for African Americans are not currently available, in a national survey conducted in 2006, approximately 17 percent of youths between the ages of twelve and seventeen reported using cigarettes, 33 percent reported using alcohol, and roughly 13 percent indicated that they used marijuana within the past year (Substance Abuse and Mental Health Services Administration, Office of Applied Studies, 2008). Research shows that early use of alcohol or any illicit substance is associated with increased risk for a number of negative outcomes in late adolescence and adulthood (Lubman, Yücel, & Hall, 2007; Teesson, Degenhardt, Lynskey, & Hall, 2005). For example, early drinking as well as early substance use has been associated with an increased likelihood of academic failure, suicidal behavior, multiple-substance use, mental illness, neuropathy, precocious sexual activity, sexual promiscuity, sexually transmitted diseases, poverty, underemployment, and even death (National Center for Health Statistics, 2007; Swahn, Bossarte, & Sullivent, 2008). Alcohol and substance use have also been linked with a number of antisocial risk behaviors and juvenile delinquency (Fisher, Eke, Cance, Hawkins, & Lam, 2008).

The toll of difficulties related to substance and alcohol abuse in the African American community has been great. The remnants of the "war against drugs" of the 1980s still have had an effect on many different groups of people. Children were forced to raise themselves as a result of having drug-addicted parents. Countless African American males found themselves incarcerated as a result of their involvement in drug dealing and gang activity. Grandparents have been required to take on additional child-care and financial responsibilities. A large proportion of African American women are struggling to negotiate and redefine female-role responsibilities. Once-vibrant neighborhoods are now littered with broken families, buildings, and dreams. Although rates of illicit substance and alcohol use among African American youth are lower than those among Caucasian youth, substantial increases in use and dependence occur once African American youth reach late adolescence and young adulthood (Hopp & Herring, 1999). Consequently, a number of social marketing efforts have been undertaken to help reshape adolescent behavioral norms as they relate to substance and alcohol use.

Although there presently is no published literature on specific social marketing campaigns to prevent substance abuse among African Americans, a number of efforts have included African American youth as a target subgroup. We briefly discuss efforts that may hold promise for intervening within African American communities, particularly those designed to assess and address the needs of program participants.

In a national study in which 10.4 percent of the sample was African American, Slater et al. (2006) utilized social marketing principles to develop an in-school campaign designed to reduce marijuana and cigarette use among middle-school-aged youth; the campaign was carried on in conjunction with a substance-abuse-prevention curriculum. At the center of campaign development was an assumption that substance-abuse initiation among youth is a result of norms and expectations based in youth social experiences within the educational and larger community environment.

Campaign developers consequently surmised that nonuse norms would also need to be articulated and reinforced at various levels of the youths' social environment if campaign efforts were to prove successful (Slater et al., 2006). The developers therefore employed community participation to mobilize media, devise communication strategies, and plan events. Drawing on primary and secondary research conducted with study participants, the authors utilized what they learned about participants' attitudes, values, and behaviors related to substance use to develop the "Be Under Your Own Influence" media campaign, which capitalized on adolescent desires for autonomy and rebellious noncompliance. The authors further conducted focus groups and individual interviews to determine the media channels and promotional items of most interest and value to participants and their peers. Based on this formative research, the promotional materials developed included posters, book covers, tray liners, T-shirts, water bottles, and lanyards. Risk-oriented images (e.g., rock climbing and four-wheeling) were also utilized in campaign materials in order to appeal to sensation-seeking youth. Mindful of the potential psychological and social-status benefits and costs associated with campaign buy-in, the researchers emphasized that substance use decreased rather than increased personal autonomy. Community-level efforts included providing half-day training workshops for community members involved in prevention activities. They learned how to identify substance-abuse-prevention strategies as well as how to use campaign promotional and media materials when working with youth.

Study results supported the effectiveness of the in-school media campaign when combined with community-level communication efforts and in-school substance-abuse prevention training. In all, student use of illicit substances was reduced by 40 percent as a result of the social marketing activities (Kelly, Comello, & Slater, 2006). Other notable multilevel social marketing campaigns have been created to reduce the use of methamphetamine (Montana Meth Project, 2009), tobacco (Evans et al., 2007; Martino-McAllister & Wessel, 2005), and alcohol (Mattern & Neighbors, 2004) in school-aged youth and young adults.

Violence

Homicide is the sixth leading cause of death among African Americans and is the primary cause of death among African American males between fifteen and twenty-four years (LaVeist, 2005; National Center for Health Statistics, 2007). Exposure to community violence is extremely common, particularly in urban communities where many African Americans reside. Farrell and Bruce (1997) found that an overwhelming majority (greater than 90 percent) of urban sixth graders interviewed reported that they had heard gunshots, had witnessed violence toward others, or had observed someone being arrested. Along with the loss of life, exposure to violence (as a victim or a witness) has been associated with a number of adjustment difficulties including psychological trauma symptoms (e.g., traumatic stress), avoidant coping behaviors (e.g., disengagement, desensitization), mood symptoms (e.g., anxiety, depression, suicidal behavior, social withdrawal), behavioral difficulties (e.g., physical and social aggression, verbal abuse, physical assault, antisocial behavior, substance use), and violence-supporting cognitive styles (e.g., hostile attributional biases, normative beliefs about violence, aggressive fantasies, expectations of positive outcomes from aggressive behavior) (Boxer et al., 2008; Lambert, Copeland-Linder, & Ialongo, 2008).

Moderate to severe levels of violence within the context of dating and intimate-partner or family relationships are also not uncommon within minority communities (Schumacher, Homish, Leonard, Quigley, & Kearns-Bodkin, 2008). As a result, several programmatic efforts have been undertaken to help increase the level of engagement in treatment among perpetrators of domestic abuse. One such effort designed to increase the recruitment of nonadjudicated, untreated, substance-abusing men with a history of male or female partner abuse is the Men's Domestic Abuse Check-Up Intervention (MDACU) research trial (Mbilinyi et al., 2008).

MDACU social marketing developers devoted eight months prior to intervention enrollment to planning and developing intervention-recruitment strategies. The researchers determined that a universal marketing approach was needed based on the fact that males who engage in domestic violence are represented in all areas of life in the United States. Campaign developers wanted to focus on males eighteen years of age and older who recognized that their substance abuse and domestic violence were causing some level of difficulty in their lives but who were not yet considering making changes. The researchers were additionally interested in targeting males who were considering changing their behavior but who were not yet ready to make a commitment to doing so.

In order to assist with the development of a marketing strategy, Mbilinyi et al. (2008) contracted with a local marketing company and enlisted the assistance of human-service intervention professionals, many of whom had extensive experience working with either abusive men or victims of abuse. Focus groups and individual interviews were also held with nine men who had successfully completed a program designed for domestic-abuse perpetrators. The consultants provided the research team with feedback regarding (1) the language, content, and appeal of the campaign's message; (2) the most effective ways of promoting the campaign's message; and (3) the general perceptions of help seeking and other attitudes among abusive men. At various points, focus-group participants additionally brainstormed about a wide number of possible campaign messages and reviewed drafts of marketing products created as a result of the consultants' input in previous planning phases. As a result of the information learned from the focus-group consultants, the researchers worked hard to avoid using images that would likely arouse defensiveness in the target group. Consequently, the research team and marketing staff reviewed approximately one hundred thousand potential images before selecting three photos for the campaign.

Because of the theory-driven and research-based approach utilized to plan and implement the marketing campaign, the research team members communicated the benefits and protections offered to receivers of the campaign's message, and they remained mindful of the intended target behaviors and the most effective methods for conveying their message. Campaign communication modes included the use of news stories, paid ads in print media, radio and bus advertisements, a website, a press conference, press kits, and brochures and flyers (Mbilinyi et al., 2008). Materials were also disseminated to community agencies, private businesses, and service outlets.

After twenty-two weeks of the campaign, marketing shifts were made based on the level of target-group interest. Some of the marketing shifts included placing new display ads that might be perceived as less threatening than the previous ads, increasing the length of radio ads, enlisting culturally specific newspapers or magazines to display campaign ads, and removing ads from displays that were not generating participant interest. The researchers shared the following insights based on their experiences: (1) the use of a universal marketing campaign is an expensive endeavor; (2) community biases, fears, and misunderstandings can potentially obstruct marketing efforts; and (3) if marketing strategies include providing radio interviews, some hosts may use attack strategies, and so requests for interviews should be evaluated to ensure that the aims of the campaign will be reached.

FUTURE DIRECTIONS

The African American population in the United States is a widely diverse group of individuals with various learning histories, economic features, regional idiosyncrasies, and cultural experiences. Much of the diversity that exists among African American people has come from the different ways in which they have progressed in society as the country has turned toward becoming a mixture of racial and ethnic groups. One would not expect that subcultural groups among all African Americans would respond in the same way to the same social marketing interventions. Thus one could conclude that the shaping of social marketing campaign messages cannot be monolithic but rather must be specifically tailored to each segment of the African American experience.

Group vs. Individual Tailoring

To this end, numerous health interventions have been developed and tested for African Americans (Resnicow, Braithwaite, Ahluwalia, & Baranowski, 1999; Resnicow, Braithwaite, Ahluwalia, & Dilorio, 2001). Almost all have been targeted interventions, in the sense that all participants receive identical messages and materials. Such interventions generally define a black audience by using cultural, behavioral, and psychological characteristics common at the group level. These group-targeted interventions have generally been more effective in changing behavior than have untargeted health messages designed for a general audience (Sellers, Chavous, & Cooke, 1998; Sellers, Rowley, Chavous, Shelton, & Smith, 1997). However, group-targeted materials generally have failed to account for individual diversity within the African American population.

Tailored interventions utilize individual-level data to customize message content based on personal variations in psychological, social, and behavioral factors.

Individually tailored interventions have been used to modify a wide range of health behaviors (Resnicow et al., 1999; Resnicow et al., 2001) across a variety of populations (Sellers et al., 1998; Sellers et al., 1997). In the few tailoring studies with African Americans, messages have generally been customized using constructs from the Transtheoretical Model, Social Cognitive Theory, and Social Support Theory (Resnicow et al., under review). In one prior study (Kreuter et al., 2005), messages were tailored on cultural constructs (religiosity, collectivism, racial pride, and time orientation), and some positive effects were observed.

Tailoring on the Basis of Ethnic Identity

Tailoring on individual Ethnic Identity (EI) has only recently been explored. EI involves the extent to which individuals identify with and gravitate to their racial/ethnic group. EI includes many elements such as racial/ethnic pride, affinity for in-group culture (e.g., food, media, language), attitudes toward the majority culture, involvement with in-group members, experience with and attitudes regarding racism, attitudes toward intermarriage, and the importance placed on preserving one's culture and aiding others of similar backgrounds. EI appears to be highly variable across African Americans. For some African Americans, their African or African American culture and heritage play a central role in their personal identity and daily psychosocial functioning, whereas for others ethnicity and race may be only peripheral elements of the self. Some African Americans define themselves in relation to Caucasians or the majority culture, while others do not view the world through a "race-tinted" lens.

An important approach to matching an intervention to the EI of participants is to begin by determining the nature of their EI. With which group do they identify? Given the degree of their identification with a specific group, it will probably be necessary to have various programs to accommodate these differences. Some aspects of the program might be similar to aspects of the dominant culture, which, within the United States, is largely European based. However, programs rooted in an Afrocentric worldview can be developed for the subgroup of African Americans for whom this is a chief component of their EI. Davis et al. (in press) have developed an instrument that segments African Americans into different EI subgroups; it can be used in designing culturally tailored messages for an African American audience. (Information available from third author.)

Applied researchers and practitioners may need to consider another aspect of EI as they go about designing and implementing prevention programs in the African American community. Some African American individuals may prefer to have an African American practitioner. Some may prefer a Caucasian service provider. Health care delivery systems should consider both measuring EI as a means of practitioner matching and querying members regarding their racial/ethnic preferences with regard to programs and providers.

It is not clear how and to what degree EI is changing as we move through the second decade of this century. Clearly, however, this construct along with other constructs (e.g., perceived hopefulness and resiliency) may have a bearing on the types of messages that we present in the African American community. Moreover, we must continue to account for the within-group heterogeneity of African Americans as it continues to evolve over time. One of the keys is that we work toward empowering the African American community in such a way that they have some control over the design and delivery of social marketing interventions so that they are culturally in sync with the evolving African American way of life. The influence of European culture on cultural characteristics derived from the African continent is a reciprocal process. Thus, it is a moving target that requires monitoring and ongoing assessment in order to identify social marketing interventions that are current and on point.

Accommodating an Increasingly Diverse African American Population

The African American community is becoming increasingly multicultural and multiracial. Thus, it will be necessary to include biracial and multiracial participants in the planning and execution of health-promotion initiatives. This has not been a problem in the past because biracial and multiracial individuals have readily identified with African American culture, but this may not always be the case as we move toward what some have referred to as a "colorless" society.

It is also not clear whether having a biracial and multiracial genetic constitution in any way affects health behavior and health status. Because race is itself a social construct, how do we determine the influence, if any, that genetic markers have on various lifestyle-related diseases and conditions such as heart disease, cardiovascular disease, stroke, cancer, and diabetes? To what degree does the changing landscape of racism affect psychological stress and related detrimental sociocultural factors? Future researchers will need to grapple with these issues as they work to diminish health disparities in the African American community.

It is likely that different subcultures and socioeconomic groups within the African American community will continue to manifest pockets of health disparities because of economic deprivation, disenfranchisement, and lack of access to quality health care. It will still be necessary to deliver appropriate services to health care consumers at the appropriate time. Social marketing technology can help to meet this need. It is not a panacea, and its misuse may cause iatrogenic effects among intervention participants.

We must therefore be constantly developing new theory-driven intervention models and intervention tools in order to keep pace with changing conditions in and composition of the African American community. Examples of these assessment methods include additional technology-driven measurement including distance-based assessment; audio-enhanced, computer-assisted structured interviewing using handheld computers; and wireless quantitative methods for classroom-based instruction. We have not fully used these technologies as a part of our social marketing strategy in the African American community.

Further, it makes sense to use all available media and organizational resources to influence the African American community in ways that promote health, such as encouraging healthy eating and weight control, regular exercise, and an appropriate number of screenings and doctor visits. Available media and organizations such as black radio, the Internet, television, community newspapers, billboards, faith-based organizations, and community organizations can be instrumental in communicating during social marketing campaigns.

Future research will need to incorporate the most rigorous designs for community-based planning and evaluation of social marketing strategies by working with community stakeholders. The integration of social marketing technology into African American and multicultural regional community coalitions through training, coaching, and consultation can be an important tool for diffusing these interventions for health areas such as substance abuse, violence, HIV, hepatitis, heart disease, and cancer prevention.

Finally, it will be necessary to groom a new cadre of African American researchers who are willing to address health disparities using social marketing tools. The cross-generational and interracial and intraracial approach to social marketing interventions that new researchers may provide is the most promising way to devise effective future interventions. African American community stakeholders will need to learn about the social marketing approach in order to appreciate the myriad ways in which it can foster health promotion and diminish the health disparities that underserved community members face.

REFERENCES

Ashley, M. (1999). Health promotion planning in African American communities. In R. Huff & M. Kline (Eds.), *Promoting health in multicultural populations: A handbook for practitioners* (pp. 223–240). Thousand Oaks, CA: Sage.

Baffour, T., Jones, M., & Contreras, L. (2006). Family health advocacy: An empowerment model for pregnant and parenting African American women in rural communities. *Family & Community Health, 29*, 221–228.

Bagozzi, R. (1975). Marketing as exchange. *Journal of Marketing, 39*, 32–35.

Barnett, E., & Casper, M. (2001). A definition of "social environment." *American Journal of Public Health, 91*, 465.

Benner, A., Graham, S., & Mistry, R. (2008). Discerning direct and mediated effects of ecological structures and processes on adolescents' educational outcomes. *Developmental Psychology, 44*, 840–854.

Boxer, P., Morris, A., Terranova, A., Kithakye, M., Savoy, S., & McFaul, A. (2008). Coping with exposure to violence: Relations to emotional symptoms and aggression in three urban samples. *Journal of Child and Family Studies, 17*, 881–893.

Bronfenbrenner, U., & Ceci, S. (1994). Nature-nurture reconceptualized in developmental perspective: A bioecological model. *Psychological Review, 101*, 568–586.

Buchanan, D., Reddy, S., & Hossain, Z. (1994). Social marketing: A critical appraisal. *Health Promotion International, 9*, 49–57.

Davis, R., Alexander, G., Calvi, J., Wiese, C., Greene, S., Nowak, M., et al. (in press). A new audience segmentation tool for African Americans: The Black Identity Classification Scale. *Journal of Health Communication*.

Diamond, A. (2009). The interplay of biology and the environment broadly defined. *Developmental Psychology, 45*, 1–8.

Evans, W., Renaud, J., Blitstein, J., Hersey, J., Ray, S., Schieber, B., et al. (2007). Prevention effects of an anti-tobacco brand on adolescent smoking initiation. *Social Marketing Quarterly, 13*, 2–20.

Farrell, A., & Bruce, S. (1997). Impact of exposure to community violence on violent behavior and emotional distress among urban adolescents. *Journal of Clinical Child Psychology, 26*, 2–14.

Fisher, H., Eke, A., Cance, J., Hawkins, S., & Lam, W. (2008). Correlates of HIV-related risk behaviors in African American adolescents from substance-using families: Patterns of adolescent-level factors associated with sexual experience and substance use. *Journal of Adolescent Health, 42*, 161–169.

Fort, J. (2007). Improving the health of African American men: Experiences from the Targeting Cancer in Blacks (TCIB) project. *Journal of Men's Health & Gender, 4*, 428–439.

Gazmararian, J., Curran, J., Parker, R., Bernhardt, J., & DeBuono, B. (2005). Public health literacy in America: An ethical imperative. *American Journal of Preventive Medicine, 28*, 317–322.

Hastings, G., & Haywood, A. (1991). Social marketing and communication in health promotion. *Health Promotion International, 6*, 135–145.

Hopp, J., & Herring, P. (1999). Promoting health among Black American populations. In R. Huff & M. Kline (Eds.), *Promoting health in multicultural populations: A handbook for practitioners* (pp. 201–222). Thousand Oaks, CA: Sage.

Icard, L., Bourjolly, J., & Siddiqui, N. (2003). Designing social marketing strategies to increase African American's access to health promotion programs. *Health & Social Work, 28*, 214–223.

Johnston, L., O'Malley, P., Bachman, J., & Schulenberg, J. (2005). *Monitoring the future national survey results on drug use, 1975–2004: Vol. 1. Secondary school students* (NIH publication no. 05-5725). Bethesda, MD: National Institute on Drug Abuse.

Kelly, K., Comello, M., & Slater, M. (2006). Development of an aspirational campaign to prevent youth substance use: "Be under your own influence." *Social Marketing Quarterly, 12*, 14–27.

Kok, G., Gottlieb, N., Commers, M., & Smerecnik, C. (2008). The ecological approach in health promotion programs: A decade later. *American Journal of Health Promotion, 22*, 437–442.

Kotler, P., & Lee, N. (2008). *Social marketing: Influencing behaviors for good* (3rd ed.). Thousand Oaks, CA: Sage.

Kotler, P., & Levy, S. (1969). Broadening the concept of marketing. *Journal of Marketing, 33*, 10–15.

Kotler, P., & Roberto, E. (1989). *Social marketing strategies for improving public health*. New York: Free Press.

Kreuter, M., Sugg-Skinner, C., Holt, C., Clark, E., Haire-Joshu, D., Fu, Q., et al. (2005). Cultural tailoring for mammography and fruit and vegetable intake among low-income African-American women in urban public health centers. *Preventive Medicine, 41*(1), 53–62.

Lambert, S., Copeland-Linder, N., & Ialongo, N. (2008). Longitudinal associations between community violence exposure and suicidality. *Journal of Adolescent Health, 43*, 380–386.

LaVeist, T. (2005). *Minority populations and health: An introduction to health disparities in the United States*. San Francisco: Jossey-Bass.

Lester, S., Meglino, B., & Korsgaard, M. (2008). The role of other orientation in organizational citizenship behavior. *Journal of Organizational Behavior, 29*, 829–841.

Lubman, D., Yücel, M., & Hall, W. (2007). Substance use and the adolescent brain: A toxic combination? *Journal of Psychopharmacology, 21*, 792–794.

Lynch, J., Smith, G., Kaplan, G., & House, J. (2000). Income inequality and mortality: Importance to health of individual income, psychosocial environment, or material conditions. *British Medical Journal, 320*, 1200–1204.

Maibach, E. (1993). Social marketing for the environment: Using information campaigns to promote environmental awareness and behavior change. *Health Promotion International, 8*, 209–224.

Marks, J., Reed, W., Colby, K., & Ibrahim, S. (2004). A culturally competent approach to cancer news and education in an inner city community: Focus group findings. *Journal of Health Communication, 9*, 143–157.

Martino-McAllister, J., & Wessel, M. (2005). An evaluation of a social norms marketing project for tobacco prevention with middle, high, and college students; use of funds from the tobacco master settlement (Virginia). *Journal of Drug Education, 35*, 185–200.

Mattern, J., & Neighbors, C. (2004). Social norms campaigns: Examining the relationship between changes in perceived norms and changes in drinking levels. *Journal of Studies on Alcohol*, 489–493.

Mbilinyi, L., Zegree, J., Roffman, R., Walker, D., Neighbors, C., & Edleson, J. (2008). Development of a marketing campaign to recruit non-adjudicated and untreated abusive men for a brief telephone intervention. *Journal of Family Violence, 23*, 343–351.

Montana Meth Project. (2009). *The Meth Project*. Retrieved January 6, 2009, from http://www.methproject.org

National Center for Health Statistics. (2007). *Health, United States, 2007, with chartbook on trends in the health of Americans*. Hyattsville, MD: Centers for Disease Control and Prevention.

Newacheck, P., Kim, S., Blumberg, S., & Rising, J. (2008). Who is at risk for special health care needs? Findings from the national survey of children's health. *Pediatrics, 122*, 347–359.

Newacheck, P., Rising, J., & Kim, S. (2006). Children at risk for special health care needs. *Pediatrics, 118*, 334–342.

Pfizer Incorporated. (2003). Eradicating low health literacy: The first public health movement of the 21st century. Retrieved December 1, 2008, from http://www.npsf.org/askme3/pdfs/white_paper.pdf.

Ratzan, S. (2001). Health literacy: Communication for the public good. *Health Promotion International, 16*, 207–214.

Resnicow, K., Braithwaite, R., Ahluwalia, J., & Baranowski, T. (1999). Cultural sensitivity in public health: Defined and demystified. *Ethnicity and Disease, 9*, 10–21.

Resnicow, K., Braithwaite, R., Ahluwalia, J., & DiIorio, C. (2001). Cultural sensitivity in public health. In R. Braithwaite & S. Taylor (Eds.), *Health issues in the black community* (2nd ed., pp. 516–542). San Francisco: Jossey-Bass.

Resnicow, K., Davis, R., Zhang, N., Saunders, E., Strecher, V., Tolsma, D., et al. (under review). Tailoring a fruit and vegetable intervention on ethnic identity: Results of a randomized study. *Health Psychology*.

Sankofa, J., & Johnson-Taylor, W. (2007). News coverage of diet-related health disparities experienced by black Americans: A steady diet of misinformation. *Journal of Nutrition Education and Behavior, 39*, S41–S44.

Schumacher, J., Homish, G., Leonard, K., Quigley, B., & Kearns-Bodkin, J. (2008). Longitudinal moderators of the relationship between excessive drinking and intimate partner violence in the early years of marriage. *Journal of Family Psychology, 22*, 894–904.

Sellers, R., Chavous, T., & Cooke, D. (1998). Racial ideology and racial centrality as predictors of African American college students' academic performance. *Journal of Black Psychology, 24*, 8–27.

Sellers, R., Rowley, S., Chavous, T., Shelton, J., & Smith, M. (1997). Multidimensional inventory of black identity: A preliminary investigation of reliability and construct validity. *Journal of Personality and Social Psychology, 73*, 805–815.

Slater, M., Kelly, K., Edwards, R., Thurman, P., Plested, B., Keefe, T., et al. (2006). Combining in-school and community-based media efforts: Reducing marijuana and alcohol uptake among younger adolescents. *Health Education Research, 21*, 157–167.

Smith, B., Tang, K., & Nutbeam, D. (2006). WHO health promotion glossary: New terms. *Health Promotion International, 21*, 340–345.

Starfield, B. (2001). Basic concepts in population health and health care. *Journal of Epidemiology and Community Health, 55*, 452–454.

Stellefson, M., & Eddy, J. (2008). Health education and marketing processes: 2 related methods for achieving health behavior change. *American Journal of Health Behavior, 32*, 488–496.

Substance Abuse and Mental Health Services Administration, Office of Applied Studies. (2008). *The NSDUH report: Quantity and frequency of alcohol use among underage drinkers*. Rockville, MD: Substance Abuse and Mental Health Services Administration.

Swahn, M., Bossarte, R., & Sullivent, E., III. (2008). Age of alcohol use initiation, suicidal behavior, and peer and dating violence victimization and perpetration among high-risk, seventh-grade adolescents. *Pediatrics, 121*, 297–305.

Teesson, M., Degenhardt, L., Lynskey, M., & Hall, W. (2005). The relationships between substance use and mental health problems: Evidence from longitudinal studies. In T. Stockwell, P. Grunewald, J. Toumbourou, & W. Loxley (Eds.), *Preventing harmful substance use: The evidence base for policy and practice* (pp. 43–51). New York: Wiley.

Van Duyn, M., McCrae, T., Wingrove, B., Henderson, K., Penalosa, T., Boyd, J., et al. (2007). Adapting evidence-based strategies to increase physical activity among African Americans, Hispanics, Hmong, and native Hawaiians: A social marketing approach. *Preventing Chronic Disease, 4*, 1–11.

Vrazel, J., Saunders, R., & Wilcox, S. (2008). An overview and proposed framework of social-environmental influences on the physical-activity behavior of women. *American Journal of Health Promotion, 23*, 2–12.

Zafirovski, M. (2003). Some amendments to social exchange theory: A sociological perspective. *International Consortium for the Advancement of Academic Publication*. Retrieved January 25, 2009, from http://theoryandscience.icaap.org

CHAPTER

27

FOSTERING A SOCIAL JUSTICE APPROACH TO HEALTH

Health Equity, Human Rights, and an Antiracism Agenda

CAMARA PHYLLIS JONES
ANTHONY HATCH
ADEWALE TROUTMAN

It is an overwhelming reality for those of African descent living in the United States that simply being black in this country conveys an increased risk of living sicker and dying younger. Yet observed differences in health outcomes are not the result of genetic, behavioral, or cultural differences but of the social injustices that have characterized the black experience in the United States for centuries (Jones, 2001). The differences between the health of black Americans and the health of white Americans that have been observed and documented over several centuries of cohabitation on this continent (Clayton & Byrd, 2000, 2002; Washington, 2006; Randall, 2006) reflect differences in social power that shape access to health-related goods and services including the social determinants of health. They are the result of systems that structure

The findings and conclusions in this chapter are those of the authors and do not necessarily represent the official position of the Centers for Disease Control and Prevention.

opportunity away from black people and that minimize the value of black people as human beings and as potential contributors to the overall society (Jones, 2003). Observing the powerful social injustices that have defined and continue to constrain the black experience in this nation, we propose a social justice approach to health to fully address health issues in the black community.

WHAT IS SOCIAL JUSTICE?

Social justice is evident when there is no systematic structuring of opportunity or assignment of value based on group membership. Social justice is evident in a society where all people can know and develop to their full potential without the constraints of artificial hierarchies based on power. Social justice is evident when there is no caste system based on group membership to constrain individual opportunity or development, when there are no barriers limiting society from accessing the full human potential of all of its members.

Social justice is foundational to the moral justification of public health, which includes concern for the least-advantaged members of society (Mathis, 2007; Powers & Faden, 2006). It involves caring not just about the health of oneself and one's family but also about the health of distant others unknown. "The leap must be made between academic discussions of justice and fairness and public understanding of these concepts when applied to health. Getting the public to see beyond individual problems and health issues is difficult at best" (Mathis, 2007, p. 291).

As sociologist Patricia Hill Collins (1998) has argued, we need to conceptualize justice at the group level and depart from traditional Eurocentric views that define justice, and therefore rights, as applying only to individuals. Although health is necessarily experienced at the individual level, we miss important aspects of how social conditions affect health if we focus only on individuals and their health attitudes and behaviors. Social justice is a group-based conception of justice that focuses on social groups and their relative position in the hierarchical power arrangements that structure access to health-related resources. When we approach health from a social justice perspective, we are necessarily concerned with the political, economic, and social arrangements that impinge on the lived experiences of social groups. In order to understand these arrangements in the case of black Americans, we have to consider how the social forces of race and racism structure opportunity and lived experience at local, national, and global levels. Stated differently, a social justice approach to health involves recognizing and contesting race and racism as systems of power that shape the life chances of black Americans.

WHAT IS HEALTH EQUITY?

In a policy environment that has seized on the elimination of racial/ethnic health disparities as a fundable agenda, there is little guidance about how to eliminate these widespread and deeply rooted disparities. Indeed, the "health disparities" agenda has focused so much on differences in health outcomes that differences in the exposures and opportunities that lead to these disparate outcomes have not always seemed pertinent or come clearly into focus. The emergence of a "health-equity" agenda is about equalizing the distributions of exposures, opportunities, resources, and risks experienced by different populations so that equal outcomes can be realized. By focusing on health equity, a social justice approach to health provides a bridge between articulating a goal to eliminate health disparities and identifying strategies for achieving that goal.

Our working definition of health equity has been developed in collaboration with members of the National Partnership for Action, Office for Minority Health and Health Disparities, Department of Health and Human Services (private communication): "Health equity is the realization by ALL people of the highest attainable level of health. Achieving health equity requires valuing all individuals and populations equally, and entails focused and ongoing societal efforts to address avoidable inequalities by [ensuring] the conditions for optimal health for all groups, particularly for those who have experienced historical or contemporary injustices or socioeconomic disadvantage."

We organize the remainder of this chapter by the main elements of this definition of health equity:

- *The realization by ALL people of the highest attainable level of health* implies health as a human right; we review the international basis for making such a claim.

- *Valuing all individuals and populations equally* launches us into a discussion of racism as a system of structuring opportunity and assigning value, a system of power that has profound and complex impacts on health. We describe the International Convention on the Elimination of All Forms of Racial Discrimination, an international treaty that provides a frame for our national antiracism efforts.

- *Focused and ongoing societal efforts to address avoidable inequalities* reminds us that racial health disparities are not natural or inevitable. A social justice approach to health provides both the motivation and specific targets for intervention in societal structures, policies, practices, norms, and values.

- *Ensuring the conditions for optimal health for all groups* expands our discussion beyond the provision of universal access to high-quality health care to address both the social determinants of health and the social determinants of equity.

- *Particularly for those who have experienced historical or contemporary injustices or socioeconomic disadvantage* highlights the importance of understanding and acknowledging history. We outline the six premises of critical race theory as they motivate an antiracism approach to improving health outcomes and eliminating health disparities.

In this chapter, we aim to foster a social justice approach to health that recognizes health as a fundamental human right and that emphasizes racism as a powerful social force that negatively impinges on the life chances of black people. By fostering a social justice approach to health, we go beyond the documentation of race-associated differences in health outcomes to expose differences in underlying exposures and opportunities, resources, and risks. We augment the call to eliminate racial health disparities with a strategy for doing so by focusing attention on the social context in which these disparities arise and are perpetuated. By fostering a social justice approach to health, we provide both a moral imperative and identifiable targets for action to eliminate health disparities and improve the health and well-being of the black community and the entire nation.

The Realization by All People of the Highest Attainable Level of Health

The principles of health as a human right, of the responsibility of government to ensure the equal application of that right, and of social justice as the foundation for creating equity have a wider acceptance in the global community than they do in the United States. The constitution of the World Health Organization (World Health Organization, 1948), which was adopted by the International Health Conference held in New York from June 19 to July 22, 1946, and which entered into force on April 7, 1948, states:

> The States Parties to this Constitution declare, in conformity with the Charter of the United Nations, that the following principles are basic to the happiness, harmonious relations and security of all peoples:
>
> ■ Health is a state of complete physical, mental, and social well-being and not merely the absence of disease or infirmity.
>
> ■ The enjoyment of the highest attainable standard of health is one of the fundamental rights of every human being without distinction of race, religion, political belief, economic or social condition.

Furthermore, the Universal Declaration of Human Rights, which was adopted and proclaimed by the United Nations on December 10, 1948 (United Nations General Assembly, 1948), states in Article 1, "All human beings are born free and equal in dignity and rights. They are endowed with reason and conscience and should act towards one another in a spirit of brotherhood." Article 2 continues, "Everyone is entitled to all the rights and freedoms set forth in this Declaration, without distinction of any kind, such as race, colour, sex, language, religion, political or other opinion, national or social origin, property, birth or other status." Article 24 further asserts, "Everyone has the right to a standard of living adequate for the health and well being of himself and his family including food, clothing, housing, and medical care."

In this context, a social justice approach to health incorporates the internationally recognized obligations of nation-states to protect and enhance the health of their populations. Public health professor Paula Braveman states that "human rights are internationally recognized norms and standards that apply equally to all people everywhere and that define obligations of governments towards individuals and groups" (quoted in Levy & Sidel, 2006, p. 405). She further delineates two broad human rights principles that need to be applied to health inequities. Government has the obligation to prohibit the direct violation of rights and to provide conditions that enable individuals to realize their rights. She sees government's role in human rights manifesting itself in three major spheres: creating legal standards and obligations, developing a conceptual framework for analysis and advocacy, and using human rights principles as guides for designing and implementing policies and programs that create equity in health.

In focusing on the future of public health, the Institute of Medicine defined the mission of public health as "fulfilling society's interest in assuring conditions in which people can be healthy" (Institute of Medicine, 1988, p. 140). Braveman flushes out this mission when she concludes that a basic element of government responsibility is the following: "The right to health reinforces government responsibility for prevention, treatment, and control of disease and for creation of conditions necessary to ensure access to health facilities, goods, and services that are essential for health. . . . Although poverty is not in and of itself a violation of human rights, government inaction leading to poverty and government failure to adequately address the conditions that create, exacerbate and perpetuate poverty and marginalization [are] often reflected or . . . closely connected with violations or denials of human rights" (quoted in Levy and Sidel, 2006, p. 407).

Valuing all Individuals and Populations Equally

Defining Race Race is the social classification of people in a race-conscious society, the social interpretation of how one looks within a caste system based on phenotype (Jones, 2001, 2003). Indeed, societies can be characterized by their "racial climate," the elements of which are the pertinence of race as a basis for social classification (as opposed to caste, religion, wealth, or other potential societal stratifiers); the rules for racial classification, including the number and names of categories and the sorting rules for placing individuals into the different categories; and the opportunities and value accorded the different "racial" groups (Jones, 2003). Race is distinct from genetic endowment and from cultural heritage.

Public health scientists have too long used race variables as proxies for socioeconomic status, culture, and genes (Jones, 2001). Although historical injustices and the contemporary structural factors that perpetuate those injustices (institutionalized racism) have created a relationship between phenotype (race) and socioeconomic status in this country, even that proxy relationship is rough. With regard to culture, each phenotypic (racial) group is culturally diverse, and there are cultural similarities across groups. With regard to genes, the few genes that determine skin color, hair texture, and facial features (the principal aspects of phenotype used to classify people into races in the United States) do not reveal anything about other aspects of the genotype at the individual level (Cavalli-Sforza, Menozzi, & Piazza, 1994, pp. 19–20).

Critical race theories understand race as having been a constitutive feature of global, social, political, economic, and cultural organization since the 1600s. Critical race theorists Michael Omi and Howard Winant define race as "a concept that signifies and symbolizes sociopolitical conflicts and interests in reference to different types of human bodies" (1994, p. 55). Race is a socially constructed category that structures the distribution of life chances, economic power, and political power across racially categorized bodies. Since the 1600s, race has given form to social inequalities in the lived experience of blacks. Omi and Winant's definition reflects the centrality of the body to critical race theories because black and brown bodies have born the brunt of racism.

Race concepts and their accompanying racisms were used to establish colonial social systems (McClintock, 1995; Stoler, 1995), modern nation-states and global political economies (Goldberg, 2002; Omi & Winant, 1994; Winant, 2001), and the human biological sciences and medicine of the eighteenth, nineteenth, and twentieth centuries (Barkan, 1992; Duster, 2003a; Graves, 2001; Reardon, 2005; Stephan, 1982). Beginning with the pioneering scholarship of W.E.B. DuBois in *The Philadelphia Negro* (DuBois, 1899), critical race theorists have long contested the construction of racial concepts and meanings in science and medicine that, in turn, influence the race-based practices of social institutions outside of science and medicine across multiple levels of society over historical time.

In other words, science and medicine are primary sites of racial formation. As many critical race scholars have observed, the meaning of race in the context of science and medicine has shifted dramatically over the past hundred years.[1] Specifically, critical race theory has contested forms of science and medicine that upheld forms of racial hierarchies and that were used to justify white supremacy—what has come to be known as "scientific racism."

Defining Racism   Jones (2003) defines racism as a system of structuring opportunity and assigning value based on the social interpretation of how one looks (which is what we call "race"); this system unfairly disadvantages some individuals and communities, unfairly advantages other individuals and communities, and saps the strength of the whole society through the waste of human resources. Indeed, this definition of racism can be seen as a specific instance of a generalized definition of social injustice as any system of structuring opportunity or assigning value based on a social assignment or group membership. Clearly classism (where opportunity is structured and value is assigned based on material possessions or social class), sexism (where opportunity is structured and value is assigned based on gender), and heterosexism (where opportunity is structured and value is assigned based on sexual orientation) join racism as organizing systems of social injustice in the United States. Indeed any caste structure, whether based on circumstances of birth or socially assigned classifications, represents social injustice in that it constrains the ability of all members of a society to both know and develop their full potential. Social injustice will always sap the strength of the whole society through the waste of human resources.

Yet among the several axes of social injustice, racism has been foundational in the establishment and growing prosperity of the United States; it can be seen in the expropriation of the land and the near genocide of American Indians; in the kidnapping, importation, and enslavement of West Africans, whose coerced, unpaid labor for centuries built this country and provided its wealth; in the exploitation of Chinese laborers in building the railroads; and in the expansion of territory through the appropriation of

Mexican lands. Racism is a core social injustice in the United States, one that is all the more pernicious because many in this country deny its continued existence. We focus on racism as a fundamental cause of social and health disparities.

Three Levels of Racism Jones (2000) has proposed an understanding of racism on three levels: institutionalized, personally mediated, and internalized. Using these levels is helpful both in developing hypotheses about how racism affects a specific health outcome and in developing interventions to address the effects of racism on health.

Institutionalized racism is defined as the system (structures, policies, practices, norms, and values) that results in differential access to the goods, services, and opportunities of society by race. Institutionalized racism is normative, sometimes legalized, and often manifests as inherited disadvantage. It is structural, having been codified in our institutions of custom, practice, and law, so there need not be an identifiable perpetrator.

Institutionalized racism manifests itself both in material conditions and in access to power. With regard to material conditions, examples include differential access to quality education, sound housing, gainful employment, appropriate medical facilities, and a clean environment. Among the most prominent ways in which opportunity is structured in the United States are residential segregation (Acevedo-Garcia, Lochner, Osypuk, & Subramanian, 2003), which facilitates the differential distribution of resources by race, and educational apartheid (Frankenberg & Orfield, 2007), which perpetuates unequal opportunity into the next generation. Unequal treatment within the justice system compounds these problems. The result is unhealthy communities that produce unhealthy individuals. With regard to access to power, examples include differential access to information (including one's own history), resources (including wealth and organizational infrastructure), and voice (including voting rights, representation in government, and control of the media). The relationship between socioeconomic status and race in the United States has its origins in discrete historical events, but it persists because of contemporary structural factors that perpetuate those historical injustices. Institutionalized racism explains why we see an association between socioeconomic status and race in this country (Jones, 2000). Institutionalized racism includes both acts of commission (doing) and acts of omission (not doing), and very often institutionalized racism manifests as inaction in the face of need.

Personally mediated racism is defined as differential assumptions about the abilities, motives, and intents of others by race, and as differential actions based on those assumptions. That is, personally mediated racism is what most people think of as racism, including prejudice (the different idea) and discrimination (the different action). It manifests as lack of respect (poor or no service, failure to communicate options); suspicion (shopkeeper vigilance, everyday avoidance including street crossing, purse clutching, empty seats on public transportation); devaluation (surprise at competence, stifling of aspirations); scapegoating, as seen for example in the Rosewood incident (Jones, Rivers, Colburn, Dye, & Rogers, 1993), the Charles Stuart case (Canellos & Sege, 1989; Jacobs, 1989; Cullen et al., 1990; Graham, 1990), and the Susan Smith case

(Davis, 1994; Terry, 1994; Harrison, 1994; Lewis, 1994); and dehumanization (police brutality, sterilization abuse, hate crimes) (Jones, 2000). Like institutionalized racism, personally mediated racism includes both acts of commission and acts of omission. In addition, personally mediated racism can be unintentional as well as intentional.

Internalized racism is defined as acceptance by members of the stigmatized races of negative messages about our own abilities and intrinsic worth. It is characterized by our not believing in others who look like us and not believing in ourselves. It involves accepting limitations to one's own full humanity, including one's spectrum of dreams, one's right to self-determination, and one's range of allowable self-expression. It manifests as embracing "whiteness" (hair straighteners and bleaching creams, skin-tone stratification within communities of color, and "the white man's ice is colder" syndrome), self-devaluation (racial slurs as nicknames, rejection of ancestral culture, and fratricide), and resignation, helplessness, and hopelessness (dropping out of school, not voting, and participating in risky health practices) (Jones, 2000).

Impacts of Racism on Health   The theoretical foundations for social and epidemiological research on the effects of racism on the health and lived experiences of black Americans have emerged through qualitative work in the late 1980s and early 1990s (Adams & Dressler, 1988; Essed, 1991; Feagin, 1991). Researchers have conceptualized discrimination within a variety of theoretical orientations. Some have focused on factors that lead to increased exposure to discriminatory experiences (Jackson, Thoits, & Taylor, 1995; Landrine & Klonoff, 1996; Schulz et al., 2000; Brown, 2001), while others have focused on factors that influence people's sensitivities and responses to discriminatory experiences (Fischer & Shaw, 1999; Van Ausdale & Feagin, 2001). Clark, Anderson, Clark, and Williams (1999) propose a biopsychosocial model of racism (discrimination attributed to race/ethnicity) that incorporates a range of factors that influence exposures to, responses to, and consequences of racism for different social groups.

Since the early 1990s, researchers from sociology and psychology have begun to disentangle the social causes and health consequences of racism for African Americans (Dressler, 1993; Krieger & Sidney, 1998; Sanders Thompson, 1996; Brown, Sellers, Brown, & Jackson, 1999; Kessler, Mickelson, & Williams, 1999; Williams, Spencer, & Jackson, 1999; Schulz et al., 2000; Brown, 2001; LaVeist, Sellers, & Neighbors, 2001). In particular, scholarship in the social epidemiology of mental health has analyzed discrimination as a source of social stress (Clark et al., 1999; Williams & Collins, 1995; Jackson et al., 1995), and discrimination has been shown to be related to poor physical and mental health outcomes (Williams & Fenton, 1994; Krieger & Sidney, 1998; Sanders Thompson, 1996; Kessler et al., 1999; Williams et al., 1999; Schulz et al., 2000; Brown, 2001; LaVeist et al., 2001).

This line of inquiry demonstrates that structural forms of racism and those that occur in everyday contexts restrict socioeconomic mobility and negatively affect black well-being. Racial health disparities exist, in large measure, because of blacks' lower relative socioeconomic positions in the class structure of U.S. society (Williams 1990;

Williams & Collins 1995). Low socioeconomic status facilitates exposure and increases vulnerability to stressful events and experiences, such as persistent financial difficulties, that are known to have deleterious effects on physical and psychological well-being (Pearlin, 1989; Williams, 1990; Williams & Collins 1995).

Studies of perceived unfair treatment typically assess three kinds of personal experience. The first is major specific instances of institutionalized discrimination such as being denied a job or being harassed by police. The second is everyday experiences of discrimination that may include being treated rudely by service workers or strangers. The third is living around members of one's own group, which might minimize exposure to racism. The essential goal of this research is to identify sources of variation in the exposure to and the perception of the ill effects of discrimination.

Kessler et al. (1999) measure two basic dimensions of discrimination: major and everyday. Their analysis of Midlife Development in the United States survey data (N = 3,032) showed that 48.9 percent of black respondents (N = 339) reported at least one discriminatory experience in their lifetimes; 89.7 percent believed that race was the main reason for these experiences. The most common incidents for black people twenty-five to sixty-four included not being hired for a job (24.4%), not being given a promotion (27.8%), being denied a bank loan (19.8%), and receiving inferior service (15.2%). Thirty-nine percent of respondents sixty-five and older reported discriminatory experiences, with the most common being not being hired for a job (5.9%), not being given a promotion (4.8%), being discouraged by a teacher from seeking higher education (2.4%), and receiving inferior service (1.7%)[2] (Kessler et al. 1999, p. 213).

Krieger and Sidney (1998) measured discrimination as reported by 2,637 black respondents in seven social contexts: at school (33%), getting a job (49%), at work (54%), finding housing (31%), obtaining medical care (14%), on the street or in a public setting (63%), and from the police or in the court system (43%) (p. 1373). Overall, 77 percent of black women and 84 percent of black men reported experiencing discrimination in at least one of these seven contexts.

Specific measures of unfair treatment may be experienced by some black people and not by others (King & Williams, 1995). Likewise, as Ruggiero and others (Ruggiero & Taylor, 1997; Ruggiero, 1999; Ruggiero & Marx, 1999; Ruggiero, Mitchell, Krieger, Marx, & Lorenzo, 2000; LaVeist et al., 2001) suggest, measures of perceived unfair treatment may not accurately reflect the actual amount of discrimination experienced by black people. Black people who may not report their personal experiences of discrimination will still recognize the existence of group-based discrimination. Additionally, their work suggests that black people may minimize the discrimination they face because it allows them "to maintain the belief that other[s] accept them for who they are, and that they have control over the outcomes they receive" (Ruggiero, 1999, p. 534).

Landrine and Klonoff (1996) assessed both the frequency of racial discrimination and respondents' evaluation of it in the past year and over the life course using the Schedule of Racist Events, an eighteen-item self-report inventory. Of their sample of 153 black people aged 15 to 70, 98.1 percent reported at least one experience of racial discrimination in the past year and 100 percent reported experiencing racial discrimination in their lifetimes. The most common discriminatory events were being discriminated against by strangers (93.7%), by people in service jobs (89.7%), by teachers and professors (81%), by institutions and their policies (80.4%), by colleagues, co-workers, or fellow students (78.1%), by employers or supervisors (69.1%), and by people in helping jobs (68.6%). Seventy-nine percent of the sample had been called a racist name at some point in their lifetime. Their results indicate that the experience of discrimination is highly prevalent in the black population, although the generalizability of these results is limited because their sample was drawn from students associated with the Black Student Union and members of the Black Faculty and Staff Group at a large university and thus did not represent a geographically or socioeconomically diverse population.

Broman, Mavaddat, and Hsu (2000, p.171) conducted a telephone survey of 495 black adults (eighteen years and over) living in Detroit in 1992 and found that nearly 60 percent reported perceiving some form of discrimination within the past three years; these incidents took place when shopping at a store (40.2%), while at work (28.8%), when getting a job (23.2%), and during encounters with police (14.5%). Younger blacks were more likely to perceive discrimination in these four key contexts and overall; 77 percent of those aged 18 to 29 compared with 24 percent of those 65 and older reported perceiving some kind of discrimination. The authors do not address the age differences; not only may older blacks have been exposed to different types of discriminatory experiences, but they may also interpret their experiences differently than do younger blacks.

Major et al. (2002) explored the relationship between ethnic-group identification and belief in individual mobility, group status (majority/minority), and perceived discrimination using both survey and experimental methodologies. Of three studies conducted, one included a sample of 421 undergraduate students including 127 black students. Perceived discrimination was measured using a single indicator: "I experience discrimination because of my ethnicity." One's belief in individual mobility was measured by four items that assessed the extent to which respondents agreed or disagreed with claims regarding the openness of American society to the advancement of individuals with various ethnic backgrounds. Similarly, four items that measured the strength and importance of ethnic-group membership as well as the closeness one felt to members of one's ethnic group assessed ethnic-group identification. Overall, minority respondents (blacks and Latinos) perceived greater personal discrimination than did whites ($B = .21$, $p < .001$), once differences in group identification and ideology were controlled. Among minority students, higher ethnic-group identification was positively associated with perceived discrimination ($B = .28$, $p < .001$); however, belief in individual mobility was not related to perceived discrimination (Major et al., 2002, pp. 278–279).

Fischer and Shaw (1999), in a study of 118 black undergraduate students, assessed the links between perceived discrimination and psychological distress. Specifically, they tested three potential moderators of this relationship: racial socialization, self-esteem, and social interactions with other black people (friends, dating partners).

In general, respondents reported relatively high exposure to racist events. The most common were being treated unfairly by people in service jobs (78%), by strangers (78%), by fellow students (57%), by institutions and their policies (50%), and by employers/supervisors (42%) (Fischer & Shaw, 1999, p. 404). The authors caution that "the data of perceptions are not ideal (i.e., they are shaped by a variety of affective and cognitive factors), but they do provide a starting point in studying the possible link between racism and mental health. We would like to state unequivocally that research on perceived discrimination should not be used to make inferences about actual racist discrimination" (p. 395). The researchers found that early racial socialization experiences and self-esteem moderate the relationship between perceived discrimination and mental health, while social interaction in black social networks was not a consistently significant moderator. They write, "Blacks who reported greater preparation by their families for racism struggles did not show a significant relation between racist events and poorer mental health, whereas those who reported lower levels of preparation did" (p. 402). Further, their results indicate that the earlier the racial socialization experiences (i.e., as a child), the more strongly they predict reports of discrimination later in life. The authors believe that early life experiences, particularly those related to living in a racist society, continue to play a role in the evaluation of discriminatory experiences later in life.

As voluminous as the research describing racial discrimination and linking it to health is, it is important to realize that racial discrimination is just one aspect of racism, a subset of what was described earlier as personally mediated racism. As Jones suggests with her "Gardener's Tale" allegory (Jones, 2000), the most profound effects of racism are likely to be the ways in which institutionalized racism structures differential access to the goods, services, and opportunities of society according to race. Although research documenting the relationship between education, income, wealth, or housing and health outcomes is often not cast as research on racism and health, it does not "just so happen" that people of color are overrepresented in poverty in this country while white people are overrepresented in wealth. Institutionalized racism explains why we see an association between socioeconomic status and race, and disproportionate poverty is an important mechanism through which racism impacts health.

Jones et al. (2008) have also provided another research strategy for examining the effects of racism on health without asking about individual experiences of discrimination. They define the variable "socially assigned race" as the response to the question "How do other people usually classify you in this country? Would you say White, Black or African American, Hispanic or Latino, Asian, Native Hawaiian or Other Pacific Islander, American Indian or Alaska Native, or some other group?" and note that this is the "on-the-street" race that is the substrate on which racism operates. They found that being perceived as white is associated with large and statistically significant advantages in self-reported general health status, even if one self-identifies with a nonwhite group. They remind us that racism results in both unfair disadvantage and its reciprocal, unfair advantage, and they encourage increased attention to the ways in which opportunity is structured and value is assigned so that "whiteness" is favored (McIntosh, 1988).

Finally, Jones (1994) has proposed that observed race-associated differences in health outcomes are due to the accelerated aging of the black population compared with the white population and that this accelerated aging is due to racism. Her "accelerated-aging hypothesis" is based on comparisons of blood pressure from national studies dating back to the first National Health Examination Survey (1959–1962) but is also supported by the observation of earlier onset of prostate cancer in black men than white men, earlier onset of breast cancer in black women than white women, earlier onset of glaucoma in black people than white people, and earlier menarche in black girls than white girls. Although doing "age-shifted analyses" to compare health outcomes among black people to health outcomes among white people who are ten years older may confirm accelerated aging with many additional health outcomes, continued development of measures of racism and vigorous investigation of the effects of racism on health are necessary to explain why we observe the accelerated-aging phenomenon.

The ample and expanding documentation of the impacts of racism on health is important for raising awareness among the general public that racism is still alive and well, for answering scientific questions about the basis of observed race-associated differences in health outcomes, and for identifying racism as a contemporary threat to the health and well-being of the whole nation. Our research efforts to name and measure racism must also provide impetus and guidance for interventions to dismantle racism and prevent its adverse impacts on health. These interventions will require strong political will and focused, concerted action. Just as there is an international framework assuring health as a human right, there is also an international convention on the elimination of all forms of racial discrimination.

International Convention on the Elimination of All Forms of Racial Discrimination
In the United States, people of African descent have long struggled for civil rights in a system that would not only deny them due process but also deny them their humanity. Although many in the United States may conclude that our unique racist history makes racism an area of peculiar interest to this country, a considerable history of naming and addressing racism exists in the international arena. In 1964, Malcolm X wrote: "The American black man is the world's most shameful case of minority oppression. What makes the black man think of himself as only an internal United States issue is just a catch-phrase, two words, 'civil rights.' How is a black man going to get 'civil rights' before first he wins his *human* rights? If the American black man will start thinking about his *human* rights, and then start thinking of himself as part of one of the world's greatest peoples, he will see he has a case for the United Nations" (X & Haley, 1965).

As arguably successful as the black struggle for civil rights has been, it appeals to the laws within the United States, which have historically been the laws of the "master" (the person in power). But what if the "master" does not feel like honoring the rights of black people today? Black Americans must recognize that they have rights that do not depend on the goodwill of the U.S. government. Universal human rights have been affirmed by the international community, and all the struggles of black Americans should reference these international human rights as well as the local rights that might or might not be protected within the U.S. legal context.

The International Convention on the Elimination of All Forms of Racial Discrimination (ICERD) was adopted by the United Nations on December 21, 1965 (United Nations General Assembly, 1965). The United States signed the treaty on September 28, 1966, but took twenty-eight years before ratifying it on October 21, 1994. Following are excerpts from the seven principal substantive articles of the ICERD:

- Article 1 (defining racial discrimination): "In this Convention, the term 'racial discrimination' shall mean any distinction, exclusion, restriction or preference based on race, color, descent, or national or ethnic origin which has the purpose or effect of nullifying or impairing the recognition, enjoyment or exercise, on an equal footing, of human rights and fundamental freedoms in the political, economic, social, cultural or any other field of public life."

- Article 2 (condemning racial discrimination): "States Parties condemn racial discrimination and undertake to pursue by all appropriate means and without delay a policy of eliminating racial discrimination in all its forms and promoting understanding among all races."

- Article 3 (condemning racial segregation): "States Parties particularly condemn racial segregation and apartheid and undertake to prevent, prohibit and eradicate all practices of this nature in territories under their jurisdiction."

- Article 4 (condemning ideas of racial superiority): "States Parties condemn all propaganda and all organizations which are based on ideas or theories of superiority of one race or group of persons of one color or ethnic origin, or which attempt to justify or promote racial hatred and discrimination in any form."

- Article 5 (promoting equality before the law): "States Parties undertake to prohibit and to eliminate racial discrimination in all its forms and to guarantee the right of everyone, without distinction as to race, color, or national or ethnic origin, to equality before the law, notably in the enjoyment of the following rights," which include equal treatment before justice, security of person and protection against bodily harm, political rights, other civil rights, and *economic, political, and cultural rights including the right to work, the right to housing, the right to public health and medical care, and the right to education.*

- Article 6 (assuring protection and remedies): "States Parties shall assure to everyone within their jurisdiction effective protection and remedies, through the competent national tribunals and other State institutions, against any acts of racial discrimination which violate his human rights and fundamental freedoms contrary to this Convention, as well as *the right to seek from such tribunals just and adequate reparation or satisfaction for any damage suffered as a result of such discrimination*" [emphasis added].

- Article 7 (education to combat prejudices): "States Parties undertake to adopt immediate and effective measures, particularly in the fields of teaching, education, culture and information, with a view to combating prejudices which lead to racial discrimination."

When ratifying the treaty, the United States specified three Reservations, an Understanding, a Declaration, and a Proviso limiting the reach of the treaty (U.S. Congress, 1994). Congress declared that the treaty would not be self-executing, thereby requiring additional implementing legislation. It also included the reservation that "with reference to Article 22 of the Convention, before any dispute to which the United States is a party may be submitted to the jurisdiction of the International Court of Justice under this article, the specific consent of the United States is required in each case."

The Committee on the Elimination of Racial Discrimination (CERD) was established in Article 8 of the ICERD as the monitoring body for compliance with the obligations laid down in the treaty. Although reports from the United States have been due to the CERD every two years starting in November 1995, the United States has so far submitted only two reports, the first in September 2000 (U.S. Department of State, 2000) and the second in April 2007 (U.S. Department of State, 2007). Each submission has been accompanied by many "shadow reports" written by nongovernmental organizations in the United States to augment the perspectives and facts presented in the official government report (U.S. Human Rights Network, 2008; Urban Justice Center, 2009).

The concluding observations of the CERD in response to the 2007 report from the U.S. government included thirty-seven concerns and recommendations, including recommendations for the prohibition of practices and legislation that may not be discriminatory in purpose but are so in effect (paragraph 10); the intensification of efforts to reduce residential segregation by race (paragraph 16); the elaboration of effective strategies to promote school desegregation and to provide equal educational opportunity (paragraph 17); the guarantee of the right to equal treatment before tribunals and all other organs administering justice (paragraph 20); the restoration of the right to vote after completion of criminal sentences (paragraph 27); the combating of de facto discrimination in the workplace (paragraph 28); the addressing of persistent health disparities (paragraph 32); and the organization of public awareness and education programs on the ICERD, including the mechanisms and procedures provided for by the treaty (paragraph 36) (United Nations Committee on the Elimination of Racial Discrimination, 2008).

Focused and Ongoing Societal Efforts to Address Avoidable Inequalities

Racial Differences Are Not Innate and Not Inevitable   Historically, race was reified as reflecting innate biological differences in order to support the enslavement of Africans and their descendants. Indeed, some diseases were described in ways that restricted them to black persons, including "drapetomania," which was defined as the insane desire to run away. Even into the second half of the twentieth century, the hypothesis that salt deficits during the Middle Passage exerted natural-selection pressure among survivors resulted in scientists seeking to explain observed differences in the prevalence of high blood pressure by searching for differences in the salt-handling ability of kidneys of black and white patients (Kaufman & Hall, 2003). Indeed, our practice of routinely documenting race-associated differences in health outcomes without vigorously investigating the root causes of those differences means that public health scientists continue to unwittingly support ideas of biologically based differences between the so-called races (Jones, 2001).

In his 1899 book, *The Philadelphia Negro: A Social Study*, W.E.B. DuBois included a detailed chapter on "The Health of Negroes" along with chapters on marital status, migration history, education and illiteracy, occupation, family, church and other social organizations, crime, poverty, the environment, and even the vote. More than a century ago, DuBois clearly recognized that health is inextricably bound to the total human condition. However, that recognition dimmed through the decades as health came to be viewed as an individual characteristic rather than the result of a broad constellation of individual and community exposures and opportunities.

The 1985 report of the Secretary's Task Force on Black and Minority Health documented the excess morbidity and premature mortality of black and other minority populations compared with white populations, disparities that were estimated to result in sixty thousand excess deaths each year (U.S. Department of Health and Human Services, 1985). In 1998, President Bill Clinton and Surgeon General David Satcher announced a national initiative to eliminate racial/ethnic health disparities by the year 2010 (White House, 1998). This initiative has sparked Congressional funding of major programs within the U.S. Department of Health and Human Services, including the Racial and Ethnic Approaches to Community Health (REACH 2010) demonstration projects in forty-one communities through the Centers for Disease Control and Prevention and the Administration on Aging, as well as projects funded through the Health Resources and Services Administration, the Agency for Healthcare Research and Quality, and the National Institutes of Health. Combined with additional efforts at the state and local level, these projects have generated a great amount of attention to racial/ethnic health disparities and ways to address them. However, the elimination of these disparities does not seem imminent as we write in 2009. Indeed, twenty years after publication of the report of the Secretary's Task Force on Black and Minority Health, the estimated number of preventable excess deaths each year caused by the black-white mortality gap had risen to 83,570 (Satcher et al., 2005). The limitation to progress on eliminating racial/ethnic health disparities does not seem to be a matter of intent but rather a matter of the types of actions that have been taken to reach that goal.

There is growing recognition that in order to rid ourselves of racial/ethnic health disparities, we will need to stop pruning the weed and attack it at its roots. As we have discussed, racism is an important aspect of our social environment that is increasingly being discussed at both national and international levels as a root cause of racial/ethnic health disparities. Documents that cite the importance of paying attention to racism and its impacts on health include the *Declaration and Programme of Action* from the third World Conference against Racism, Racial Discrimination, Xenophobia, and Related Intolerance, convened by the United Nations in 2001 (United Nations General Assembly, 2002); the report Unequal Treatment: Confronting Racial and Ethnic Disparities in Health Care, sponsored by the Institute of Medicine in 2003 (Smedley, Stith, & Nelson, 2003); and the resolution "Research and Intervention on Racism as a Fundamental

Cause of Ethnic Disparities in Health," adopted as public policy by the American Public Health Association in 2001 (American Public Health Association, 2002).

Scientific racism consists of ideas of race based on presumed physiological, biological, or genetic differences, and the deployment of such ideas as explanations for racial stratification and oppression. Scientific racism emerged as an ad hoc justification of colonial subjugation and slavery in the eighteenth century and is most easily associated with the social practices of eugenics and Nazi racial hygiene in the nineteenth and early-to-mid-twentieth centuries. Racial-formation theorist Winant argues that scientific racism severs the effects of racism from the causes of white capitalist supremacy by attributing systematic racial inequalities to "the nature of things," to "science" (2001, p. 296).

By the 1950s, however, the UNESCO statements on race signaled the emerging scientific consensus that race concepts were socially constructed and were without foundation in human biology or nature (Reardon, 2005). Yet, in contemporary biomedical theory and practice, racial categories are still assumed to be proxies for genetic or biological variation (Jones, LaVeist, & Lillie-Blanton, 1991; Institute of Medicine, 2003). Many interpreters have agreed, describing these emerging biomedical theories and research practices as "the biological reification" or "biological rewriting" of race (Duster, 2005; Fausto-Sterling, 2004; Gannett, 2004; Thompson, 2006). Writing at the onset of what he calls the "new genetic prism," Troy Duster argues that racial categories are increasingly used to discern the respective influence of environmental and genetic factors in the causation and distribution of multifactorial disease; in these new interpretations, racial differences in disease are explained as the consequence of inherent, group-based genetic susceptibilities (Duster, 2005, p. 1050). Duster argues that social, economic, and political interests profoundly influence the production of scientific knowledge about race and the racial distribution of disease more than any specific biological or genetic understandings about the etiology or course of disease. Thus, understanding the interrelationships of sociopolitical processes, scientific practices, and racially categorized bodies is fundamental to understanding what remains contested and problematic about the concept of race in science (Duster, 2003b).[3] Racial differences in health are not inherent in our bodies but in the racialization of those bodies. They are thus amenable to change through attention to social justice.

Social Justice as Both a Motivation and a Guide for Action   The fact that social justice in health is a yet-unrealized goal is a severe problem. The results are the shortened life expectancy and the reality of inferior health and health care services for black people, the absence of a national affirmation that health is a human right, and a negation of the role of the social determinants of health. The myopic focus on the medical model extends even to the public health community, in which upstream, systemic, and structural causes for the poor health of black people are denied.

Former Seattle–King County Public Health Director Alonzo Plough states, "The major challenge of public health practice is to move theoretical knowledge about the relationship of social injustice to increased health risks and poor health outcomes into broad and sustainable changes in agency policies and practices" (quoted in Levy & Sidel, 2006, p. 424). However, "no national performance standards or performance measures explicitly deal with the promotion of social justice as a public health practice core capacity" (p. 419). Plough describes public health as a "social enterprise" with a mandate to align the technical tools of epidemiology and assessment with effective community partnerships and advocacy (p. 423). Public health professionals must engage with their communities in challenging social injustices that impinge on health. Indeed, all citizens of this nation have a stake and a role in confronting health inequities as part of a moral commitment to group-based social justice.

The ethos of American "rugged individualism," the overwhelming attention in this country to "market justice," and an unnatural separation of social factors from their impacts on health and illness all play a critical role in understanding some public views of inequities in health. When health is seen as the sole responsibility of the individual, society will be deemed to have no role in addressing health inequities. Social justice, however, argues that the societal influences on the health of individuals and groups are significant. These influences are structural, systemic, and historic. Therefore, intervention on a societal scale is required to ensure the right to health and to eliminate health inequities.

Among the other factors that continue to support the existence of health inequities are the continued overwhelming effects of race and racism and the role of the social determinants of health on personal and community health status. The reliance on the medical model of health, which denies these factors, has dramatically contributed to the current status of "black folk on the critical list." Added to this formula is a national adoration of high-tech, expensive diagnostics and the growth of a tertiary-care focus. There is an upside down pyramid of health and health care in which specialists dominate and prevention and primary care are almost afterthoughts.

If racism structures opportunity and assigns value based on race, a social justice approach to improving the health of the black community will involve examining and intervening in structures, policies, practices, norms, and values (Jones, 2003). Structures are the "who," "what," "when," and "where" of decision making. They include who is at the decision-making table and who is not, what is on the agenda and what is not. Policies are the written "how" of decision making and are perhaps the easiest point at which to investigate and intervene. Practices and norms are the unwritten "how" of decision making, and values are the all-important "why." Attention to what exists and what is lacking with regard to all these aspects of our racist system are necessary in order to dismantle it and replace it with a system in which all are able to both know and develop to their full potential.

Following is a description of four kinds of policy that are among the mechanisms of institutionalized racism (Jones, 2003):

■ Policies that allow the segregation of resources and risks by race. These include redlining, zoning, and other environmental policies that permit the segregation of residential resources and risks by race; policies mandating the use of local property taxes to fund public education, which perpetuate segregation of educational resources by race; and institutional policies allowing discretion in hiring or lending or medical treatment, which permit and condone the expression of personally mediated racism in these arenas.

■ Policies that create inherited group disadvantage (or its reciprocal inherited group advantage) by race. These include the lack of social security for children, the intergenerational transfer of wealth through estate inheritance, and the lack of reparations for historical injustices.

■ Polices that favor the differential valuation of human life by race. These include curriculum policies that teach certain histories and not others. They also include societal blindness to racism, which denies the continued existence of an unfair system, and the myth of meritocracy, which devalues those who are not successful in it.

■ Policies that limit self-determination. These include policies that affect representation on school boards, policies that result in disproportionate incarceration and subsequent disenfranchisement, and "majority rules" as the only mode of decision making when there is a fixed minority. We conceptualize self-determination as including the power to decide, the power to act, and control of resources.

Ensuring the Conditions for Optimal Health for All Groups

Addressing the Social Determinants of Health   The U.S. health system currently identifies individual behaviors as the principal determinants of health status (Mokdad, Marks, Stroup, & Gerberding, 2004). Smoking, drinking, sedentary lifestyle, overeating, risky sexual practices, and illicit drug use have all been in the public eye as health risks and targets for medical and public health action (Satcher, 2006). However, there is growing recognition that individual behaviors do not arise in a vacuum but are conditioned by the social and physical environments in which we live (Link and Phelan, 1995, 2000). Therefore, in addition to focusing on individual behaviors, we must widen our gaze to acknowledge and address the social determinants of health (Jones, Jones, Perry, Jones, & Barclay under review).

The social determinants of health are those determinants of health that are outside the individual; they are beyond genetic endowment and beyond individual behaviors. They are, in fact, the context in which individual behaviors arise and in which individual behaviors convey risk. The social determinants of health include individual resources, neighborhood (place-based) or community (group-based) resources, hazards and toxic exposures, and opportunity structures (Jones et al., under review). Individual resources include individual education, occupation, income, and wealth, all aspects of individual socioeconomic position. Neighborhood or community resources include the quality of the housing stock, the range of food choices, the level of public safety, the availability of transportation, the accessibility of parks and recreation, and the level of political clout. Hazards and toxic exposures include pesticides, lead, and reservoirs of infection that can be differential by place, occupation, or group membership. Opportunity structures include quality schools, meaningful jobs, and equal justice (Jones et al., under review).

Addressing the social determinants of health involves the medical care and public health systems but also requires collaboration with nonhealth sectors, including education, housing, labor, justice, transportation, environment, agriculture, and immigration. Addressing the social determinants of health is necessary if we are to achieve sustained improvements in health outcomes (National Association of County and City Health Officials, 2006). Unlike attending to individual health behaviors, addressing the social determinants of health involves more than individual action and an individual sense of efficacy. Individuals need to accept and embrace their interconnectedness with others and join together in collective action to affect structures and policies outside themselves (Robinson, 2005). Indeed, the very act of joining with others in collective action may provide a sense of collective efficacy, which can be empowering (Jones et al., under review).

Addressing the Social Determinants of Equity When describing the contexts in which individual behaviors arise as the social determinants of health, we are led to the further questions of why we see the range of contexts that we do and why we see different populations differentially distributed into those contexts. We must enlarge our conceptualization of the determinants of health beyond seeing individual behaviors at the center and the contexts in which the individual behaviors arise (the social determinants of health) as a surrounding ring. We must acknowledge an additional outer ring, the societal determinants of context, which are the forces that create and distribute contexts. We describe these forces as the social determinants of equity (Jones et al., under review).

The social determinants of equity are systems of power that determine the range of social contexts and the distribution of populations into those social contexts. They include our economic system, which creates class structure through the private ownership of the means of production. They include racism, which structures opportunity and assigns value based on the social interpretation of how one looks (Jones, 2003). And they include homophobia, sexism, and other "isms" that structure opportunity and assign value based on gender, sexual orientation, and other axes of difference from those in power. If the social determinants of health are the contexts that answer the question "Why do we see this distribution of behaviors?", then the social determinants of equity are the forces that answer the question "Why do we see this distribution of contexts?" (Jones et al., under review).

Addressing the social determinants of equity involves monitoring for inequities along axes of societal power. It involves examining and intervening in structures, policies, practices, norms, and values. Addressing social determinants of equity is necessary if we are to eliminate health disparities and achieve health equity (Jones et al., under review).

Particularly for Those Who Have Experienced Historical or Contemporary Injustices or Socioeconomic Disadvantage

The Importance of Attention to History Americans tend to be ahistorical; they often do not realize how history structures the present and explains the current inequitable distribution of exposures, opportunities, resources, and risks in this nation

(Jackson, 2001). A social justice approach to health does not pretend that the currently observed unequal playing field just happened to appear; this approach understands that historical injustices need to be addressed before contemporary equity can be achieved (Robinson, 2000). In addition, attention must be paid to the contemporary structural factors that perpetuate the initial historical injustices. If we do not acknowledge and dismantle those contemporary structural factors, which include the mechanisms of institutionalized racism, even magically providing equitable living conditions by race today would not ensure that racial disparities in living conditions would not reappear within a generation.

Critical Race Theory and an Antiracism Agenda   Critical race theory is a historical and contemporary body of scholarship that aims to interrogate the discourses, ideologies, and social structures that produce and maintain conditions of racial injustice. At the broadest level, critical race theories analyze how race and racism are foundational elements in historical and contemporary social structures and in the life experiences of people living in racialized societies. Critical race theories understand racism as a vast and complicated system of institutionalized practices that structure the allocation of social, economic, and political power in unjust and racially coded ways.

While some race theorists have examined racism as a form of maligned individual prejudice, critical race theorists tend to embrace a more institutional understanding of racism (Bonilla-Silva, 1997, 2003) that aims to identify how racism is embedded in the racially patterned practices of social institutions (Carmichael & Hamilton, 1967). In examining the institutionalized aspects of racism, critical race theorists challenge the idea that people of color are responsible for their own oppression (Brown, Carnoy, Currie, & Duster, 2003). These theories continue to challenge entrenched racial inequalities in health, education, criminal injustice, political representation, and social class (Brown et al., 2003; Guiner & Torres, 2002; Shapiro, 2004).

The six premises of critical race theory (Matsuda, Lawrence, Delgado, & Crenshaw, 1993, pp. 1–7) are:

1. Racism is endemic to American life, not aberrational.

2. Dominant claims about neutrality, objectivity, and colorblindness should be met with skepticism.

3. Current racial inequalities are linked to laws and practices imposed during periods of overt discrimination.

4. Racial disparities will not be eliminated unless we incorporate the experiential knowledge of people of color into research and practice.

5. Addressing racial inequality demands interdisciplinarity and intersectionality over single-axis approaches.

6. Measure progress on the elimination of racial disparity using yardsticks that demonstrate fundamental social transformation.

Acceptance of these premises suggests that those pursuing a social justice approach to improving health outcomes and eliminating health disparities must include an anti-racism agenda in their toolbox. We propose that the three basic elements of an antiracism action agenda are naming racism, asking the question "How is racism operating here?", and organizing and strategizing to act.

Naming racism means putting racism (not just race or cultural competence or disparities or diversity) on the agenda and keeping it there. It includes identifying racism as a force that determines the distribution of other social determinants of health, including education, employment, income, and wealth. In the scientific realm it involves routinely monitoring for differential exposures, opportunities, and outcomes by race, where the differences in outcomes are our well-documented racial "disparities" while the differences in exposures and opportunities are the racial "inequities" that lead to those disparities. We need to name racism as the system that makes race have meaning. We need to combat the notion that racism is a thing of the past and name racism as both a historical and a contemporary threat to the health and well-being of the nation.

Asking the question "How is racism operating here?" provides a guide to how to intervene to dismantle the system of racism. After all, racism is not a miasma nor formless cloud, but a system of power that is institutionalized in our laws, customs, and norms. We can get traction on how to dismantle this system by identifying the mechanisms of institutionalized racism in our structures, policies, practices, norms, and values. Attending to values is particularly important, even as we work to change structures and policies, because values will continue to guide decisions going forward. And as we ask the question "How is racism operating here?" in all the aspects of our lives, we need to attend to both what exists and what is lacking.

Organizing and strategizing to act involves a shift from being passive consumers to being active citizens. After identifying one or more of the mechanisms of institutionalized racism operating in our work or school or community, we have a responsibility to take targeted action. Although we may feel that addressing racism is too large a task for one person, we must realize that we do not have to act alone. In addition to our sense of individual efficacy, we can develop a sense of collective efficacy by stepping out of our bubble and joining with others. We don't even need to go out and announce that we are going to be antiracist today. We simply need to join in grassroots organizing around the conditions of people's lives and then identify the structural factors creating and perpetuating those conditions. By linking with similar efforts across the country and around the world, we will share our experiences and learn from the successes and failures of others (Jones, 1999).

CONCLUSION

A social justice approach to health provides a moral foundation for rejecting the structuring of opportunity and assigning of value based on group membership. A social justice approach to health provides a path forward from a disparities focus on outcomes to an equity focus on exposures and opportunities. By taking a social justice approach to health, we traverse the terrain from human rights to health equity to critical race theory and an antiracism agenda for improving the health of the black community. Describing his comprehensive study of the "Philadelphia Negro," DuBois later wrote (1940), "It revealed the Negro group as a symptom, not a cause; as a striving, palpitating group, and not an inert, sick body of crime; as a long historic development and not a transient occurrence." Motivated by fairness, acknowledging historical injustices, and insisting on intervention, we aim to foster a social justice approach to health that will identify and target the underlying causes of black dis-ease in the United States and preserve for black Americans our full humanity.

REFERENCES

Acevedo-Garcia, D., Lochner, K., Osypuk, T., & Subramanian, S. (2003). Future directions in residential segregation and health research: A multilevel approach. *American Journal of Public Health*, *93*(2), 215–221.

Adams, J., & Dressler, W. (1988). Perceptions of injustice in a black community: Dimensions and variation. *Human Relations*, *41*(10), 753–767.

American Public Health Association. (2002). Research and intervention on racism as a fundamental cause of ethnic disparities in health (Public Policy 2001-7). *American Journal of Public Health*, *92*(3), 458–460.

Barkan, E. (1992). *The retreat of scientific racism: Changing concepts of race in Britain and the United States between the World Wars*. New York: Cambridge University Press.

Bonilla-Silva, E. (1997). Rethinking racism: Toward a structural interpretation. *American Sociological Review*, *62*, 465–480.

Bonilla-Silva, E. (2003). *Racism without racists: Color-blind racism and the persistence of racial inequality in the United States*. Lanham, MD: Rowman & Littlefield.

Broman, C., Mavaddat, R., & Hsu, S. (2000). The experience and consequences of perceived racial discrimination: A study of African Americans. *Journal of Black Psychology*, *26*(2), 165–180.

Brown, M., Carnoy, M., Currie, E., Duster, T., Oppennheimer, D., Shultz, M., & Wellman, D. (2003). *Whitewashing race: The myth of a colorblind society*. Berkeley: University of California Press.

Brown, T. (2001). Exposure to all black contexts and psychological well-being: The benefits of racial concentration. *African American Research Perspectives*, *7*(1).

Brown, T., Sellers, S., Brown, K., & Jackson, J. (1999). Race, ethnicity, and culture in the sociology of mental health. In C. Aneshensel & J. Phelan (Eds.), *Handbook of the sociology of mental health* (pp. 167–182). New York: Kluwer Academic/Plenum.

Canellos, P., & Sege, I. (1989, October 24). Couple shot after leaving hospital: Baby delivered. *Boston Globe*, Metro/Region sec., 1.

Carmichael, S., & Hamilton, C. (1967). *Black power: The politics of liberation in America*. New York: Vintage Books.

Cavalli-Sforza, L., Menozzi, P., & Piazza, A. (1994). *The history and geography of human genes*. Princeton, NJ: Princeton University Press.

Clark, R., Anderson, N., Clark, V., & Williams, D. (1999). Racism as a stressor for African Americans: A biopsychosocial model. *American Psychologist*, *54*(10), 805–816.

Clayton, L., & Byrd, W. (2000). *An American health dilemma: A medical history of African Americans and the problem of race, beginnings to 1900*. New York: Routledge.

Clayton, L., & Byrd, W. (2002). *An American health dilemma: Race, medicine, and health care in the United States, 1900–2000*. New York: Routledge.

Collins, P. H. (1998). *Fighting Words: Black Women and the Search for Justice*. Minneapolis: University of Minnesota Press.

Cooper, R., Kaufman, J., & Ward, R. (2003). Race and genomics. *New England Journal of Medicine*, *348*(12), 1166–1170.

Cullen, K., Murphy, S., Barnicle, M., et al. (1990, January 5). Stuart dies in jump off Tobin Bridge after police are told he killed his wife: The Stuart murder case. *Boston Globe*, Metro/Region sec., 1.

Davis, R. (1994, October 27). Prayers lifted up for abducted boys: Tots whisked off in S.C. carjacking Tuesday. *USA Today*, 10A.

Dressler, W. (1993). Health in the African American community: Accounting for health inequalities. *Medical Anthropology Quarterly, 7*, 325–345.

DuBois, W. (1899). *The Philadelphia Negro: A social study*. Philadelphia: University of Pennsylvania Press.

DuBois, W. (1940). *Dusk of dawn: An essay toward an autobiography of a race concept*. New York: Schocken Books.

Duster, T. (2003a). *Backdoor to eugenics*. New York: Routledge. (Orig. pub. 1990.)

Duster, T. (2003b). Buried alive: The concept of race in science. In A. Goodman, D. Heath, & M. Lindee (Eds.), *Genetic nature/culture: Anthropology and science beyond the two-culture divide* (pp. 258–277). Berkeley and London: University of California Press.

Duster, T. (2005). Race and reification in science. *Science, 307*, 1050–1051.

Essed, P. (1991). *Understanding everyday racism: An interdisciplinary theory*. Newbury Park, CA: Sage Publications.

Fausto-Sterling, A. (2004). Refashioning race: DNA and the politics of health care. *differences: A Journal of Feminist Cultural Studies, 15*, 1–37.

Feagin, J. (1991). The continuing significance of race: Antiblack discrimination in public places. *American Sociological Review, 56*, 101–116.

Fischer, A., & Shaw, C. (1999). African-Americans' mental health and perceptions of racist discrimination: The moderating effects of racial socialization experiences and self-esteem. *Journal of Counseling Psychology, 46*(3), 395–407.

Frankenberg, E., & Orfield, G. (Eds.). (2007). *Lessons in integration: Realizing the promise of racial diversity in American schools*. Charlottesville: University of Virginia Press.

Gannett, L. (2001). Racism and human genome diversity research: The ethical limits of "population thinking." *Philosophy of Science, 68*, S479–S492.

Gannett, L. (2004). The biological reification of race. *British Journal for the Philosophy of Science, 55*, 323–345.

Goldberg, D. (2002). *The racial state*. Malden, MA: Blackwell.

Graham, R. (1990, January 11). Hoax seen playing on fear, racism: The Stuart murder case. *Boston Globe*, Metro/Region sec., 1.

Graves, J., Jr. (2001). *The emperor's new clothes: Biological theories of race at the millennium*. New Brunswick, NJ: Rutgers University Press.

Guiner, L., & Torres, G. (2002). *The miner's canary: Enlisting race, resisting power, transforming democracy*. Cambridge, MA: Harvard University Press.

Harding, S. (1993). *The "racial" economy of science: Toward a democratic future*. Bloomington: Indiana University Press.

Harrison, E. (1994, November 9). Accused child killer's family apologizes to blacks. Race relations: Susan Smith's brother says that his sister's false claim that an African American man kidnapped her sons was a "terrible misfortune." *Los Angeles Times*, A9.

Institute of Medicine, Committee for the Study of the Future of Public Health. (1988). *The future of public health*. Washington, DC: National Academies Press.

Institute of Medicine, Committee on Assuring the Health of the Public in the 21st Century. (2003). *The future of the public's health in the 21st century*. Washington, DC: National Academies Press.

Jackson, J., Jr. (2001). *A more perfect union: Advancing new American rights*. New York: Welcome Rain.

Jackson, P., Thoits, P., & Taylor, H. (1995). Composition of the workplace and psychological well-being: The effects of tokenism and America's black elite. *Social Forces, 74*(2), 543–557.

Jacobs, S. (1989, December 29). Stuart is said to pick out suspect. *Boston Globe*, Metro/Region sec., 1.

Jones, C. (1994). *Methods for comparing distributions: Development and application exploring "race"-associated differences in systolic blood pressure*. Unpublished doctoral dissertation, Johns Hopkins School of Hygiene and Public Health, Baltimore, MD.

Jones, C. (1999). *Maori-Pakeha health disparities: Can treaty settlements reverse the impacts of racism?* 1999 Ian Axford Fellowship Report. Wellington, New Zealand: New Zealand–United States Educational Foundation.

Jones, C. (2000). Levels of racism: A theoretic framework and a Gardener's Tale. *American Journal of Public Health, 90*(8), 1212–1215.

Jones, C. (2001). "Race", racism, and the practice of epidemiology. *American Journal of Epidemiology, 154*(4), 299–304.

Jones, C. (2003). Confronting institutionalized racism. *Phylon, 50*(1–2), 7–22.

Jones, C., Jones, C., Perry, G., Jones, C., & Barclay, G. (under review). The social determinants of children's health: A cliff analogy. *Journal of Health Care for the Poor and Underserved.*

Jones, C., LaVeist, T., & Lillie-Blanton, M. (1991). "Race" in the epidemiologic literature: An examination of the *American Journal of Epidemiology,* 1921–1990. *American Journal of Epidemiology, 134*(10), 1079–1084.

Jones, C., Truman, B., Elam-Evans, L., Jones, C., Jones, C., Jiles, R., et al. (2008). Using "socially assigned race" to probe white advantages in health status. *Ethnicity and Disease, 18*(4), 496–504.

Jones, M., Rivers, L., Colburn, D., Dye, R., & Rogers, W. (1993). A documented history of the incident which occurred at Rosewood, Florida, in January 1923. Available at State Library, Tallahassee, Florida. Additional information retrieved July 9, 2009, from http://dlis.dos.state.fl.us/fgils/rosewood.html

Kaufman, J., & Hall, S. (2003). The slavery hypertension hypothesis: Dissemination and appeal of a modern race theory. *Epidemiology, 14*(1), 111–118.

Kessler, R., Mickelson, K., & Williams, D. (1999). The prevalence, distribution, and mental health correlates of perceived discrimination in the United States. *Journal of Health and Social Behavior, 40*(3), 208–230.

King, G., & Williams, D. (1995). Race and health: A multidimensional approach to African American health. In B. Amick III, S. Levine, D. Walsh, & A. Tarlov (Eds.), *Society and health* (pp. 93–130). Oxford: Oxford University Press.

Krieger, N., & Sidney, S. (1998). Racial discrimination and blood pressure: The CARDIA study of young black and white adults. *American Journal of Public Health, 86*(10), 1370–1378.

Landrine, H., & Klonoff, E. (1996). The schedule of racist events: A measure of racial discrimination and a study of its negative physical and mental health consequences. *Journal of Black Psychology, 22*(2), 144–168.

LaVeist, T., Sellers, R., & Neighbors, H. (2001). Perceived racism and self and system blame attribution: Consequences for longevity. *Ethnicity and Disease, 11,* 711–721.

Levy, B., & Sidel, V. (Eds.). (2006). *Social injustice and public health.* New York: Oxford University Press.

Lewis, C. (1994, November 16). The game is to blame the blacks. *Philadelphia Inquirer,* A15.

Link, B., & Phelan, J. (1995). Social conditions as fundamental causes of disease. *Journal of Health and Social Behavior* [extra issue], 80–94.

Link, B., & Phelan, J. (2000). McKeown and the idea that social conditions are fundamental causes of disease. *American Journal of Public Health, 92*(5), 730–732.

Major, B., McKoy, S., Schmader, T., Gramzow, R., Levin, S., & Sidanius, J. (2002). Perceiving personal discrimination: The role of group status and legitimizing ideology. *Journal of Personality and Social Psychology, 82*(3), 269–282.

Mathis, R. (2007). Health care and philosophy: Adding justice to the debate [Book Review]. *Health Affairs, 26*(1), 291–292.

Matsuda, M., Lawrence, C., III, Delgado, R., & Crenshaw, K. (1993). *Words that wound: Critical race theory, assaultive speech, and the First Amendment.* Boulder, CO: Westview Press.

McClintock, A. (1995). *Imperial leather: Race, gender, and sexuality in the colonial context.* New York: Routledge.

McIntosh, P. (1988). *White privilege and male privilege: A personal account of coming to see correspondences through work in women's studies* (Working Paper 189). Wellesley, MA: Wellesley College Center for Research on Women.

Mokdad, A., Marks, J., Stroup, D., & Gerberding J. (2004). Actual causes of death in the United States, 2000. *Journal of the American Medical Association, 291*(10), 1238–1245.

National Association of County and City Health Officials. (2006). *Tackling health inequities through public health practice: A handbook for action* (R. Hofrichter, Ed.). Washington, DC: Author.

Omi, M., & Winant, H. (1994). *Racial formation in the United States.* New York: Routledge.

Ossorio, P., & Duster, T. (2005). Race and genetics: Controversies in biomedical, behavioral, and forensic sciences. *American Psychologist, 60,* 115.

Paul, D. (1998). *The politics of heredity: Essays on eugenics, biomedicine, and the nature-nurture debate.* Albany: State University of New York Press.

Pearlin, L. (1989). The sociological study of stress. *Journal of Health and Social Behavior, 30,* 241–256.

Powers, M., & Faden, R. (2006). *Social justice: The moral foundations of public health and health policy.* New York: Oxford University Press.

Rabinow, P., & Rose, N. (2003). Some thoughts on biopower today. In *Vital politics: Health, medicine, and bio-economics into the twenty first century*. London: London School of Economics.

Randall, V. (2006). *Dying while black: An in-depth look at a crisis in the American healthcare system*. Dayton, OH: Seven Principles Press.

Reardon, J. (2005). *Race to the finish: Identity and governance in an age of genomics*. Princeton, NJ: Princeton University Press.

Robinson, R. (2000). *The debt: What America owes to blacks*. New York: Dutton.

Robinson, R. (2005). Community development model for public health applications: Overview of a model to eliminate population disparities. *Health Promotion Practice, 6*(3), 338–346.

Ruggiero, K. (1999). The personal/group discrimination discrepancy: Extending Allport's analysis of targets. *Journal of Social Issues, 55*(3), 519–536.

Ruggiero, K., & Marx, D. (1999). Less pain and more to gain: Why high-status group members blame their failure on discrimination. *Journal of Personality and Social Psychology, 77*(4), 774–784.

Ruggiero, K., Mitchell, P., Krieger, N., Marx, D., & Lorenzo, M. (2000). Now you see it, now you don't: Explicit versus implicit measures of the personal/group discrimination discrepancy. *Psychological Science, 11*(6), 511–514.

Ruggiero, K., & Taylor, D. (1997). Why minority group members perceive or do not perceive the discrimination that confronts them: The role of self-esteem and perceived control. *Journal of Personality and Social Psychology, 72*(2), 373–389.

Sanders Thompson, V. (1996). Perceived experiences of racism as stressful life events. *Community Mental Health Journal 32*(3), 223–233.

Satcher, D. (2006). The prevention challenge and opportunity. *Health Affairs, 25*(4), 1009–1011.

Satcher, D., Fryer, G., Jr., McCann, J., Troutman, A., Woolf, S., & Rust, G. (2005). What if we were equal? A comparison of the black-white mortality gap in 1960 and 2000. *Health Affairs, 24*(2), 459–464.

Schulz, A., Williams, D., Isreal, B., Becker, A., Parker, E., James, S. & Jackson, J. (2000). Unfair treatment, neighborhood effects, and mental health in the Detroit metropolitan area. *Journal of Health and Social Behavior, 41*, 314–332.

Shapiro, T. (2004). *The hidden costs of being African American: How wealth perpetuates inequality*. New York: Oxford University Press.

Smedley, A., & Smedley, B. (2005). Race as biology is fiction, racism as a social problem is real. *American Psychologist, 60*, 16–26.

Smedley, B., Stith, A., & Nelson, A. (Eds.). (2003). *Unequal treatment: Confronting racial and ethnic disparities in health care*. Washington, DC: National Academies Press.

Stephan, N. (1982). *The idea of race in science*. Hamden, CT: Archon Books.

Stoler, L. (1995). *Race and the education of desire: Foucault's history of sexuality and the colonial order of things*. Durham, NC: Duke University Press.

Terry, D. (1994, November 6). A woman's false accusation pains many blacks. *New York Times*, sec. 1, 32.

Thompson, C. (2006). Race science. *Theory, Culture, and Society, 23*, 547–548.

United Nations Committee on the Elimination of Racial Discrimination. (2008, May 8). *Consideration of reports submitted by states parties under Article 9 of the Convention: Concluding observations of the Committee on the Elimination of Racial Discrimination, United States of America*. CERD/C/USA/CO/6. Retrieved April 14, 2009, from http://www.state.gov/documents/organization/107361.pdf

United Nations General Assembly. (1948, December 10). *The Universal Declaration of Human Rights*. General Assembly resolution 217 A (III). Retrieved April 14, 2009, from http://www.un.org/Overview/rights.html

United Nations General Assembly. (1965, December 21). *International Convention on the Elimination of All Forms of Racial Discrimination*. General Assembly resolution 2106 (XX). Retrieved April 14, 2009, from http://www2.ohchr.org/english/law/cerd.htm

United Nations General Assembly. (2002, January 25). *Report of the World Conference Against Racism, Racial Discrimination, Xenophobia and Related Intolerance*. Document A/CONF.189/12. Retrieved April 2, 2009, from http://www.un.org/WCAR/aconf189_12.pdf

Urban Justice Center, Human Rights Project. (2009). *The CERD Implementation Project*. Retrieved April 14, 2009, from http://www.hrpujc.org/CERDShadowReporting.html

U.S. Congress. (1994, June 24). Senate ratification of the International Convention on the Elimination of All Forms of Racial Discrimination. *Congressional Record* 140 (daily edition), S7634-02. Retrieved April 14,

2009, from http://frwebgate1.access.gpo.gov/cgi-bin/TEXTgate.cgi?WAISdocID=727357378640+14+1+0& WAISaction=retrieve; also at http://www1.umn.edu/humanrts/usdocs/racialres.html

U.S. Department of Health and Human Services, Task Force on Black and Minority Health. (1985). *Report of the Secretary's Task Force on Black and Minority Health: Vol. 1. Executive summary*. Washington, DC: U.S. Government Printing Office.

U.S. Department of State. (2000, October 10). *Committee on the Elimination of Racial Discrimination. Reports submitted by states parties under Article 9 of the Convention: Third periodic reports of states parties due in 1999; Addendum; United States of America*. CERD/C/351/Add.1. Retrieved April 14, 2009, from http://www.state.gov/documents/organization/100306.pdf

U.S. Department of State. (2007, April). *Periodic report of the United States of America to the U.N. Committee on the Elimination of Racial Discrimination concerning the International Convention on the Elimination of All Forms of Racial Discrimination*. Retrieved April 14, 2009, from http://www.state.gov/documents/organization/83517.pdf

U.S. Human Rights Network. (2008). *2008 CERD Shadow Report Summary*. Retrieved April 15, 2009, from http://www.ushrnetwork.org/

Van Ausdale, D., & Feagin, J. (2001). *The First R: How Children Learn Race and Racism*. Lanham, MD: Rowman and Littlefield.

Washington, H. (2006). *Medical apartheid: The dark history of medical experimentation on black Americans from colonial times to the present*. New York: Doubleday.

White House. (1998, February 21). President Clinton announces new racial and ethnic health disparities initiative (fact sheet). Washington, DC: US Department of Health and Human Services Press Office.

Williams, D. (1990). Socioeconomic differentials in health: A review and redirection. *Social Psychology Quarterly*, *53*(2), 81–99.

Williams, D., & Collins, C. (1995). US socioeconomic and racial differences in health: Patterns and explanations. *Annual Review of Sociology*, *21*, 349–386.

Williams, D., & Fenton, B. (1994). The mental health of African Americans: Findings, questions, and directions. In I. Livingston (Ed.), *Handbook of black American health: The mosaic of conditions, issues, policies, and prospects* (pp. 253–269). Westport, CT: Greenwood Press.

Williams, D., Spencer, M., & Jackson, J. (1999). Race, stress, and physical health: The role of group identity. In R. Contrada & R. Ashmore (Eds.), *Self, social identity, and physical health: Interdisciplinary explorations* (pp. 71–100). New York: Oxford University Press.

Winant, H. (2001). *The world is a ghetto: Race and democracy since World War II*. New York: Basic Books.

World Health Organization (1948). *Constitution of the World Health Organization*. Retrieved April 14, 2009, from http://www.who.int/gb/bd/PDF/bd46/e-bd46_p2.pdf

X, Malcolm, & Haley, A. (1965). *The Autobiography of Malcolm X*. New York: Grove Press.

Zack, N. (2002). *Philosophy of science and race*. London: Routledge.

---

[1]Since the late 1980s a voluminous body of work on the history, philosophy, and politics of race in science has been published. Some outstanding sources on these issues are Duster (2003a); Graves (2001); Harding (1993); Paul (1998); Stephan (1982); Zack, (2002).

[2]The history and philosophy of race in science is an interdisciplinary body of scholarship from epidemiology, sociology, biology, philosophy, legal studies, and anthropology (Cooper, Kaufman, & Ward, 2003; Duster, 2003a, 2005; Fausto-Sterling, 2004; Gannett, 2001, 2004; Ossorio & Duster, 2005; Rabinow & Rose, 2003; Smedley & Smedley, 2005).

[3]The total sample included blacks, whites, and other races.

CHAPTER

28

CLOSING THE GAP

Eliminating Health Disparities

HENRIE M. TREADWELL
RONALD L. BRAITHWAITE
SANDRA E. TAYLOR

As indicated in the opening chapter, the United States is reported by the United Nations Development Program (UNDP) to be a developed nation according to the most widely used indices of both global and national well-being, the Human Development Index (HDI). This status indicates high levels of population health and longevity, knowledge and education, and standard of living. Despite the favorable overall international HDI ranking and UNDP classification, a closer examination of the U.S. population reveals the health and longevity of blacks to be comparable to those of people in medium-development countries, such as Colombia and occupied Palestine (see Table 1.1 in Chapter One) (Gadson, 2006).

On a national level, racially and ethnically, U.S. whites have the highest HDI ranking, second only to Asians, whose earning potential is slightly higher and whose health and educational advantages are vastly greater than those of whites (Burd-Sharps, Lewis, & Martins, 2008). Despite ranking third in income and education, blacks have the lowest HDI ranking because of their poor health status. The health status of blacks has for the past hundred years resulted in the shortest life expectancy of any U.S. racial or ethnic group; currently black life expectancy is five years less than that of Native Americans, who have the second lowest health ranking, and thirteen years less than that of Asians, who have the highest health ranking (Burd-Sharps, Lewis, & Martins, 2008; Gadson, 2006).

THE CASE FOR CHANGE

In an effort to understand and explain the vast health differences between blacks and whites, we, as the editors of this third edition, invited nationally known public health and medical professionals to contribute chapters that directly address five of the ten leading causes of death among blacks (cancer, diabetes, homicide, HIV/AIDS, and kidney disease); five contributing health and behavioral factors (hypertension, substance abuse, nutrition and obesity, alcohol, and smoking) for seven of the leading causes of death among blacks; four types of disparities (racial, stigma, environmental, and incarceration) that contribute to the diminished health status of blacks; and five strategies (physical activity, chiropractic, faith communities, community health workers, and social marketing) for ameliorating or preventing various unfavorable health outcomes. We also give attention to high-risk populations (black men, women, children, and elderly) and other health issues of major concern (lupus and oral health) for blacks.

The chapters dedicated to leading causes of death discuss cancer, the second leading cause of death for blacks, whites, and the nation; diabetes, the fourth leading cause of death for blacks and the sixth leading cause of death for whites and the nation; and kidney disease, the ninth leading cause of death for blacks, whites, and the nation (see Table 1.2 in Chapter One). Chapters are also dedicated to two additional leading causes of death for blacks that do not rank among the top ten causes of death for whites or the nation—homicide, the sixth leading cause of death among blacks, and HIV/AIDS, the seventh leading cause of death among blacks. All these chapters report disproportionately higher rates of incidence and prevalence of morbidity and mortality for black men, women, children, and elderly when they are compared with their white counterparts.

Chapters also cover the primary risk factors for many of the leading causes of death in the black community; hypertension, substance abuse, and nutrition and obesity help to explain the disproportionate occurrence of disease and negative health outcomes among blacks. Hypertension, which is more prominent among blacks than whites, is a serious and chronic condition in its own right; it is known to contribute to or cause such health conditions as diabetes, stroke, kidney disease, and heart disease. Substance abuse (drug or alcohol abuse) is known to lower sexual inhibitions and foster unsafe drug-use behaviors (needle sharing), and it has contributed to the spread of HIV/AIDS, the impact of which has been greatest in the black community (Centers for Disease Control and Prevention, 2007, 2008a, 2008b). Poor nutrition and obesity have been shown to cause or to aggravate conditions such as diabetes, hypertension, and stroke—all of which are most prevalent among blacks.

Chapters on nutrition and obesity, physical activity, faith communities, community health workers, and social marketing address strategies that are capable of diminishing various negative health outcomes among blacks. These chapters describe the protective and ameliorating effect of physical activity and nutrition on disease, the proven effectiveness of church-based interventions and community health workers, as well as the effectiveness of properly marketed health messages directed to the black community. However, various disparities (e.g., insurance coverage) have undermined or stalled the development of new and/or more efficacious programs and strategies and have fostered the inequitable distribution of current health services.

The following excerpt from Chapter Thirteen effectively acknowledges the disproportionate burden of disease on blacks as well as systemic social and health care factors that contribute to this burden.

Reasons for the disproportionate burden of . . . [disease] among African Americans include inadequate access to health care or preventive services and higher rates of overall health problems relative to white Americans (NCI 1999; Haynes & Smedley, 1999; Smedley, Stith, & Nelson, 2003; Gross et al., 2008; Virnig et al., 2009). In the "Unequal Treatment" report issued by the United States Institute of Medicine (IOM), [the authors] discussed barriers within the health system and in patient-physician clinical encounters. Examples of health care system barriers cited in the IOM report include linguistic and cultural barriers on the part of providers, lack of a stable relationship between patient and provider (mistrust), financial limitations of poor and minority patients, and fragmentation of the health care system. These factors, along with disproportionate employment in high-risk occupations and exposure to prejudice and discrimination, may contribute to higher rates of [disease] incidence and mortality among African American populations (Bacquet & Ringen, 1986; Jones, 1989; Smedley et al., 2003).

Although education and wealth were somewhat protective for medium- to high-income blacks, who fared better than low-income blacks; overall blacks still fared worse than their white counterparts with access to the same resources (DeNavas-Walt, Proctor, & Smith, 2008). As identified in the preceding chapters, the compromised health status of blacks is in some respects a result of a biased and non-culturally-sensitive medical system. Compared with whites, blacks are less likely to get the same care and are also less likely to receive the advantageous medical procedures that are given to whites at the same disease stage (Smedley, Stith, & Nelson, 2003). The IOM has cited race and ethnicity, rather than disease stage, income, and insurance, as the factors that determine who receives the most advantageous and appropriate care.

The unequal treatment of blacks by medical professionals has led to calls for the education of additional black physicians and for increased cultural sensitivity among nonblack physicians. Such sensitivity would include understanding that blacks are not all the same and that their residential environments and economic circumstances may have a bearing on their health risk. For example, lack of exercise may be a result of residing in a violent neighborhood; poor nutrition may be due to monetary constraints. (These cultural differences are discussed in prior chapters.) In addition to physician bias and cultural insensitivity, the increased likelihood that blacks will be underinsured or uninsured contributes to their poor health (DeNavas-Walts, Proctor, & Smith, 2008). The United States is home to over forty-five million uninsured persons, including over eight million children (DeNavas-Walts, Proctor, & Smith, 2008). Eighty percent of the uninsured are working class. The high numbers of uninsured and underinsured are often by-products of unaffordable health care (Kohn, Corrigan, &

Donaldson, 2000). Since the turn of this century, health insurance premiums, which are rising 3.7 times faster than wages, have doubled resulting in co-pays and deductibles high enough to threaten health care access (Kaiser Family Foundation, 2008).

FLAWS IN U.S. HEALTH CARE

Although the United States has the world's most expensive health care system, it is by far not the best. When compared with other countries, the United States consistently underperforms on most dimensions. In a 2007 international comparison conducted by the Commonwealth Fund, the U.S. health care system ranked last or next to last in quality, access, efficiency, equality, and healthy lives, the five dimensions of a high-performance health care system, when compared with five other developed nations—Australia, Canada, Germany, New Zealand, and the United Kingdom (Davis et al., 2007). The United States was the only nation (among those to which it was compared) without universal health insurance, and its poor performance ratings were attributed partly to this fact.

As seen in Figure 28.1, the overall health care ranking of the United States was last (sixth place) (Davis et al., 2007). In the quality-of-care subcategories the United States ranked first on provision and receipt of preventive care, a dimension of the subcategory of right care. However, the United States had poor scores on the other subcategories—safe care (fourth), coordinated care (third), and patient-centered care (third). The result was a second-to-last overall quality of care ranking (fifth place). The poor ranking was partly attributable to the fact that the United States is not as advanced as the other nations in the use of information technology and team approaches, which enhance physicians' ability to identify and monitor patients with chronic conditions.

The findings from the Commonwealth Fund international comparison are reminiscent of findings reported by the IOM and the U.S. Department of Health and Human Services (HHS). The IOM report concurs with the conclusions stated in the Commonwealth Fund report—the U.S. health care system is not technology advanced. Despite the obvious benefits that would follow from adopting a technologically advanced record system, the U.S. health care system allocates a quarter of its funding to the support of antiquated paper-based record and information systems, on which it relies; it also covers administrative and overhead costs that have been deemed needless expenses (Kohn et al., 2000). The ineffective allocation of funds relates to another performance dimension, efficiency, on which the United States ranked last because of its poor performance on health expenditures, administrative costs, use of information technology and multidisciplinary teams, as well as the likelihood that sick people will use emergency rooms to treat conditions that could have been treated by a community physician, if one had been available (Davis et al., 2007).

The report by the HHS's Agency for Healthcare Research and Quality (AHRQ) cited two major factors for health disparities—substandard quality of care and inadequate access to care (Agency for Healthcare Research and Quality [AHRQ], 2006). In the HHS report, the United States is said to have substandard care on the basis of

FIGURE 28.1 *Overall Rankings in an International Comparison of Health Care Systems.*

Country Rankings						
1.00–2.66						
2.67–4.33						
4.34–6.00						

	Australia	Canada	Germany	New Zealand	United Kingdom	United States
Overall Ranking (2007)	3.5	5	2	3.5	1	6
Quality Care	4	6	2.5	2.5	1	5
Right Care	5	6	3	4	2	1
Safe Care	4	5	1	3	2	6
Coordinated Care	3	6	4	2	1	5
Patient-Centered Care	3	6	2	1	4	5
Access	3	5	1	2	4	6
Efficiency	4	5	3	2	1	6
Equity	2	5	4	3	1	6
Healthy Lives	1	3	2	4.5	4.5	6
Healthy Expenditures per Capita, 2004	$2,876*	$3,165	$3,005*	$2,083	$2,546	$6,102

*2000 data.
Source: Davis et al. (2007). Figure ES-1: Overall ranking. Calculated by the Commonwealth Fund based on the Commonwealth Fund 2004 International Health Policy Survey, the Commonwealth Fund 2005 International Health Policy Survey of Sicker Adults, the 2006 Commonwealth Fund International Health Policy Survey of Primary Care Physicians, and the Commonwealth Fund Commission on a High Performance Health System National Scorecard.

patient-provider miscommunication and provider discrimination, stereotyping, and/or prejudice. The HHS's conclusions are the same as those drawn by several authors in this book, who not only identify various kinds of substandard care received by black Americans but also discuss the impact of such care on them. The concerns raised by these authors and echoed in the HHS report have serious consequences. It is estimated that substandard, flawed health care results in one hundred thousand deaths annually in the United States (Kohn et al., 2000). According to the HHS report, access to care (receipt of appropriate and effective care) for minorities remains relatively unchanged even when access barriers (e.g., economic, geographic, linguistic, cultural, and financial), health insurance, and education were held constant (AHRQ, 2006).

In the absence of a universal health care system, many Americans go without needed health care services more often than do people in countries with a universal health care system. Americans cite costs as the primary reason for not seeking care

(Davis et al., 2007). However, properly insured Americans report rapid access to specialized health care services, an advantage over some countries with universal health care such as the United Kingdom and Canada. There, health care costs are a nonissue, but long waits for specialized services are common. In the international health care comparison report generated by the Commonwealth Fund, the United States and Canada ranked sixth and fifth out of six developed nations (see Figure 28.1). Both these countries fall short on the promptness and accessibility of physician appointments. Patients in the United States and Canada reported wait times upward of six days for "needed" appointments. In the United States, the overutilization of emergency room services is the result (Davis et al., 2007).

The United States ranked last in the final two performance dimensions, equity and healthy lives. More than two-thirds of adult Americans with below-average incomes reported not visiting a physician when sick; not getting a recommended test, treatment, or follow-up care; not filling a prescription or not seeing a dentist when needed because of cost (Davis et al., 2007). In regard to healthy lives, the United States had much higher death rates (25 percent to 50 percent higher than Canada, which ranked third, and Australia, which ranked first) from conditions amenable to medical care.

The flaws in the U.S. health care system, revealed in the international comparison, further validate the conclusions drawn in the preceding chapters of this book. The findings from the international Commonwealth Fund report, supported by independent findings from the IOM and the HHS, undermine those who argue that the state of health care in the United States is sufficient or that health disparities are a product of economics rather than race and ethnicity (Smedley et al., 2003). These reports echo the editors' as well as the chapter authors' call for action.

UNIVERSAL HEALTH CARE

Universal health care is characterized by some form of governmental action aimed at extending access to health care to as many people as possible. Known originally as National Health Service, universal health care was first established in the United Kingdom in 1948. Universal health care is implemented through legislation and regulation, which determine what care to provide to whom and on what basis, and through taxation, which covers the bulk if not all of the cost.

In universal health care systems, despite varying structure and funding mechanisms, most medical, dental, and mental health costs are covered by a single payer—the government. Although universal health care systems have been implemented in all other wealthy, industrialized countries and in some developing countries, the United States has yet to implement such a system (Institute of Medicine [IOM], 2004).

Despite recommendations by the IOM that the United States adopt a universal health care system by 2010, the country has yet to do so. In its urgings, the IOM has argued that the institutionalization of a universal health care system would extend coverage, lower costs, and improve quality, thus effectively reducing the direct and hidden costs, shared by all, associated with uninsured persons (IOM, 2004). Those in favor of universal health care point to the fact that the United States has a lower life expectancy and higher infant mortality rates than do other industrialized nations—such as Australia, the United Kingdom, Canada, and Sweden—with a universal health care system (Central Intelligence Agency [CIA], 2009).

Using the same argument, opponents of universal health care state that life expectancy and infant mortality rates cannot be used to indicate quality of care (Hogberg, 2006); they believe such correlations are inaccurate because of factors such as alternative causality and variations in data collection and statistical reporting across countries (CIA, 2009). Opponents go on to argue that the United States has the same health care system that it had when it led the world in life expectancy in the 1980s and that it is the surge in obesity that has lowered life expectancy, not the lack of universal care (Olshansky et al., 2005). Those against universal health care feel that such a program restricts individual freedom by not allowing people to opt out of health insurance, imposes financial burdens because of increased taxes, and ultimately increases utilization and reduces quality of care.

To summarize, the common arguments forwarded by supporters of universal health care systems include:

- Health care is a basic human right or entitlement.

- Ensuring the health of all citizens benefits a nation economically. About 60 percent of the U.S. health care system is already publicly financed with federal and state taxes, property taxes, and tax subsidies; a universal health care system would merely replace private/employer spending with taxes. Total spending would go down for individuals and employers.

- A single-payer system could save $286 billion a year in overhead and paperwork costs (Public Citizen, 2004). Administrative costs in the U.S. health care system are substantially higher than those in other countries and than in the public sector in the United States; one estimate put the total administrative costs at 24 percent of U.S. health care spending (Reinhardt, Hussey, & Anderson, 2004).

- Several studies have shown a majority of taxpayers and citizens across the political divide would prefer a universal health care system to the current U.S. system.

- Wastefulness and inefficiency in the delivery of health care would be reduced.

- The United States spends a far higher percentage of GDP on health care than any other country but has worse ratings on such criteria as quality of care, efficiency of care, access to care, safe care, equity, and wait times, according to the Commonwealth Fund (Davis et al., 2007).

- A universal system would increase productivity, encourage preventive care, and improve the management of chronic conditions.

- The profit motive adversely affects the cost and quality of health care. If managed care programs and their concomitant provider networks are abolished, then doctors would no longer be guaranteed patients solely on the basis of their membership in a provider group and regardless of the quality of care they provide. Theoretically, quality of care would increase as true competition for patients was restored.

■ A 2008 poll of two thousand U.S. doctors found that 59 percent supported universal health care and 32 percent opposed it. In 2002 the figures were 49 percent in support and 40 percent in opposition. By specialty, of those who were polled 83 percent of psychiatrists supported a universal system, 69 percent of emergency medicine specialists, 65 percent of pediatricians, 64 percent of internists, 60 percent of family physicians, and 55 percent of general surgeons. The reasons given were the current inability of doctors to make decisions about patient care and the plight of patients who are unable to afford care (Fox, 2008).

Common arguments forwarded by opponents of universal health care systems include:

■ Health care is not a right, and therefore it is not the responsibility of government to provide health care.

■ Universal health care would result in increased wait times, which could result in unnecessary deaths.

■ Unequal access and health disparities still exist in universal health care systems.

■ The performance of administrative duties by doctors results from medical centralization and overregulation and may reduce charitable provision of medical services by doctors.

■ Many problems that universal health care is meant to solve are caused by limitations on the free market. Free-market solutions have greater potential to improve care and coverage.

■ The widely quoted health care system ranking by the World Health Organization, in which the United States ranked below other countries, used biased criteria, giving a false sense of those countries' superiority.

■ Empirical evidence on the Medicare single-payer insurance program demonstrates that the cost exceeds the expectations of advocates (Blevins, 2003). As an open-ended entitlement, Medicare does not weigh the benefits of technologies against their costs. Paying physicians on a fee-for-service basis also leads to spending increases. As a result, it is difficult to predict or control Medicare's spending. Large market-based public program such as the Federal Employees Health Benefits Program (FEHBP) and CalPERS (the agency that manages pension and health benefits for California public employees) can provide better coverage than Medicare while still controlling costs.

At the heart of both sets of arguments is the question of whether health care is a fundamental right. A survey of the American people failed to yield a clear consensus on universal health care (Bodenheimer, 2005). The survey showed that although most Americans were in support of expanding health care coverage many were opposed to increasing taxes to do so. Overall, most Americans reported being satisfied with their own health care. Regardless of which side one chooses, the sad truth is that the current U.S. health care system has in many ways caused or contributed to current health disparities and has done little to alleviate these disparities. Although it is clear that greater and more consistent coverage and medical treatment are needed, what it is not clear is the method by which to achieve these goals.

The plan proposed by President Barack Obama attempts to strike a balance between the two extremes, universal insurance and private insurance, by emphasizing the strengths and minimizing the drawbacks of both systems. The plan is intended to strengthen employer coverage, hold insurance companies accountable, and ensure patient choice of doctors and care without governmental interference. In an effort to provide affordable and accessible health care to all, the Obama plan will build on the existing system, using existing providers, doctors, and plans, to enable patients to make health care decisions with their doctors unimpeded by the insurance company bureaucracy. It will require preventive coverage (including cancer screenings), lower the cost of health care (by as much as $2,500 per year) without forcing people to change plans or coverage if they are happy with their current plan, and provide new, affordable insurance for those without it. The new $50–65 billion reform effort will be funded by increasing the taxes of Americans earning more than $250,000 per year (Obama & Biden, 2008).

Currently, inefficiencies in the U.S. health care system cost the nation $50 to $100 billion a year with billions more being wasted on administrative and overhead costs because of system inefficiencies (Commonwealth Fund, 2006; Woolhandler, Campbell, & Himmelstein, 2003). The Obama plan will redesign the U.S. health care system to reduce inefficiency and waste and improve quality, thus driving down individual and family cost.

The Obama plan addresses several of the dimensions of care determined to be subpar in reports generated by the Commonwealth Fund, the IOM, and the HHS. The plan is responsive to the conclusion, made in the international health care system comparison report generated by the Commonwealth Fund and seconded by the Institute of Medicine, that the poor quality of care is partly attributable to the lack of technological advancement and team management of chronic disease (Davis et al., 2007; IOM, 2004). The Obama plan calls for the investment of $10 billion a year, over the next five years, in a standards-based electronic information system that will include electronic medical records (Obama & Biden, 2008). Transitioning to such a system will reduce medical errors by eliminating the difficulty of coordinating care and measuring quality of care with paper records, a system that costs twice as much to maintain as electronic records (Girosi, Meili, & Scoville, 2005, p. 79).

In regard to the team management of chronic disease, the plan seeks to require insurance providers participating in the new public plan, Medicare, or the FEHBP to utilize proven disease-management programs. The plan will also encourage outside providers to install care-management programs and provide team care to improve coordination and integration of care for those with chronic conditions (Centers for Medicare and Medicaid Services, 2007). Considering that $1.7 trillion, over 75 percent of all health care dollars, are spent on the more than 133 million American patients with one or more chronic conditions, the mandates for improving the standard of care at a lower patient cost may yield outcomes that equal those of nations, such as the United Kingdom, with similar mandates in place.

The Obama health care plan also addresses another issue present in reports by the IOM and reflected in the preceding chapters of this book: provider delivery of care and its role in creating health disparities. The proposed plan will ensure provider delivery of quality care by promoting patient safety; instituting incentives for excellence; incorporating comparative effectiveness reviews and research; tackling disparities in health care; and reforming medical malpractice while preserving patient rights. In an effort to promote patient safety, the Obama plan will require providers to report all prevention efforts and will support hospital and physician improvements to prevent future errors. Such a mandate may greatly reduce the 100,000 lives lost annually because of substandard or flawed health care service (Kohn et al., 2000).

The Obama health care plan proposes to move away from the common practice of both public and private insurers of paying providers based on volume of services rather than the quality or effectiveness of that service (Lambrew, 2007). Under this scheme, physicians seeing patients enrolled in the new public plan, the National Health Insurance Exchange, Medicare, or FEHBP will be encouraged to adopt best practices because reimbursement will be based on the provision of high-quality care and the achievement of performance thresholds on physician-validated outcome measures. To aid in the development and dissemination of best-practice approaches and to work toward the elimination of waste and missed opportunities, the plan will establish an independent institute to guide reviews and research on comparative effectiveness and to provide accurate and objective information on the basis of which patients and their physicians can make good decisions.

The Obama health care plan, acknowledging an overwhelming body of evidence demonstrating certain populations to be significantly more likely to receive a lower quality of health care than others, proposes to tackle the root causes of the resulting health disparities by addressing differences in access to health coverage and promoting disease prevention and public health. The plan hopes to reduce or eliminate health disparities caused by provider delivery of care by challenging the medical system to eliminate inequities in health care by requiring hospitals and health plans to collect, analyze, and report health care quality data for different populations. The hospitals and health plans would then be held accountable for any differences found in health services. The plan, like several of the authors in this book, calls for the diversification of the medical workforce to ensure culturally effective care, the implementation and funding of evidence-based interventions, such as patient navigation programs, and the support and expansion of safety-net institutions' capacity; these institutions currently provide a disproportionate amount of care for underserved populations with inadequate funding and technical resources. To ensure provider delivery of quality care, the plan will call for the strengthening of antitrust laws to prevent insurers from overcharging physicians for malpractice insurance. The plan will also call for the promotion of new models for addressing physician error, which in turn will improve patient safety, strengthen doctor-patient relationships, and reduce the need for malpractice suits.

Although only time will reveal the effectiveness of the Obama health care plan, it does appear to be promising. It focuses on many aspects of care, including quality, access, and delivery, that have been the source of the current health disparities suffered by most U.S. minorities, particularly blacks. Despite aspiring to do so, the plan will not cover everyone; however, it will extend affordable coverage to many of the uninsured and underinsured. The plan hopes to close population health gaps not only by achieving increased coverage but also by requiring uniform access to and delivery of health services dedicated to disease prevention and management more than to treatment.

One of the concerns surrounding the Obama-Biden health care plan is the fact that the plan is an innovation for the United States, despite already being used by other countries. Even though the United States has spent over $250 billion verifying the effectiveness of health care innovations, it has not implemented innovations well (Nembhard, Alexander, Hoff, & Ramanujam, 2009). In fact, implementation failure has been so great that the lack of improvement in the health care industry relative to other U.S. industries has been attributed to this shortfall. It is a shortfall the Obama-Biden health care plan will have to avoid if it is to be successful in its efforts to improve access to and quality of care.

CALL TO ACTION

The Challenge

The United States is continually evolving into a more diverse nation. The 2000 Census documented a 13 percent increase in population growth in the previous decade, during which minority communities experienced the most growth (U.S. Census Bureau, 2000). As the fastest growing U.S. groups, racial and ethnic minorities are projected to constitute 40 percent of the total population by 2030 (U.S. Census Bureau, 2006, p. 2). These figures indicate that in the next twenty years, if effective actions are not taken to close the current health gaps, nearly half of the U.S. population will suffer with or die (prematurely) from diseases that could have been prevented or whose impact could have been minimized with adequate access to preventive care and disease-management services. One of the key players in the efforts to eliminate health disparities is the Office of Minority Health (OMH), a federal office within HHS. OMH's mission is to improve the health of racial and ethnic minority populations through the development of policies and programs that aid in the elimination of health disparities. These efforts include providing health services to underserved communities, sponsoring community-based health education and communication campaigns and programs, and supporting biomedical, behavioral, and social science research and health-services and community-based prevention research; the OMH has also devised a five-component strategic framework for prioritizing, addressing, and reducing/eliminating health disparities (see Figure 28.2).

FIGURE 28.2 *General Structure of the Office of Minority Health Strategic Framework.*

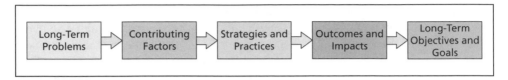

Note: Developing a strategic framework using a logic model development process emphasizes five steps, which correspond to each of the components in Figure 28.2: (1) examination of the long-term problems that OMH and others are trying to address; (2) review of the major factors known to contribute to or cause the long-term problems; (3) identification of promising, best, and/or evidence-based strategies and practices known to impact the causal or contributing factors; (4) presentation of measurable outcomes and impacts that might be expected from the strategies and practices; and (5) assessment of the extent to which long-term objectives and goals have been achieved.
Source: Office of Minority Health (2008). *Figure 1: A graphic depiction of the general structure of the framework.*

Suggested Framework

The first component of the OMH framework, long-term problems, identifies minority health issues with preventable morbidity and premature mortality; working to resolve these problems requires a systems approach. Using its five-component framework, details of which are presented in Figure 28.3, the OMH has identified high blood pressure, diabetes, cancer, prenatal care, and health insurance as health disparities of primary importance for which immediate actions are needed (OMH, 2008). High blood pressure occurs 40 percent more often among blacks than among whites and is the major risk factor for coronary heart disease, stroke, kidney disease, and heart failure—all of which are among the top ten leading causes of death for all races. Hypertension is a preventable and manageable disease whose impact could have easily been curtailed through education, preventive screening, diet, and exercise. The cost of hypertension prevention is nil compared with the cost of treating the disease and its associated diseases. In that hypertension disproportionately affects blacks, attempts to treat it would benefit greatly from the services of trained community health workers able to bridge the gap between the medical community and the black community.

Considering the vast health needs of the black community and its equally as great distrust of the medical community, community health workers are a valuable and underutilized resource. Another underutilized method for relaying valuable health messages and providing venues for preventive screenings is through the black churches. Given their ability to convene large samples from the targeted or high-risk population, churches and faith-based functions have been shown to be effective sites for health screenings and health marketing, yet many health initiatives have not included black churches in their intervention plans.

Diabetes, the second minority health issue with preventable morbidity and premature mortality in need of a systems approach, occurs 2.1 times more often in blacks than in

FIGURE 28.3 *A Strategic Framework for Improving Racial/Ethnic Minority Health and Eliminating Racial/Ethnic Health Disparities.*

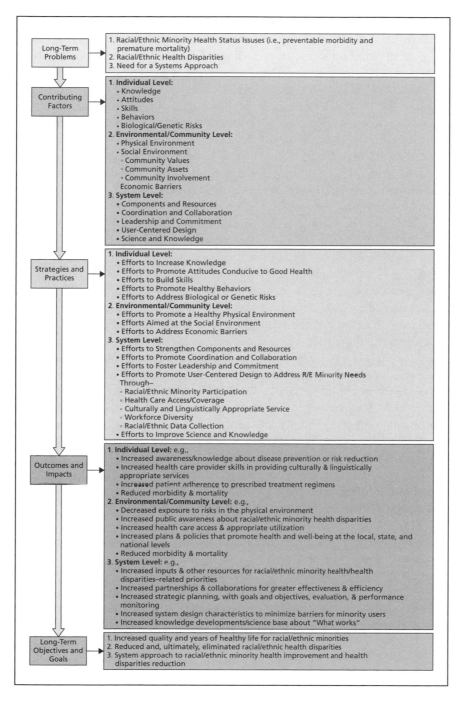

Source: Office of Minority Health (2008). Chart: A strategic framework for improving racial/ethnic minority health and eliminating racial/ethnic health disparities.

whites and 1.7 times more often in Hispanics than in whites. Like hypertension, diabetes is a preventable and manageable disease that has been allowed to escalate to the point of crisis. It can be prevented or managed through simple and low-cost efforts such as education, screenings, and diet and exercise. Therefore, it is likely that diabetes is a disease that also can be greatly affected by community health workers and faith-based intervention efforts.

Cancer, the third area of concern identified using the criteria detailed in the OMH strategic framework (see Figure 28.3), is admittedly not as easily addressed as the previous two diseases. The complexities of this disease (no true known and/or common etiology) increase the need for an effective systems approach. Blacks are 21 percent more likely to die from all forms of cancer than are whites and are 50 percent more likely to die of prostate cancer and 36 percent more likely to die of breast cancer than are whites. The key to overcoming cancer-related disparities may lie in early-detection efforts tailored to minority communities. This method would again call for the use of trained community health workers and the cooperation and involvement of black churches.

The fourth health disparity of concern identified by the OMH is prenatal care. Mexican and black mothers are 2.5 times more likely to initiate such care in the third trimester or to go without any prenatal care than are white mothers (National Center for Health Statistics, 2001, Table 7.). This practice among Mexican and black mothers can lead to birth defects for the child and health complications for the mother (such as pregnancy-induced hypertension or diabetes).

The underutilization of prenatal care by Mexican and black mothers may be a by-product of the final health disparity in need of immediate action identified by the OMH—lack of health coverage. Among those aged 18 to 64 years, 49 percent of Hispanics and 28 percent of blacks, compared with 21 percent of whites and 18 percent of Asians, reported being uninsured in 2006 (Beal, Doty, Hernandez, Shea, & Davis, 2007). Forty-three percent of Hispanics and 21 percent of blacks, compared with 15 percent of whites and 16 percent of Asians, reported the lack of a regular health care provider; thus, blacks and Hispanics were more likely to experience differential access to doctors and care (Beal et al., 2007).

Although efforts, in the form of the Obama-Biden health care reform, are currently being taken to overcome some of the health consequences related to limited or no access to care and differential treatment, additional efforts are needed to meet the demands and needs of the underserved. The higher prevalence of Hispanics and blacks with no or insufficient prenatal care may speak to a lack of education on the importance of prenatal care or access to care. This is again a health concern that would benefit from community health workers with an inherent knowledge of the populations' cultural concerns and financial limitations.

Recommendations

As the editors of this book, we agree with the OMH's identification of the five disparities of greatest urgency and share their belief that a strategic approach, starting with these five disparities, is needed to maximize limited resources. It is possible that the utilization of a divided approach (each agency working independently or in small groups in the fight against their own identified disparity) rather than a collective approach (all agencies, regardless of their primary disparity focus, working together to address the collective targeted disparities—those which have been identified by the OMH) has contributed to the slow to no progress in the fight to eliminate health disparities. Our first recommendation, therefore, is that a nationwide initiative targeting all private, state, governmental, nonprofit, grassroots, and legislative entities with any experience or desire to work toward the limitation of health disparities, be initiated and led by the OMH. Second, we call for the legitimatization of community health workers and an increase in their numbers. We believe that initially federal funding should be used to sponsor training institutes for community health workers, but ultimately public health and social work schools should be encouraged to institute certificate programs in order to bring recognition to community health workers as trained public health/social-service professionals. Third, we recommend encouraging the inclusion of community-based churches in the development and delivery of health interventions by requiring federally funded programs working with minority populations to partner with at least one church. Finally, we recommend improved efforts to provide health care to the disenfranchised with special care being given to gender disparities (e.g., coverage for poor men of color). Although the Obama-Biden plan would extend coverage to the full-time working class, it will do little to provide health care to the homeless or part-time workers. The provision of mobile health clinics by hospitals and clinics would provide semi-regular primary-care homes, which have been noted as essential in preventive care and early detection.

CONCLUSION

The call to action has been issued, on more than one occasion, but little headway has been made. The lack of progress may have little to do with the lack of action and more to do with a lack of concentrated effort. History has shown that the current strategy of divided effort is not working, given the limited resources and reach of individual health initiatives. The time has come for a single, collective approach. Therefore, this is not a call to action but rather an enlistment call to duty. If we are to gain, grow, and eventually overcome the enemy, health disparities, those in the fight must band together as one army under one rule with a shared systemic approach.

REFERENCES

Agency for Healthcare Research and Quality (AHRQ). (2006). *National healthcare disparities report 2006*. Rockville, MD: Author.

Beal, A., Doty, S., Hernandez, S., Shea, K., & Davis, K. (2007, June). *Closing the divide: How medical homes promote equality in health care: Results from the Commonwealth Fund 2006 Health Care Quality Survey*. New York: Commonwealth Fund.

Blevins, S. (2003, April). Universal healthcare won't work—witness Medicare. Retrieved June 10, 2009, from the Cato Institute website: http://www.cato.org/pub_display.php?pub_id=3057

Bodenheimer, T. (2005). The political divide in health care: A liberal perspective. *Health Affairs, 24*(6), 1426–1435.

Burd-Sharps, S., Lewis, K., & Martins, E. (2008). *The measures of America: American human development report 2008–2009*. New York: Columbia University Press.

Centers for Disease Control and Prevention. (2007). Racial and ethnic disparities in diagnoses of HIV/AIDS—33 states, 2001–2005. *MMWR Morbidity Mortality Weekly Report, 59*(09), 189–193.

Centers for Disease Control and Prevention. (2008a, August). *HIV and AIDS in the United States: A picture of today's epidemic* [revised fact sheet]. Atlanta: Author.

Centers for Disease Control and Prevention. (2008b). HIV prevalence estimates—United States, 2006. *MMWR Morbidity Mortality Weekly Report, 57*(39), 1073–1076.

Centers for Medicare and Medicaid Services, Office of the Actuary. (2007, February). *National Health Expenditures.* Retrieved February 10, 2009, from http://www.cms.hhs.gov/NationalHealthExpendData/downloads/proj2007.pdf

Central Intelligence Agency [CIA]. (2009). *The World Factbook: Country comparison: Life expectancy at birth.* Retrieved March 2, 2009, from https://www.cia.gov/library/publications/the-world-factbook/rankorder/2102rank.html.

Commonwealth Fund. (2006, September). *Why not the best? Results from a national scorecard on U.S. health system performance.* Retrieved February 10, 2009, from http://www.commonwealthfund.org/Content/Publications/Fund-Reports/2008/Jul/Why-Not-the-Best--Results-from-the-National-Scorecard-on-U-S--Health-System-Performance--2008.aspx

Davis, K., Schoen, C., Schoenbaum, S., Doty, M., Holmgren, A., Kriss, J., & Shea, K. (2007). *Mirror, mirror on the wall: An international update on the comparative performance of American health care,* vol. 59. New York: Commonwealth Fund.

DeNavas-Walt, C., Proctor, B., & Smith, J. (2008). Income, poverty, and health insurance coverage in the United States: 2007, In U.S. Census Bureau, *Current population reports,* P60-235. Washington, DC: U.S. Government Printing Office. Also available at http://www.census.gov/prod/2008pubs/p60-235.pdf.

Fox, M. (2008, April 11). *Doctors support universal health care: Survey.* New York: Thomson Reuters.

Gadson, S. (2006). The third world health status of black American males. *Journal of the National Medical Association, 98*(4), 488–491.

Girosi, F., Meili, R., & Scoville, R. (2005). *Extrapolating evidence of health information technology saving and costs.* Santa Monica, CA: RAND.

Hogberg, D. (2006). Don't fall prey to propaganda: Life expectancy and infant mortality are unreliable measures for comparing the US health care system to others. *National Policy Analysis, 547,* 1–6.

Institute of Medicine at the National Academy of Sciences [IOM]. (2004). *Insuring America's health: Principles and recommendations.* Washington, DC: National Academy of Sciences.

Kaiser Family Foundation and Health Research & Education Trust. (2008). *Employer Health Benefits 2008.* Retrieved September 2008 from http://kff.org/insurance/7527/index.cfm.

Kohn, L., Corrigan, J., & Donaldson, M. (Eds.), Committee on Quality of Health Care in America, Institute of Medicine. (2000). *To Err is Human.* Washington, DC: National Academies Press.

Lambrew, J. (2007, April). *A wellness trust to prioritize disease prevention.* The Hamilton Project, Brookings Institution. Retrieved February 3, 2009, from http://www3.brookings.edu/views/papers/200704lambrew.pdf.

National Center for Health Statistics. (2001). *Healthy people 2000 final review.* Hyattsville, MD: Public Health Service.

Nembhard, I., Alexander, J., Hoff, T., & Ramanujam, R. (2009). Why does the quality of health care continue to lag? Insights from management research. *Academy of Management Perspectives, 23,* 25–42.

Obama, B., & Biden, J. (2008). *Barack Obama and Joe Biden's plan to lower health care costs and ensure affordable, accessible health coverage for all.* Retrieved February 20, 2009, from http://barackobama.com/pdf/issues/HealthCareFullPlan.pdf.

Office of Minority Health. (2008). *A strategic framework for improving racial/ethnic minority health and eliminating racial/ethnic health disparities.* Washington, DC: Author.

Olshansky, S., Passaro, D., Hershow, R., Layden, J., Carnes, B., Brody, J., et al. (2005). A potential decline in life expectancy in the United States in the 21st century. *New England Journal of Medicine, 352*(11), 1138–1145.

Public Citizen. (2004). Physicians for a national health program. Washington, DC: Author.

Reinhardt, U., Hussey, P., & Anderson, G. (2004). U.S. health care spending in an international context. *Health Affairs, 23*(3), 10-25.

Smedley, B., Stith, A., & Nelson, A. (Eds.). (2003). *Unequal treatment: Confronting racial and ethnic disparities in healthcare.* Washington, DC: National Academies Press.

U.S. Census Bureau. (2000). Resident population of the 50 states, the District of Columbia, and Puerto Rico: April 1, 2000 (Census 2000) and April 1, 1990 (1990 Census) and State Rank as of 2000 and State Rank as of 1990. Published December 28, 2000, at http://www.census.gov/population/cen2000/tab04.txt.

U.S. Census Bureau. (2006). *Population profile of the United States: Dynamic version.* Last updated January 2006. Retrieved February 10, 2009, from http://www.census.gov/population/www/pop-profile/profiledynamic.html

Woolhandler, S., Campbell, T., & Himmelstein, D. (2003). Costs of health care administration in the United States and Canada. *New England Journal of Medicine, 349*(8), 768–775.

AFTERWORD

GAIL C. CHRISTOPHER

When will we enter a post-health-disparities era? With so many unprecedented events and changes in American society, journalists and pundits are quick to ascribe "post" prefixes to core aspects of our existence. Some suggest we are now in a post-racialist era because Barack Obama has become the first African American to be elected president. There is also the idea that the days of irresponsible executives, widening inequalities, and corporate greed are behind us. Some say we are entering an era of post-excess, where less is more. Not so fast.

Simply put, the United States cannot close the gap in health status between African Americans and whites until we have effectively addressed the issue of structural and institutional racism and its consequences. Racism is a societal pathology that privileges some and disadvantages others. The election of the first African American president does not herald the beginning of a post-racialist nation. Nor does the collapse of the financial sector and unprecedented economic crisis herald a post-excess era. In fact, the economic crisis will continue to exacerbate structural racism and its attendant social conditions, which contribute to health disparities.

For example, unemployment rates are highest in the African American community at all times, but unemployment for African Americans during the 2009 recession is twice as high as for whites. The most significant loss of wealth from the mortgage crisis is in the African American and Latino communities. And the closing of retail stores and factories has a disproportionate effect on low-income minority communities. Job losses reverberate in loss of health insurance, and the already high numbers of uninsured African Americans and Latinos increase once again.

Current and historic effects of a racially biased social and economic structure touch individuals, communities, and institutions. On the individual level, reactions to uncertainty and to discrimination cause physiological and biochemical stress responses. These bodily stress reactions, cumulatively known as allostatic load, over time contribute to negative health outcomes such as hypertension and other chronic conditions. Uncertainty and discrimination also lead to high levels of residential segregation and isolation by race and poverty. Evidence is growing about the relationship between segregation and one of the most persistent health disparities: infant mortality. Over 40 percent of black child-bearing women live in hypersegregated areas. Residential segregation is a global construct with five distinct dimensions of spatial separation within a metropolitan area: exposure (the probability that blacks have contact with black neighbors), unevenness (the degree to which each neighborhood incorporates the same proportions of blacks and whites as the metropolitan area overall), clustering (the tendency of black neighborhoods to cluster together), centralization (the degree to which black neighborhoods are at the center of the metropolitan area), and concentration (population density). "A high level of segregation with regard to any one dimension may be harmful, but since blacks experience high segregation across multiple dimensions simultaneously (hypersegregation), the detrimental effects of segregation multiply," according to researchers Theresa Osypuk and Dolores Acevedo-Garcia. They have demonstrated that living in a hypersegregated metropolitan area has a more pronounced association with preterm births among older black women and that racial disparities in preterm births are larger in hypersegregated areas among older mothers.[1]

On the institutional level, disproportionate minority confinement in the juvenile justice and prison systems illustrates the effects of historic and contemporary racism. Little substantive progress has been made in resolving the nationwide crisis in disproportionate minority confinement since 1974, when the U.S. Congress mandated that states address overrepresentation of youth of color in the juvenile justice system.[2] In fact, the years following this mandate saw Congress enact harsh mandatory minimums and racially disparate drug sentencing laws that brought us to the point where one in ten black men aged 25 to 29 was in jail in 2008.

Given the multidimensional relationship of race, society and health, it is clear that we require a comprehensive, systemic approach to end health disparities. If the new "post-racialist America" mantra is allowed to persist, it could distract us from and undermine the kinds of interventions that are required to end health disparities. This powerful book on health disparities can serve as a needed reality check, preventing our descent into denial of facts, consequences, implications, and feelings about racism in the United States and its most potent marker—life for some and death for others.

The editors and authors provide a valuable, timely contribution at a moment when so much is at stake. As this nation grapples with the possibility of reforming a long-broken health care system, the contributors to this book elucidate the historically unmet challenge of closing the health gap between minorities and whites. They use a scholarly, data-laden, objective approach that is tempered by a passion for knowing deeply the nuances of communities of color and their histories. The contributors paint thoughtful, caring portraits of faces and bodies too often neglected or euphemized by statistical phrases like infant mortality and domestic violence. These authors take you beyond the hands that strike and the body that bends into the hearts that ache from dreams deferred. And through their commitment, readers glean hope and concrete recommendations for bringing about a post-health-disparities era.

---

[1]Theresa L. Osypuk and Dolores Acevedo-Garcia, "Are Racial Disparities in Preterm Birth Larger in Hypersegregated Areas?" *American Journal of Epidemiology*, *167*(2008), 1296, 1298.
[2]See the 1988 Amendments to the Juvenile Justice and Delinquency Prevention Act of 1974.

When will we enter that era? The hope for creating such a time in this country rests on mobilizing a comprehensive, multisectoral strategy that is commensurate with a challenge that has roots in this country's very genetic code. All sectors have contributions to make. First, the African American community must continue to demonstrate the agency that has underpinned its survival to date. Second, the government must radically expand its treatment of the health-disparities issue to encompass a social determinants perspective. Third, the often-neglected private sector has a role to play, as it will benefit from a healthier and more productive workforce and consumer base. Finally, the philanthropic sector has played a catalytic role and can be even more effective given its ability to convene and direct resources across multiple issue areas.

THE AFFECTED COMMUNITIES

The introductory chapters of this third edition of *Health Issues in the Black Community* provide context and historic appreciation of the "agency" of African Americans who help themselves by identifying health disparities, attributing them to social conditions, and mobilizing community institutions to overcome injustice.

The African American community lost one of its giants in 2009. John Hope Franklin, at age 94, made his transition in March 2009. He was a tireless champion of equality who contributed to every major civil rights battle over the last century and finally lived to see the Obamas become the first family of the United States. He was a revered historian and icon who authored the seminal book *From Slavery to Freedom: A History of Negro Americans*. Dr. Franklin understood that the incredible resilience of black people would ensure our survival but that we cannot do it alone. This shared responsibility was captured in the recommendations of approximately thirty black leaders convened by Dr. Franklin and Eleanor Holmes Norton in 1986. Their report, entitled "Black Initiative and Governmental Responsibility," concluded with the following statement:

1. The black community has always been an agent for its own advancement.

2. The "self-help" tradition is so embedded in the black heritage as to be virtually synonymous with it.

3. We must reach more broadly and more deeply to levels of participation that include the poorest blacks and that draw them closer to blacks who have been more fortunate.

4. Persistent poverty has eroded but not destroyed the strong, deep value framework that for so long has sustained black people.

5. The black community must take the lead in defining the new and continuing problems it faces, in communicating the urgency of these problems, and in both prescribing and initiating solutions.

6. Many fruitful strategies are in place and should be expanded. Many of the most pressing problems of the black community are well beyond its capacity or that of any community to resolve.

7. We urge a concentrated effort by government to invest first in models and then in programs and strategies for human development that will facilitate economic independence and encourage the poor to take charge of their own lives.

8. The inexcusable disparities between blacks and whites . . . can be eradicated only if the government assumes its appropriate role in a democratic, humane, and stable society.[3]

Although these leaders were not referring specifically to the issue of health disparities, they were describing the constellation of social dislocations that burden African Americans and other communities of color. Disproportionate poverty, premature death, and excess incarceration are issues of which health disparities are but a symptom. They remind us of the resilience and inherent agency that has enabled African Americans to survive in the United States. Dr. Franklin and the other leaders called for concentrated efforts on the part of the government. Clearly, there is still a critical role for government in closing the gap in health status between African Americans and whites. In addition to tackling major disease disparities using a medical model, the government role is to address the "opportunity gap" by ameliorating the negative social determinants of health disparities.

GOVERNMENT

Governments—federal, state, county, and local—must enact and enforce policies that foster equity in opportunities. Examples include living-wage ordinances, transportation investments that connect isolated residents to hubs of employment, commercial, and food opportunities, as well as access to affordable housing in integrated neighborhoods with successful schools and quality health care. Air quality and risk for vulnerability to climate-related disasters must also be addressed.

Many are hopeful that the United States will soon join other developed nations in the world by providing some form of universal access to health care. It is likely that a unique national health-insurance system will be based on some of the dynamics of the current private/public system. There is, however, a very strong probability that racial health disparities will persist within the new framework of national health insurance unless that system emphasizes the primacy of health in all areas of public policy. The new health care model will require coordination among multiple public agencies and all levels of government. It will need to engage public health and medical care providers in partnership with local leaders to implement community- and place-based efforts

---

[3]Quoted in Donna L. Franklin, *Ensuring Inequality: The Structural Transformation of the African-American Family* (New York: Oxford University Press, 1997), 235–236.

that transform the health of communities and their residents. The new system must leverage longstanding efforts of many public health groups to champion a health-promotion and disease-prevention focus. Such efforts empower local communities to take ownership of creating the conditions for healthy living by all age groups.

PRIVATE SECTOR

The private sector—employers and businesses marketing to communities of color—is rarely enlisted in social justice efforts, and yet it must be. Local employers, businesses, and private-sector leaders have important roles to play in closing the health-disparities gap. Improving conditions in workplaces and assuring health insurance coverage for all workers are critical factors. But business leaders can play even more pivotal roles by becoming champions for equitable development, transportation, living-wage ordinances, equitable financing of schools, and the equitable distribution of resources for healthy living. Enlightened self-interest may be the incentive for increased private-sector engagement. A healthy workforce is more productive and less costly than an unhealthy one in the short and long term.

PHILANTHROPY

Finally, there is a growing awareness within the philanthropic sector, particularly among health funders, about the necessity of enlarging the model or lens for addressing health disparities. Major funders such as Atlantic Philanthropies, the California Endowment, the Annie E. Casey Foundation, and the W. K. Kellogg Foundation recognize that health equity can be achieved only when the lingering effects of racism and discrimination are addressed. These effects include harmful social, environmental, economic, and community conditions, including limited access to affordable, quality health care and persistent segregation and poverty. Grantmakers In Health, the oldest and largest philanthropic affinity group, published Issue Brief No. 33 in March 2009. Entitled "Effective Community Programs to Fight Health Disparities," it acknowledges that the Healthy People 2010 deadline for eliminating health disparities is upon us and the gap persists in many areas. The importance of engaging communities in sustainable efforts is addressed throughout the report.

■ Ensure strong governing support and participation in efforts to fight health disparities. Boards and organizations must have a willingness to learn new things, take risks when necessary, provide adequate funding, and be patient to stay the course for long-term success.

■ Encourage advocacy for public and private policies that address the broad determinants of health, as well as for specific disparities-related issues.

■ Consider the creation of a Surgeon General's report on health equity in the United States. A high-level declaration of the costs of ignoring health equity among all populations, not just low-income groups, could be an important statement.

- Listen! Funders must realize that they cannot unilaterally make decisions about what is needed in a community or about the strategies that should be employed. Instead, a planning process should be funded with an assessment of the stakeholders to include in designing and implementing initiatives.

- Tackle agency and organizational silos, which can allow for increased communication and mutual goal setting across federal, state, and local agencies. Allowing more flexible spending of current health funding may also help break down silos and increase cross-sectoral collaborations.

Racism and inequality are part of the genetic code of the United States and nothing reflects their continued influence more accurately than the persistent gap in health status and health outcomes between minorities and whites. Despite the election of a new, progressive president, and despite the crash of the "spend-driven economy" as we know it, racial health inequities remain, and, without focused heroic efforts, are likely to increase in the near future. The real "post" era we risk experiencing is rushing headlong into a time of myopia, past realistic appreciation of the systemic privilege and injustices that define and predict morbidity and mortality based on physical characteristics such as skin color. The authors of this third edition of *Health Issues* provide much of what is "known" about the complexities of health disparities and invite an acceleration of collective efforts to end them once and for all.

INDEX

NOTE: Page numbers in *italics* refer to figures; page numbers followed by "*t*" refer to tables; page numbers followed by *n* refer to notes.